Mayo Clinic
Gastroenterology and Hepatology
Board Review

Second Edition

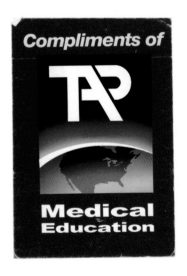

Mayo Clinic
Gastroenterology and Hepatology
Board Review

Second Edition

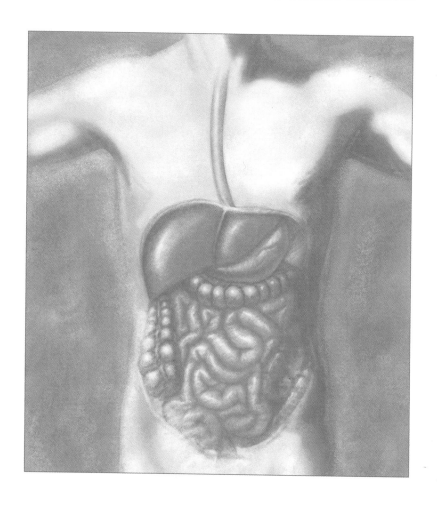

Editor
Stephen C. Hauser, M.D.

Co-Editors
Darrell S. Pardi, M.D.
John J. Poterucha, M.D.

MAYO CLINIC SCIENTIFIC PRESS

AND INFORMA HEALTHCARE USA, INC.

ISBN 0849370183

For order inquiries, contact: Informa Healthcare, Kentucky Distribution Center, 7625 Empire Dr., Florence, KY 41041

www.informahealthcare.com

Catalog record is available from the Library of Congress.

Care has been taken to confirm the accuracy of the information presented and to describe generally accepted practices. However, the authors, editors, and publisher are not responsible for errors or omissions or for any consequences from application of the information in this book and make no warranty, express or implied, with respect to the contents of the publication. This book should not be relied on apart from the advice of a qualified health care provider.

The authors, editors, and publisher have exerted efforts to ensure that drug selection and dosage set forth in this text are in accordance with current recommendations and practice at the time of publication. However, in view of ongoing research, changes in government regulations, and the constant flow of information relating to drug therapy and drug reactions, the reader is urged to check the package insert for each drug for any change in indications and dosage and for added warnings and precautions. This is particularly important when the recommended agent is a new or infrequently employed drug.

Some drugs and medical devices presented in this publication have Food and Drug Administration (FDA) clearance for limited use in restricted research settings. It is the responsibility of the health care providers to ascertain the FDA status of each drug or device planned for use in their clinical practice.

10 9 8 7 6 5 4 3 2

Printed in Canada

DEDICATION

To the many persons who have taught, encouraged, and inspired us.

PREFACE

The specialty of gastroenterology and hepatology encompasses a vast anatomical assortment of organs with diverse structure and function, potentially afflicted by a multiplicity of disease processes. To assist physicians in training preparing for the gastroenterology board examination as well as a growing number of gastroenterologists awaiting recertification, we designed the Mayo Clinic Gastroenterology and Hepatology Board Review course and produced the second edition of this book. The book is not intended to replace the many more encyclopedic textbooks of gastroenterology, hepatology, pathology, endoscopy, nutrition, and radiology now available, nor is it intended to serve as an update to physicians looking for the newest advances in the science and art of gastroenterology and hepatology. Instead, this book provides a core of essential knowledge in gastroenterology, hepatology, and integral related areas of pathology, endoscopy, nutrition, and radiology. Clinical knowledge related to diagnostic and therapeutic approaches to patient management is emphasized. Case-based presentations and multiple board-examination–type, single-best–answer questions with annotated answers are featured. As such, this text also is intended to be used by medical students and residents for their clerkships on internal medicine and gastroenterology rotations and by gastroenterology fellows in training. Physicians in practice should find this book to be a practical review to consolidate their knowledge in gastroenterology and hepatology.

The book is organized along subspecialty topics, including esophageal disorders, gastrointestinal disorders, small-bowel disease and nutrition, miscellaneous disorders, colonic disorders, liver disease, and pancreaticobiliary disease. Many color and black-and-white figures are included in the text. Each subspecialty section concludes with questions and answers (materials in the questions and answers are not included in the index). The faculty responsible for this book are all Mayo Clinic gastroenterologists and hepatologists who spend the majority of their time caring for patients and have a commitment to teaching medical students, house officers, fellows, nurses, and physicians. The faculty's particular interests in subspecialty areas of clinical gastroenterology and hepatology provide broad expertise to the book's content.

We thank the staffs of the Section of Scientific Publications, Media Support Services, and Mayo School of Continuing Medical Education at Mayo Clinic for their contributions. The support of the publisher, Taylor & Francis Group, also is greatly appreciated. We give special thanks to our secretaries and to Keith Lindor, M.D., for his ongoing enthusiasm and support for our faculty and teaching mission.

Stephen C. Hauser, M.D.

LIST OF CONTRIBUTORS

Jeffrey A. Alexander, M.D.
Consultant, Division of Gastroenterology and Hepatology, Mayo Clinic; Assistant Professor of Medicine, Mayo Clinic College of Medicine; Rochester, Minnesota

Todd H. Baron, Sr., M.D.
Consultant, Division of Gastroenterology and Hepatology, Mayo Clinic; Professor of Medicine, Mayo Clinic College of Medicine; Rochester, Minnesota

Adil E. Bharucha, M.B.B.S., M.D.
Consultant, Division of Gastroenterology and Hepatology, Mayo Clinic; Associate Professor of Medicine, Mayo Clinic College of Medicine; Rochester, Minnesota

Lisa A. Boardman, M.D.
Consultant, Division of Gastroenterology and Hepatology, Mayo Clinic; Assistant Professor of Medicine, Mayo Clinic College of Medicine; Rochester, Minnesota

David J. Brandhagen, M.D.
Consultant, Division of Gastroenterology and Hepatology, Mayo Clinic; Assistant Professor of Medicine, Mayo Clinic College of Medicine; Rochester, Minnesota

Michael Camilleri, M.D.
Consultant, Division of Gastroenterology and Hepatology, Mayo Clinic; Atherton and Winifred W. Bean Professor, and Professor of Medicine and of Physiology, Mayo Clinic College of Medicine; Rochester, Minnesota

Suresh T. Chari, M.D.
Consultant, Division of Gastroenterology and Hepatology, Mayo Clinic; Associate Professor of Medicine, Mayo Clinic College of Medicine; Rochester, Minnesota

Michael R. Charlton, M.B.B.S.
Consultant, Division of Gastroenterology and Hepatology, Mayo Clinic; Associate Professor of Medicine, Mayo Clinic College of Medicine; Rochester, Minnesota

Albert J. Czaja, M.D.
Consultant, Division of Gastroenterology and Hepatology, Mayo Clinic; Professor of Medicine, Mayo Clinic College of Medicine; Rochester, Minnesota

Gregory J. Gores, M.D.
Consultant, Division of Gastroenterology and Hepatology, Mayo Clinic; Professor of Medicine and of Physiology, Mayo Clinic College of Medicine; Rochester, Minnesota

John B. Gross, Jr., M.D.
Consultant, Division of Gastroenterology and Hepatology, Mayo Clinic; Associate Professor of Medicine, Mayo Clinic College of Medicine; Rochester, Minnesota

Gavin C. Harewood, M.D.
Senior Associate Consultant, Division of Gastroenterology and Hepatology, Mayo Clinic; Associate Professor of Medicine, Mayo Clinic College of Medicine; Rochester, Minnesota

Stephen C. Hauser, M.D.
Consultant, Division of Gastroenterology and Hepatology, Mayo Clinic; Assistant Professor of Medicine, Mayo Clinic College of Medicine; Rochester, Minnesota

J. Eileen Hay, M.B.,Ch.B.
Consultant, Division of Gastroenterology and Hepatology, Mayo Clinic; Professor of Medicine, Mayo Clinic College of Medicine; Rochester, Minnesota

Patrick S. Kamath, M.D.
Consultant, Division of Gastroenterology and Hepatology, Mayo Clinic; Professor of Medicine, Mayo Clinic College of Medicine; Rochester, Minnesota

Darlene G. Kelly, M.D., Ph.D.
Consultant, Division of Gastroenterology and Hepatology, Mayo Clinic; Associate Professor of Medicine, Mayo Clinic College of Medicine; Rochester, Minnesota

Mark V. Larson, M.D.
Consultant, Division of Gastroenterology and Hepatology, Mayo Clinic; Assistant Professor of Medicine, Mayo Clinic College of Medicine; Rochester, Minnesota

Paul J. Limburg, M.D.
Consultant, Division of Gastroenterology and Hepatology, Mayo Clinic; Assistant Professor of Medicine, Mayo Clinic College of Medicine; Rochester, Minnesota

Keith D. Lindor, M.D.
Chair, Division of Gastroenterology and Hepatology,
Mayo Clinic; Professor of Medicine, Mayo Clinic College
of Medicine; Rochester, Minnesota

G. Richard Locke III, M.D.
Consultant, Division of Gastroenterology and Hepatology,
Mayo Clinic; Associate Professor of Medicine, Mayo
Clinic College of Medicine; Rochester, Minnesota

Edward V. Loftus, Jr., M.D.
Consultant, Division of Gastroenterology and Hepatology,
Mayo Clinic; Associate Professor of Medicine, Mayo
Clinic College of Medicine; Rochester, Minnesota

Thomas F. Mangan, M.D.
Consultant, Division of Gastroenterology and Hepatology,
Mayo Clinic; Assistant Professor of Medicine, Mayo
Clinic College of Medicine; Rochester, Minnesota

Joseph A. Murray, M.D.
Consultant, Division of Gastroenterology and Hepatology,
Mayo Clinic; Professor of Medicine, Mayo Clinic College
of Medicine; Rochester, Minnesota

Darrell S. Pardi, M.D.
Consultant, Division of Gastroenterology and Hepatology,
Mayo Clinic; Assistant Professor of Medicine, Mayo
Clinic College of Medicine; Rochester, Minnesota

Randall K. Pearson, M.D.
Consultant, Division of Gastroenterology and Hepatology,
Mayo Clinic; Assistant Professor of Medicine, Mayo
Clinic College of Medicine; Rochester, Minnesota

Bret T. Petersen, M.D.
Consultant, Division of Gastroenterology and Hepatology,
Mayo Clinic; Assistant Professor of Medicine, Mayo
Clinic College of Medicine; Rochester, Minnesota

John J. Poterucha, M.D.
Consultant, Division of Gastroenterology and Hepatology,
Mayo Clinic; Associate Professor of Medicine, Mayo
Clinic College of Medicine; Rochester, Minnesota

Yvonne Romero, M.D.
Consultant, Division of Gastroenterology and Hepatology,
Mayo Clinic; Assistant Professor of Medicine, Mayo
Clinic College of Medicine; Rochester, Minnesota

William J. Sandborn, M.D.
Consultant, Division of Gastroenterology and Hepatology,
Mayo Clinic; Professor of Medicine, Mayo Clinic College
of Medicine; Rochester, Minnesota

John A. Schaffner, M.D.
Consultant, Division of Gastroenterology and Hepatology,
Mayo Clinic; Associate Professor of Medicine, Mayo
Clinic College of Medicine; Rochester, Minnesota

Vijay H. Shah, M.D.
Consultant, Division of Gastroenterology and Hepatology,
Mayo Clinic; Associate Professor of Medicine, Mayo
Clinic College of Medicine; Rochester, Minnesota

Nicholas J. Talley, M.D., Ph.D.
Consultant, Division of Gastroenterology and Hepatology,
Mayo Clinic; Professor of Medicine, Mayo Clinic College
of Medicine; Rochester, Minnesota

William J. Tremaine, M.D.
Consultant, Division of Gastroenterology and Hepatology,
Mayo Clinic; Professor of Medicine, Mayo Clinic College
of Medicine; Rochester, Minnesota

Santhi S. Vege, M.D.
Consultant, Division of Gastroenterology and Hepatology,
Mayo Clinic; Professor of Medicine, Mayo Clinic College
of Medicine; Rochester, Minnesota

Thomas R. Viggiano, M.D.
Consultant, Division of Gastroenterology and Hepatology,
Mayo Clinic; Professor of Medicine, Mayo Clinic College
of Medicine; Rochester, Minnesota

Kenneth K. Wang, M.D.
Consultant, Division of Gastroenterology and Hepatology,
Mayo Clinic; Associate Professor of Medicine, Mayo
Clinic College of Medicine; Rochester, Minnesota

TABLE OF CONTENTS

CHAPTER 1

Study Design and Statistics for the Boards

Gavin C. Harewood, M.D.

TYPES OF STUDY DESIGN

Most clinical studies fall into one of two categories: case-control study or cohort study.

Case-Control Study

Two groups of patients are identified, one with the disease being studied (cases) and one without the disease (controls) (Fig. 1). Both groups are analyzed to determine whether they have a specific risk factor or exposure. For example, patients with gastroesophageal reflux disease (GERD) (cases) and patients without GERD (controls) could be analyzed to determine whether they are cigarette smokers (exposure). The findings would allow comparison of the proportion of smokers among patients with GERD and those without GERD. Case-control studies are generally retrospective.

Cohort Study

Two groups of patients are identified, one with exposure (cases) and one without exposure (controls) (Fig. 1). Both groups are followed prospectively to determine whether a specific disease develops. For example, patients with asbestos exposure (cases) and those without asbestos exposure (controls) could be followed prospectively to determine whether pancreatic cancer develops (outcome). The findings would allow comparison of the proportion of those exposed to asbestos and those not exposed in whom pancreatic cancer develops. Cohort studies are prospective.

In treatment cohort studies (i.e., clinical trials comparing disease outcomes in patients receiving a new medication [cases] vs. untreated patients [controls]), desirable features of the study design include the following:

Placebo-control: untreated patients receive a nonactive treatment (placebo) indistinguishable from the active treatment

Randomization: each patient has an equal likelihood of receiving active treatment or placebo

Double blinding: neither patient nor investigator is aware of whether active treatment or placebo is given to each study subject

Concealed allocation: investigator enrolling patients is unaware of treatment arm (active treatment vs. placebo) to which each recruited subject is assigned

BASIC STATISTICS

The 2×2 Table

The 2×2 table is the fundamental building block used to solve many statistical questions in the board examination. It requires allocation of patients in one of four boxes (Fig. 2). By convention,

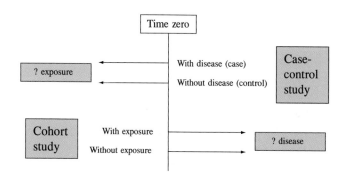

Fig. 1. Comparison of case-control study and cohort study.

1

the two columns are used to designate patients with and without disease, and the two rows represent patients with positive and negative test results. This table allows all patients to be assigned as 1) true positive (TP), positive test result in the setting of disease; 2) true negative (TN), negative test result in the absence of disease; 3) false positive (FP), positive test result in the absence of disease; or 4) false negative (FN), negative test result in the setting of disease.

Definitions to Remember

Some epidemiology and statistical definitions that may be helpful for the board examination are the following:

Incidence: proportion of a population initially free of disease in whom disease subsequently develops over time

Prevalence: proportion of a population with disease at a single point in time

Sensitivity: proportion of patients with disease who have a positive test result, true positive/(true positive + false negative)

Specificity: proportion of patients without disease who have a negative test result, true negative/(true negative + false positive)

Positive predictive value (PPV): proportion of patients with a positive test result who have disease, true positive/(true positive + false positive)

Negative predictive value (NPV): proportion of patients with a negative test result without disease, true negative/(true negative + false negative)

Clinical Examples

The application of the terms defined above is best illustrated with clinical examples.

Question 1

A new test has been developed to detect colon cancer. Its sensitivity is 80%, and its specificity is 90%. If the prevalence of colon cancer in the population is 5%, what are the PPV and NPV of this new test?

Step 1: Construct a 2×2 table using a hypothetical population of 1,000 people (Fig. 3) (disease present and absent in the columns; text positive or negative in rows, by convention)

Step 2: The prevalence of 5% informs us that 50 of the 1,000 people have colon cancer (i.e., 950 are cancer-free)

Step 3: The test sensitivity of 80% (true positive/[true positive + false negative]) indicates the true-positive value (40) and the false-negative (10) value. Similarly, the test specificity of 90% (true negative/[true negative + false positive]) indicates the true-negative value (855) and the false-positive (95) value.

Step 4: With the formulas for PPV (TP/TP + FP) and NPV (TN/TN + FN) numerical values can be calculated:

$$PPV = 40/(40+95) = 29.6\%$$
$$NPV = 855/(10+855) = 98.8\%$$

Question 2

If the new test for colon cancer is now applied to a higher-risk population with a 50% risk of colon cancer, how do the PPV and NPV change?

Again, a 2×2 table is constructed. However, in this case the prevalence of colon cancer has increased to 50%; that is, in our population of 1,000 people, 500 have colon cancer and 500 are cancer-free (Fig. 4). Steps 1 through 4 are applied again, yielding the following:

$$PPV = 400/(400 + 50) = 88.9\%$$
$$NPV = 450/(100 + 450) = 81.8\%$$

- As prevalence of disease changes, sensitivity and specificity remain constant. However, PPV and NPV change. As prevalence increases, PPV increases and NPV decreases; as prevalence decreases, PPV decreases and NPV increases.

Other Statistical Terms

Type I (alpha) error: a difference between treatment and placebo is erroneously reported when no difference actually exists. For most studies, the alpha level is set a priori at 0.05; that is, for a difference to be statistically significant, a 1 in 20 chance, no more, exists that this difference occurred by chance alone ($P < .05$).

Type II (beta) error: a difference between treatment and placebo is erroneously not detected when one actually does

	Disease present	Disease absent
Test (+)	TP	FP
Test (−)	FN	TN

Fig. 2. A 2×2 table. FN, false-negative result; FP, false-positive result; TN, true-negative result; TP, true-positive result.

	Colon ca	No colon ca	
Test (+)	40	95	95
Test (−)	10	855	865
	50	950	1,000

Fig. 3. A 2×2 table used to determine the negative predictive value and the positive predictive value of a test to detect colon cancer (ca) in a population of 1,000 people; the prevalence of colon cancer is 5%.

	Colon ca	No colon ca	
Test (+)	400	50	450
Test (−)	100	450	550
	500	500	1,000

Fig. 4. A 2×2 table used to determine the negative predictive value and the positive predictive value of a test to detect colon cancer (ca) in a population of 1,000 people; the prevalence of colon cancer is 50%.

exist. If a type II error occurs, it usually is due to an insufficient number of patients enrolled in the study to detect the difference (i.e., the study was underpowered).

Common Statistical Tests

χ^2 Analysis
This is used to compare noncontinuous data (e.g., sex, only two are possible). This test compares the proportions of noncontinuous variables (e.g., the proportion of males in group A vs. the proportion of males in group B).

t Test
This is used to compare continuous data (e.g., age, this is a number that can fall anywhere along a spectrum of values). This test compares the mean of continuous variables between two groups (e.g., the mean age of patients in group A vs. the mean age in group B). When a continuous variable is being compared among three or more groups, analysis of variance (ANOVA) is used.

EVALUATING DATA ON TREATMENT
Other definitions that are useful include the following:

Relative risk reduction (RRR): the reduction in bad outcomes achieved in the treated patients expressed as a proportion of the bad outcomes in the untreated group

Absolute risk reduction (ARR): the actual decrease in bad outcomes in the treated group compared with the untreated group

Number needed to treat (NNT): 1/ARR: the number of patients who would be required to be treated to prevent one bad outcome

Clinical Example
The application of these terms is illustrated in the example below.

Question 3
In a double-blinded, randomized, placebo-controlled trial assessing the effect of β-adrenergic blockers on esophageal varices, 1,000 patients with varices are enrolled: 500 patients receive β-blockers and 500 patients receive placebo. During the subsequent 12 months, hematemesis develops in 5 patients in the β-blocker group and 20 patients in the placebo group. What are the ARR for β-blockers and the NNT?

Step 1: Calculate ARR

Bad outcomes (hematemesis) in placebo group: 20/500 = 4%

Bad outcomes (hematemesis) in β-blocker group: 5/500 = 1%

Therefore, ARR is 4% − 1% = 3%

Step 2: Calculate NNT

NNT = 1/ARR = 1/0.03 = 33.3 (i.e., 33 patients with varices need to be treated with β-blockers to avoid one hematemesis developing in one patient)

Step 3: Calculate RRR

RRR = ARR/bad outcome rate in placebo group = 0.03/0.04 = 75%

SECTION I

Esophagus

CHAPTER 2

Gastroesophageal Reflux Disease

Joseph A. Murray, M.D.

Gastroesophageal reflux is the reflux of gastric contents other than air into or through the esophagus. Gastroesophageal reflux disease (GERD) refers to reflux that produces frequent symptoms or results in damage to the esophageal mucosa or contiguous organs of the upper aerodigestive system and occasionally the lower respiratory tract.

ETIOLOGY

Gastroesophageal reflux results from several factors that lead to symptoms or injury of the mucosa of the esophagus or the airway by reflux of corrosive material from the stomach (Table 1). These factors include a weak or defective sphincter, transient lower esophageal sphincter relaxations (TLESRs), hiatal hernia, poor acid clearance from the esophagus, diminished salivary flow, increased acid production, delayed gastric emptying of solids, and obstructive sleep apnea (Fig. 1). The relative contribution of these varies from patient to patient.

FACTORS CONTRIBUTING TO GASTROESOPHAGEAL REFLUX DISEASE

Barrier Function of the Lower Esophageal Sphincter

The lower esophageal sphincter (LES) and its attached structures form a barrier to reflux of material across the esophagogastric junction and is the central protection against pathologic reflux of gastric contents into the esophagus. This barrier has several components, including the smooth muscle LES, the gastric sling fibers, and the striated muscle crural diaphragm. The

Table 1. Etiologic Factors of Gastroesophageal Reflux Disease

Motility disorders
Transient lower esophageal relaxations*
Weak lower esophageal sphincter*
Weak esophageal peristalsis
Scleroderma and CREST
Delayed gastric emptying
Damaging factors
Increased gastric acid production
Bile and pancreatic juice
Resistance factors
Reduced saliva and HCO_3 production
Diminished mucosal blood flow
Growth factors, protective mucus
Others
Hiatal hernia*
Obstructive sleep apnea

CREST, calcinosis cutis, Raynaud phenomenon, esophageal dysfunction, sclerodactyly, and telangiectasia.
*Major/common factors.

LES maintains tone at rest and relaxes with swallowing and gastric distention as a venting reflex. This latter relaxation has been termed "transient lower esophageal sphincter relaxation" (TLESR). In persons with mild reflux disease, acid liquid contents instead of air alone are vented, resulting in many episodes of acid reflux. In patients with severe reflux, the LES resting pressure usually is diminished and easily overcome.

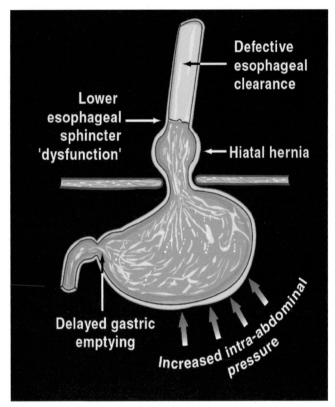

Fig. 1. Causes of increased exposure of the esophagus to gastric refluxate. (From www.astrazeneca.com. Used with permission.)

The presence of hiatal hernia has an important role in defective barrier function, both by removing the augmentation that the crural diaphragm provides the LES and lowering the threshold for TLESRs to occur.

Acid Clearance

The clearance of acid from the esophagus is a combination of mechanical volume clearance (gravity and peristalsis) and chemical neutralization of the lumen contents (saliva and mucosal buffering). This may be delayed in patients with reflux because of either impaired esophageal peristalsis or reduced buffering effects of swallowed saliva. The defective peristalsis can be a primary idiopathic motor disorder or, occasionally, it can result from a connective tissue disorder such as CREST (calcinosis cutis, Raynaud's phenomenon, esophageal dysfunction, sclerodactyly, and telangiectasia) syndrome or scleroderma. Many drugs and Sjögren's syndrome can decrease salivary flow. Salivary flow normally is decreased at night; thus, if reflux occurs during the night when the person is supine, acid will not be cleared by either gravity or saliva. This is why episodes of reflux at night are long-lasting and have a greater chance of causing severe injury to the mucosa.

Intrinsic Mucosal Factors

The mucosa of the esophagus has intrinsic factors that protect the esophageal lining against acid damage. These include the stratified squamous mucosa, intercellular tight junctions, growth factors, buffering blood flow, and production of mucin, bicarbonate, and epidermal growth factors. When these factors are overcome, GERD causes reflux esophagitis (Fig. 2 and 3).

Gastric Factors

Delayed gastric emptying or increased gastric production of acid is less frequently part of GERD. Reflux esophagitis is rarely a manifestation of Zollinger-Ellison syndrome. The availability of corrosive gastric contents in the cardia of the stomach is necessary for reflux to occur during TLESR or when a defective LES is overcome during recumbency or abdominal straining. The cardia is often submerged under liquid gastric contents when a subject is in the right lateral decubitus position. It has been suggested recently that what differentiates patients with GERD from normal subjects is not the number of actual reflux events but the reflux of acidic gastric contents instead of the release of air. The timing of reflux is also important. Because gastric acid is buffered by food during the first hour after eating, normal physiologic reflux that may occur during maximal gastric distension is not as harmful as the reflux that occurs later after the stomach pH has again decreased. Any obstruction of the outflow from the stomach increases the propensity to reflux, although this is often associated with nausea and vomiting. Pure bile reflux may occur in patients who have had gastric surgery. More common is pathologic reflux associated with a restrictive bariatric procedure such as vertical-banded gastroplasty. If too much acid-producing mucosa is present above the restrictive band, pathologic reflux may occur.

Helicobacter pylori and GERD

Whether chronic *Helicobacter pylori* infection protects against GERD is a matter of controversy. Duodenal ulcers and distal gastric cancer (both caused by *H. pylori*) are becoming rare, and adenocarcinoma of the proximal stomach and esophagus is becoming more common as the carriage rates of *H. pylori* decrease. Patients with GERD symptoms may be less likely to carry *H. pylori* than the population without GERD symptoms. Reports that symptoms of GERD developed after the eradication of *H. pylori* have led to a reexamination of those treatment trials of duodenal ulcers, which included *H. pylori* eradication, for the new development of GERD symptoms. The evidence is conflicting whether the symptoms of GERD are more common in those in whom *H. pylori* eradication has been successful or in those with persistent infection. In some persons, *H. pylori* infection may cause chronic atrophic gastritis that affects the corpus of the stomach, resulting in diminished acid secretion. It is this relative hypochlorhydria that protects against GERD. Indeed, it has been suggested that acid suppression heals reflux esophagitis faster in patients with *H. pylori* infection (Fig. 4). Other explanations for

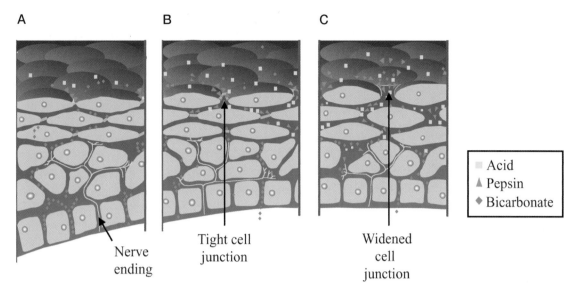

Fig. 2. Mechanism of action of refluxate in gastroesophageal reflux disease. The sequence of events hypothesized to lead to symptoms and tissue damage in gastroesophageal reflux disease is as follows: *A* and *B*, Acid-peptic attack weakens cell junctions and, *C*, widens the cell gaps, thus allowing acid penetration. Exposure to gastric acid and pepsin can cause microscopic damage to the esophageal mucosa, which may not be visible endoscopically but still result in heartburn. (From www.astrazeneca.com. Used with permission.)

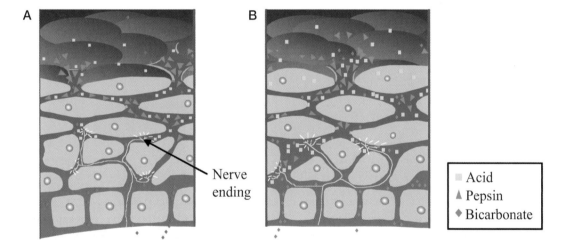

Fig. 3. Mechanism of action of refluxate in gastroesophageal reflux disease. *A*, Penetration of acid and pepsin into the mucosa allows contact of acid with epithelial nerve endings (which may result in heartburn). *B*, Additional influx of acid and pepsin into the mucosa triggers a cascade of events ultimately leading to cell rupture and mucosal inflammation. (From www.astrazeneca.com. Used with permission.)

the apparent occurrence of GERD after the eradication of *H. pylori* may include unrecognized GERD injury or symptoms present before eradication, rebound acid secretion after cessation of potent acid suppression, or other unrelated factors.

Connective Tissue Disease

Scleroderma, CREST syndrome, or mixed connective tissue diseases are rare causes of reflux, but these should be considered in young women who have Raynaud's phenomenon or subtle cutaneous features of scleroderma in the hands or face. Occasionally, GERD may be the first manifestation of these disorders. Esophageal manometry usually demonstrates a low-pressure LES and decreased amplitude of contractions in the esophagus (Fig. 5).

Mechanism of Extraesophageal Symptoms

The mechanism for extraesophageal manifestations of GERD, such as wheeze or cough, may not always be direct aspiration or

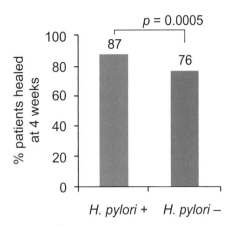

Fig. 4. The efficacy of proton pump inhibitor therapy may be greater in patients with gastroesophageal reflux disease who are positive for *Helicobactor pylori* (*H. pylori* +) than in those negative for *H. pylori* (*H. pylori* –).

damage of mucosa in the respiratory tract but a vagally mediated reflex triggered by acidification of the distal esophageal mucosa. Subglottic stenosis and granuloma of the vocal cords are very serious consequences of reflux caused by direct contact injury of the delicate mucosa of the airway, resulting in stridor, cough, or dysphonia (Fig. 6).

EPIDEMIOLOGY OF GERD

GERD can be defined as chronic symptoms of heartburn, acid regurgitation or dysfunction, or injury to the esophagus or other organs because of abnormal reflux of gastric contents. Symptoms suggestive of GERD are common: 40% of the adult population in the United States reports heartburn monthly and 18% report it weekly (Fig. 7). GERD becomes more common with increasing age (Fig. 8). GERD and its complications once were rare in China, Japan, and other Asian countries, but this is changing rapidly with the adoption of a Western diet. A protective role of *H. pylori*–induced hypochlorhydria has been suggested as a protective influence in countries with high carriage rates of infection. However, actual organ damage is observed less frequently, and fewer than 50% of patients who present for medical attention for reflux symptoms have esophagitis. Of patients who have endoscopy for GERD, 10% have benign strictures and only 3% to 4% have Barrett's esophagus; an extremely small number have adenocarcinoma. Complications of GERD may be more common in males. Whether reflux is becoming more common is not clear, but it certainly is diagnosed more frequently than in the past. Also, because of direct-to-consumer advertising and public education campaigns, the public is more aware of GERD.

For patients with GERD, the quality of life may be impaired even more than for those with congestive heart failure or diabetes

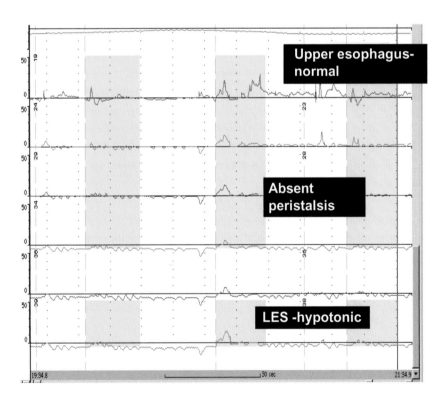

Fig. 5. Esophageal manometric tracing illustrating complete absence of peristalsis or absence of lower esophageal sphincter (LES) pressure consistent with scleroderma involvement of the esophagus.

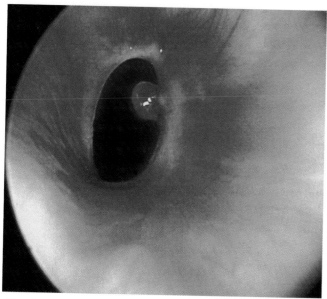

Fig. 6. Laryngeal stenosis. (Courtesy of Dr. Dana Thompson, Otorhinolaryngology/Pediatric Otolaryngology, Mayo Clinic.)

mellitus (Fig. 9). Treatment of GERD has important health economic effects because, currently, proton pump inhibitors are among the most commonly prescribed and most expensive drugs.

PRESENTATION

The classic symptoms of GERD, that is, heartburn and acid regurgitation, are common in the general population and usually are readily recognized. GERD may be manifested in a wide array of esophageal and extraesophageal symptoms. GERD may contribute to many clinical syndromes, either as a common factor or a rare culprit (Table 2).

SYMPTOMS

Esophageal Symptoms

The cardinal symptoms of GERD are heartburn (defined as retrosternal burning ascending toward the neck) and acid regurgitation (the unpleasant return of sour or bitter gastric contents to the pharynx). This is to be differentiated from the nonacid (bland) regurgitation of retained esophageal contents in an obstructed esophagus, as occurs in achalasia or the almost volitional regurgitation of recently swallowed food which is remasticated and again swallowed that typifies rumination. Patients may report relief of symptoms with antacids or milk. The symptoms of heartburn and especially acid regurgitation are specific for GERD. Their presence alone usually suffices to justify medical therapy. Objective confirmation is required before recommending surgery or endoscopic treatment. Although regurgitation of acid is a specific symptom highly suggestive of GERD, heartburn may have many different meanings for patients, and, indeed, patients may use different and imprecise terms to describe their symptoms, such as "indigestion," "stomach upset," and "sour stomach." Less common symptoms suggestive of but not diagnostic of GERD include water brash (hypersalivation associated with an episode of esophageal acid exposure), dysphagia (difficulty swallowing), odynophagia (painful swallowing), and chest discomfort not identified as heartburn. Reflux is more common after eating. Although reflux symptoms can occur at any time, they tend to aggregate in the period 1 to 3 hours after eating, when acid production overcomes the buffering effects of food (Fig. 10). It has been reported recently that a layer of acid may remain

Table 2. Symptoms of Gastroesophageal Reflux Disease

Esophageal symptoms
    Heartburn
    Acid regurgitation
    Odynophagia
    Dysphagia
    Angina-like chest pain
    Water brash (hypersalivation)
Airway symptoms
    Cough
    Wheezing
    Hoarseness
    Throat clearing
    Globus
    Tracheal stenosis
    Aspiration pneumonia
    Pulmonary fibrosis
    Apnea in infants

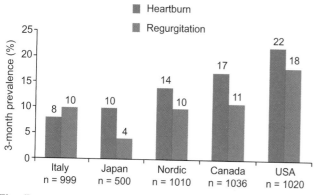

Fig. 7. Prevalence of gastroesophageal reflux disease worldwide. Note that the prevalence varies markedly from country to country, largely because of differences in physicians' awareness and understanding of the condition.

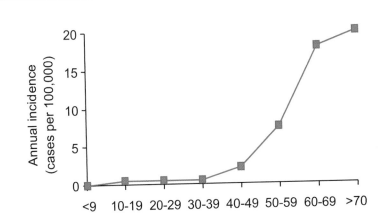

Fig. 8. Incidence of gastrointestinal reflux disease increases with age. Note that the incidence increases markedly after age 40 years. (From Brunnen PL, Karmody AM, Needham CD. Severe peptic oesophagitis. Gut. 1969;10:831-7. Used with permission.)

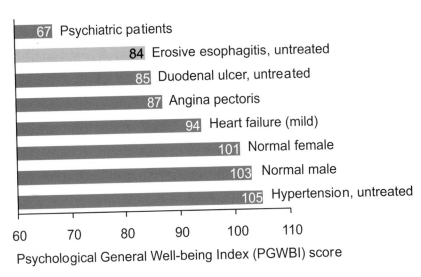

Fig. 9. Gastroesophageal reflux disease has a greater effect on quality of life than other common diseases. Quality of life, assessed by the PGWBI, was compared between patients with untreated gastroesophageal reflux disease and those with other disorders. For example, the mean PGWBI score of patients with untreated erosive esophagitis is similar to that of patients with untreated duodenal ulcer and lower (i.e., worse) than that of patients with angina pectoris or mild heart failure. Normal scores are 101 for women and 103 for men, but they vary slightly from country to country. (Modified from Dimenäs E. Methodological aspects of evaluation of Quality of Life in upper gastrointestinal diseases. Scand J Gastroenterol Suppl. 1993;199:18-21. Used with permission.)

unbuffered on the surface of the gastric meal contents. Reflux may occur also at night or when a person with a weak LES is supine or, especially, in the right lateral decubitus position.

Esophageal Chest Pain

GERD is the most common esophageal cause of noncardiac chest pain. The pain may be referred to any point on the anterior or posterior chest, with radiation to the neck, arm, or back. It may be indistinguishable from cardiac pain. Because of the potential fatal significance of cardiac pain, it is imperative that cardiac investigation precede esophageal investigation. Frequently, patients who have both cardiac and esophageal diseases cannot distinguish between reflux-associated pain and real angina. GERD may decrease the threshold for coronary ischemia, further confusing the clinical picture. This emphasizes the importance of first investigating the heart.

Extraesophageal Symptoms

GERD may be a frequent contributor of symptoms originating in other areas of the upper aerodigestive system. These symptoms, which can occur without the classic symptoms of heartburn and acid regurgitation, include cough, wheeze, hoarseness, sore throat, repetitive throat clearing, postnasal drip, neck or throat pain, globus, apnea, or otalgia. They are not specific for GERD. Indeed, GERD is only one of many causes of most of these symptoms. Like GERD, cough and wheezing are very common and likely to coexist by chance alone. Whether these symptoms are due to GERD needs to be confirmed by investigation or by the response to an empiric trial of potent acid-blocking therapy. Ideally, the demonstration of a pathologic degree of GERD and a response of the atypical symptoms to an adequate antireflux regimen is needed to conclude that GERD is the cause. GERD may produce extraesophageal symptoms in one of two ways. The first is by direct irritation or inflammation of the delicate mucosa of the larynx, trachea, or bronchi. The second is by reflex-mediated changes in function. Both mechanisms may operate in some patients.

ESTABLISHING A DIAGNOSIS

Therapeutic Trial

Several studies have investigated the usefulness of empiric trials of acid-suppressive therapy with proton pump inhibitors (Table 3).

Typical GERD Symptoms

Patients who present with typical symptoms without "alarm" symptoms should be given acid-suppression therapy. Complete resolution of the symptoms with treatment and relapse when treatment is discontinued confirm the diagnosis and suggest the need for a long-term management strategy. However, even in these patients, the specificity of a response to potent acid suppression is not specific for GERD because other acid peptic disorders respond to acid suppression therapy. If symptomatic improvement is limited, either an increase in dose or additional diagnostic testing is needed. If there is little or no symptomatic improvement with acid-suppression therapy, further investigation is indicated.

Atypical GERD Symptoms

GERD may cause or contribute to many different clinical syndromes. The more common causes of these syndromes should be evaluated first. For example, patients with asthma or chronic hoarseness should be evaluated for asthma or laryngeal neoplasm, respectively. If GERD is a possible cause, a therapeutic trial of acid suppression may be attempted. For esophageal symptoms such as chest pain, a 2-week trial of therapy usually is sufficient. For extraesophageal symptoms, a more prolonged therapeutic trial (2 to 3 months) may be necessary.

The acid-suppression test uses a potent regimen of acid suppression, for example, proton pump inhibitors (omeprazole, 40 mg in the morning and 20 mg in the evening). If the symptoms resolve, the patient should receive long-term treatment, with an attempt at dose reduction or cessation. For atypical symptoms, it is important to consider that they may have had alternative causes that resolved spontaneously. However, if there are reversible factors that are altered and if GERD is the major cause, the symptoms are likely to recur when therapy is discontinued. If the symptoms do not resolve completely, further evaluation with upper endoscopy or 24-hour ambulatory esophageal pH

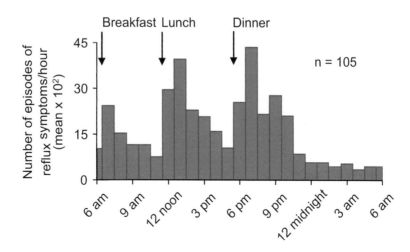

Fig. 10. Distribution of symptoms of gastroesophageal reflux disease over 24 hours in 105 patients who took their major meals at the same time of day. Note that food intake was associated with marked increase in the number of symptom episodes and relatively few episodes occurred during the night. (From Johnsson L, Adlouni W, Johnsson F, Joelssson B. Timing of reflux symptoms and esophageal acid exposure. Gullet. 1992;2:58-62. Used with permission.)

Table 3. Empiric Trials of Acid-Suppressive Therapy
With Proton Pump Inhibitors for Diagnosis

Symptom	Treatment	Sensitivity,* %	Specificity, %
Heartburn and regurgitation	Omeprazole twice daily for 7 d	80	56
Noncardiac chest pain	Omeprazole twice daily for 14 d	75	85
Extraesophageal	Proton pump inhibitor twice daily for 3 mo	?	?

*For the confirmation of gastroesophageal reflux disease.

monitoring with symptom-reflux correlation (or both) is indicated. If GERD is confirmed, chronic acid-suppression therapy is indicated. If symptoms persist, ambulatory esophageal pH monitoring may be repeated to document that the esophagus is no longer exposed to acid.

DIAGNOSTIC TESTS FOR GERD

Diagnostic tests are unnecessary for most persons with GERD. Investigations should be conducted in patients who have alarm symptoms, equivocal results on a treatment trial, or atypical symptoms of sufficient importance to warrant confirmation of GERD and those undergoing surgical or endoscopic therapy for GERD. For most patients, the endoscopic demonstration of esophagitis is sufficient proof of GERD and further investigation is unnecessary. However, more than 50% of patients with symptoms typical of GERD have normal endoscopic findings, and additional tests are required to identify increased esophageal exposure to acid either directly by ambulatory pH monitoring or indirectly by showing the reflux of a detectable material such as barium or a radiolabeled compound during a provocative maneuver or by reproducing symptoms through instillation of acid (Table 4).

Endoscopic Examination

Endoscopic examination allows direct visualization of the esophageal mucosa. In reflux esophagitis, the characteristic finding is linear erosions in the distal esophagus. These usually start at the esophagogastric junction and extend for various distances. The degree of severity varies. By their appearance alone, these erosions usually are readily differentiated from rarer infectious, allergic (eosinophilic), or corrosive causes of

inflammation. If the diagnosis is in question, biopsy specimens should be obtained not primarily to confirm reflux but to identify alternative pathologic conditions.

Several grading schemas, generally based on the extent of involvement, have been used. The Los Angeles classification system is the one used most commonly worldwide (Fig. 11). Erythema and increased vascularity are nonspecific features, and a break in the mucosa is required to make the diagnosis of reflux esophagitis. Careful scrutiny of the esophagogastric junction with adequate air insufflation is needed to examine the mucosa in its entirety. Endoscopy identifies the esophageal complications of GERD, including esophageal ulceration and stricture, Barrett's esophagus, and esophageal adenocarcinoma. Alarm symptoms that suggest these complications include long duration (more than 10 years) of typical symptoms, dysphagia, hematemesis or melena, and weight loss. The presence of these symptoms is a strong indication for diagnostic testing, especially endoscopy. Male sex, middle age, and nocturnal heartburn may be associated with a higher risk of esophagitis and its complications.

Barium Upper Gastrointestinal Tract Series

The barium contrast study, a readily available test, is sometimes used in the evaluation of patients with GERD. Its major usefulness in GERD is in identifying strictures and large hiatal hernias. It is insensitive for detecting erosions or superficial

Table 4. Uses of Diagnostic Tests for Gastroesophageal Reflux Disease

Endoscopy
    Direct identification of reflux esophagitis
    Biopsy Barrett's esophagus, adenocarcinoma
    Dilate strictures
    Endoscopic therapy (?)
Contrast radiography
    Hiatal hernia
    Identify strictures
    Reproduce reflux of barium (?)
Ambulatory 24-hour pH studies
    Quantify acid reflux in the absence of esophagitis
    Determine temporal correlation between gastroesophageal
      reflux and atypical symptoms
Bernstein test
    Provoke symptoms with acid
Gastroesophageal scintigraphy
    Quantify gastroesophageal reflux
    Identify aspiration

mucosal changes. The ability to reflux barium while at rest or in response to a provocative maneuver or postural change is not a sensitive test for GERD because most patients have a normal-pressure LES. In patients with extraesophageal symptoms, reflux of barium to or above the level of the aortic arch suggests the possibility of proximal reflux. The contrast study has limited value in detecting mucosal changes other than the most pronounced inflammation, which requires a double contrast study. The sensitivity for GERD is only 20%. When provocative maneuvers are added, the sensitivity increases but at great cost to specificity. A barium contrast study may be useful in delineating postoperative anatomical relationships and the intactness of an antireflux repair.

Prolonged Ambulatory Esophageal pH Monitoring Studies

Ambulatory pH monitoring of the esophageal lumen, a well-established test, was introduced in the early 1970s. It provides objective evidence of the degree of GERD and its timing. For most patients with symptoms of GERD and in whom the diagnosis is not in doubt, this test is not needed. The indications for ambulatory esophageal pH monitoring are listed in Table 5. The test is performed with a probe that has a pH sensor at its tip. The tip is placed 5 cm above the proximal border of the LES. Accurate location of the LES is critical because normal values for acid exposure apply only if the distance between the pH probe and the LES is 5 cm. The LES position is usually determined manometrically with a standard stationary esophageal manometry study or with a combined single water-perfused

pressure transducer with a pH probe that can accurately locate the proximal border of the LES and requires only a single intubation. Other methods such as endoscopic measurement and pH step-up on withdrawal are not sufficiently accurate for the placement of the nasoesophageal probe. The pH is recorded by a small portable recorder. A newer method uses a tubeless pH capsule that is pinned to the distal esophagus 6 cm above the endoscopically determined squamocolumnar junction. It transmits the pH measurements to a recorder worn on the chest. Its advantages are that it can record for prolonged periods and patients may eat more normally without the discomfort of the nasal tube. The patient should maintain his or her usual diet, activity, and habits during the study to allow the assessment of findings relative to the patient's normal lifestyle. The recorders have a patient-activated event button (or buttons) to indicate meals, changes in posture, and symptom events. The duration of the recording must be long enough to reflect all periods of the day, especially postprandial periods. Ideally, 20 hours or more of analyzable recordings are made.

The recordings are analyzed initially by visual inspection of the graphs and then by computer-assisted quantitative analysis of the number and duration of reflux episodes and the relation to any symptoms the patient may have recorded (Fig. 12). "Reflux of acid" is defined as a decrease in intraesophageal pH below 4.0 that lasts longer than 5 seconds. The six most commonly reported measurements are 1) the percentage of total time that pH is less than 4.0, 2) the percentage of upright time that pH is less than 4.0, 3) the percentage of recumbent time that pH is less than 4.0, 4) the total number of reflux events, 5) the

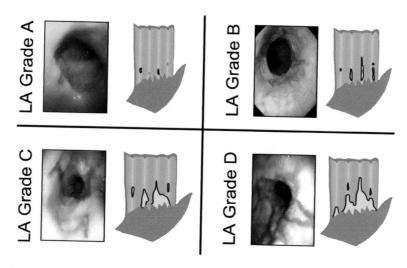

Fig. 11. Erosive esophagitis. Summary of the Los Angeles (LA) classification. Grade A, one or more mucosal breaks not more than 5 mm in maximal length. Grade B, one or more mucosal breaks more than 5 mm in maximal length, but not continuous between the tops of two mucosal folds. Grade C, mucosal breaks that are continuous between the tops of two or more folds but involve less than 75% of esophageal circumference. Grade D, mucosal breaks that involve at least 75% of esophageal circumference. (From www.astrazeneca.com. Used with permission.)

Table 5.   Indications for Ambulatory Esophageal pH Monitoring

Atypical symptoms: respiratory, ear, nose, and throat
Frequent atypical chest pain
Refractory symptoms in well-established GERD
Preoperative confirmation of GERD

GERD, gastroesophageal reflux disease.

number of reflux episodes that last longer than 5 minutes, and 6) the longest episode of reflux (in minutes). The first three measurements of acid exposure are used most frequently in everyday practice, and combined, they have a reported sensitivity of 85% and a specificity greater than 95% for diagnosing GERD associated with esophagitis. Another important strength of ambulatory esophageal pH monitoring is its ability to determine whether a temporal relation exists between the patient's recorded symptoms and acid reflux. This determination is made initially by examining the tracing on which the symptom events have been marked and then performing a semiquantitative analysis.

Several measures have been used to calculate the correlation between symptoms and reflux, including the symptom index (i.e., the percentage of symptom events that occur at the time of an acid reflux event). A symptom index greater than 50% usually is regarded as significant. The symptom sensitivity index is the percentage of reflux events associated with symptoms. A symptom sensitivity index greater than 5% usually is regarded to indicate an association between symptoms and acid reflux. More recently, the symptom association probability has been used as a more robust test for association. The ability to determine whether a temporal association exists depends on the number of symptom events and the amount of reflux that occurs. The patient must record his or her symptoms diligently and accurately during the study. If the symptoms occur once a week, there is little use in performing pH testing.

The 24-hour ambulatory esophageal pH monitoring test has limitations. Absolute values for sensitivity and specificity have been estimated because no standards exist for comparison with prolonged ambulatory pH monitoring. Also, pH monitoring may give false-negative results in 17% of patients with proven erosive esophagitis. This may reflect day-to-day variability in reflux or patients may have limited their diet or activities that would lead to reflux. Even simultaneous recording of pH from adjacent sensors may give different results in 20% of subjects. Some patients have a physiologic degree of acid reflux but have a strong correlation between the short-lived

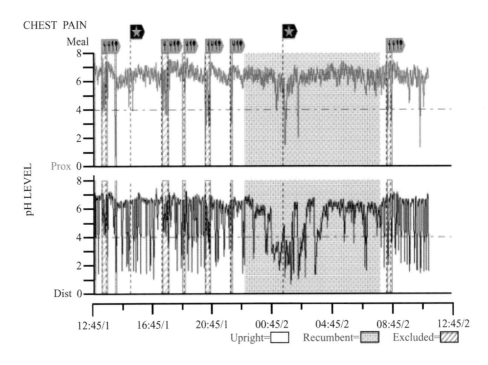

Fig. 12. Typical traces of 24-hour pH monitoring. Test was performed in patient with chest pain. Upper trace, Electrode placed 20 cm above lower esophageal sphincter. Lower trace, Electrode placed in distal esophagus, 5 cm above lower esophageal sphincter. Traces were recorded simultaneously. Esophageal pH must be less than pH 4 to be categorized as acid reflux. Marker flags, symptom episodes. Both episodes of chest pain occurred during reflux episodes (symptom index = 100%). Abnormal upright and recumbent esophageal acid exposure occurs in distal esophagus, suggesting both daytime and nightime reflux.

reflux events and symptoms. This may be due to a hypersensitive esophagus. Patients who frequently have symptoms of heartburn but no corresponding acid reflux may have what is termed "functional heartburn."

Generally, pH monitoring is performed when the patient is not taking any acid-suppressing medication. However, occasionally and for specific indications, pH monitoring may be performed when a patient is taking these medications. These indications include frequent typical reflux symptoms that are refractory to what should be adequate acid-suppressive therapy with usual doses of proton pump inhibitors. Another indication is persistent extraesophageal symptoms despite high-dose proton pump inhibitor therapy in patients with confirmed reflux disease. Usually, a prerequisite for performing the test is that the diagnosis of GERD is fairly certain and the intent is to verify that the suppression of acid reflux is complete.

Establishing a temporal correlation between symptoms and acid reflux events may be a secondary aim of the study. However, heartburn and regurgitation may occur in the absence of acid reflux. This may be due to nonacid reflux, gastric dyspepsia, or an unrelated process. A newer technique that measures both pH and intraluminal impedance may be able to detect nonacid reflux, but its role is not fully accepted and its clinical usefulness has not been demonstrated. Often, gastric pH is measured simultaneously to assess the degree of gastric acid suppression. Approximately one-third of patients receiving regular doses of proton pump inhibitors have marked production of acid in the stomach at night, but this breakthrough acid production does not always produce symptoms or actual esophageal acid reflux.

Gastroesophageal Scintigraphy

Gastroesophageal scintigraphy rarely is used to demonstrate gastroesophageal reflux or aspiration. The technique involves feeding the patient a technetium 99m sulfur colloid-labeled meal and obtaining postprandial images with a gamma camera. Delayed images obtained the following morning may show scintigraphic activity within the lung fields, demonstrating aspiration (usually, gross aspiration is needed). The test may be more useful in patients who have concomitant symptoms of delayed gastric emptying.

Bernstein Test

The Bernstein test is a provocative test in which acid (0.1N HCL) and water are infused alternately through a nasoesophageal tube into the midesophagus, with the patient unaware of the order of infusion. Of patients with GERD, 70% complain of heartburn within a few minutes after the start of the infusion of acid. Ideally, the symptom is relieved promptly when water is instilled. Because of low sensitivity and poor tolerance of the infusion, this test is not performed frequently. Great care must be taken to ensure that the tube is not in the airway,

because instillation of acid into the lungs may have severe consequences.

TREATMENT

Patient- or physician-initiated empirical treatment for presumed GERD has become commonplace. Indeed, guidelines for primary care have supported this approach for patients who do not have alarm symptoms. Treatment options for GERD are summarized in Table 6. Potent acid suppression with proton pump inhibitors is effective and heals reflux esophagitis after only a few weeks of therapy. This has resulted in a shift in the disease as it presents to endoscopists. It is rare to find severe disease in patients who have been treated with proton pump inhibitors. This practice poses a problem when symptoms do not resolve as expected. Perhaps there is partial improvement in symptoms. Although the diagnosis of GERD was suggested at the time of presentation and initiation of proton pump inhibitor therapy, the disease cannot be confirmed by the usual method without stopping the medications for a substantial time, and this may not be acceptable to patients in whom proton pump inhibitors have healed their esophagitis. A careful reexamination of the pretreatment symptoms may reveal that what the patient

Table 6. Summary of Treatment Options for Gastroesophageal Reflux Disease

Treatment	Options	Healing rate, %
Lifestyle modifications	Elevate the head of the bed Avoid eating within 3 hours before going to bed Moderate size and fat content of meals Reduce intake of caffeine, chocolate Stop smoking	20-30
Acid neutralization	Antacids Chewing gum Alginate preparations	20-30
Acid suppression	H_2 blockers	50
	Proton pump inhibitors	≥80
Prokinetics	Metoclopramide (not useful) Others in development	30-40
Mechanical prevention of reflux	Laparoscopic surgery	≥80
	Endoscopic therapies	≥50

thought was GERD may have been something else, for example, dyspepsia.

Acid-suppression therapy is the cornerstone of the treatment of GERD. It provides excellent healing and relief of symptoms in patients with esophagitis or classic heartburn. The relief appears to be related directly to the degree of acid suppression achieved.

Long-term maintenance therapy is needed for most patients. Lifestyle modifications alone may produce remission in 25% of patients with symptoms, but only a few patients are compliant with the restrictions. The same principles that apply to short-term therapy apply also to long-term therapy. Less acid equals less recurrence.

Histamine₂ Receptor Blockers

Histamine$_2$ (H$_2$) receptor blockers act by blocking the histamine-induced stimulation of gastric parietal cells. H$_2$ blockers provide moderate benefit when given in moderate doses (cimetidine, 400 mg twice daily; famotidine, 20 mg twice daily; nizatidine, 150 mg twice daily; and ranitidine, 150 mg twice daily) and heal esophagitis in 50% of patients. Higher doses suppress acid more rapidly. Lower doses are less effective, and nighttime-only dosing misses all the daytime reflux that predominates. A particular role for H$_2$ blockers may be to augment proton pump inhibitors when given at night to block nocturnal acid breakthrough; however, nocturnal H$_2$ blockade does not produce sustained nocturnal acid suppression because of tachyphylaxis.

Proton Pump Inhibitors

Proton pump inhibitors are absorbed rapidly and taken up and concentrated preferentially in parietal cells. They irreversibly complex with the H$^+$-K$^+$-ATPase pump, which is the final step in acid production. To produce acid, parietal cells must form new pumps, a process that takes many hours. Proton pump inhibitors are more potent than H$_2$ blockers as suppressors of acid reflux. The healing of esophagitis and the relief of symptoms are more rapid with proton pump inhibitors than with H$_2$ blockers. With proton pump inhibitor therapy, esophagitis heals within 4 weeks in more than 80% of patients and in virtually 100% by 8 weeks. However, the rate of complete relief from symptoms is less than the rate of healing.

Whether a proton pump inhibitor should be given as initial therapy and then replaced with H$_2$ blocker therapy or whether H$_2$ blocker therapy should precede proton pump inhibitor therapy is debated. Economic analysis, which takes into account the patient's quality of life, suggests that the latter approach is preferred. It is well established that therapy can sometimes be "stepped down" successfully after treatment with a proton pump inhibitor or switched to on-demand therapy, although this is rarely suitable for patients with substantial complications of GERD. This approach is not recommended unless cost considerations are paramount.

Although routine doses of proton pump inhibitors (esomeprazole, 40 mg/d; lansoprazole, 30 mg/d; omeprazole, 20 mg/d; pantoprazole, 40 mg/d; rabeprazole, 20 mg/d) are adequate for most patients with GERD, some may require higher or more frequent dosing to suppress GERD completely. Recent data have demonstrated that proton pump inhibitors are not entirely effective in blocking nocturnal production of acid in the stomach. Complete acid blockade can be achieved by dose escalation or by adding a nocturnal H$_2$ blocker. However, the latter strategy does not have a sustained effect.

Incomplete blockade may be the result of differences in metabolism or bioavailability. Omeprazole is absorbed more readily on an empty stomach and is most effective if the stomach parietal cells are stimulated. This is achieved by having patients eat within an hour after taking the medication.

With maintenance proton pump inhibitor therapy, the rate of relapse of esophagitis is 20% or less, which is lower than for H$_2$ blockers (Fig. 13). A slight escalation in dose may be needed with long-term therapy. Also, maintenance proton pump inhibitor therapy is more effective than H$_2$ blockers in reducing the need for redilatation in patients with reflux-associated benign strictures.

Proton pump inhibitor therapy causes a clinically insignificant increase in the serum level of gastrin. Although this has caused concern about a theoretical risk of carcinoid, the risk has not been realized after more than 10 years of long-term use of these agents. The increase in serum levels of gastrin and parietal cell mass may lead to rebound acid secretion after the therapy is stopped. The same effect also occurs, but for a shorter time, after H$_2$ blocker therapy is stopped.

Prokinetics

The idea that a motility disorder is the genesis of GERD made a prokinetic approach intellectually enticing. Drugs such as metoclopramide and, formerly, cisapride, which increase LES tone and esophageal clearance and accelerate gastric emptying, have been used to treat reflux. However, the healing rate and safety of these drugs have been questioned. Cisapride has been withdrawn from use in the United States, and the long-term use of metoclopramide is associated with so many side effects that it is rarely prescribed for GERD unless that is incidental to its use for gastroparesis. Several prokinetic agents are being studied for the treatment of GERD, but the lower efficacy of prokinetics compared with that of proton pump inhibitors limits their potential usefulness. Drugs that target the TLESRs also have been used, including baclofen, which probably can reduce reflux but is not approved or widely used for that indication.

Refractory Reflux

"Refractory reflux disease" can be defined as symptoms of GERD that are refractory to treatment with regular dosages of

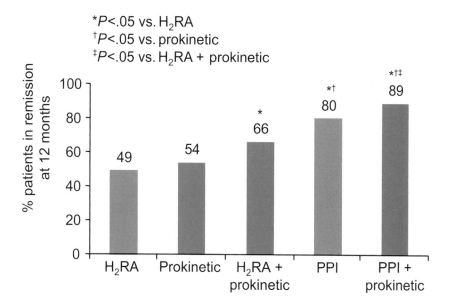

Fig. 13. Proton pump inhibitors (PPI) are the most effective drugs for maintenance therapy of gastroesophageal reflux disease. Although the remission rate was slightly higher with PPI + prokinetic than with PPI alone, the difference was not significant. H_2RA, histamine$_2$ receptor antagonist. (Data from Vigneri S, Termini R, Leandro G, Badalamenti S, Pantalena M, Savarino V, et al. A comparison of five maintenance therapies for reflux esophagitis. N Engl J Med. 1995;333:1106-10.)

proton pump inhibitors. The many common causes of refractory reflux symptoms are listed in Table 7.

Functional Chest Pain

Many patients who complain the most bitterly of severe reflux often have very little reflux on 24-hour pH monitoring and have no endoscopic features of reflux. This condition has been termed "nonerosive reflux disease." As with other functional gastrointestinal tract problems, females are overrepresented. Features of anxiety, panic, hyperventilation, and somatization may be clues to the diagnosis. Antacid therapies may help reduce the frequency of the symptoms, but they rarely relieve them completely. Therapies aimed at reducing visceral hypersensitivity may be helpful, for example, a low dose of an antidepressant.

Surgical and Endoscopic Antireflux Procedures

What is the role of laparoscopic and endoscopic methods of therapy? Medical therapy has been reduced to acid neutralization or suppression of acid production. Surgeons and endoscopists have focused on the role of the mechanical or functional failure of the antireflux barrier, and this has become the prime target of various approaches for preventing the reflux of gastric contents into the esophagus.

For many years, antireflux surgery was performed through a transabdominal or transthoracic approach, with considerable morbidity. Surgical treatment was reserved for intractable reflux that the available weak medical therapy failed to cure. With the advent of proton pump inhibitors, even severe degrees of reflux came to be well controlled, although the therapy is expensive. With the advent of minimally invasive surgery, surgical treatment has had a renaissance. The laparoscopic antireflux procedure has become a staple of the community surgeon. Its outcomes are similar to those of the open approach. With well-chosen patients and experienced surgeons, an 80% to 90% success rate is expected. The success rate decreases remarkably if the patients have symptoms refractory to proton pump inhibitor therapy or poorly documented reflux disease and if the procedure is performed by less experienced surgeons. A substantial number of these patients resume taking acid-blocking medications, often for unclear reasons. Preoperatively, it is important to verify that the patient's symptoms in fact are due to reflux. This is accomplished by documenting reflux esophagitis and a response to proton pump inhibitor therapy or by confirming the pathologic degree of reflux with a 24-hour pH assessment while the patient is not receiving therapy. If the patient belches frequently, he or she should be informed that belching may not be possible after the operation and gas bloat may result. Preoperative esophageal manometry has been widely recommended. It identifies a severe motility disturbance such as achalasia or connective tissue disease, and some surgeons want confirmation of a weak LES sphincter (if present).

Table 7. Causes of Refractory Reflux Symptoms in Patients Receiving Proton Pump Inhibitor Therapy

Incorrect initial diagnosis
   Nonreflux esophagitis—pill injury, skin diseases, eosinophilic esophagitis, infection
   Heart disease
   Chest wall pain
   Gastric pain
Additional diagnoses
   Dyspepsia—delayed gastric emptying, gastritis, peptic ulcer disease, nonulcer dyspepsia
   Above diagnoses
Inadequate acid suppression
   Noncompliance
   Rapid metabolizers
   Dose timing
   Too low a dose
   Zollinger-Ellison syndrome
Adenocarcinoma in Barrett's esophagus
   Postoperative reflux—partial gastrectomy, vertical-banded gastroplasty
Esophageal dysmotility
   Spasm
   Achalasia
   Nutcracker esophagus
Functional chest pain
   Hypersensitive esophagus
   Somatic features of depression
Free regurgitation
   Absence of lower esophageal sphincter tone
   Large hiatal hernia
   Achalasia
   Regurgitation

Postoperatively, 20% of patients have some dysphagia, but this persists in only 5%. Gas bloat, diarrhea, and dyspepsia may occur or become more evident postoperatively and may be troubling to patients. As many as one-third of the patients may still require proton pump inhibitor therapy postoperatively for persistent reflux or dyspepsia. Patients who have respiratory symptoms, free regurgitation, or simple but severe heartburn without gastric symptoms seem to have the best response to antireflux surgery. Female sex, lack of objective evidence of pathologic reflux, and failure to respond to proton pump inhibitor therapy all predict a poor response to surgery. Patient selection and operator experience seem to be the main determinants of a favorable surgical outcome. Reflux surgery is superior to long-term treatment with H_2 blockers to maintain the healing of GERD; however, follow-up for more than 10 years has shown an unexplained increase in mortality, predominantly due to cardiovascular disease, in the surgical group.

Who Not to Send to Surgery
It would be prudent to reconsider carefully the wisdom of sending to surgery a patient who has symptoms that are refractory to proton pump inhibitors. A hypersensitive esophagus or gastric dysmotility may be worse after fundoplication. Also, symptoms of irritable bowel syndrome may worsen postoperatively.

Endoscopic Methods of Therapy
Several endoscopic methods have been cleared as reasonably safe by the U.S. Food and Drug Administration, and several other methods are in development for the treatment of GERD. Radiofrequency ablation of the muscularis propria causes burning and subsequent scarring (Fig. 14), which results in a slightly increased resting pressure at the esophagogastric junction and a decrease in the number of TLESRs that occur postprandially. The total acid exposure time decreases, and many patients are able to stop taking acid-blocking drugs. Several weeks may be needed for the ablation to take effect. Radiofrequency ablation is relatively simple to perform, and the side effects are related to injury of the esophageal wall. Long-term benefits and adverse effects have not been reported. Trials are ongoing.

Several endoscopic methods to alter the shape or to tighten the esophagogastric junction are in various stages of development. These consist of inserting sutures or other devices into the gastric wall to generate a mechanical barrier or "speed bump" to reflux (Fig. 15). Although some of these methods are already in clinical use, evidence for long-term efficacy is lacking. Injections of nonabsorbable beads into the esophagogastric junction or the placement of more substantial mechanical barriers endoscopically has been achieved, although long-term durability has not been demonstrated for most of these methods. Some require considerable endoscopic skill, and although some patients appear to have less need for acid-blocking medication, the benefits are modest. Side effects are rare but have included bleeding, perforation, and embolization. These methods are likely to be refined, with improvement in effect. However, they are likely to reach the market with efficacy data that, compared with those for well-proven drug therapy, are slim to nonexistent.

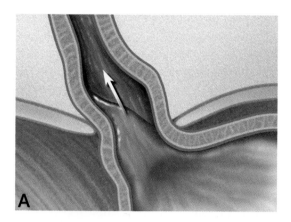

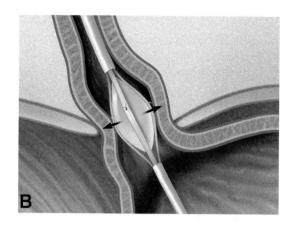

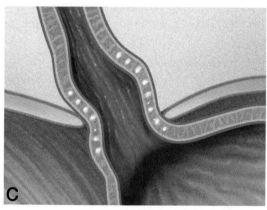

Fig. 14. Stretta procedure. *A*, Most episodes of reflux occur because of inappropriate relaxation of the lower esophageal sphincter (*arrow*, direction of reflux). *B*, Electrodes are deployed against the interior surface of the lower esophageal sphincter by inflating a small balloon in a specially designed endoscopic instrument. *C*, Current passed through the electrodes creates thermal lesions (*white circles*) in lower esophageal sphincter. The lesions disrupt nerve pathways and lead to tissue remodelling. This may reduce inappropriate relaxations of lower esophageal sphincter. (From www.astrazeneca.com. Used with permission.)

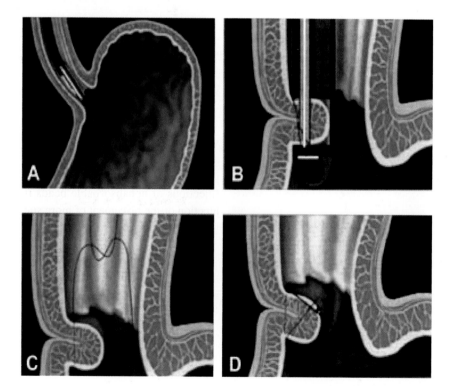

Fig. 15. Endoscopic gastroplication. The objective is to tighten the lower esophageal sphincter and form a barrier to reflux. *A*, Endoscope is advanced into the gastric cardia. *B*, A vacuum is applied, tissue is captured, and a stitch is placed. *C*, Suture material is knotted. *D*, The knot is drawn tight, forming a gastroplication. Typically, two to three plications are performed 1 cm below the Z line, with each plication requiring two stitches. (From Litin SC, editor. Endoscopic fundoplication for gastroesophageal reflux disease. Clinical Update. 2000;16[3]:1-3. By permission of Mayo Foundation for Medical Education and Research.)

RECOMMENDED READING

Dent J. Patterns of lower esophageal sphincter function associated with gastroesophageal reflux. Am J Med. 1997;103:29S-32S.

Dent J, Brun J, Fendrick AM, Fennerty MB, Janssens J, Kahrilas PJ, et al. An evidence-based appraisal of reflux disease management: the Genval Workshop Report. Gut. 1999;44 Suppl 2:S1-S16.

DeVault KR, Castell DO, the Practice Parameters Committee of the American College of Gastroenterology. Updated guidelines for the diagnosis and treatment of gastroesophageal reflux disease. Am J Gastroenterol. 1999;94:1434-42.

Fletcher J, Wirz A, Young J, Vallance R, McColl KE. Unbuffered highly acidic gastric juice exists at the gastroesophageal junction after a meal. Gastroenterology. 2001;121:775-83.

Furuta T, Ohashi K, Kosuge K, Zhao XJ, Takashima M, Kimura M, et al. CYP2C19 genotype status and effect of omeprazole on intragastric pH in humans. Clin Pharmacol Ther. 1999;65:552-61.

Gillen D, Wirz AA, Ardill JE, McColl KE. Rebound hypersecretion after omeprazole and its relation to on-treatment acid suppression and *Helicobacter pylori* status. Gastroenterology. 1999;116:239-47.

Hogan WJ, Shaker R. Supraesophageal complications of gastroesophageal reflux. Dis Mon. 2000;46:193-232.

Holtmann G, Cain C, Malfertheiner P. Gastric *Helicobacter pylori* infection accelerates healing of reflux esophagitis during treatment with the proton pump inhibitor pantoprazole. Gastroenterology. 1999;117:11-6.

Kahrilas PJ, Shi G, Manka M, Joehl RJ. Increased frequency of transient lower esophageal sphincter relaxation induced by gastric distention in reflux patients with hiatal hernia. Gastroenterology. 2000;118:688-95.

Katzka DA, Paoletti V, Leite L, Castell DO. Prolonged ambulatory pH monitoring in patients with persistent gastroesophageal reflux disease symptoms: testing while on therapy identifies the need for more aggressive anti-reflux therapy. Am J Gastroenterol. 1996;91:2110-3.

Klauser AG, Schindlbeck NE, Muller-Lissner SA. Symptoms in gastro-oesophageal reflux disease. Lancet. 1990;335:205-8.

Klinkenberg-Knol EC, Nelis F, Dent J, Snel P, Mitchell B, Prichard P, et al. Long-term omeprazole treatment in resistant gastroesophageal reflux disease: efficacy, safety, and influence on gastric mucosa. Gastroenterology. 2000;118:661-9.

Locke GR III, Talley NJ, Fett SL, Zinsmeister AR, Melton LJ III. Prevalence and clinical spectrum of gastroesophageal reflux: a population-based study in Olmsted County, Minnesota. Gastroenterology. 1997;112:1448-56.

Orlando RC. Why is the high grade inhibition of gastric acid secretion afforded by proton pump inhibitors often required for healing of reflux esophagitis? An epithelial perspective. Am J Gastroenterol. 1996;91:1692-6.

Stanghellini V: Three-month prevalence rates of gastrointestinal symptoms and the influence of demographic factors: results from the Domestic/International Gastroenterology Surveillance Study (DIGEST). Scand J Gastroenterol Suppl. 1999;231:20-8.

Tobey NA. How does the esophageal epithelium maintain its integrity? Digestion. 1995;56 Suppl 1:45-50.

Tobey NA. Systemic factors in esophageal mucosal protection. Digestion. 1995;56 Suppl 1:38-44.

Vakil N, Kahrilas P, Magner D. Does baseline Hp status impact erosive esophagitis (EE) healing rates? [Abstract.] Am J Gastroenterol. 2000;95:2438-9.

Vigneri S, Termini R, Leandro G, Badalamenti S, Pantalena M, Savarino V, et al. A comparison of five maintenance therapies for reflux esophagitis. N Engl J Med. 1995;333:1106-10.

CHAPTER 3

Barrett's Esophagus

Yvonne Romero, M.D.

DEFINITIONS

Barrett's esophagus is clinically relevant only because of its strong association with esophageal adenocarcinoma (Fig. 1). Barrett's esophagus requires endoscopic and pathologic criteria for diagnosis. To meet the criteria for Barrett's esophagus, endoscopy must demonstrate salmon-colored mucosa in the tubular esophagus (Fig. 2) and biopsy specimens must show intestinal metaplasia with goblet cells (so-called *specialized* intestinal metaplasia) (Fig. 3).

Arbitrarily, "long-segment Barrett's esophagus" refers to salmon-colored segments of specialized intestinal metaplasia at least 3 cm long (Fig. 4). Essentially all the literature before 1989 refers to this type. "Short-segment Barrett's esophagus" refers to macroscopic segments or tongues of salmon-colored epithelium less than 3 cm long seen at endoscopy (Fig. 4). Biopsy specimens from these segments demonstrate intestinal metaplasia with goblet cells. "Intestinal metaplasia of the cardia" refers to the histologic finding of intestinal metaplasia with goblet cells at a normally located and normal-appearing squamocolumnar junction (the so-called zig-zag or Z-line) (Fig. 4). This also has been termed "focal intestinal metaplasia of a normal-appearing Z-line." Neither intestinal metaplasia of the cardia nor focal intestinal metaplasia of a normal-appearing Z-line is classified as Barrett's esophagus.

PATHOPHYSIOLOGY

Barrett's esophagus is an acquired disorder in which columnar epithelium replaces the stratified squamous epithelium that normally lines the distal esophagus. It is thought to occur in response to years of reflux of gastric contents into the distal esophagus. Patients with Barrett's esophagus, compared with normal healthy controls and patients with erosive esophagitis, more frequently have hiatal hernias, weaker lower esophageal sphincter tone, and abnormal distal esophageal acid exposure, by 24-hour pH testing. Currently, it is presumed that hiatal

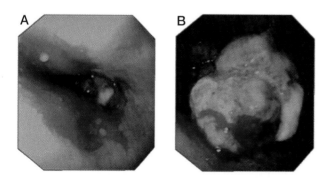

Fig. 1. Squamous epithelium, Barrett's esophagus, and the consequence, esophageal adenocarcinoma. *A*, Endoscopic view of three types of mucosa: icy pink squamous epithelium, salmon-colored mucosa, which is diagnostic of Barrett's esophagus if biopsy specimen shows intestinal metaplasia with goblet cells, and the mushroom-like growth of esophageal adenocarcinoma. *B*, Close-up view of exophytic esophageal adenocarcinoma in a field of Barrett's esophagus.

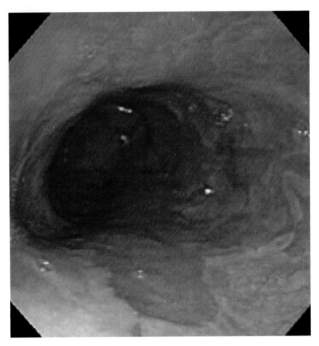

Fig. 2. Barrett's esophagus. (Courtesy of Drs. Kenneth K. Wang and Louis M. Wong Kee Song, Gastroenterology and Hepatology, Mayo Clinic.)

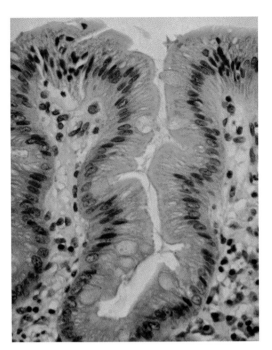

Fig. 3. Intestinal metaplasia with goblet cells. (Courtesy of Dr. Thomas C. Smyrk, Anatomic Pathology, Mayo Clinic.)

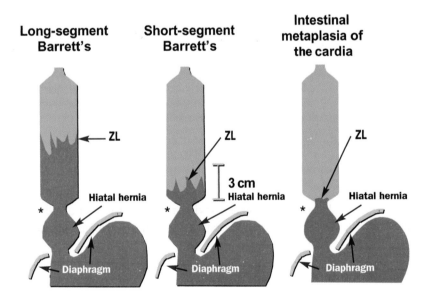

Fig. 4. Patients with long-segment or short-segment Barrett's esophagus have salmon-colored mucosa extending up into the tubular esophagus. Biopsy specimens must demonstrate intestinal metaplasia with goblet cells. If intestinal metaplasia with goblet cells is found at a normally located zig-zag line (ZL), the patient has intestinal metaplasia of the cardia, which confers a lower cancer risk. *End of tubular esophagus and beginning of stomach.

herniation and weak lower esophageal sphincter tone predispose to more severe reflux and that chronic reflux initiates the metaplastic change from a squamous to a columnar epithelial lining.

The length of the salmon-colored mucosal segment seen endoscopically does not change over time in patients with long-segment Barrett's esophagus. In one study, the segmental length remained constant in 21 patients who had repeat examinations at least 5 years apart (mean, 7.3 years). It is not clear if this also is true of short-segment Barrett's esophagus. With the common use of proton pump inhibitors, and thus notable acid suppression, islands of squamous epithelium often are identified within the segment of Barrett's esophagus.

EPIDEMIOLOGY OF BARRETT'S ESOPHAGUS

Barrett's esophagus is associated with reflux symptoms, advancing age, male sex, and white race.

Population Prevalence of Barrett's Esophagus

Olmsted County, Minnesota, is one of a rare handful of enumerated populations in the world. Enumerated populations allow confident epidemiologic estimates to be calculated because the denominator is known and all members are accounted for. As of January 1, 1987, the *clinically* diagnosed age- and sex-adjusted prevalence of long-segment Barrett's esophagus was 22.6 per 100,000 persons, and by January 1, 1998, it had increased to 80.3 per 100,000, almost a fourfold increase. The number of new cases of long-segment Barrett's esophagus diagnosed per 100,000 population per year increased from 0.37 in 1965-1969 to 10.5 in 1995-1997, a 28-fold increase. Initially, it was thought that the prevalence of long-segment Barrett's esophagus had increased over three decades. However, during the same period, the number of upper endoscopic examinations performed on Olmsted County residents had increased from 65 to 1,461 per 100,000 population per year, a 22-fold increase. Currently, in Olmsted County, long-segment Barrett's esophagus is diagnosed more frequently than it was in the past partly because more persons undergo endoscopy now than previously. Also, endoscopists are now probably more aware of this clinical entity and, hence, less likely to overlook or miss it.

European investigators have another opinion. Prach et al, in a brief report from Dundee, Scotland, found that the incidence of long-segment Barrett's esophagus increased from 1 per 100,000 population in 1980-1981 to 48 per 100,000 per year in 1992-1993. They found that for the same years the rate of detection of long-segment Barrett's esophagus increased from 1.4 to 16.5 per 1,000 endoscopic examinations performed (including only cases with histologic confirmation). Other investigators have surmised that the increased prevalence of esophageal adenocarcinoma in the United Kingdom during the past three decades most likely reflects an increased prevalence of Barrett's esophagus. Currently, however, the evidence does not clearly show an increased prevalence of Barrett's esophagus in Europe.

Population-based information on the incidence and prevalence of short-segment Barrett's esophagus is limited. Before 1989, most endoscopists disregarded small tongues of salmon-colored mucosa of the distal esophagus and did not obtain biopsy specimens. Mayo Clinic physicians were not aware of short-segment Barrett's esophagus until 1989. As awareness of this entity grew, so did its documentation at endoscopy, with concomitant indexing of "short-segment Barrett's esophagus" as a recognized diagnosis. By 1998, the prevalence of short-segment Barrett's esophagus in Olmsted County was 33 per 100,000 population, with a 2:1 male predominance. Population estimates of prevalence are not available for intestinal metaplasia of the cardia.

Prevalence of Long-Segment Barrett's Esophagus at Autopsy

In 1990, an autopsy study was performed to estimate the population prevalence of long-segment Barrett's esophagus. The esophagus and proximal stomach were removed as a single segment from consecutive autopsy subjects for daily review by a single endoscopist. Histologic sections were made whenever the squamocolumnar junction appeared to lie 3 cm above the gastroesophageal junction. Hence, conclusions could not be drawn about the prevalence of short-segment Barrett's esophagus and intestinal metaplasia of the cardia. Of 733 consecutive unselected autopsies of Olmsted County residents, 7 had long-segment Barrett's esophagus. Thus, in 1990, the age- and sex-adjusted prevalence of long-segment Barrett's esophagus was 376 per 100,000 population. No other studies with this design have been conducted, and it is not known whether the prevalence of long-segment Barrett's esophagus has changed since 1990.

Prevalence of Barrett's Esophagus Among Patients Having Endoscopy

The prevalence of long-segment Barrett's esophagus in consecutive patients undergoing endoscopy for any indication is approximately 1%. In an Italian multicenter study, 0.74% of 14,898 patients having endoscopy had long-segment Barrett's esophagus. In Olmsted County, long-segment Barrett's esophagus was reported in 1% of patients 25 years and older.

In 1998 in Olmsted County, a comparison of the prevalence rate of Barrett's esophagus and the number of patients with clinically diagnosed Barrett's esophagus showed that the diagnosis had been made in only 1 of 7 of those who had the disease. Recently, a systematic review reported that fewer than 5% of patients with both Barrett's esophagus and esophageal adenocarcinoma documented in a surgical resection specimen had been given the diagnosis of Barrett's esophagus before seeking medical care for symptoms of cancer (dysphagia, weight loss of unclear origin, or anemia).

Short-segment Barrett's esophagus is found in 10% to 15% of white adults who have elective endoscopy, regardless of the indication for the procedure. Because the 3-cm criterion for diagnosis of long-segment Barrett's esophagus was selected arbitrarily, the occurrence of shorter, endoscopically visible tongues of salmon-colored mucosa consisting of specialized intestinal metaplasia is not surprising. What was not expected initially was the demonstration of small foci of specialized intestinal metaplasia in 15% to 18% of people with normal-appearing Z-lines who had endoscopy for any indication. As mentioned above, this condition is now known as "intestinal metaplasia of the cardia."

Risk Factors for Barrett's Esophagus

Age

Barrett's esophagus is an acquired disorder. Thus, the prevalence of long-segment Barrett's esophagus increases with age (Fig. 5). The mean age at time of diagnosis is 63 years. Long-segment Barrett's esophagus is rare in children. In the Mayo Clinic experience spanning more than 20 years, only 377 of 51,000 children who had upper endoscopy had long-segment Barrett's esophagus.

Male Sex

In a Mayo Clinic study of patients who had endoscopy between 1976 and 1989, long-segment Barrett's esophagus was twice as common in males as in females, and in a large multicenter Italian study (patients enrolled from 1987 to 1989), it was 2.6 times more common in males than in females. Higher male-to-female ratios have been reported in studies of military populations in which females were in the extreme minority. Recently, the prevalence data have been updated for Olmsted County residents. Although the number of males and females who had endoscopy was almost equal, the prevalence of long-segment Barrett's esophagus in January 1998 was 148 males per 100,000 population, fourfold greater than for females, 36 per 100,000 population. Possibly, male predominance in prevalence of Barrett's esophagus has increased with time. Also, women may seek health care more often than men and, hence, have endoscopy for fewer symptoms.

Geography and Ethnicity

Long-segment Barrett's esophagus is frequently described in Western countries but apparently is rare in other countries, such as Japan. However, this seems to be changing. In South Africa, long-segment Barrett's esophagus is found more commonly in whites than in blacks. In an American study, long-segment Barrett's esophagus was found in 6.5% of 611 white patients who had endoscopy compared with 0 of 200 African Americans. This finding has been confirmed by others. In another study, the overall rate of Barrett's esophagus of any length was similar for non-Hispanic whites and Hispanics; however, the majority of Hispanics had short-segment Barrett's esophagus and most non-Hispanic whites had long segments of intestinal metaplasia with goblet cells.

Reflux Symptoms

The symptoms of gastroesophageal reflux disease (GERD) include heartburn, which is described as substernal burning pain, and acid regurgitation, which is a bitter or sour taste that travels to the mouth. About 15% to 20% of adults in the United States report experiencing heartburn at least once a week, and 7% report having symptoms daily. Of adults with symptoms of GERD, long-segment Barrett's esophagus is diagnosed at endoscopy in 3.5% to 7% (an age- and sex-adjusted estimate). In contrast, long-segment Barrett's esophagus is found at endoscopy in only 1% of adults who say they do not have symptoms of GERD.

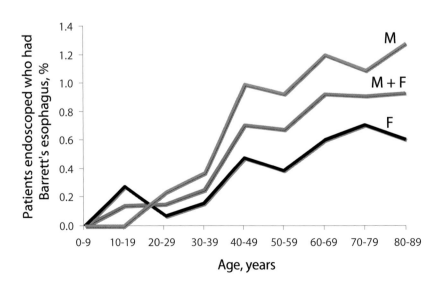

Fig. 5. Prevalence of Barrett's esophagus increased with age up to seventh decade. Half the maximum prevalence was reached by about age 40. Mean age at diagnosis was 63 years. (Courtesy of Dr. Alan J. Cameron, Emeritus, Mayo Clinic.)

Risk-factor estimates for short-segment Barrett's esophagus are based mainly on cohort or case-control studies, which increase the possibility of overestimation of risk because of study design limitations. In a study in which all subjects reported heartburn at least twice a week, short-segment Barrett's esophagus was diagnosed in 7 of 378 (1.8%) consecutive patients who had endoscopy for various indications. In a case-control study, patients with short-segment Barrett's esophagus were more likely to have reflux symptoms than controls without this condition who had endoscopy for another indication.

Intestinal Metaplasia of the Cardia

Before 1994, biopsy of a normal-appearing zig-zag line (the junction of the cardia and the pale stratified squamous lining of the distal esophagus) was not common. It was presumed that biopsy specimens from this junction would demonstrate gastric cardia-type mucosa or, if the specimen was from an adjacent area, fundic mucosa. In 1994, Spechler et al reported on 143 consecutive patients who did not have endoscopic evidence of Barrett's esophagus but in whom biopsy specimens were obtained from the squamocolumnar junction according to protocol. Histologic evidence of intestinal metaplasia was found in 18% of these patients. Intestinal metaplasia with goblet cells at a normal-appearing Z-line has been demonstrated repeatedly by numerous investigators. For all patients who have endoscopy for any indication, the prevalence estimates range from 6% to 36%. The prevalence increases with age, suggesting that it is an acquired condition. However, unlike long- or short-segment Barrett's esophagus, intestinal metaplasia of the cardia is found equally in males and females and in whites and blacks, regardless of whether the symptoms of GERD are present. Intestinal metaplasia of the stomach is associated with *Helicobacter pylori*. The role of *H. pylori* in the development of intestinal metaplasia of the cardia is debated.

CANCER RISK

Barrett's Esophagus

Reports of long-term follow-up of patients with long-segment Barrett's esophagus suggest that one cancer develops per 180 to 208 patient-years; that is, annually, esophageal adenocarcinoma develops in 0.5% of patients with Barrett's esophagus. Although a patient with Barrett's esophagus has a 40- to 125-fold higher risk of the disease progressing to adenocarcinoma than someone without this premalignant lining, the absolute risk of cancer is approximately 0.005 cancer per patient annually, which is quite low. Thus, a 50-year-old man with Barrett's esophagus and otherwise normal life expectancy has a 3% to 10% lifetime risk (cumulative incidence) of developing esophageal adeno-carcinoma.

The rate of neoplastic transformation is less for patients with shorter segments of specialized intestinal metaplasia. The findings from three series suggest that one cancer develops in short segments every 293 patient-years (i.e., of 293 patients with 1 year of follow-up, 1 will have progression to esophageal adenocarcinoma). Rudolph et al demonstrated that the most important risk factor for predicting neoplastic progression is the degree of dysplasia and not the length of Barrett's esophagus. Although length was not an independent risk factor for neoplastic progression, there was a trend toward significance, suggesting that perhaps this study was underpowered to address this specific outcome. It may be beneficial for a patient to have a shorter segment of Barrett's esophagus. Because short-segment Barrett's esophagus is more common than long-segment Barrett's esophagus, the former is highly relevant from a societal perspective.

Intestinal Metaplasia of the Cardia

Esophageal cancer is uncommon. For the general population, the prevalence of esophageal adenocarcinoma is 3 or 4 per 100,000 persons per year. This rate includes people with undiagnosed long-segment Barrett's esophagus who develop adenocarcinoma. Population follow-up studies of patients with intestinal metaplasia of the cardia are not available, but the practical conclusion seems clear. If one in five adults has intestinal metaplasia of the cardia, the risk that a person with this finding will develop adenocarcinoma must be extremely small.

SURVEILLANCE

Because Rudolph et al showed that transformation to neoplasia depends more on the degree of dysplasia than on mucosal length, the current practice is to offer the same surveillance regimen to patients with short-segment or long-segment Barrett's esophagus.

The guidelines of the American College of Gastroenterology recommend that the initial diagnostic endoscopic examination measure the proximal extent of salmon-colored mucosa and the distal end of the tubular esophagus–proximal extent of the gastric folds and biopsy specimens be collected as follows: 1) from any suspicious lesions (e.g., nodules, raised edges of an ulcer, stricture, erosions) and 2) four-quadrant biopsy specimens every 2 cm along the length of the segment.

Currently, dysplasia is the best indicator of cancer risk. Surveillance endoscopy should be recommended to patients deemed eligible for intervention when an early lesion is identified. If no dysplasia is found at initial endoscopy, surveillance endoscopy is recommended in 1 year to exclude incident cancers or dysplasia. If dysplasia of any degree of severity is identified, with the exception of cancer, the Updated Guidelines for the Diagnosis, Surveillance, and Therapy of Barrett's Esophagus, published in late 2002 by the American

College of Gastroenterology, recommend that additional acid-suppression medications be administered before endoscopy is repeated, preferably in 6 to 12 weeks. Inflammation commonly causes "reactive atypia," a cellular response to inflammation that can be easily overinterpreted as dysplasia. On repeat endoscopy, focused biopsy specimens should be collected from the level at which dysplasia was initially detected in addition to the usual four-quadrant biopsy specimens obtained at every 2-cm interval for follow-up of low-grade dysplasia or at 1-cm intervals for high-grade dysplasia. The American College of Gastroenterology recommends consideration of endoscopic resection of the mucosa of any focal lesion to obtain more tissue for more accurate staging of disease. All slides should be reviewed by at least two gastrointestinal pathologists who are experts at staging Barrett's esophagus.

Low-Grade Dysplasia

If low-grade dysplasia is the most severe grade of dysplasia detected and follow-up endoscopy shows that it persists, endoscopy every 6 months ×2 is recommended, followed by surveillance endoscopy annually ×2. If low-grade dysplasia still persists or if there is no evidence of dysplasia, surveillance endoscopy then can be performed every 3 to 5 years.

High-Grade Dysplasia

If at least two subspecialty, expert pathologists agree on the presence of focal high-grade dysplasia (dysplasia involving five or fewer crypts), options for the patient include 1) observation, while the patient receives high-dose acid-suppression medications, and endoscopy every 3 months following the intense biopsy protocol described above; 2) esophagectomy, the standard of care for otherwise physically fit patients; or 3) experimental treatment with photodynamic therapy or other ablative modalities. Patients interested in pursuing esophagectomy should be referred to high-volume centers. Perioperative mortality rates for this complex procedure vary greatly from less than 3% to 20%, depending on the experience of the center.

For patients with diffuse or multifocal high-grade dysplasia, options include esophagectomy and photodynamic therapy. The American College of Gastroenterology has less confidence in the safety of simple observation for patients with multifocal high-density dysplasia.

RECOMMENDED READING

Cameron AJ, Kamath PS, Carpenter HA. Prevalence of Barrett's esophagus and intestinal metaplasia at the esophagogastric junction (abstract). Gastroenterology. 1997;112 Suppl 4:A82.

Conio M, Cameron AJ, Romero Y, Branch CD, Schleck CD, Burgart LJ, et al. Secular trends in the epidemiology and outcome of Barrett's oesophagus in Olmsted County, Minnesota. Gut. 2001;48:304-9.

Dulai GS, Guha S, Kahn KL, Gornbein J, Weinstein WM. Preoperative prevalence of Barrett's esophagus in esophageal adenocarcinoma: a systematic review. Gastroenterology. 2002;122:26-33.

Lagergren J, Bergstrom R, Lindgren A, Nyren O. Symptomatic gastroesophageal reflux as a risk factor for esophageal adenocarcinoma. N Engl J Med. 1999;340:825-31.

Locke GR III, Talley NJ, Fett SR, Zinsmeister AR, Melton LJ III. Prevalence and clinical spectrum of gastroesophageal reflux: a population based study in Olmsted County, Minnesota. Gastroenterology. 1997;112:1448-56.

Prach AT, MacDonald TA, Hopwood DA, Johnston DA. Increasing incidence of Barrett's oesophagus: education, enthusiasm, or epidemiology? Lancet. 1997;350:933.

Rudolph RE, Vaughan TL, Storer BE, Haggitt RC, Rabinovitch PS, Levine DS, et al. Effect of segment length on risk for neoplastic progression in patients with Barrett esophagus. Ann Intern Med. 2000;132:612-20.

Sampliner RE. Updated guidelines for the diagnosis, surveillance, and therapy of Barrett's esophagus. Am J Gastroenterol. 2002;97:1888-95.

Shaheen NJ, Crosby MA, Bozymski EM, Sandler RS. Is there publication bias in the reporting of cancer risk in Barrett's esophagus? Gastroenterology. 2000;119:333-8.

Shaheen NJ, Ransohoff DF. Gastroesophageal reflux, Barrett esophagus, and esophageal cancer: scientific review. JAMA. 2002;287:1972-81.

Spechler SJ. Clinical practice: Barrett's esophagus. N Engl J Med. 2002;346:836-42.

Spechler SJ, Zeroogian JM, Antonioli DA, Wang HH, Goyal RK. Prevalence of metaplasia at the gastro-oesophageal junction. Lancet. 1994;344:1533-6.

CHAPTER 4

Esophageal Cancer

Kenneth K. Wang, M.D.

EPIDEMIOLOGY OF ESOPHAGEAL TUMORS

Currently, the most common histologic type of esophageal cancer in the United States is adenocarcinoma, which is related to Barrett's esophagus and heartburn. This is unexpected because more than a decade ago it was believed that the esophagus did not commonly develop adenocarcinoma. Adenocarcinoma was thought to involve only 2% to 4% of esophageal cancers and even these were suspect because they were thought to be related to gastric cancers that had migrated proximally. Case control epidemiologic studies of nutritional factors have implicated less-than-average intake of fresh fruits and vegetables in the pathogenesis of esophageal adenocarcinoma. Specific nutrients that have been found to be important in the development of esophageal cancers include vitamins A, B$_6$, C, E, and folate. Also, fiber is protective against the development of esophageal adenocarcinoma. Even though adenocarcinoma is now the most common cancer of the esophagus in the United States, cancers of the esophagus are not common. The incidence of cancer within Barrett's esophagus is thought to be approximately 0.4% to 0.5% per patient-year. This is far less than the previously suspected cancer incidence of 10% to 15%.

Worldwide, squamous cell cancers are the most common cancer of the esophagus (30%-40%) and are related to the use of tobacco and alcohol. Rare causes include Plummer-Vinson syndrome, achalasia, lack of trace metals (including selenium), tylosis, lye ingestion, ionizing radiation, human papilloma virus, and drinking of maté (South American beverage made from yerba maté [maté herb]). Nutritional deficiencies in vitamins A and C also are associated with squamous cell cancers, and providing supplemental β-carotene, vitamin C, and selenium to patients at high risk for esophageal cancer can decrease cancer risk. Squamous cell cancers of the esophagus arise primarily in females. However, esophageal cancers are still more common in males, with a male-to-female ratio of 3:1. Squamous cell cancers occur most commonly in the sixth decade of life. The differential diagnosis of mass lesions that occur in the distal esophagus of young patients must also include possible metastatic disease.

Rare primary cancers of the esophagus include small cell cancer, choriocarcinoma, melanoma, sarcoma, and lymphoma. The overall incidence of esophageal cancer is about 3/100,000 persons in the United States.

The location of malignancies in the esophagus can often help predict the type of tumor present. Esophageal tumors in the upper and middle one-third of the esophagus are likely squamous cell cancers and those in the distal third are generally adenocarcinoma. Most rare tumors (sarcoma, melanoma, choriocarcinoma) tend to occur in the distal esophagus.

- Typical board questions about the epidemiology of esophageal cancer could be radiographs of a distal esophageal cancer being matched with a male with chronic heartburn, a proximal cancer matched with a chronic smoker, and a smooth intramural lesion matched with a patient who previously had melanoma.

MOLECULAR MECHANISMS OF ESOPHAGEAL CANCER

The most common abnormalities found in squamous cell cancer are mutations in the cyclin D1 gene, which is involved in cell cycling with the cyclin-dependent kinases. This complex phosphorylates the product of the retinoblastoma gene (*Rb*), which is a major negative regulator of the G_1 phase of the cell cycle and thus leads to increased cell cycling. With inactivation of this gene product, the number of cells entering the cell cycle from the G_1 phase increases, as does proliferation. It also has been noted that abnormalities in the E-cadherin/β-catenin complex increase the ability of cells to metastasize. Tumor angiogenesis factors such as vascular endothelial growth factor and growth factors such as epidermal growth factor are also involved in tumor invasion.

In adenocarcinomas, the mechanism is thought to occur through inactivation of the *p16* gene through hypermethylation of its promoter region. The loss of this cell checkpoint gene also leads to increased cell cycling and genetic instability, resulting in the formation of *p53* mutations and subsequently to aneuploidy (widespread chromosomal abnormalities). This genetic instability also results in cancer formation.

CANCER PREVENTION

The elimination of risk factors is recommended for all patients, including the elimination of tobacco use and control of gastroesophageal reflux disease. Multiple single-center studies have shown that antireflux procedures do not eliminate the risk of cancer in patients with reflux disease. Also, the avoidance of foods known to provoke reflux symptoms, such as dietary fat, chocolate, mints, coffee, onions, citrus fruit, or tomatoes, does not have any protective effect against the development of cancer. A recent epidemiologic study from Sweden showed that surgical control of gastroesophageal reflux disease did not offer any significant protection against esophageal adenocarcinoma. The only epidemiologic evidence for prevention of esophageal cancer comes from studies that have found a 90% reduction in cancer risk in patients who routinely take aspirin. Chemoprevention with cyclooxygenase-2 inhibitors is currently being investigated.

PRESENTING SYMPTOMS

The primary presenting symptoms for esophageal tumors are the development of dysphagia, present in 90% of patients, and odynophagia, present in 50%. Typically, the symptoms occur with solid foods such as steak or breads and gradually worsen to involve even liquids. Rare presenting symptoms include back pain (possible mediastinal involvement), hematemesis, nausea, or hoarseness (involvement of the recurrent laryngeal nerve). Dysphagia associated with esophageal cancer usually signals an advanced stage of cancer, typically T3.

STAGING OF ESOPHAGEAL CANCER

Esophageal cancer is staged according to internationally accepted standards (Table 1). The staging of esophageal tumors is related

Table 1. Staging of Esophageal Cancer

Primary tumor		
	Tx	Primary tumor cannot be assessed
	T0	No evidence of primary tumor
	Tis	Carcinoma in situ
	T1	Tumor invades submucosa or lamina propria
	T2	Tumor invades muscularis propria
	T3	Tumor invades adventitia
	T4	Tumor invades adjacent structures
Lymph nodes		
	Nx	Regional lymph nodes cannot be assessed
	N0	No regional lymph nodes
	N1	Regional lymph node metastasis
Distant metastasis		
	Mx	Distant metastasis cannot be assessed
	M0	No distant metastasis
	M1	Presence of distant metastasis
	M1a	Nodal metastasis in the celiac region for adenocarcinoma
	M1b	Other distant metastasis
Staging		
	Stage 0	Tis N0 M0
	Stage I	T1 N0 M0
	Stage IIA	T2 or T3 N0 M0
	Stage IIB	T1 or T2 N1 M0
	Stage III	T3 or T4 N1 M0
	Stage IV	Any T, Any N, M1

directly to the probability of nodal metastasis. Because the lymphatic system of the esophagus penetrates close to the mucosa, even a cancer that penetrates to the lamina propria can have up to a 20% chance of regional metastasis. Thus, disease that can be treated endoscopically is limited to very superficial tumors.

ENDOSCOPIC ULTRASONOGRAPHIC STAGING

Endoscopic ultrasonography (EUS) uses specially modified endoscopes and probes to image the esophageal wall. Typically, endoscopes can image using ultrasound frequencies of 7.5 to 20 MHz, whereas probes are designed to image more superficial lesions and use frequencies of 5 to 30 MHz. Generally, higher ultrasound frequencies allow higher resolution imaging of lesions closer to the endoscope and lower ultrasound frequencies allow increased penetration of tissue and imaging of distant lesions. These modalities have been used extensively in the esophagus because of the ease of their application in this region. Instruments are available that can image 360 degrees radially in a plane perpendicular to the endoscope or linearly in a plane roughly 180 degrees parallel with the endoscope (most commonly used for fine-needle aspiration). The muscularis propria is seen as the hypoechoic layer most distal from the esophageal lumen. This is a critical region because tumors that extend to this level are classified ultrasonographically as T2 and are associated with a significant risk of nodal metastasis compared with lesions (T1) that do not extend to this region. Whereas T3 lesions extend outside the wall of the esophagus, T4 lesions involve adjacent structures such as the pleura, pericardium, or aorta. Several studies on ultrasonographic staging of esophageal cancer have shown that the accuracy of EUS for staging primary esophageal cancer (T staging) is approximately 90% and for lymph node staging, about 80%. EUS is seldom used as a single staging modality because it cannot detect distant metastases. Also, it often understages T2 lesions and overstages T3 lesions. This may be explained by inflammatory changes that can occur with esophageal cancer. Several studies have shown that the use of dilatation to accommodate passage of the instrument is safe. EUS procedures do not produce more bacteremia than standard gastrointestinal endoscopy.

COMPUTED TOMOGRAPHIC STAGING

Computed tomographic (CT) staging of esophageal cancer is common and provides the most information about distant spread of cancer. CT staging of esophageal cancer is less accurate than EUS staging; CT accurately determines the T stage in about 60% of patients. EUS staging is more accurate because the EUS instrument is close to the target lesion and can obtain fine-needle aspirates of suspected lymph nodes. CT is useful primarily for detecting distant disease and excluding T4 status if the fat plane between a tumor and adjacent structures is preserved. CT is used routinely to examine the chest and upper abdominal area.

POSITRON EMISSION TOMOGRAPHY

The use of positron emission tomography (PET) has been proposed for staging esophageal cancer. Unlike EUS and CT, PET is a functional test that does not demonstrate anatomical changes. It involves the administration of fluorine 18 fluorodeoxyglucose, which is concentrated in rapidly metabolizing cells. In clinical practice, PET often is paired with CT to create a so-called fusion image that allows the CT image to be correlated with the nuclear scan. PET is used primarily to detect metastatic disease. PET is limited by the inability to determine T stage and by false-negative results obtained if metastatic lesions are smaller than 1 cm. Also, with PET, the anatomic structure in which the metastasis occurs cannot be discerned. The use of fusion images has improved the detection ability of PET. Currently, PET appears to be of more value in detecting

nodal metastasis, with greater sensitivity and specificity for tumor involvement. PET excels in the detection of residual cancer after chemotherapy and radiotherapy, which currently are the standard of care in the United States for regionally advanced disease.

TREATMENT OF ESOPHAGEAL CANCER

Surgery

Esophagectomy is the primary treatment for esophageal cancer. However, about only half of the patients who undergo surgical exploration for possible esophageal resection actually have a curative resection because distant metastasis is found at the time of surgery. The procedure (Ivor-Lewis esophagogastrectomy) generally is performed through the right chest and upper abdomen to allow greater exposure of the upper esophagus and anastomosis of the stomach to the esophagus in the upper chest. The overall mortality rate of this procedure is approximately 10%, with specialized centers having rates less than 5%. Morbidity is related primarily to leakage from the anastomosis (10% of cases), pulmonary problems (30%-40% of cases), and cardiac events (15% of cases). A transhiatal approach has been advocated because it avoids opening the chest. The incidence of complications and results of this approach are similar to those of the Ivor-Lewis procedure. With laparoscopic-assisted esophagectomy, the abdominal portion of the procedure can be completed without a major incision. Thoracoscopic assistance with the esophageal portion has been reported to decrease the need for the large incisions that have been required previously. However, no studies have compared the superiority of these potentially less invasive techniques with traditional open procedures. The survival rate for esophagectomy is about 20% for 1 year and 5% for 5 years.

- Primary surgical resection for esophageal cancer is indicated for stage I or II tumors. No study has found that the addition of adjuvant therapy affects outcome in this group of patients. Possible board questions could include CT or PET scans or EUS pictures demonstrating a large esophageal mass without regional lymph nodes and questions about possible treatment of the cancer.

Radiotherapy

Radiation is seldom used as monotherapy for esophageal cancer. Instead, it is combined with chemotherapy to enhance the effect. As monotherapy, radiation has been reported to have survival rates similar to those for surgical resection. There is no evidence that the addition of radiotherapy to surgery, either preoperatively or postoperatively, increases survival. One of the most important effects of radiotherapy is the elimination of dysphagia in half of the patients treated. Side effects include acute dysphagia, fibrosis, myelitis, and pulmonary fibrosis.

Chemotherapy

Chemotherapy based on cisplatin as monotherapy for esophageal cancer has produced a response in 42% to 64% of treated patients. In stage IV disease, combination chemotherapy is preferred without radiotherapy because the cancer presumably is disseminated throughout the body. Definitive chemotherapy usually involves cisplatin and fluorouracil or newer medications such as the taxanes and irinotecan. Side effects include leukopenia, bleeding, nausea, vomiting, paresthesias, and altered sense of taste.

Combined Chemotherapy and Radiotherapy

Combined neoadjuvant therapy increases survival of patients with regional metastasis. The combination is usually cisplatin and fluorouracil with 4,400 cGy of radiation administered over 6 weeks before the operation. With this regimen, the response rate is approximately 30% and median survival time is 1 to 2 years. This has become the standard regimen for locally advanced tumors even though several studies have not confirmed these results. Newer agents that have been considered for the treatment of esophageal cancer include carboplatin and paclitaxel.

Endoscopic Curative Therapy

With the development of high-frequency endoscopic ultrasound probes, the staging of early esophageal cancers has increased the possibility of treating early cancers with endoscopic mucosal resection. This technique was popularized in Japan, where early esophageal and gastric cancers often are detected in screening studies. The basic technique involves creating a submucosal fluid "blister" to elevate the target lesion, which is converted into a pseudopolyp by various methods. With the first method, a dual channel endoscope and forceps were used to lift the lesion so it could be resected with a snare. With the second method, a polyp was created with a variceal ligation device. Recently, a suction cap fitted to the end of the endoscope has been used to create a polyp that is resected with a snare. These techniques can remove pieces of mucosa at least 1 cm in diameter down to the level of the deep submucosa. These methods can eliminate superficial cancer in about 94% of cases. Other curative endoscopic therapies include photodynamic therapy, currently approved by the US Food and Drug Administration for palliation of esophageal cancer and treatment of Barrett's esophagus with high-grade dysplasia.

Palliation of Esophageal Cancer

The standard of care for esophageal cancer has evolved to include expandable metal esophageal stents. These self-expandable devices are placed in a constrained position. The stents are positioned fluoroscopically and released within the lumen of the tumor. Over a period of several days, the stent expands to its maximal diameter. Previously, the tumor had to be dilated immediately to accommodate plastic stents 18 mm or more in diameter; this led to difficulties with perforation and bleeding. Devices used for palliation have not been compared directly, although a prospective study has found that expandable metal stents were superior to laser therapy for palliation of malignant dysphagia. Stents are probably best suited for mid-esophageal tumors. With cervical cancers, it can be difficult to position a stent without interfering with the cricopharyngeal muscle. Stents that penetrate the lower esophageal sphincter can be used for palliation of distal tumors, but they create free reflux from the stomach. Although antireflux stents have been developed to decrease reflux of gastric contents, they tend to become obstructed with food debris. Complications that can be anticipated with stent placement include poor stent position, esophageal perforation, pain (can be severe), bleeding, and compression of the bronchi or trachea. Late complications include stent migration, occlusion, fistula formation, and perforation. The estimated mortality rate for stent placement is 1% to 2%.

Laser therapy can also be attempted for palliation. This generally entails the use of a thermal laser such as the Nd:YAG laser. Although this is capable of providing palliation for more than 90% of patients initially, dysphagia recurs within 1 to 2 months in most patients. Argon plasma coagulation has been used, but it has limited depth of penetration, which decreases efficacy (but increases safety). Thermal therapies depend considerably on the skill of the operator and can cause perforation, bleeding, and fistula formation. Other thermal therapies such as multipolar coagulation have been attempted but require substantial time. Photodynamic therapy has been approved recently for providing palliation when no other method succeeds. This treatment entails the use of a drug that is administered intravenously and then activated 48 hours later by red light. This therapy is easy to apply; however, because of cutaneous photosensitivity, patients have to be protected from sunlight for 30 to 90 days after the drug is administered. Photodynamic therapy can cause pain, nausea, and, rarely, fistula formation.

- Dyspnea in a patient with esophageal cancer can result from tracheal compression by the tumor or stent, formation of a tracheoesophageal fistula, or recurrent aspiration because of near-complete obstruction. If dyspnea occurs in relation to a large midesophageal lesion, bronchoscopy may be indicated before placement of a stent.

RECOMMENDED READING

Baron TH. Expandable metal stents for the treatment of cancerous obstruction of the gastrointestinal tract. N Engl J Med. 2001;344:1681-7.

Buttar NS, Wang KK, Lutzke LS, Krishnadath KK, Anderson MA. Combined endoscopic mucosal resection and photodynamic therapy for esophageal neoplasia within Barrett's esophagus. Gastrointest Endosc. 2001;54:682-8.

Devesa SS, Blot WJ, Fraumeni JF Jr. Changing patterns in the incidence of esophageal and gastric carcinoma in the United States. Cancer. 1998;83:2049-53.

Inoue H. Treatment of esophageal and gastric tumors. Endoscopy. 2001;33:119-25.

Kim K, Park SJ, Kim BT, Lee KS, Shim YM. Evaluation of lymph node metastases in squamous cell carcinoma of the esophagus with positron emission tomography. Ann Thorac Surg. 2001;71:290-4.

Lerut T, Flamen P, Ectors N, Van Cutsem E, Peeters M, Hiele M, et al. Histopathologic validation of lymph node staging with FDG-PET scan in cancer of the esophagus and gastroesophageal junction: a prospective study based on primary surgery with extensive lymphadenectomy. Ann Surg. 2000;232:743-52.

Mallery S, Van Dam J. EUS in the evaluation of esophageal carcinoma. Gastrointest Endosc. 2000;52 Suppl 6:S6-S11.

Miller DL. Clinical trials for esophageal carcinoma. Chest Surg Clin N Am. 2000;10:583-90.

Morgan G, Vainio H. Barrett's oesophagus, oesophageal cancer and colon cancer: an explanation of the association and cancer chemopreventive potential of non-steroidal anti-inflammatory drugs. Eur J Cancer Prev. 1998;7:195-9.

Narayan S, Sivak MV Jr. Palliation of esophageal carcinoma: laser and photodynamic therapy. Chest Surg Clin N Am. 1994;4:347-67.

Nijhawan PK, Wang KK. Endoscopic mucosal resection for lesions with endoscopic features suggestive of malignancy and high-grade dysplasia within Barrett's esophagus. Gastrointest Endosc. 2000;52:328-32.

Ye W, Chow WH, Lagergren J, Yin L, Nyren O. Risk of adenocarcinomas of the esophagus and gastric cardia in patients with gastroesophageal reflux diseases and after antireflux surgery. Gastroenterology. 2001;121:1286-93.

CHAPTER 5

Normal and Abnormal Esophageal Motility

Nicholas J. Talley, M.D., Ph.D.

Swallowing is a complex neuromuscular process that depends on intact motor and sensory innervation. The oropharyngeal phase of swallowing is under voluntary control, but once the bolus is moved into the pharynx, the process becomes involuntary, with the initiation of an integrated pattern of esophageal motor activity. Difficulty swallowing ("dysphagia") can occur with uncoordinated or failed peristalsis.

ANATOMY

Shaped like a funnel, the pharynx joins the mouth to the esophagus and trachea. The upper esophagus consists of striated muscle. The upper esophageal sphincter (UES) is composed of the cricopharyngeus muscle, which is formed by muscle thickening of three overlapping sheets of striated muscle at the pharyngoesophageal junction. The esophagus is a relatively simple neuromuscular tube containing an inner circular layer of muscle and an outer longitudinal layer of muscle. At approximately the level of the aortic arch, which is 22 to 24 cm from the incisors, the striated muscle begins to be replaced by smooth muscle in the transition zone. Fifty percent of the esophagus is entirely smooth muscle. A ring of thickened smooth muscle at the esophagogastric junction marks the lower esophageal sphincter (LES). Between swallows, the UES and LES protect from esophagopharyngeal and gastroesophageal reflux, respectively, because they keep the esophageal lumen closed.

SWALLOWING PHYSIOLOGY

After the lips are closed and the teeth are clenched, the tongue is elevated against the palate (from anterior to posterior), forcing the bolus to the pharynx under conscious control. However, entry of the bolus into the pharynx triggers the swallowing reflex, which is involuntary. The soft palate is elevated against the posterior pharyngeal wall, sealing the oropharynx and preventing nasopharyngeal reflux. The larynx is also elevated, and the laryngeal inlet is closed, which prevents aspiration. The long axis of the pharynx shortens, removing the recesses formed by the piriform sinuses, valleculae, and laryngeal vestibule. Behind the bolus follows peristaltic contraction of the pharyngeal muscles. As this contraction approaches, the cricopharyngeus muscle relaxes and elevation of the larynx actively pulls open the UES. As the contraction passes, the UES closes tightly. The LES relaxes long before the peristaltic contraction reaches the esophagogastric junction and remains relaxed until the bolus has entered the stomach, at which time the LES closes.

Relaxation of the UES occurs through the release of nitric oxide from myenteric neurons that innervate the UES. Myenteric neurons are also important in maintaining the resting basal tone of the upper esophagus. Peristaltic contractions are under local control of the myenteric plexus. The release of acetylcholine (excitatory effect) and nitric oxide (inhibitory effect) from neurons that supply the circular smooth muscle are involved in this process, activated by swallowing.

Figures 1 through 7 originally appeared in a chapter authored by Jeffrey L. Conklin, M.D., in the first edition of the book *Mayo Clinic Gastroenterology and Hepatology Board Review*.

The smooth muscle of the esophagus is innervated by axons in cranial nerve X (vagus nerve) that originate in the dorsal motor nucleus of the vagus and synapse on myenteric plexus neurons in the esophagus. The striated muscle of the pharynx, the UES, and striated muscle in the proximal esophagus are innervated by cranial nerves IX (glossopharyngeal nerve) and X.

UPPER ESOPHAGEAL SPHINCTER (CRICOPHARYNGEUS) DISORDERS

Disease that affects striated muscle causes oropharyngeal motor dysfunction and oropharyngeal dysphagia. These disorders can occur at the level of the muscle, peripheral nerves, or central nervous system.

To diagnose oropharyngeal dysphagia, consider the following important hints from the history:

- True dysphagia is present
- Food bolus transfer from the pharynx or hypopharynx is impaired (difficulty starting to swallow, food caught in the throat, unusual head or neck maneuvers during swallowing)
- Nasopharyngeal regurgitation is common (regurgitation of swallowed liquids through the nose)
- Aspiration is common (coughing or choking when swallowing, difficulty breathing when eating)

Neurologic disease can cause oropharyngeal incoordination, whereas muscle disease can result in weak pharyngeal contractions. The causes of oropharyngeal dysphagia are listed in Table 1.

Investigations

Oropharyngeal dysphagia is best assessed with videofluoroscopy. For this test, patients swallow boluses of different texture. The test is best conducted in the presence of a speech therapist working with a radiologist. The following can be identified with videofluoroscopy:

- An uncoordinated tongue, which will impair bolus transmission
- Soft palate dysfunction, which can lead to nasopharyngeal regurgitation
- Poor laryngeal closure, which can lead to aspiration
- Poor pharyngeal peristalsis causing residue in the valleculae or piriform sinuses

Identifying the presence of a cricopharyngeal bar is important. This is an indentation of the cricopharyngeal muscle seen as barium passes by slowly and the muscle relaxes poorly during swallowing. A cricopharyngeal bar can be the primary cause of oropharyngeal dysphagia in the absence of other neuromuscular disease, but the latter must be excluded. A

Table 1. Causes of Oropharyngeal Dysphagia

Brain—cerebrovascular accident, head injury, Parkinson's disease, brainstem disease, multiple sclerosis, motor neuron disease, phenothiazines

Muscle or nerve—dermatomyositis, poliomyelitis, muscular dystrophies, myasthenia gravis

Cricopharyngeal dysfunction
> Inadequate opening from fibrosis resulting in Zenker's diverticulum
> Reduced muscle compliance leading to a cricopharyngeal bar

pharyngeal or esophageal diverticulum ("Zenker's diverticulum") needs to be looked for carefully. It results from abnormal opening of the UES and can be due to localized muscle disease. Most patients who present with Zenker's diverticulum are older than 50 years.

The presence of Zenker's diverticulum increases the risk of perforation by esophagogastroduodenoscopy or nasogastric tube placement, so it is important that intubation be performed under direct vision if the history is suggestive of oropharyngeal dysphagia. This is another reason videofluoroscopy should be the initial test of choice.

Computed tomography (CT) of the neck can be helpful for excluding rare structural causes of oropharyngeal dysphagia such as malignancy or cervical osteophytes. An ears-nose-throat evaluation may detect malignancy missed by other tests if the diagnosis is unclear. Esophageal manometry has a limited role and is generally unhelpful.

Treatment

The underlying neuromuscular disease, if present, should be treated. Speech therapy can be useful; learning new swallowing maneuvers can aid the process despite underlying abnormalities. If malnutrition is an issue and the patient has no improvement with speech therapy, placement of a percutaneous endoscopic gastrostomy tube should be considered. If Zenker's diverticulum is present, a surgical diverticulectomy with UES myotomy is the treatment of choice. Endoscopic myotomy is an alternative to surgery; also, botulinum toxin can be injected into the UES.

SMOOTH MUSCLE DISORDERS

Disorders of esophageal motility can be identified with manometry. An example of a normal manometric recording of primary peristalsis is shown in Figure 1. After a water swallow, peristaltic progression occurs at a rate of 2 to 8 cm per second, followed by complete relaxation of the LES. The LES is

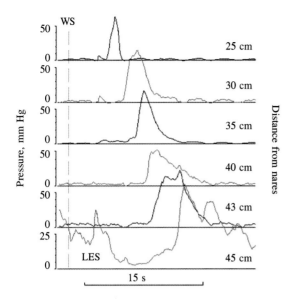

Fig. 1. Normal esophageal motor function. Manometric recording of normal esophageal peristalsis and relaxation of the lower esophageal sphincter (LES). The most distal sensor (bottom trace) is in the LES, which is defined as a region of elevated pressure near the gastroesophageal junction that decreases with swallowing. A peristaltic sequence is recorded in the sensors above the LES. WS, occurrence of a wet swallow.

tonically closed at rest, with a normal mean pressure of 20 mm Hg (range, 10-45 mm Hg). However, a water swallow can alter subsequent swallows for up to 20 to 30 seconds, so it is important to note the time intervals between the water swallows provided on a tracing. The normal distal wave amplitude is 30 to 180 mm Hg.

CLINICAL ASSESSMENT

Esophageal motility disorders classically present with dysphagia for both liquids and solids. Symptoms typically are intermittent. Chest pain is common.

CLASSIFICATION OF ESOPHAGEAL MOTILITY DISORDERS

A classification of esophageal motility disorders is summarized in Table 2.

ACHALASIA

Definition

Unlike most esophageal motility disorders, achalasia is a well-accepted neuropathic disease. "Achalasia" literally means "failure to relax." Its primary features are failure of peristalsis and failure of relaxation or incomplete relaxation of the LES.

Pathophysiology

The hallmark pathologic feature of achalasia is a reduced number of nonadrenergic noncholinergic inhibitory ganglion cells. The cause of achalasia is unknown. Infection, especially varicella zoster, has been implicated. A similar disease pathologically is Chagas' disease, which is due to infection by *Trypanosoma cruzi*. In Chagas' disease, a parasitic antigen that is similar to a protein on myenteric neurons produces an immunologic attack against the myenteric plexus. Achalasia has a possible genetic component. Myenteric neuronal antibodies have been identified in up to 60% of patients with achalasia. However, whether this is an epiphenomenon or is causally related to the disease is unclear.

Clinical Presentation

Any age group can be affected by achalasia, but it typically occurs in the third to fifth decades. Men and women are affected equally. Often, there is a long history before the correct diagnosis is made. Virtually all patients have dysphagia for solids and two-thirds of them have dysphagia for liquids. The dysphagia typically fluctuates, which is a hint. Regurgitation occurs in 60% to 90% of patients. Heartburn is common, not only from acid reflux but also from fermentation of food in the aperistaltic esophagus. Approximately one-third of patients report chest pain, although the mechanism is unclear. Weight loss may occur. Patients may have cough and pulmonary symptoms from aspiration.

Diagnosis

Barium swallow with fluoroscopy is an excellent screening test for achalasia. If the classic bird's beak appearance with a dilated esophagus is seen and typical symptoms are present, the diagnosis of achalasia is virtually certain (Fig. 2). However, pseudoachalasia needs to be actively excluded.

Manometrically, aperistalsis occurs with incomplete or failed relaxation of the LES after a swallow (Fig. 3). Increased LES pressure is common but not diagnostic. Low-amplitude

Table 2. Esophageal Motility Disorders

Inadequate LES relaxation: achalasia (aperistalsis), atypical disorders
Uncoordinated contractions: diffuse esophageal spasm
Hypercontractile: nutcracker esophagus, isolated hypertensive LES
Hypocontractile: ineffective motility (nonspecific motility disorder)

LES, lower esophageal sphincter.
From Spechler SJ, Castell DO. Classification of oesophageal motility abnormalities. Gut. 2001;49:145-51. Used with permission.

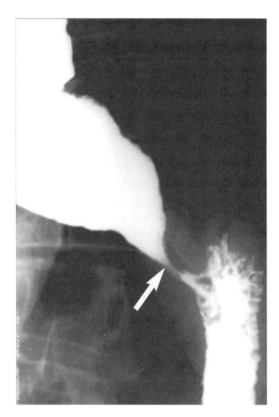

Fig. 2. Barium swallow study in a patient with achalasia. Note the dilated esophagus and tapering ("bird's beak") (*arrow*) at the gastroesophageal junction.

simultaneous contractions may be seen. Intraesophageal pressure is usually increased because the esophagus is behaving as a common cavity. Consider the esophagus as though it were a sausage-shaped balloon filled with either liquid or air and containing a manometry catheter. If you squeeze the balloon anywhere (without blocking the lumen), an increase in pressure will be recorded nearly everywhere simultaneously in the balloon. In vigorous achalasia, simultaneous repetitive high-amplitude contractions occur in the esophagus. However, this manometric change does not have any clear clinical correlate.

Differential Diagnosis

It is essential to exclude malignancy-causing pseudoachalasia. This can occur through infiltration of the neural plexus directly by tumor, the presence of a large constricting mass in the esophagus, or rarely from antineuronal nuclear autoantibodies. Manometry cannot distinguish between pseudoachalasia and achalasia. Although presentation at older age, short duration of symptoms, and rapid weight loss all suggest pseudoachalasia, the history alone is insufficient for making the diagnosis. Endoscopy is essential in examining for evidence of malignancy. Other conditions that can cause pseudoachalasia include amyloidosis, sarcoidosis, postvagotomy, chronic intestinal pseudo-obstruction, neurofibromatosis, and even pancreatic pseudocyst.

Management

The four major options for management are drugs, botulinum toxin, pneumatic dilatation, and surgical myotomy.

Drugs

All drugs for achalasia have very limited efficacy. Nifedipine (10-30 mg), a calcium channel antagonist, was shown in a small crossover trial of 10 patients to reduce dysphagia and LES pressure in achalasia, although the overall results were not impressive. Sublingual isosorbide dinitrate (a nitric oxide donor) can relax the LES. Sildenafil (which increases cyclic guanosine monophosphate) also may have some benefit for LES relaxation.

Botulinum Toxin

Injection of botulinum toxin into the LES is effective. The toxin binds to the presynaptic cholinergic receptors and inhibits release of acetylcholine from the presynaptic terminals of the neuromuscular junctions. The injection decreases LES pressure by more than 30% and induces a clinical response in 60% to 75% of patients. However, symptoms usually recur within 3 to 12 months, leading to the need for repeated injections. Furthermore, antibodies develop against the botulinum toxin, usually resulting in its loss of efficacy. Although botulinum toxin can cause fibrosis, pain, or rash after injection, it generally is well tolerated. This treatment is not a contraindication to surgery even though it potentially can cause tissue reactions

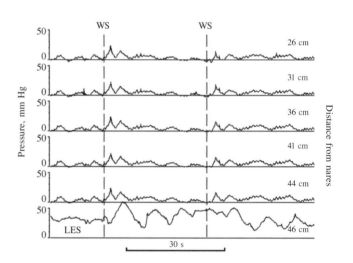

Fig. 3. Manometric recording from a patient with classic achalasia. The most distal sensor (bottom trace) is in the lower esophageal sphincter (LES). Note that the LES does not relax with wet swallows (WS). Wet swallows do not produce peristaltic pressure waves in the esophagus; instead, there are low-amplitude, simultaneous pressure waves with a nearly identical configuration.

that obscure fascial planes. Botulinum toxin is a useful option for "buying time" in achalasia, if this is needed. It is the optimal approach for frail elderly patients who are not candidates for surgery or pneumatic dilatation.

Pneumatic Dilatation

Pneumatic dilatation has more than a 60% and up to a 90% good response rate in achalasia. The forceful dilatation disrupts the LES, and this is believed to be the mechanism producing the benefit. If patients do not have a response to a second dilatation, they are less likely to have a response to additional dilatations, but some physicians attempt pneumatic dilatation one more time after other options have been discussed with the patient. The response tends to be better in patients who are older and have a long history of achalasia. The poorest response occurs when patients are younger than 40 years and the postdilatation LES pressure is greater than 20 mm Hg.

Treatment should begin with the smallest (3-cm diameter) achalasia balloon (e.g., Microvasive Rigiflex). The dilatation should be done under fluoroscopic guidance. The balloon should be inflated gradually until the indentation at the esophagogastric junction is obliterated (7-10 psi) for 60 seconds. If dysphagia has not improved in 4 to 8 weeks, then a 3.5-cm balloon should be used. The largest balloon is 4 cm.

A major disadvantage of pneumatic dilatation is the risk of complications. The reported rate of esophageal perforation is approximately 3%, with half of the patients requiring surgical repair. The overall procedure mortality rate is less than 0.5%. Because of this risk, it is important to give water-soluble contrast after dilatation and observe patients for 6 hours before discharge. Small contained perforations can be treated conservatively by not allowing any oral intake and administering antibiotics and by close observation with a surgical colleague. Gastroesophageal reflux disease (GERD) can develop after pneumatic dilatation (3%-15% of patients). After a patient has pneumatic dilatation, annual quantitative barium esophageal studies can be useful to quantify esophageal emptying.

Standard bougienage has been compared with pneumatic dilatation in a study of 18 patients with Chagas' disease. The results suggested that dilatation of the esophagus by bougienage has no long-term value, although patients may report brief improvement of symptoms.

Surgical Myotomy, Open or Laparoscopic

Currently, laparoscopic surgical myotomy is the procedure of choice. The previous use of botulinum toxin or pneumatic dilatation is not a contraindication to surgery. Data suggest that patients have the best symptom response rate (90%) and durability with surgery. Postoperatively, up to one-half of patients may require acid suppression for GERD.

If dysphagia recurs after being treated successfully with pneumatic dilatation or surgery, the literature provides little guidance about the optimal next step in management. However, pneumatic dilatation or repeat myotomy can be performed after myotomy fails, with a success rate better than 50%. In very severe disease unresponsive to all the above-mentioned approaches, esophagectomy is the only option.

Long-term Outcome

Patients with achalasia have a 2% to 7% increased risk of squamous cell carcinoma. However, routine surveillance is not standard practice. If new or worsening dysphagia develops in a patient with a history of achalasia, repeat upper endoscopy is indicated. Aspiration pneumonia is a well-recognized complication of achalasia.

ESOPHAGEAL SPASTIC DISORDERS

Diffuse Esophageal Spasm

This is a relatively rare disease, and the manometric findings correlate poorly with symptoms. Approximately 3% to 10% of patients with noncardiac chest pain or unexplained dysphagia may have esophageal spasm. In about 3% to 5% of patients, esophageal spasm progresses to achalasia. Diffuse esophageal spasm may improve spontaneously in some patients during follow-up. Whether esophageal spasm results from an imbalance of inhibitory and excitatory motor innervation of the esophagus is unclear.

The esophagogram may be abnormal (Fig. 4), but manometry is usually required to make the diagnosis. The manometric definition of esophageal spasm is that more than 30% of wet swallows have simultaneous pressure waves (Fig. 5). A prolonged duration of the wet swallows (>6 seconds), normal peristalsis, and normal relaxation of the LES support the diagnosis. Vigorous achalasia is a combination of diffuse esophageal spasm and failure of the LES to relax.

Nutcracker Esophagus

This manometric condition is characterized by high-pressure peristaltic contractions greater than 180 mm Hg. Importantly, the peristaltic contractions propagate normally in the esophagus; also the LES relaxes normally. It is unclear whether this is a "real" disease.

Treatment

In a crossover study of 22 patients with nutcracker esophagus, diltiazem (60 and 90 mg 4 times daily) versus placebo was tested. Diltiazem significantly lowered mean distal esophageal peristaltic pressure compared with placebo and also had a tendency to reduce chest pain scores, but the results were not

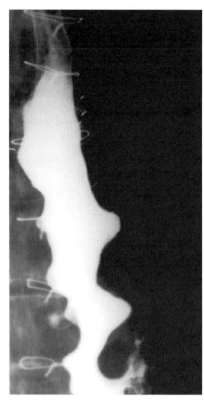

Fig. 4. Barium swallow study in a patient with diffuse esophageal spasm. Note the irregular border of the esophagus ("corkscrew esophagus"), suggesting uncoordinated contractile activity.

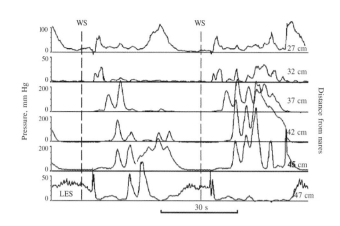

Fig. 5. Manometric recording from a patient with diffuse esophageal spasm. The most distal sensor (bottom trace) is in the lower esophageal sphincter (LES). WS, occurrence of a wet swallow.

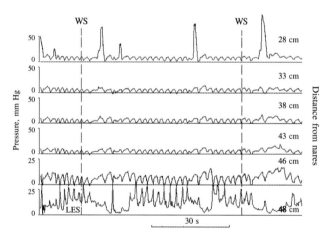

Fig. 6. Manometric recording from a patient with scleroderma. The most distal sensor (bottom trace) is in the lower esophageal sphincter (LES). Typical manometric findings of scleroderma include low-amplitude or absent peristaltic pressure waves in the smooth muscle part of the esophagus and a low-pressure LES. Generally, the striated muscle part of the esophagus (top trace) functions normally. WS, occurrence of a wet swallow.

impressive. Use of other therapies for esophageal spastic disorders is largely anecdotal. Nitrates and sildenafil may provide some benefit. Tricyclic antidepressants may reduce noncardiac chest pain, but this is irrespective of the underlying manometric findings (which may reflect that the manometric findings are irrelevant). In uncontrolled studies, botulinum toxin has been helpful.

Spastic esophageal disorders can be triggered by underlying GERD. Thus, aggressive treatment of documented gastroesophageal reflux is reasonable. Pneumatic dilatation of the esophagus has not been demonstrated to improve diffuse esophageal spasm. Long myotomy for refractory diffuse esophageal spasm is effective in 50% to 70% of patients.

HYPOMOTILITY OF THE ESOPHAGUS

This is characterized by a decreased or absent resting LES and reduced or absent peristaltic wave pressures. Sometimes it is difficult to distinguish between esophageal hypomotility and achalasia. Scleroderma and other connective tissue diseases can present with esophageal hypomotility (Fig. 6). Muscular dystrophies and familial visceral myopathies also may present in this way.

NONSPECIFIC ESOPHAGEAL MOTOR ABNORMALITY

In the esophageal manometry laboratory, about half of the patients with dysphagia have nonspecific motor abnormalities, which may or may not occur in relation to reflux disease. These abnormalities are not associated with dysphagia and are not specific. Diseases such as diabetes mellitus, amyloidosis, or hypothyroidism can be associated with a nonspecific esophageal motor abnormality.

EOSINOPHILIC ESOPHAGITIS

Patients presenting with unexplained solid-food dysphagia or intermittent food impaction may have eosinophilic esophagitis. This is most common in young, typically male patients who do not have symptoms of GERD. Endoscopic examination may show a corrugated ("ringed") esophagus, particularly in the proximal middle esophageal region. Increased intraepithelial eosinophils (>20/high-power field) are seen in biopsy specimens. There are no distinct underlying esophageal motility findings, although abnormalities may be seen on manometry. Many adult patients have a response to corticosteroids applied topically for 6 weeks. Montelukast also has been used successfully.

POST FUNDOPLICATION MOTOR DISORDERS

Several abnormalities are detected with esophageal manometry after fundoplication. The resting LES pressure may be higher than normal or the LES may not relax normally in response to swallowing. Also, the intrabolus pressure may increase just before the peristaltic pressure wave ("proximal escape") (Fig. 7). Dilatation of the esophagus for persistent dysphagia after fundoplication can be helpful.

SUMMARY

Generally, asymptomatic esophageal manometric findings should be ignored. Achalasia is the best established esophageal motility disorder. Most other esophageal motility disorders have questionable associations with clinical presentations. GERD is a common cause of dysphagia, and this can be secondary to motor dysfunction. Disorders of the UES produce oropharyngeal dysphagia, which clinically is quite distinct from the symptoms of distal esophageal motor disorders. An algorithm for assessing dysphagia is given in Figure 8.

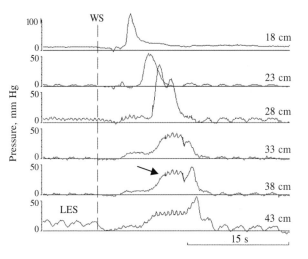

Fig. 7. Manometric recording from a patient with Nissen fundoplication. All the sensors are within the esophagus. Note that in the distal esophagus the pressure waves are biphasic. The first pressure wave (*arrow*) is the pressure in the bolus, preceding the peristaltic contraction; this is the intrabolus pressure. The second is the pressure wave accompanying the peristaltic contraction. Normally, the intrabolus pressure is seen during esophageal manometry, but it is of lower amplitude. The intrabolus pressure in this example is increased because of the distal esophageal obstruction produced by a tight fundoplication. LES, lower esophageal sphincter; WS, occurrence of a wet swallow.

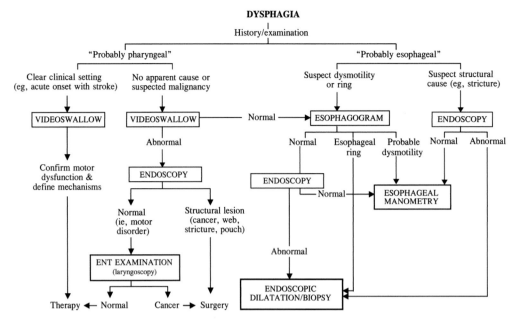

Fig. 8. Management of dysphagia. ENT, ear-nose-throat. (Modified from Cook I. Difficult swallowing and painful swallowing. In: Talley NJ, Martin CJ, editors. Clinical gastroenterology. A practical problem-based approach. Sydney: MacLennan & Petty; 1996. Used with permission.)

RECOMMENDED READING

Annese V, Bassotti G, Coccia G, Dinelli M, D'Onofrio V, Gatto G, et al. A multicentre randomised study of intrasphincteric botulinum toxin in patients with oesophageal achalasia: GISMAD Achalasia Study Group. Gut. 2000;46:597-600.

Cook IJ. Treatment of oropharyngeal dysphagia. Curr Treat Options Gastroenterol. 2003;6:273-81.

Croese J, Fairley SK, Masson JW, Chong AK, Whitaker DA, Kanowski PA, et al. Clinical and endoscopic features of eosinophilic esophagitis in adults. Gastrointest Endosc. 2003;58:516-22.

Eherer AJ, Schwetz I, Hammer HF, Petnehazy T, Scheidl SJ, Weber K, et al. Effect of sildenafil on oesophageal motor function in healthy subjects and patients with oesophageal motor disorders. Gut. 2002;50:758-64.

Lacima G, Grande L, Pera M, Francino A, Ros E. Utility of ambulatory 24-hour esophageal pH and motility monitoring in noncardiac chest pain: report of 90 patients and review of the literature. Dig Dis Sci. 2003;48:952-61.

Mikaeli J, Fazel A, Montazeri G, Yaghoobi M, Malekzadeh R. Randomized controlled trial comparing botulinum toxin injection to pneumatic dilatation for the treatment of achalasia. Aliment Pharmacol Ther. 2001;15:1389-96.

Nastos D, Chen LQ, Ferraro P, Taillefer R, Duranceau AC. Long myotomy with antireflux repair for esophageal spastic disorders. J Gastrointest Surg. 2002;6:713-22.

Potter JW, Saeian K, Staff D, Massey BT, Komorowski RA, Shaker R, et al. Eosinophilic esophagitis in adults: an emerging problem with unique esophageal features. Gastrointest Endosc. 2004;59:355-61.

Spechler SJ, Castell DO. Classification of oesophageal motility abnormalities. Gut. 2001;49:145-51.

Sperandio M, Tutuian R, Gideon RM, Katz PO, Castell DO. Diffuse esophageal spasm: not diffuse but distal esophageal spasm (DES). Dig Dis Sci. 2003;48:1380-4.

Storr M, Allescher HD, Rosch T, Born P, Weigert N, Classen M. Treatment of symptomatic diffuse esophageal spasm by endoscopic injections of botulinum toxin: a prospective study with long-term follow-up. Gastrointest Endosc. 2001;54:754-9.

Straumann A, Spichtin HP, Grize L, Bucher KA, Beglinger C, Simon HU. Natural history of primary eosinophilic esophagitis: a follow-up of 30 adult patients for up to 11.5 years. Gastroenterology. 2003;125:1660-9.

Vaezi MF, Baker ME, Achkar E, Richter JE. Timed barium oesophagram: better predictor of long term success after pneumatic dilation in achalasia than symptom assessment. Gut. 2002;50:765-70.

Vela MF, Richter JE, Wachsberger D, Connor J, Rice TW. Complexities of managing achalasia at a tertiary referral center: use of pneumatic dilatation, Heller myotomy, and botulinum toxin injection. Am J Gastroenterol. 2004;99:1029-36.

Williams RB, Grehan MJ, Hersch M, Andre J, Cook IJ. Biomechanics, diagnosis, and treatment outcome in inflammatory myopathy presenting as oropharyngeal dysphagia. Gut. 2003;52:471-8.

Esophagus

Questions and Answers

Multiple Choice (choose the one best answer)

1. A 45-year-old man was referred by his primary care physician because of new onset of dysphagia of 4 weeks' duration. The patient has had a history of smoking, 5-pack years, in high school and a history of heartburn self-medicated with over-the-counter antacids. An upper gastrointestinal tract study by the primary care physician showed a mass lesion in the distal esophagus. Which of the following statements is incorrect?
   a. The lesion is most likely produced by metastatic cancer
   b. The patient probably has had Barrett's esophagus
   c. Biopsy specimens from the gastroesophageal junction of this patient would show adenocarcinoma
   d. Squamous cell cancer is unlikely in this location
   e. Most patients with this cancer would likely be male

2. You performed endoscopy, with biopsy of the mass, in the patient in question 1. The results confirm your suspicions. You now wish to begin to stage the mass. Which of the following would be the first procedure of choice?
   a. Positron emission tomography
   b. Computed tomography of the chest and upper abdomen
   c. Endoscopic ultrasonography, with fine-needle aspiration if lymph nodes are present
   d. Video-assisted thoracoscopy, with biopsy
   e. Flow cytometry of the endoscopically acquired biopsy specimen

3. The patient in questions 1 and 2 was found to have positive celiac-axis lymph nodes as well as periesophageal lymph nodes. The primary tumor is seen to penetrate the muscularis propria but does not involve other organs. No other signs of metastatic disease are noted. What would be the stage of the patient's cancer?
   a. Stage IIA
   b. Stage IIB
   c. Stage I
   d. Stage IV
   e. Stage V

4. The patient in questions 1-3 is referred back to you for palliation of dysphagia during his treatment. The patient has begun to lose weight but is functionally good. Which palliative therapy is likely to produce the longest lasting relief of dysphagia for this patient?
   a. Photodynamic therapy
   b. Nd:YAG laser therapy
   c. Expandable metal stent
   d. Percutaneous gastrostomy
   e. Argon plasma coagulation

5. A patient is referred to you for treatment of a cancer of the distal esophagus found during surveillance endoscopy for Barrett's esophagus. The cancer is still said to be intramucosal, and no lymph nodes are detected with endoscopic ultrasonography. The patient asks about success rate in eliminating the cancer with endoscopic therapy. Which of the following is most accurate?
   a. 60%
   b. 70%
   c. 80%

d. 90%

e. 100%

6. A 50-year-old woman reports a 1-month history of dysphagia. She finds that solid foods seem to stick in the midneck area, and she has difficulty starting to swallow. She often coughs or chokes when she swallows and has difficulty because liquids regurgitate into her nose. She has a history of Parkinson's disease. The next step in management is:

   a. Ear, nose, and throat evaluation

   b. Esophagogastroduodenoscopy

   c. Video swallow

   d. Esophageal manometry

   e. Computed tomography of the neck

7. A 31-year-old woman presents with a 6-month history of dysphagia and recurrent central chest pain. These symptoms followed a laparoscopic Nissen fundoplication for nonerosive gastroesophageal reflux disease. She has difficulty swallowing after every meal and has the sensation of food sticking in the lower retrosternal area. Dysphagia has been progressive and occurs with solids and liquids. Esophagogastroduodenoscopy has shown an intact fundoplication with no evidence of esophagitis or stricture. Esophageal manometry showed no peristalsis, a lower esophageal sphincter tone of 29 mm Hg, and no relaxation in response to any wet swallows. The most likely diagnosis in this case is:

   a. Failed antireflux surgery

   b. Nutcracker esophagus

   c. Nonspecific motility disorder of the esophagus due to fundoplication

   d. Achalasia

   e. Pseudoachalasia

8. Which of the following symptoms is *not* a side effect of laparoscopic Nissen fundoplication?

   a. Diarrhea

   b. Dysphagia

   c. Gas bloat

   d. Constipation

   e. Recurrence of reflux

9. A 25-year-old man presents with a history of intermittent food impaction for which he has undergone two previous esophagogastroduodenoscopies to treat the problem. The esophagus has been reported to look normal on these examinations. He has dysphagia for solids, only occasionally, and no liquid dysphagia. He now presents with his third episode of food impaction in the past year. Your next step in management would be:

   a. Repeat upper endoscopy, with random biopsies

   b. Esophageal manometry testing

   c. Empiric trial of proton pump inhibitor therapy

   d. Trial of empiric corticosteroid therapy

   e. Reassurance and dismiss

10. A 59-year-old lawyer presents with intermittent episodes of chest pain unrelated to exertion. The pain often occurs after meals but is erratic. It can last for minutes to hours and is always in the retrosternal region. He has had a full cardiac work-up, including coronary angiography that has been negative. The next test that is likely to have the highest diagnostic yield is:

   a. Esophagogastroduodenoscopy

   b. 24-Hour esophageal pH monitoring

   c. Esophageal manometry

   d. Upper abdominal ultrasonography

   e. Computed tomography of the chest

ANSWERS

1. Answer a

The only choice that is incorrect is that metastatic cancer would be a likely cause of a distal esophageal tumor. Metastatic cancer most commonly obstructs in the middle of the esophagus. Most distal esophageal cancers are adenocarcinomas related to Barrett's esophagus and a chronic history of reflux disease. Adenocarcinomas generally affect males, with a male-to-female ratio of 4:1.

2. Answer b

The upper abdomen and chest are the most likely locations for metastasis from a distal esophageal cancer. Although cost-efficacy studies have suggested that endoscopic ultrasonography (EUS) and fine-needle aspiration may be a more appropriate starting point, it would depend on the availability of experienced EUS-trained endoscopists in the area. Positron-emission tomography (PET)–computed tomography (CT) fusion scans have become an early diagnostic study, but their place in routine staging is still debatable. Medicare should reimburse for PET scans, but the need for a PET scan may be obviated should CT show distal metastases. Video-assisted thoroscopy or video-assisted thoracic surgery is not routinely performed for staging but mainly for diagnosis of enlarged nodes before attempted resection. Flow cytometry may be of value in determining patients at risk for cancer development, but the value for staging a known cancer has not been determined.

3. Answer d

The penetration of the muscularis propria makes the lesion a T2 tumor. Involvement of celiac-axis lymph nodes makes it a T3/M1a lesion that is a stage IV cancer, although there is a suggestion that these celiac nodes should be classified as N1 lesions or regional nodes for distal cancers according to the 2002 American Joint Commission for Cancer (AJCC) tumor classification. Thus, stage III may be a reasonable alternative, but it is not one of the choices. Stage IIB with N1 nodal disease may also be a possibility but would not apply with T3 disease. There is no stage V in the AJCC classification system.

4. Answer c

Palliation is best achieved with expandable metal stents that are relatively easy to place and have a prolonged duration of palliation. Endoluminal ablative therapies such as photodynamic therapy, Nd:YAG laser, or argon plasma coagulation rarely offer effective palliation for more than a month. Percutaneous gastrostomy is not indicated for palliative care unless the patient is undergoing chemotherapy or radiotherapy to help control the tumor.

5. Answer d

Most studies that have investigated photodynamic therapy, endoscopic mucosal resection, or a combination have reported success rates of 84% to 95% for treating intramucosal cancers. Thus, 90% would be the most reasonable choice.

6. Answer c

This patient has a history consistent with oropharyngeal dysphagia associated with Parkinson's disease. Videofluoroscopy is the initial assessment of choice for any patient with oropharyngeal dysphagia. Esophagogastroduodenoscopy is likely to offer little diagnostic information. Computed tomography of the neck is useful to exclude rare structural causes in the oropharyngeal area, as is an ear-nose-throat evaluation. Usually, esophageal manometry is not helpful.

7. Answer d

This patient has had a laparoscopic Nissen fundoplication for reflux disease, but regardless of this, the esophageal manometric findings are now classic for achalasia, with aperistalsis and failure of lower esophageal sphincter relaxation. Esophagogastroduodenoscopy did not show any evidence of malignancy, making pseudoachalasia unlikely. Furthermore, her young age also suggests that pseudoachalasia is highly unlikely. Possibly, the initial diagnosis of reflux disease was not correct and she originally had achalasia. Achalasia can cause heartburn not only from acid reflux but also from fermentation of food in the aperistaltic esophagus. However, there have been reports of achalasia rarely developing after fundoplication when the initial esophageal manometric findings were normal.

8. Answer d

Constipation is not a well-recognized complication of fundoplication. However, diarrhea can occur, particularly in patients who may have a history of underlying irritable bowel syndrome. Dysphagia is common, affecting at least 20% of patients after the operation, with 5% having persistent dysphagia. Gas bloat is common and a difficult problem for some patients. Recurrence of reflux can be an early or late complication of fundoplication. After fundoplication, up to 50% of patients may still require acid-suppression medication.

9. Answer a

This patient has a history that could be suggestive of eosinophilic esophagitis. With the patient's history, esophageal manometry is unlikely to yield a cause. Some patients with eosinophilic esophagitis respond to treatment with topical corticosteroids, but a diagnosis is needed first.

10. Answer b

The most prevalent cause of noncardiac chest pain is gastroesophageal reflux disease. Reflux esophagitis is relatively uncommon in this population, and thus the yield of endoscopy is relatively low. However, it is often the first test performed to exclude not only esophagitis but also an atypical presentation of peptic ulcer disease (now also relatively uncommon).

Esophageal manometry usually is not helpful because esophageal spasm or achalasia as a cause of chest pain in this setting is relatively rare. An alternative to testing would be an empiric trial of high-dose proton pump inhibitor therapy, but in view of this patient's age, investigations would be reasonable before taking this approach.

SECTION II

Stomach

CHAPTER 6

Peptic Ulcer Disease

Thomas F. Mangan, M.D.

Peptic ulcers are defects in the gastrointestinal mucosa that extend through the muscularis mucosae (Fig. 1). They persist because of peptic acid effects from gastric juice. The incidence has decreased in the last half century, but peptic ulcer disease still affects 200,000 to 400,000 people annually and accounts for 10% of medical costs for digestive diseases. The discovery of *Helicobacter pylori* infection has dramatically changed our understanding of the pathophysiology of ulcer disease and its treatment.

ETIOLOGY AND PATHOPHYSIOLOGY

The long-held dictum "no acid–no ulcer" still applies. Compared with age-matched controls, patients with duodenal ulcers secrete 70% more acid during the day and 150% more at night. The balance between peptic acid secretion and gastroduodenal mucosal defense includes stimulatory and inhibitory mechanisms that involve multiple lines of defense (Fig. 2). The balance between aggressive and defensive factors may be disrupted and lead to the development of mucosal injury. Exogenous factors, such as nonsteroidal anti-inflammatory drugs (NSAIDs), alcohol, and *H. pylori*, and endogenous factors, such as bile, acid, and pepsin, may alter the lines of defense, allowing back diffusion of hydrogen ions and subsequent injury of epithelial cells.

Although mucosal abnormalities are consistently present with *H. pylori* infection (active gastritis) and NSAID use (prostaglandin inhibition), a clinical ulcer develops in only a small number of patients. The protective factors, including mucus, mucosal blood flow, tight intercellular junctions, and cell restitution and epithelial renewal, seem to prevent the development of ulcers. Thus, other pathogenic factors must have a role in the formation of ulcers. Other covariables may include high levels of acid secretion, low levels of sodium bicarbonate secretion, gastric metaplasia, and cigarette smoking.

ETIOLOGY

The most common etiologic factors for peptic ulcer disease are *H. pylori* infection and NSAID use. Uncommon causes are hypersecretory states such as Zollinger-Ellison syndrome, antral G-cell hyperplasia, mastocytosis, and basophilic leukemias. Viral infections with herpes simplex virus type 1 and cytomegalovirus also cause gastroduodenal ulceration, as may Crohn's disease.

Helicobacter pylori

H. pylori is a gram-negative spiral-shaped bacterium containing four to six unipolar flagella (Fig. 3). These bacteria occur only in the gastric epithelium, and when found in the duodenum, they are associated with metaplastic gastric epithelium. They produce urease and mucolytic proteases that help them survive the hostile environment of the stomach. Urease is responsible for the resistance of *H. pylori* to acid.

H. pylori organisms are found in otherwise healthy persons. The infection is acquired typically in childhood. In developed countries such as the United States, the prevalence may vary depending on ethnic group and socioeconomic status. There is evidence that the organism is transmitted from person to person. Currently, the specific mode of transmission—fecal-oral, oral-oral, or gastric-oral—is not known.

H. pylori causes a chronic active gastritis that involves predominantly the antrum. The presence of these bacteria in the

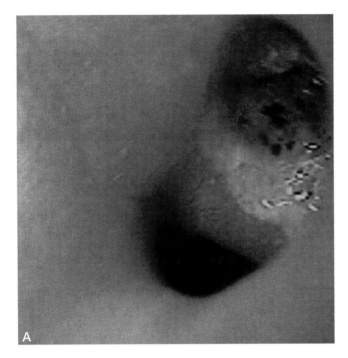
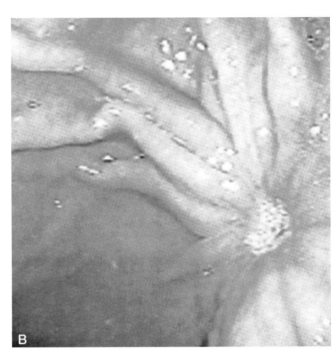

Fig. 1. Stomach with peptic ulcer (*A*) and healing peptic ulcer (*B*). (From Emory TS, Carpenter HA, Gostout CJ, Sobin LH. Atlas of gastrointestinal endoscopy & endoscopic biopsies. Washington, DC: Armed Forces Institute of Pathology, American Registry of Pathology; 2000.)

antrum leads to a loss of D cells, which release somatostatin, and allows the antral G cells to release gastrin without inhibition. This, in turn, leads to increased gastric acid secretion and ulcer formation. In addition, *H. pylori* is important in the development of duodenitis and gastric metaplasia of the duodenum, which is thought to contribute importantly to duodenal ulceration (Fig. 4). These bacteria also release enzymes and cytotoxic substances that disrupt the protective gastric mucus barrier.

Supportive evidence for a pathogenic role of *H. pylori* in duodenal ulcer includes the following: 1) Antibiotic therapy heals duodenal ulcers at the same rate histamine$_2$ (H$_2$)-receptor antagonists do. 2) The recurrence rate of duodenal ulcers is lower after *H. pylori* eradication than after conventional ulcer treatment. 3) Ulcer recurrence is always associated with failure to eradicate *H. pylori*. *H. pylori*-negative ulcers require one to be certain that *H. pylori* status has been assessed appropriately (false-negative test resulting from the recent use of proton pump inhibitors [PPIs] or antibiotics) or that it is caused by surreptitious use of aspirin or NSAIDs.

The critical role of *H. pylori* in the development of peptic ulcer disease is clear. What is not clear is why so few patients with *H. pylori* develop clinical ulcerations. Host immune responses, genetic predisposition, bacterial virulence factors, and other environmental factors have been implicated.

Nonsteroidal Anti-inflammatory Drugs

NSAIDs are responsible for the majority of peptic ulcers not caused by *H. pylori*. Because 40% of patients may not report

using these drugs, clinicians need a high index of suspicion. NSAIDs disrupt the mucosal defense mechanism by both topical and systemic effects. Topical injury occurs within the stomach as a direct injury to the gastric epithelium. The inhibition of prostaglandins disrupts mucosal blood flow, alters mucus secretion, and inhibits bicarbonate secretion, all of which lead to increased hydrogen ion back diffusion and mucosal injury. Prostaglandin inhibition also leads to alteration in the tight intercellular junctions and to trapping of neutrophils within the capillaries. These neutrophils release cytokines, increasing the inflammatory reaction.

Duodenal ulcers occur in approximately 10% of persons taking NSAIDs long term. Risk factors associated with ulcer formation and gastrointestinal tract bleeding include age older than 60 years, personal history of peptic ulcer disease, past history of gastrointestinal tract hemorrhage, taking more than one NSAID concomitantly, taking anticoagulants concurrently with NSAIDs, and comorbid conditions, primarily cardiovascular disease.

Attempts have been made to avoid gastrointestinal ulceration through the use of newer agents that preferentially inhibit the COX-2 isoform. Although these agents appear to be less ulcerogenic, this class of drug is not without risk and the incidence of ulcer among those taking these drugs appears to be about 3% to 5%. The potential gastroduodenal-sparing effects of COX-2 agents are lost with the concurrent use of aspirin. Recently, several drugs from this class have been removed from the U.S. market because of increased risk of stroke and cardiovascular disease. Prophylactic therapy with

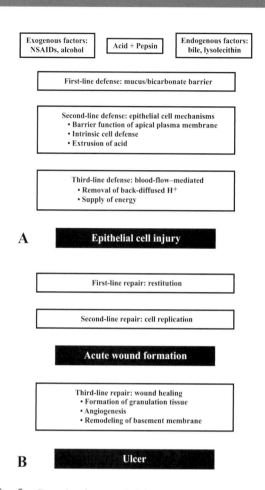

A

B

Fig. 2. Cascade of mucosal defense (*A*) and repair (*B*) mechanisms. Damaging effects on epithelial cells of exogenous and endogenous factors are amplified by peptic acid activity. If the three sets of lines of defense mechanisms fail, epithelial cell injury occurs that is repaired by restitution and cell replication. If these repair mechanisms fail, an acute wound forms. Ulcers form only with failure of acute wound healing mechanisms. NSAID, nonsteroidal anti-inflammatory drug. (From Soll AH. Peptic ulcer and its complications. In: Feldman M, Sleisenger MH, Scharschmidt BF, editors. Sleisenger & Fordtran's gastrointestinal and liver disease: pathophysiology, diagnosis, management. Vol 1. 6th ed. Philadelphia: WB Saunders Company; 1998. p. 620-78. Used with permission.)

a high-dose H_2-receptor antagonist or PPI may be as effective as misoprostol in preventing gastroduodenal ulcers caused by NSAIDs.

ACID HYPERSECRETORY STATES

Classically, acid hypersecretory states have been associated with multiple ulcerations, some of which occur in unusual locations (beyond the first portion of the duodenal bulb) (Tables 1 and 2). These conditions are associated with secretion of a large volume of acid that disrupts the normal digestion-absorption process and may be associated with diarrhea and malabsorption.

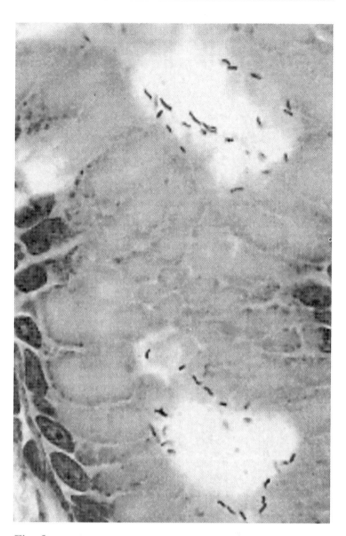

Fig. 3. Section of stomach showing *Helicobacter pylori*. (Wenger-Angritt stain.) (From Emory TS, Carpenter HA, Gostout CJ, Sobin LH. Atlas of gastrointestinal endoscopy & endoscopic biopsies. Washington, DC: Armed Forces Institute of Pathology, American Registry of Pathology; 2000.)

Patients with hypergastrinemia have uninhibited gastric acid secretion, leading to secretion rates of more than 15 mEq/h. The serum level of gastrin is the most sensitive and specific method for identifying patients who have gastrinoma. The average gastrin level is 50 to 60 pg/mL (upper level, 100 pg/mL). In patients with gastrinoma, the average level is 1,000 pg/mL. If patients have a fasting gastrin level of 1,000 pg/mL, gastric acid hypersecretion, and the appropriate clinical features, the diagnosis is Zollinger-Ellison syndrome (Fig. 5). Provocative tests with secretin have been helpful in identifying the syndrome in patients who do not have markedly elevated fasting gastrin levels. In response to intravenously administered secretin, patients with Zollinger-Ellison syndrome have an increase in serum gastrin of at least 200 pg/mL. Other tests include intravenous infusion of calcium and a standard protein

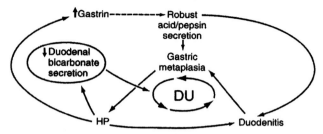

Hypothesis: DU pathogenesis?

Fig. 4. Hypothesis for the relation of acid hypersecretion with gastric metaplasia, duodenitis, duodenal *Helicobacter pylori* (HP), and bicarbonate secretion. It appears that the robust (high-normal or elevated) acid secretion that characterizes duodenal ulcer (DU) promotes and sustains gastric metaplasia in the duodenum, caused either by direct epithelial damage or inflammation secondary to this damage. These areas with gastric metaplasia provide a site for HP adherence; the adherent organism then exacerbates inflammation. A critical mass of HP may be necessary for it to thrive. By causing inflammation and epithelial injury, HP may expand gastric metaplasia. Another factor is that HP appears to decrease duodenal bicarbonate secretion, thereby compromising defenses against peptic acid injury. HP infection, by increasing gastrin secretion, in some subjects may contribute to the robust levels of acid secretion. These factors may contribute to the vicious cycle that promotes duodenal ulcer formation. (From Soll AH. Peptic ulcer and its complications. In: Feldman M, Sleisenger MH, Scharschmidt BF, editors. Sleisenger & Fordtran's gastrointestinal and liver disease: pathophysiology, diagnosis, management. Vol 1. 6th ed. Philadelphia: WB Saunders Company; 1998. p. 620-78. Used with permission.)

Table 1. Conditions That May Accompany Gastric Acid Hypersecretion

Duodenal ulcers
   Numerous
   Recurrent
   Resistant
   Complicated
   Not associated with *Helicobacter pylori* infection or use
      of nonsteroidal anti-inflammatory drugs
Ulcers in unusual sites
Ulcers and kidney stones
Ulcers and endocrinopathies
Any patient undergoing gastric surgery for ulcer disease
Large nasogastric output after gastric surgery
Ulcers after gastric surgery
Chronic watery diarrhea
Malabsorption

Table 2. Causes of Hypergastrinemia

Low acid output
   Gastric atrophy
   Helicobacter pylori gastritis
   Pernicious anemia type I
   Associated with other autoimmune diseases
   Antisecretory medications
Intermediate acid output
   H. pylori gastritis
   Vagotomy (total or highly selective)
   Pheochromocytoma (occasionally)
   Chronic renal failure
High acid output
   Zollinger-Ellison syndrome
   Sporadic
   Associated with multiple endocrine neoplasia
   Retained gastric antrum
   Chronic gastric outlet obstruction
   G-cell hyperfunction
   H. pylori gastritis
   Short-gut syndrome

meal. In the calcium infusion test, a positive response is an increase in gastrin of more than 400 pg/mL. With the standard protein meal, the increase in gastrin may be from minimal to more than 200%. This test is less sensitive.

Gastrinomas may be either sporadic or part of the multiple endocrine neoplasia (MEN)-1 syndrome. Sporadic gastrinomas are solitary and located with almost equal frequency in the pancreas or duodenum (Fig. 6). They are malignant in approximately 60% of patients, as determined by metastatic disease. These lesions typically metastasize to local lymph nodes and the liver.

Gastrinomas associated with MEN-1 syndrome are multiple and usually in the duodenum. They, too, are malignant in 60% of patients, with local metastasis to lymph nodes but rarely to the liver.

With the availability of potent acid-suppressant medications, the principal threat to the life of patients with Zollinger-Ellison syndrome is malignant invasion by the tumor. The optimal form of treatment is surgical resection of the gastrinoma. Preoperative testing should attempt to localize the tumor. In approximately 90% of cases, the gastrinoma is located preoperatively, with a cure rate of approximately 40%. The role for surgery in MEN-1 has been a matter of controversy because the tumors are multiple and multifocal. Recent, improved surgical results, however, have led to recommendations that all patients with Zollinger-Ellison syndrome without liver metastases be evaluated with the intent to resect.

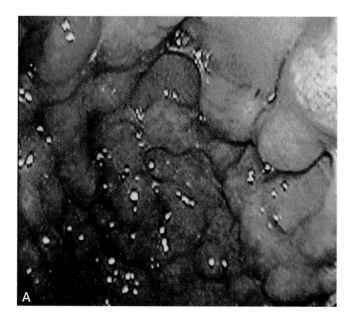
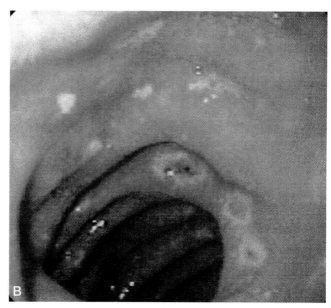

Fig. 5. *A*, Hypertrophic gastropathy. *B*, Multiple erosions in postbulbar duodenum. (From Emory TS, Carpenter HA, Gostout CJ, Sobin LH. Atlas of gastrointestinal endoscopy & endoscopic biopsies. Washington, DC: Armed Forces Institute of Pathology, American Registry of Pathology; 2000.)

Systemic Mastocytosis

This is a disorder associated with mast cell infiltration of multiple organs, including the skin, gastrointestinal tract, lymph nodes, bone marrow, and liver. Hypersecretion of acid, produced by increased histamine levels, is found in approximately 30% of the patients. H_2-Receptor antagonists have been successful in treating this condition.

Antral G-cell Hyperplasia

This condition has been described in a cluster of patients who have a familial history of peptic ulcer disease and an increased number of antral G cells. These patients have increased basal hypergastrinemia and acid hypersecretion. A secretin stimulation test can distinguish between antral G-cell hyperplasia and Zollinger-Ellison syndrome. In antral G-cell hyperplasia, the response to secretin stimulation is a decrease, no change, or a slight increase (<200 pg/mL).

Management of antral G-cell hyperplasia should begin with ruling out *H. pylori* infection. If this infection is identified, the organism should be eradicated. If *H. pylori* infection is not found, gastrinoma needs to be ruled out.

Retained Antrum Syndrome

Antral exclusion is a rare form of hypergastrinemia in patients who have had a Billroth II operation. If a small cuff of antrum remains and is excluded from the gastric acid, the gastrin-producing G cells will release gastrin without negative feedback, leading to hypersecretion of acid in the remaining stump. Ulcers develop postoperatively in these patients because of

hypergastrinemia. The results of a secretin stimulation test in patients with retained antrum syndrome are negative.

CLINICAL FEATURES

The clinical features of peptic ulcer disease range from silent ulceration presenting with active gastrointestinal tract hemorrhage or perforation to the classic symptoms of acid dyspepsia

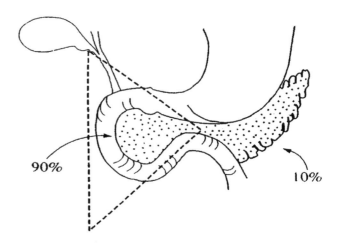

Fig. 6. Gastrinoma triangle (*dashed lines*). More than 90% of gastrinomas are found within the limits of this anatomic triangle. (From Stabile BE, Morrow DJ, Passaro E Jr. The gastrinoma triangle: operative implications. Am J Surg. 1984;147:25-30. Used with permission.)

and epigastric pain. In classic peptic ulcer, pain occurs 2 to 3 hours after a meal, improves with food or antacids, and awakens the patient several hours after the patient goes to sleep.

With uncomplicated ulcer disease, the physical examination findings tend to be normal except for occasional minimal epigastric tenderness. Clinical features of complicated disease include hematemesis, vomiting associated with gastric outlet obstruction, or an acute abdomen associated with perforation.

DIAGNOSIS

Because the signs and symptoms of peptic ulcer disease are not specific, making the diagnosis on the basis of medical history and physical examination findings alone is difficult. The diagnosis usually is based on the results of an upper gastrointestinal tract radiographic study or esophagogastroduodenoscopy (EGD). The findings of these two tests correlate in about 80% to 90% of cases. EGD is the preferred method for evaluating suspected duodenal ulcer disease because the upper gastrointestinal tract radiographic series is not as effective in detecting small ulcers. Also, EGD allows biopsy of the antrum for *H. pylori*, biopsy of gastric ulcers to differentiate benign from malignant ulcers, and evaluation of infiltrative, granulomatous, neoplastic, or infectious causes of ulceration.

Diagnostic testing for *H. pylori* has become important in the diagnosis and management of peptic ulcer disease. Tests that require samples of gastric mucosa include histologic examination for evidence of chronic active gastritis and the presence of *H. pylori*. Biopsy with histologic examination is the reference standard for the diagnosis of *H. pylori* infection. It is recommended that two biopsy specimens be taken from the gastric antrum, two from the gastric fundus, and one from the angularis. Standard staining with hematoxylin and eosin is excellent for detecting infection and the associated chronic gastritis. If the number of bacteria is small, a silver stain (Warthin-Starry) is often necessary.

Mucosal biopsy specimens can also be tested for urease with the urease test, called the "CLO (*Campylobacter*-like organism) test." It is imperative to be aware that recent therapy with PPIs or antibiotics or a recent gastrointestinal tract hemorrhage can produce false-negative results.

Tests that do not require mucosal sampling include serologic tests (IgG antibody), *H. pylori* stool assays, and the urea breath test. Serologic tests are as sensitive and specific as biopsy and are very useful in the initial diagnosis of *H. pylori* infection. However, they are less helpful in confirming cure after treatment because a marked loss of titers may take 6 to 12 months after therapy. The *H. pylori* stool assay appears to be highly accurate. It is a noninvasive, simple, and cost-effective test that is used to diagnose *H. pylori* infection in symptomatic adults and to monitor response to therapy. The urea breath test is performed by labeling urea with either carbon 13 or carbon 14 (Fig. 7).

If urease is present in the stomach, labeled carbon dioxide is split off and absorbed and then easily measured in expired breath. This test is accurate, but if a small number of bacteria occur in the stomach or the patient has recently had antibiotic or PPI therapy, the results can be false-negative. The urea breath test is the test of choice to confirm eradication of *H. pylori*. This test should be performed 4 weeks after treatment with antibiotics or PPIs has been discontinued.

In summary, for patients in whom endoscopy is indicated, the rapid urease test is the least expensive form of diagnosis. If the results are negative, other samples of tissue obtained at the time of biopsy can be stained to examine specifically for *H. pylori*. For patients in whom EGD is contraindicated or unnecessary, serologic tests are quick, inexpensive, and accurate. However, the urea breath test or stool antigen study can better reflect the current status of the infection and is most helpful in confirming eradication of the organism.

TREATMENT

The treatment of peptic ulcer disease has changed remarkably since *H. pylori* infection has been identified and associated with peptic ulcer disease. The recurrence rate of peptic ulcer disease has decreased from approximately 90% at 1 year to 1% to 2% after eradication of the organism. It is imperative that *H. pylori* initially be considered the cause of ulcer disease in all patients. The pretest probability of *H. pylori* infection as the cause must be considered and, if the test is negative, the negative result must be confirmed with a second test or biopsy. If the test results are in fact negative, alternative explanations, such as NSAIDs or hypersecretory states, are considered.

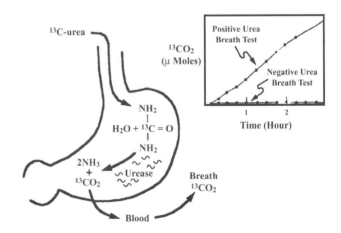

Fig. 7. The urea breath test. (From Walsh JH, Peterson WL. The treatment of *Helicobacter pylori* infection in the management of peptic ulcer disease. N Engl J Med. 1995;333:984-91. Used with permission.)

Historically, bed rest, milk, and a bland diet were prescribed for peptic ulcer disease. Dietary change is no longer advised. The only general measures recommended are to discontinue cigarette smoking and to avoid NSAIDs. Although certain foods, such as spicy foods and sauces, may increase the dyspeptic complaints of patients, they do not cause ulcer disease or interfere with healing.

Antacids

Antacids containing aluminum and magnesium hydroxide effectively heal ulcers by binding bile and inhibiting pepsin. Antacids also promote angiogenesis in injured mucosa. However, at least seven 30-mL doses daily are needed to heal ulcers. This high dose can produce such adverse side effects as diarrhea (magnesium-containing agents), constipation (aluminum-containing agents), and sodium overload. Calcium-containing antacids can cause acid stimulation and acid rebound.

H$_2$-Receptor Antagonists

In the mid-1970s, H$_2$-receptor antagonists were shown to heal ulcers in 70% to 85% of patients after 4 to 6 weeks of therapy. Currently, four H$_2$-receptor antagonists (cimetidine, famotidine, nizatidine, ranitidine) are available. Although their potency, bioavailability, and side effect-profiles differ, they are overall one of the safest classes of drugs available. Cimetidine produces gynecomastia and impotence in a time-dependent fashion. It also binds to the cytochrome P-450 mixed oxidase system and may affect the metabolism of certain drugs, including warfarin, theophylline, and phenytoin. Central nervous system side effects include confusion, restlessness, somnolence, agitation, headache, and dizziness. These symptoms have been seen more frequently in elderly patients in intensive care units. Rare side effects have included a mild increase in liver aminotransferase levels and cardiac rhythm disturbance.

Single nocturnal dosing is at least as effective as twice-daily dosing regimens (same total daily dose) in suppressing 24-hour gastric acid secretion and in healing duodenal ulcers. All H$_2$-receptor antagonists have healing rates of 90% to 95% at 8 weeks of therapy.

Sucralfate

This is a sulfated polysaccharide that is complexed with aluminum hydroxide. It prevents acute ulceration and heals chronic ulcers without affecting the secretion of gastric acid or pepsin. Like aluminum-containing antacids, sucralfate promotes angiogenesis and the formation of granulation tissue. Because binding of this drug to the ulcer is enhanced at a pH < 3.5, it should be administered 30 to 60 minutes before meals. From 3% to 5% of this drug is absorbed, and, because of potential aluminum toxicity, it should be prescribed with caution for patients with renal failure.

Prostaglandins

Misoprostol (prostaglandin E$_1$ analogue) exerts a mucosal protective effect by stimulating the secretion of mucus and bicarbonate and by enhancing mucosal blood flow and epithelial cell restitution. From 20% to 30% of patients have a dose-dependent diarrhea from stimulation of the cyclic adenosine monophosphate system. Prostaglandins are uterotropic and induce bleeding, cramps, and spontaneous abortion in pregnant women. Hence, they should not be administered to women of childbearing age. The primary role of misoprostol is prevention of NSAID-induced gastroduodenal injury.

Proton Pump Inhibitors

PPIs (lansoprazole, omeprazole, pantoprazole, rabeprazole) are prodrugs that are acid labile and inactivated when exposed to gastric juice. They are enteric coated to dissolve at a pH > 6. After absorption, they become concentrated in the secretory canaliculus of the parietal cell and irreversibly inactivate the hydrogen-potassium adenosine triphosphatase (ATPase) system—the final common pathway for acid secretion. PPIs are the most powerful drugs available to suppress gastric acid secretion. Several important features of clinical relevance need to be stressed:

1. Because of the lag time to peak antisecretory effectiveness, PPIs should not be administered on an "as needed" basis.
2. Because PPIs effectively inhibit only stimulated parietal cells, their effectiveness may be diminished by the coadministration of H$_2$-receptor antagonists.
3. Because PPIs are most effective when taken shortly before a meal, they should be taken 30 minutes before breakfast.

PPIs have an excellent safety profile. Although prolonged acid inhibition, hypergastrinemia, and enterochromaffin-like cell hyperplasia have caused concern, they have not proved to be clinically important in humans.

H. pylori and Ulcer Treatment

Treatment regimens for *H. pylori* have evolved over the past decade from monotherapy to combinations of antisecretory and antibiotic therapy (Table 3). A 10- to 14-day course of therapy with bismuth and antibiotics or with a PPI and antibiotics is as effective for inducing ulcer healing as a 4-week course of PPI therapy. Combination therapy enhances the cure of *H. pylori* infection, shortens the treatment period, and has a 90% cure rate at 1 week.

Bacterial resistance has been a concern. Both metronidazole- and clarithromycin-resistant strains of *H. pylori* have been encountered. Resistance has not been found to amoxicillin, tetracycline, or bismuth. The addition of a PPI to metronidazole-based therapy lessens the effect of metronidazole resistance. No clarithromycin regimen has been shown to reliably treat clarithromycin-resistant organisms. If patients are thought to

Table 3. *Helicobacter pylori* Eradication Rates and 95% Confidence Interval Limits (CL) for Each Treatment Regimen in the MACH I Study*

| | Eradication rate (%) (95% CL) | | |
| | All patients | Per | Intention to |
Treatment	treated	protocol	treat
OAC250	83.8	85.1	79.5
	(76.9-90.6)	(78.3-91.8)	(72.2-86.8)
OAC500	96.4	90.0	90.6
	(92.9-99.9)	(95.4-100)	(85.3-95.9)
OMC250	94.6	94.3	89.7
	(90.4-98.8)	(89.9-98.7)	(84.3-95.2)
OMC500	89.8	92.5	85.5
	(84.4-95.3)	(87.4-97.5)	(79.3-91.7)
OAM	79.0	81.6	75.8
	(71.7-86.3)	(74.5-88.7)	(68.3-83.3)
OP	0.9	0.9	0.8
	(0.0-2.6)	(0.0-2.7)	(0.0-2.5)

A, amoxicillin, 1,000 mg bid; bid, twice daily; C, clarithromycin, 250 or 500 mg bid; M, metronidazole, 400 mg bid; O, omeprazole, 20 mg bid; P, placebo.
*All regimens were given for 7 days.
From Lind T, Veldhuyzen van Zanten S, Unge P, Spiller R, Bayerdorffer E, O'Morain C, et al. Eradication of Helicobacter pylori *using one-week triple therapies combining omeprazole with two antimicrobials: the MACH I Study. Helicobacter. 1996;1:138-44. Used with permission.*

have clarithromycin resistance, they should receive a metronidazole-based regimen.

The development of an *H. pylori* vaccine has generated widespread interest. A long-term worldwide solution to *H. pylori*-related disease is prevention. Currently, the problem in vaccine development is finding an acceptable mucosal adjuvant to introduce the stimulating antigen to the immune system. Systemic immunization does not produce protective immunity against the bacteria.

RECOMMENDED READING

Brandt LJ, editor. Clinical practice of gastroenterology. Philadelphia: Current Medicine, 1999.

Emory TS, Carpenter HA, Gostout CJ, Sobin LH. Atlas of gastrointestinal endoscopy & endoscopic biopsies. Washington, DC: Armed Forces Institute of Pathology, American Registry of Pathology; 2000.

Feldman M, Sleisenger MH, Scharschmidt BF, editors. Sleisenger & Fordtran's gastrointestinal and liver disease: pathophysiology, diagnosis, management. 6th ed. Philadelphia: WB Saunders Company; 1998.

Graham DY, Genta RM, Dixon MF, editors. Gastritis. Philadelphia: Lippincott Williams & Wilkins; 1999.

Isenberg J, McQuaid KR, Laine L, Walsh JH. Acid-peptic disorders. In: Yamada T, editor. Textbook of gastroenterology. Vol 1. 2nd ed. Philadelphia: JB Lippincott Company; 1995. p. 1347-1430.

Lanas AI, Remacha B, Esteva F, Sainz R. Risk factors associated with refractory peptic ulcers. Gastroenterology. 1995;109:1124-33.

Marshall BJ, editor. *Helicobacter pylori*. Part I. Gastroenterol Clin N Am. 2000;29(3):559-757.

Marshall BJ, editor. *Helicobacter pylori*. Part II. Gastroenterol Clin N Am. 2000;29(4):759-950.

Savage RL, Moller PW, Ballantyne CL, Wells JE. Variation in the risk of peptic ulcer complications with nonsteroidal antiinflammatory drug therapy. Arthritis Rheum. 1993;36:84-90.

Silverstein FE, Faich G, Goldstein JL, Simon LS, Pincus T, Whelton A, et al. Gastrointestinal toxicity with celecoxib vs nonsteroidal anti-inflammatory drugs for osteoarthritis and rheumatoid arthritis: the CLASS study: a randomized controlled trial: Celecoxib Long-term Arthritis Safety Study. JAMA. 2000;284:1247-55.

CHAPTER 7

Gastritis

Thomas F. Mangan, M.D.

INTRODUCTION

Gastritis, or inflammation of the gastric mucosa, is a group of disorders associated with inflammatory changes that have different clinical features, causative mechanisms, and histologic characteristics.

"Gastritis" has been a vague and ambiguous term to histopathologists for years. Its use has led to confusion in comparing studies. Since the discovery of *Helicobacter pylori* and the associated gastritis, attempts have been made to resolve the confusion. A group of pathologists met in Houston, Texas, in 1994 to establish a terminology. The result is the Sydney System, a classification based on topography, morphology, and etiology (Table 1).

Gastritis has a broad histologic appearance that leads to specific patterns of disease. It has been divided into acute, chronic, and special forms.

ACUTE GASTRITIS

Acute gastritis has two forms: acute hemorrhagic or erosive gastritis and acute neutrophilic gastritis.

Acute hemorrhagic gastritis generally is defined as a diffuse reaction to irritants or chemical injury (Fig. 1). Substances such as alcohol, aspirin, corticosteroids, and nonsteroidal anti-inflammatory drugs (NSAIDs) have been implicated. Also, it has been associated with major trauma, surgery, sepsis, burns, and hypothermia.

Acute neutrophilic gastritis is associated with *H. pylori* infection (Fig. 2), marked neutrophilic infiltration, and epithelial degeneration.

Acute hemorrhagic gastritis is the result of an imbalance between aggressive and defensive factors that maintain mucosal integrity. Some of these factors are discussed below.

1. Stress and shock—These conditions lead to underperfusion of the tissue, with accumulation of vasoactive amines and leukotrienes. The mucosal barrier is impaired and allows back diffusion of hydrogen ions, leading to further damage.

2. NSAIDs—These agents can cause a topical injury that allows back diffusion of hydrogen ions. NSAIDs also have a systemic effect through the prostaglandin system that decreases bicarbonate release, diminishes mucus formation, and affects mucosal blood flow, which is needed to maintain mucosal integrity and repair by the process of restitution.

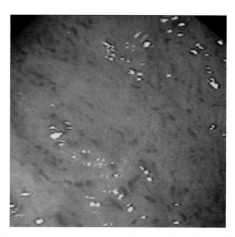

Fig. 1. Stomach—Acute hemorrhagic gastritis. (From Emory TS, Carpenter HA, Gostout CJ, Sobin LH. Atlas of gastrointestinal endoscopy & endoscopic biopsies. Washington, DC: Armed Forces Institute of Pathology, American Registry of Pathology; 2000. p. 101.)

Table 1. Sydney System of Classification of Chronic Gastritis Based on Topography, Morphology, and Etiology

Type of gastritis	Etiologic factors	Gastritis synonyms
Nonatrophic	*Helicobacter pylori*	Superficial
	Other factors (?)	Diffuse antral gastritis
		Chronic antral gastritis
		Interstitial-follicular
		Hypersecretory
		Type B
Atrophic	Autoimmunity	Type A
	H. pylori (?)	Diffuse corporeal
Autoimmune	*H. pylori*	Pernicious anemia–associated
	Environmental factors	Type B, type AB
Multifocal atrophic		Environmental
		Metaplastic
		Atrophic pangastritis
		Progressive intestinalizing pangastritis
Special forms		
Chemical	Chemical irritation	Reactive
	Bile	Reflux
	Nonsteroidal anti-inflammatory drugs	
	Other agents (?)	
Radiation	Radiation injury	
Lymphocytic	Idiopathic (?)	Varioliform
	Autoimmune mechanisms (?)	Celiac disease–associated
	Gluten (?)	
	Drugs (ticlopidine)	
	H. pylori (?)	
Noninfectious granulomatous	Crohn's disease	Isolated granulomatous
	Sarcoidosis	
	Wegener's granulomatosis	
	Foreign substances	
	Idiopathic (?)	
Eosinophilic	Food sensitivity	Allergic
	Other allergies (?)	
Other infectious gastritides	Bacteria (other than *H. pylori*)	Phlegmonous, syphilitic
	Viruses	Cytomegalovirus
	Fungi	Anisakiasis
	Parasites	

From Graham DY, Genta RM, Dixon MF. Gastritis. Philadelphia: Lippincott Williams & Wilkins; 1999. Used with permission.

3. Alcohol—It has long been known to cause acute gastritis. The severity of damage has been associated directly with the concentration of alcohol and the duration of exposure. The key event in alcohol-associated gastritis is disruption of the mucosal microvasculature. Capillary congestion with increased vascular permeability and adhesion of polymorphonuclear leukocytes sets the stage for inflammatory modulation and free radical formation, causing injury.

Acute gastritis is an important clinical condition for which therapy is incomplete. Prostaglandin analogues represent a major advance in treatment of NSAID-induced gastritis, but they have their own set of side effects. Acid suppression and supportive measures are the principal treatment options.

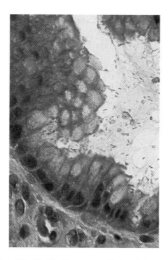

Fig. 2. Stomach with *Helicobacter pylori*. (From Emory TS, Carpenter HA, Gostout CJ, Sobin LH. Atlas of gastrointestinal endoscopy & endoscopic biopsies. Washington, DC: Armed Forces Institute of Pathology, American Registry of Pathology; 2000. p. 91.)

CHRONIC GASTRITIS

Nonatrophic Gastritis (Type B)
In nonatrophic gastritis, inflammation is more intense in the gastric antrum than in the corpus (Fig. 3). This form of gastritis is associated with *H. pylori* infection and is characterized by surface degeneration, foveolar hyperplasia, hyperemia with lamina propria edema, neutrophilic infiltration, and chronic inflammatory cell infiltration (Fig. 4). Special stains may or may not demonstrate the organism in biopsy specimens.

Atrophic Gastritis (Type A)
The two forms of atrophic gastritis are autoimmune gastritis (Fig. 5) and multifocal atrophic gastritis.

Autoimmune Gastritis
Autoimmune gastritis is defined as chronic gastritis that is restricted to the corpus-fundal mucosa and associated with severe diffuse atrophy of the acidophilic glands, leading to achlorhydria. This gastritis is associated with anti-intrinsic factor antibodies and antiparietal cell antibodies that lead to loss of intrinsic factor and achlorhydria.

Autoimmune gastritis differs from atrophic gastritis of *H. pylori* in that it lacks bacterial colonization, mature parietal cells, and a monomorphous lymphocytic cell infiltrate. In addition to pernicious anemia, gastric parietal cell antibodies have been detected in patients who have an autoimmune endocrinopathy such as Hashimoto's thyroiditis, thyrotoxicosis, myxedema, Addison's disease, diabetes mellitus, or Sjögren's syndrome.

Clinical manifestations of autoimmune gastritis include achlorhydria, hypergastrinemia, and anemia due to both iron deficiency and malabsorption of vitamin B_{12}.

Autoimmune gastritis is associated with an increased risk of gastric neoplasia. Associated with this form of gastritis are hyperplastic and adenomatous polyps, carcinoma, malignant lymphoma, and endocrine tumors.

Multifocal Atrophic Gastritis
In this form of atrophic gastritis, inflammation is similar in the antrum and corpus (Fig. 6). Multifocal atrophic gastritis is seen in association with *H. pylori* infection.

When obtaining biopsy specimens from a stomach with suspected *H. pylori* infection, it is imperative to obtain two specimens from the antrum and two from the corpus. Specimens from the corpus are important because the patient may have received proton pump inhibitor therapy, which causes the organism to disappear from the antrum and to relocate in tissue of the corpus. In addition, a fifth biopsy specimen should be obtained from the incisura because this is the site most likely to first show atrophic gastritis and the premalignant dysplasia associated with *H. pylori*.

Special Forms of Gastritis

Reactive Gastritis
The endoscopic appearance of reactive gastritis is associated with the topical effects of such substances as alcohol, NSAIDs, and bile. This is seen often in patients who have duodenal gastric reflux

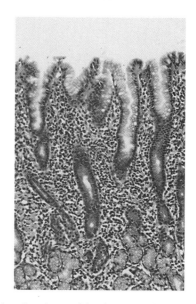

Fig. 3. Active chronic gastritis of antrum of stomach. (From Emory TS, Carpenter HA, Gostout CJ, Sobin LH. Atlas of gastrointestinal endoscopy & endoscopic biopsies. Washington, DC: Armed Forces Institute of Pathology, American Registry of Pathology; 2000. p. 90.)

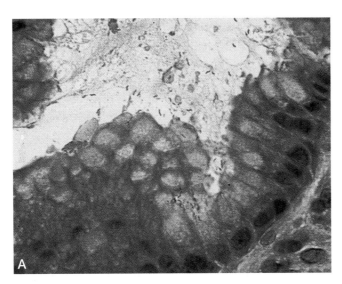
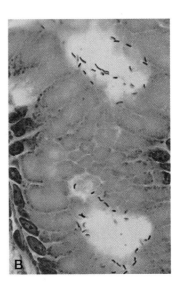

Fig. 4. *Helicobacter pylori* infection of stomach. Sections stained with, *A*, hematoxylin and eosin and, *B*, Wenger-Angritt stain. (From Emory TS, Carpenter HA, Gostout CJ, Sobin LH. Atlas of gastrointestinal endoscopy & endoscopic biopsies. Washington, DC: Armed Forces Institute of Pathology, American Registry of Pathology; 2000. p. 91.)

associated with pyloric dysfunction or previous gastric surgery. It tends to involve the antrum but may spread proximally. The chief histologic finding is a decrease in mucin. These findings are commonly referred to as "reactive gastropathy."

Lymphocytic Gastritis

Lymphocytic gastritis is characterized by a dense infiltration of lymphocytes (Fig. 7). Histologically, the epithelial surface is crowded with small lymphocytes that have scant cytoplasm and cleaved nuclei. The bulk of the infiltration lies in the superficial epithelium, with few cells seen within the glands. Previously, this form of gastritis was called "varioliform gastritis." Lymphocytic gastritis is thought to belong to a group of pathologic disorders that include gastric involvement by celiac disease. The infiltration is always present in the body as well as the antrum and consists of T lymphocytes, mostly CD8 cells.

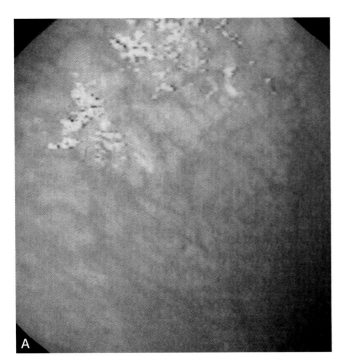
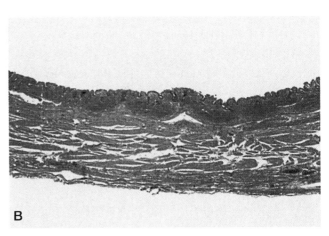

Fig. 5. Chronic atrophic autoimmune gastritis. *A*, Gross appearance. *B*, Section through corpus. (Hematoxylin and eosin.) (From Emory TS, Carpenter HA, Gostout CJ, Sobin LH. Atlas of gastrointestinal endoscopy & endoscopic biopsies. Washington, DC: Armed Forces Institute of Pathology, American Registry of Pathology; 2000. p. 94.)

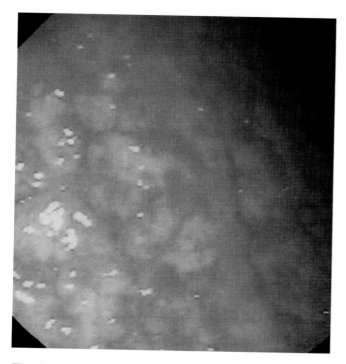

Fig. 6. Multifocal atrophic gastritis. (From Emory TS, Carpenter HA, Gostout CJ, Sobin LH. Atlas of gastrointestinal endoscopy & endoscopic biopsies. Washington, DC: Armed Forces Institute of Pathology, American Registry of Pathology; 2000. p. 93.)

Although spontaneous healing is possible, lymphocytic gastritis usually has a protracted course. Improvement has been noted in patients who receive omeprazole therapy. Certainly, improvement would be expected while patients follow a gluten-free diet.

Infectious Gastritis

H. pylori is the major cause of gastritis worldwide. Acute gastritis associated with this organism is rarely encountered clinically because the acute illness is mild, transient, and, oftentimes, completely asymptomatic. The acute gastritis of *H. pylori* infection is characterized by degenerative changes of the epithelium, including mucin depletion, cellular exfoliation, and infiltration by polymorphonuclear leukocytes. Spiral organisms are identified with hematoxylin and eosin stain, special stains such as the modified Giemsa stain, the Warthin-Starry silver stain, and specific immunostaining.

Viral Infections

Cytomegalovirus (CMV) may infect any cell within the gastrointestinal tract. CMV gastritis is diagnosed when an erosive or ulcerative process occurs in the presence of immunodeficiency (Fig. 8 *A*). Characteristic cytomegalic cells in the biopsy specimen are a classic feature (Fig. 8 *B*), and a CMV antigen is present on immunohistochemistry.

Microscopic findings include mucosal hemorrhage, erosion, and ulceration. Rarely, gross nodular mucosa, called "pseudo-tumors," may be seen. The identification of cytomegalic cells provides unequivocal evidence of tissue infection. Patients with acquired immunodeficiency syndrome (AIDS) are prone to this infection when the CD4 count is less than 100 cells/mm^3. The infection may also occur after kidney, liver, bone marrow, or heart transplantation. The treatment of choice is ganciclovir. However, because ganciclovir suppresses the virus but does not eliminate it, relapse is common.

Bacterial Gastritis

As mentioned above, *H. pylori* is the most common form of bacterial gastritis. However, several other species of bacteria may reside in the stomach after antrectomy or in association with achlorhydria. *Streptococcus*, *Staphylococcus*, *Lactobacillus*, *Bacteroides*, *Klebsiella*, and *Escherichia coli* have all been cultured from gastric juice. These organisms reside within the oral cavity and are thought to be swallowed. They rarely have clinical significance. However, under special circumstances, for example, ischemia or immunosuppression, they may produce marked morbidity. "Phlegmonous gastritis" is a life-threatening condition characterized by purulent necrosis that invades the full thickness of the gastric wall. When associated with a gas-forming organism, this form of gastritis is called "emphysematous gastritis."

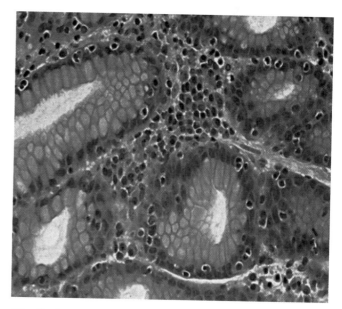

Fig. 7. Lymphocytic gastritis. (From Emory TS, Carpenter HA, Gostout CJ, Sobin LH. Atlas of gastrointestinal endoscopy & endoscopic biopsies. Washington, DC: Armed Forces Institute of Pathology, American Registry of Pathology; 2000. p. 96.)

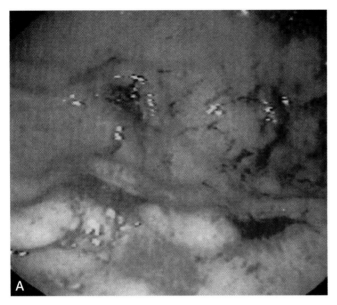
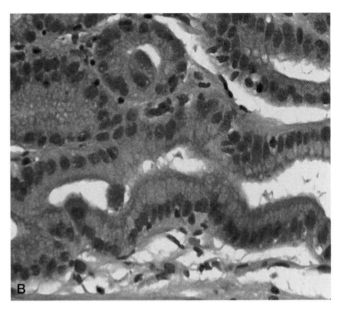

Fig. 8. Cytomegalovirus (CMV) infection of stomach. *A*, Gross appearance of CMV ulcers. *B*, CMV gastropathy. (From Emory TS, Carpenter HA, Gostout CJ, Sobin LH. Atlas of gastrointestinal endoscopy & endoscopic biopsies. Washington, DC: Armed Forces Institute of Pathology, American Registry of Pathology; 2000. p. 123.)

Mycobacterium

Mycobacteria can involve the stomach of patients with disseminated tuberculosis. Histologically, necrotizing granulomas are seen. In persons with AIDS and systemic *Mycobacterium avium-intracellulare* complex infection, the stomach may be infected by mycobacteria. Histologically, there is an accumulation of foamy histiocytes that stain positive for acid-fast bacilli.

Syphilitic Gastritis

This is an infection of the stomach by *Treponema pallidum*. The infection is associated with the second and third stages of syphilis. The gross appearance of the stomach is that of erosive antral gastritis. In some cases, thick gastric folds develop from infiltration by mononuclear plasma cells. Spirochetes are difficult to identify. During tertiary syphilis, an infiltrative process may have an appearance that suggests linitis plastica or lymphoma.

Fungal Infection

Although *Candida* species colonize gastric ulcers, they are not thought to cause primary gastritis. Rare opportunistic fungi have caused severe necrotizing gastritis, including mucormycosis in patients with diabetes mellitus. *Torulopsis glabrata* and *Cryptococcus neoformans* may infect immunosuppressed patients.

Parasitic Gastritis

The stomach is not a preferred site for parasitic infection.

Strongyloides stercoralis may rarely infect the stomach. *Cryptosporidium* and *Giardia* are seen in the stomach but are not thought to have a pathologic role. Anisakiasis may cause gastritis in persons with a history of ingesting raw fish.

Granulomatous Gastritis

Granulomas result from the direct toxic effect of certain substances or infection. A granuloma is a compact collection of mature monocytic phagocytes (Fig. 9). In most instances, the morphologic changes provide no clue to the cause. Clinical and laboratory information is needed to make a firm diagnosis. Infectious causes include tuberculosis, syphilis, and histoplasmosis. Foreign body granulomas may be associated with food trapped within an ulcer or, rarely, with mucin-producing adenocarcinoma. Granulomas may be seen in sarcoidosis, Crohn's disease, Wegener's granulomatosis, or anisakiasis.

Eosinophilic Gastritis

Eosinophilic gastritis is associated with extensive eosinophilic infiltration that may involve all layers of the stomach (Fig. 10). The antrum is involved more often than the body or fundus. Thick mucosal folds or nodules may be seen macroscopically. Corticosteroid therapy has controlled the symptoms of abdominal pain, nausea, and vomiting.

Vascular Gastropathies

These are characterized by abnormalities in the gastric tissue involving the mucosal vessels with little or no inflammation. The two most important clinical conditions are gastric antral vascular

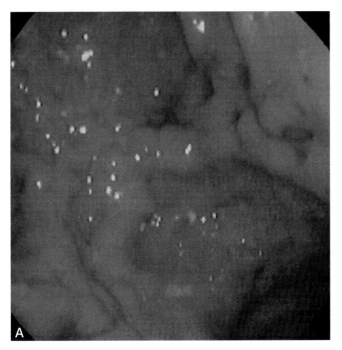

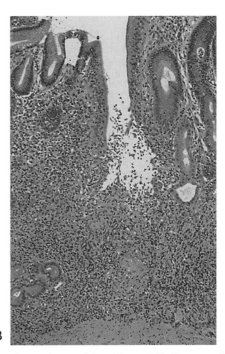

B

Fig. 9. Granulomatous gastritis. *A*, Gross appearance. *B*, Histologic appearance of granuloma. (From Emory TS, Carpenter HA, Gostout CJ, Sobin LH. Atlas of gastrointestinal endoscopy & endoscopic biopsies. Washington, DC: Armed Forces Institute of Pathology, American Registry of Pathology; 2000. p. 98, 99.)

ectasia (GAVE), or "watermelon stomach," and portal hypertensive gastropathy.

GAVE

Grossly, GAVE is characterized by longitudinal columns of continuous blood vessels that cross the antrum and converge on the pylorus (Fig. 11 *A*). These lesions appear to predominate in females and in association with achlorhydria and atrophic gastritis. Histopathologic examination of the lesions demonstrates little inflammation in the lamina propria but shows fibromuscular hyperplasia (Fig. 11 *B*). In addition, there are marked dilated mucosal capillaries. For patients who are transfusion-dependent, treatment includes Nd-YAG laser or argon plasma coagulation. Patients who cannot undergo this

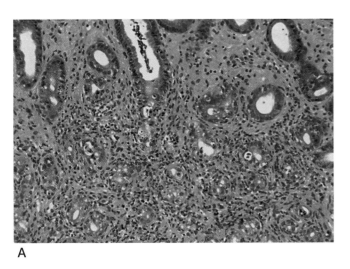

A

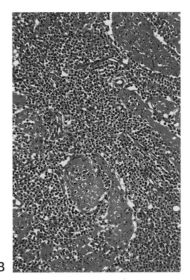

B

Fig. 10. Eosinophilic gastritis. Note marked eosinophilic infiltration. *A*, High-power and, *B*, low-power views. (From Emory TS, Carpenter HA, Gostout CJ, Sobin LH. Atlas of gastrointestinal endoscopy & endoscopic biopsies. Washington, DC: Armed Forces Institute of Pathology, American Registry of Pathology; 2000. p. 97.)

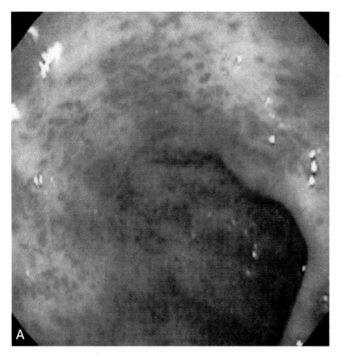

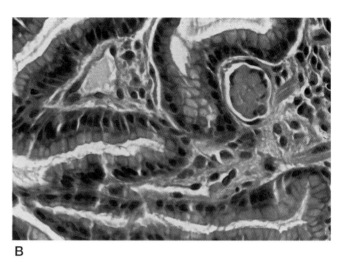

Fig. 11. "Watermelon" stomach (antrum). *A*, Gross specimen, and, *B*, histologic section showing thick-walled ectatic vessels. (From Emory TS, Carpenter HA, Gostout CJ, Sobin LH. Atlas of gastrointestinal endoscopy & endoscopic biopsies. Washington, DC: Armed Forces Institute of Pathology, American Registry of Pathology; 2000. p. 118.)

form of therapy or who do not have a response to it may benefit from antrectomy.

Portal Hypertensive Gastropathy

Portal hypertensive gastropathy (Fig. 12) is characterized by a mosaic pattern of the mucosa that is more pronounced in the fundus and body of the stomach. The histologic changes are also more prominent in the proximal stomach. Compared with GAVE, the vascular abnormalities are better defined in the deeper submucosal vessels, which are characterized by dilatation, irregularity, and tortuosity. This form of gastropathy is treated with β-blockers, transjugular intrahepatic portosystemic shunt, or portal decompression surgery.

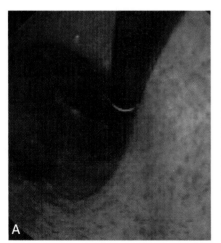

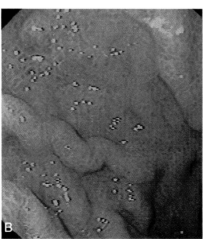

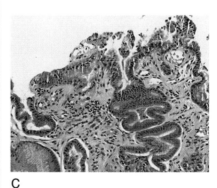

Fig. 12. Portal hypertensive gastropathy. *A* and *B*, Gross specimen showing the mosaic mucosal pattern. *C*, Histologic section showing dilated tortuous blood vessels. (From Emory TS, Carpenter HA, Gostout CJ, Sobin LH. Atlas of gastrointestinal endoscopy & endoscopic biopsies. Washington, DC: Armed Forces Institute of Pathology, American Registry of Pathology; 2000. p. 116.)

RECOMMENDED READING

Brandt LJ, Daum F. Clinical practice of gastroenterology. Philadelphia: Current Medicine; 1999.

Cryer B. Nonsteroidal anti-inflammatory drugs and gastrointestinal disease. In: Feldman M, Scharschmidt BF, Sleisenger MH, editors. Sleisenger & Fordtran's gastrointestinal and liver disease: pathophysiology/diagnosis/management. Vol 1. 6th ed. Philadelphia: WB Saunders; 1998. p. 343-57.

Emory TS, Carpenter HA, Gostout CJ, Sobin LH. Atlas of gastrointestinal endoscopy & endoscopic biopsies. Washington, DC: Armed Forces Institute of Pathology, American Registry of Pathology; 2000.

Graham DY, Genta RM, Dixon MF. Gastritis. Philadelphia: Lippincott Williams & Wilkins; 1999.

Kamath PS, Lacerda M, Ahlquist DA, McKusick MA, Andrews JC, Nagorney DA. Gastric mucosal responses to intrahepatic portosystemic shunting in patients with cirrhosis. Gastroenterology. 2000;118:905-911.

Marshall BJ, editor. *Helicobacter pylori*. Part I. Gastroenterol Clin North Am. 2000;29(3).

Marshall BJ, editor. *Helicobacter pylori*. Part II. Gastroenterol Clin North Am. 2000;29(4).

Scheiman JM. Clinical implications of cyclooxygenase inhibition for gastrointestinal disease. Gastroenterol Clin North Am. 2001;30(4).

Sleisenger MH, Fordtran JS, Feldman M, Scharschmidt B, editors. Sleisenger & Fordtran's gastrointestinal and liver disease: pathophysiology, diagnosis, management. 6th ed. Philadelphia: WB Saunders; 1998.

Watanabe T, Tada M, Nagai H, Sasaki S, Nakao M. *Helicobacter pylori* infection induces gastric cancer in mongolian gerbils. Gastroenterology. 1998;115:642-8.

CHAPTER 8

Gastric Neoplasms

Mark V. Larson, M.D.

GASTRIC CANCER

Epidemiology

Gastric carcinoma is the second most common cancer worldwide, with more than 750,000 new cases reported annually. It is also the second most common cause of cancer-related death, behind only lung cancer. In the United States, it was the leading cause of cancer-related mortality until the 1930s. Since then, the incidence has been decreasing; it has been estimated that about 22,000 new cases of gastric cancer are discovered in the United States each year. In this country, gastric cancer ranks eighth in cancer-related mortality for men and tenth for women.

The incidence of gastric carcinoma varies widely throughout the world and is highest in Japan, China, Thailand, South America, and Eastern Europe. In Japan, gastric carcinoma is the most frequently occurring cancer in both sexes, with an annual incidence of 78/100,000 men and 34/100,000 women, which is about eightfold higher than the incidence in the United States.

The incidence of gastric cancer increases with age. Relatively few cases are reported in persons younger than 30 years, but the incidence increases sharply after age 50. The risk of gastric cancer continues to be greatest in lower socioeconomic groups. Although the importance of race has not been determined, the decrease in gastric cancer mortality rate has been less pronounced in the black than in the white population. Some authors have suggested that this is the result of delayed diagnosis rather than specific factors that may make blacks more susceptible to this malignancy.

In the early decades of the 1900s, most cases of gastric carcinoma in the United States occurred in the distal stomach (gastric body and antrum). The significant decrease in the incidence of gastric cancer primarily reflects a decrease in distal stomach lesions. In contrast, data from the Surveillance, Epidemiology, and End Results (SEER) program have demonstrated a sharply rising increase in the incidence of adenocarcinoma involving the proximal stomach and gastroesophageal junction. A recent review examined the incidence of adenocarcinoma in 10 European countries from 1968 to 1995 and noted an increase in the incidence of adenocarcinoma of the gastric cardia and gastroesophageal junction, accompanied by a decrease in malignancies of the noncardia portion of the stomach. These findings suggest that gastroesophageal and proximal gastric adenocarcinoma may have a common pathogenesis, and one that is different from that of distal gastric cancers.

Etiology and Predisposing Conditions

Because gastric cancer has remained a major source of morbidity and mortality globally, considerable effort has been made to understand its causes. The current belief is that gastric cancer does not have a single cause but rather multiple etiologic factors, including diet, exogenous chemicals, infectious agents, and genetic factors. Of these, the most extensively studied have been dietary habits and *Helicobacter pylori* infection.

Environmental Factors

Although dietary habits may influence the development of gastric cancer, population studies and case-control studies are far from perfect scientific tools and isolating specific dietary elements remains elusive. Nonetheless, a few dietary themes have emerged. Food substances rich in nitrates, nitrites, and secondary amines have been shown to be gastric carcinogens. Before the era of refrigeration, nitrates and nitrites were used in food preservation. Consumption of preserved meats and vegetables has been linked consistently to increased risk for the development of gastric cancer. In developed countries, where home refrigeration is widely available, consumption of preserved meats and vegetables has markedly declined. This has been postulated as a critical factor in the decreased incidence of gastric cancer in North America and Europe. High intake of carbohydrates and salt has also been suggested to increase the risk of gastric cancer. In experimental animals, a high salt diet has been associated with atrophic gastritis, a preneoplastic condition.

The risk of gastric cancer has been shown in case-control studies to be lower in persons who consume a diet high in fresh fruits and vegetables. Whether this is due to a protective effect of certain vitamins in fresh fruit and vegetables or whether these vitamins act through various mechanisms, such as antioxidant effects or the inhibition of nitrosamine conversion, has not been determined.

Genetic Factors

Considerable evidence supports the role of various genetic factors in gastric carcinogenesis. Families with clusters of members with gastric carcinoma have been described, and gastric neoplasms are a relatively frequent component of the cancer family syndrome (Lynch syndrome II). First-degree relatives of patients with gastric cancer have a twofold to threefold greater incidence of this malignancy. Case-control studies have shown that the familial clustering of gastric cancer potentially could be explained by common environmental or dietary exposures rather than a strictly genetic predisposition.

Microsatellite instability, a form of genomic instability, is present in up to nearly one-half of gastric cancers. Gastric cancers with microsatellite instability phenotypes tend to have certain clinicopathologic characteristics, such as location in the antrum, and generally are associated with a better prognosis. A single gene defect or a dominating genetic pattern formation has not been identified, and multiple genetic abnormalities may be required for its development.

Infection with *Helicobacter pylori*

H. pylori is an organism found in the mucus layer of the human stomach, and not only is the association well established between this organism and gastric and duodenal ulcerations but also with gastric cancer. Chronic inflammation and gastric atrophy appear to be precursors of some gastric cancers. Infection with *H. pylori* is the most common known cause of chronic gastritis, and in 1994, the World Health Organization and International Agency for Research on Cancer consensus group stated that the epidemiologic and histologic evidence was sufficient to classify *H. pylori* as a group I carcinogen. The data pooled from case-control studies have suggested that the combined odds ratio for gastric cancer in *H. pylori*–infected subjects (compared with those not infected) is 1.92 (95% CI, 1.32-2.78). The association of *H. pylori* with gastric cancer is particularly strong in young infected persons. The odds ratio increased from 1.05 at age 70 to 9.29 at age 29 or younger.

Although the exact relation between the acquisition of *H. pylori* and the development of gastric cancer has not been determined, it is well established that *H. pylori* infection leads to chronic gastritis. This typically appears first in the antral mucosa and, with time and increasing age, can extend to involve most of the body of the stomach. The damage can be exacerbated by the host immune response to the infection. Chronic inflammation reduces the mucus layer overlying mucosal cells, thus exposing these cells to a greater degree to various substances such as nitrites and free radicals generated by inflammatory cells. Chronic infection with *H. pylori* can result eventually in the destruction of the gastric mucosa, which leads to atrophic gastritis, a premalignant condition. *H. pylori*–related carcinogenesis has been associated most strongly with cancers in the distal portion of the stomach and is not associated with cancers involving the gastroesophageal junction and cardia.

Many questions persist about the potential causal relation between *H. pylori* infection and gastric cancer. The fact that so many people globally, especially in underdeveloped countries, are infected with *H. pylori* and yet a relatively small percentage develop gastric cancer suggests that various cofactors in combination with *H. pylori* are required to promote carcinogenesis. First-degree relatives of patients with noncardia gastric cancers should be tested for *H. pylori* infection and, although data are not available to support this recommendation, should be treated if infected with *H. pylori*.

Pernicious Anemia

Pernicious anemia is an autoimmune-type atrophic gastritis, often limited to the body of the stomach. Patients with this condition appear to be at increased risk for the development of gastric cancer, perhaps a twofold to threefold excess risk. An excess risk of carcinoid tumors has also been reported in these patients. The carcinoid tumors that develop may be the result of prolonged acid suppression, with subsequent hypergastrinemia and neuroendocrine hyperplasia.

Partial Gastrectomy for Benign Disease

Whether patients who have had partial gastrectomy for peptic ulcer disease have an increased incidence of gastric carcinoma has been debated for decades, but a review of 58 studies concluded that the risk was increased only slightly. In this setting, the risk of gastric cancer developing remains low for 15 to 20 years after a distal stomach resection and appears to increase thereafter. However, reports do not suggest that persons who have had a partial gastric resection warrant frequent endoscopic surveillance.

Gastric Polyps

Gastric polyps are uncommon, almost always asymptomatic, and usually discovered incidentally during an endoscopic or radiologic examination. Most gastric polyps are benign and without malignant potential. The most frequent among these are hyperplastic polyps, which account for up to 80% of all gastric polyps.

When multiple gastric polyps are encountered in the fundus of the stomach, they usually are dilated fundic glands, which appear as small polypoid nodules. They do not cause any specific symptoms. Diffuse fundic gland polyposis may occur in adenomatous polyposis coli. These fundic gland polyps are not associated with gastrointestinal polyposis syndrome. These polyps are usually small, occur in large numbers, and do not cause specific symptoms.

Adenomatous polyps are less common but pathologically more important because they may give rise to and coexist with gastric adenocarcinoma. Adenomatous polyps usually occur in areas of chronic atrophic gastritis. They tend to grow larger and to exhibit progressively more advanced pathologic features. Because they have malignant potential, they should be removed under most circumstances. This usually can be accomplished endoscopically, but with larger (e.g., >2.0 cm) sessile lesions, surgical resection sometimes is required.

Hypertrophic Gastropathy (Ménétrier's Disease)

Ménétrier's disease is a rare, idiopathic condition characterized by rugal fold hypertrophy, hypochlorhydria, and protein-losing enteropathy. Gastric cancer reportedly occurs in up to 10% of patients with this disease, suggesting that it may be a premalignant condition.

Pathologic Features

Approximately 95% of all gastric cancers are adenocarcinomas, and the rest are lymphomas, carcinoids, and sarcomas. Distinguishing between adenocarcinoma and lymphoma is critical because the prognosis and treatment of these two malignancies differ considerably. Grossly, gastric adenocarcinoma can take many forms and may appear as an exophytic, polypoid mass or as an irregular, infiltrating lesion with surface nodularity or ulceration.

Gastric cancer localization has etiologic importance. Distal cancers (gastric body and antrum) are more common in areas with a high incidence of gastric cancer, whereas cardia cancers are more prevalent in whites from populations with a low background incidence of gastric cancer. Distal cancers may be related closely to chronic *H. pylori* infection, whereas cardia and gastroesophageal junction cancers may arise as a consequence of chronic gastroesophageal reflux disease and Barrett's esophagus. As mentioned above, the decrease in incidence of gastric cancer is a result of the marked decline in the incidence of distal gastric cancers. In contrast, the incidence of gastroesophageal carcinomas is increasing in the United States and many other developed countries.

The linitis plastica lesion occurs in up to 10% of adenocarcinomas. This is typically an infiltrating tumor, consisting of highly anaplastic cells, that evokes a strong desmoplastic response. The tumor tends to spread diffusely throughout the stomach, resulting in a nondistensible stomach that can be appreciated both radiographically and endoscopically. This pattern of growth is poorly contained, and metastatic disease invariably is present at the time of diagnosis.

Microscopically, several histologic classifications of gastric adenocarcinoma have evolved. The most widely used and accepted classification was proposed by Lauren (see Recommended Reading). This classification divides gastric adenocarcinomas into intestinal and diffuse types. The intestinal type of carcinoma is characterized by epithelial cells that form discrete glands, microscopically resembling colonic adenocarcinoma. Typically, the intestinal type is better circumscribed than the diffuse type, and it may be polypoid, or ulcerated, or both (Fig. 1). The intestinal type is the more frequent variety in countries with a high incidence of stomach cancer. It often arises within an area of intestinal metaplasia.

The diffuse type of carcinoma is characterized by sheets of epithelial cells. Glandular structure is rarely present. The diffuse type extends widely, with no distinct margins. Mucus-producing signet ring cells often are present. The diffuse type occurs more commonly in younger persons, is less likely to be seen in a setting of intestinal metaplasia, and tends to be infiltrating and poorly differentiated. The diffuse type is generally associated with a poor prognosis, whereas the intestinal type has a somewhat better prognosis.

Extensive observational studies have strongly suggested that gastric cancer is usually a multistep progression, beginning with chronic gastritis, followed by atrophic gastritis, then

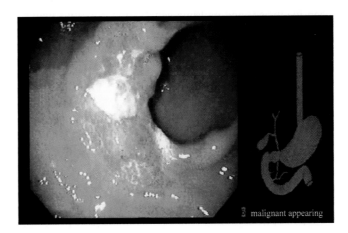

Fig. 1. Well-circumscribed, ulcerated adenocarcinoma arising in the distal stomach.

intestinal metaplasia, and ultimately dysplasia and cancer (Fig. 2). *H. pylori* infection may be the initial event in the development of many, if not most, gastric cancers.

Clinical Features

The clinical features of gastric cancer are typically vague and nonspecific and thus rarely lead to an early diagnosis. Patients may complain of epigastric pain, early satiety, abdominal bloating, or meal-induced dyspepsia. Weight loss, nausea, and anorexia are common with advanced lesions. In patients with cancer involving the distal antrum or pylorus, vomiting may be due to gastric outlet obstruction. Occult bleeding may be present, resulting in microcytic anemia. With advanced, ulcerated lesions, overt bleeding in the form of hematemesis may occur. Dysphagia may be the main symptom associated with lesions involving the gastric cardia. No physical findings are associated with early gastric cancer, and the presence of a palpable abdominal mass generally indicates an advanced tumor mass and often regional extension.

Gastric carcinoma spreads by direct extension through the stomach wall to perigastric tissue, and it can invade adjacent structures such as the pancreas, colon, spleen, kidney, or liver. Lymphatic metastases occur early, and local and regional nodes are the first to be involved. Via lymphatic vessels, the disease spreads to more distant intra-abdominal lymph nodes as well as to supraclavicular (Virchow's node) and periumbilical nodes, or it may result in peritoneal carcinomatosis with malignant ascites. The liver is the most common site of hematogenous spread, followed by the lung, bones, and brain.

Patients with gastric cancer occasionally present with a paraneoplastic syndrome such as acanthosis nigricans or venous thrombi (Trousseau's syndrome). Laboratory tests are nonspecific and may demonstrate anemia, hypoproteinemia, or abnormal liver function tests if metastatic disease is present.

Diagnostic Studies

Contrast radiography of the upper gastrointestinal tract may be the first diagnostic test performed to evaluate symptoms related to the upper gastrointestinal tract. Obviously, the detection of a large luminal mass is suggestive of malignancy, whereas a more subtle finding, such as decreased distensibility of the stomach, may be the only indication of a diffuse, infiltrative carcinoma. Small or relatively flat lesions can be missed on a contrast study; it also can be difficult to differentiate the underlying cause of a gastric ulcer radiographically, that is, whether it is associated with a benign or a malignant process. Endoscopy with biopsy should always be performed if a contrast study suggests that a gastric malignancy may be present.

Fiberoptic endoscopy with biopsy of a suspicious mass or lesion is the diagnostic gold standard, and the accuracy increases with the number of biopsy specimens obtained. Endoscopically,

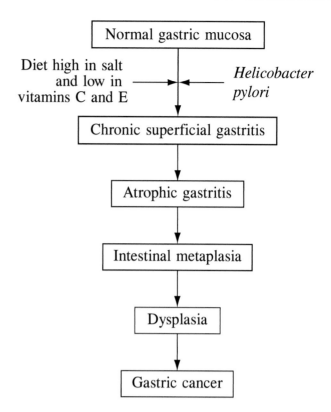

Fig. 2. Probable sequence of gastric carcinogenesis.

an advanced adenocarcinoma generally presents as a large (>2 cm), exophytic, ulcerated mass with an irregular margin. Diffusely infiltrative carcinomas can produce large, thickened folds or a nondistensible stomach (or both). Classically, a malignant ulcer is raised above the mucosal level, the margins are firm and friable, and the surrounding tissue may be thickened or nodular. Because endoscopic biopsy specimens may demonstrate only inflammation or necrotic tissue, multiple specimens (at least eight) should be obtained from both the base and the rim of a malignant-appearing ulcer. With the submucosal location of lymphoid neoplasms, deep or larger snare biopsy specimens may be needed to detect gastric lymphoma and to differentiate lymphoma from carcinoma.

Computed tomography (CT) of the abdomen can be used to diagnose the primary tumor and to determine the extent of spread and the presence of nodal metastases. Because CT is not able to distinguish between layers of the gastric wall, it is unable to determine the depth of tumor invasion. Its sensitivity for detecting extragastric invasion is relatively low (50%-75%). CT is used primarily to determine if distant lymph node or liver metastases are present. Generally, CT tends to understage gastric cancer, but it is useful for identifying advanced-stage disease that may not be suitable for curative surgical resection.

Endoscopic ultrasonography (EUS) can delineate clearly all five layers of the gastric wall and accurately determine the T stage of gastric malignancy. EUS generally is more accurate than CT in determining the nature of regional lymph nodes, although it is not suitable for assessing distant metastases because of its limited penetration. Even though EUS is highly operator dependent, it has become the most accurate tool for determining tumor and nodal status (T and N stage, respectively) of gastric malignancies. Where high-quality EUS examinations are available, CT is reserved for determining if distant or liver metastases (or both) are present.

Staging and Prognosis

The clinical and pathologic stage of gastric cancer at the time of diagnosis is critical for making decisions about patient management. The TNM staging classification (T = tumor invasion, N = lymph node involvement, M = metastasis to other organs) is widely used in the evaluation of gastric cancer. The extent of disease at the time of diagnosis is the most important factor for determining whether potential curative excision of the tumor is possible. Early gastric cancer, stages 0 and IA, has a favorable prognosis, with a 5-year survival rate of 90% and 80%, respectively. The prognosis for stage IB disease (T1 N1 M0 or T2 N0 M0) is less favorable, with about 80% survival at 5 years. However, most patients do not present with early-stage disease, but rather with stage III (a T4 tumor or T2/T3 tumor with regional lymph node metastases) or stage IV (extensive regional or distant metastases) disease. The 5-year survival rate is 13% to 20% for stage III disease and only 3% to 5% for stage IV disease. The current overall 5-year and 10-year survival rates in the United States for patients with gastric cancer are about 28% and 20%, respectively, reflecting the substantial proportion of tumors that are diagnosed at an advanced stage.

Treatment

Surgery is the mainstay of treatment for gastric cancer. Complete surgical removal of a gastric tumor, with resection of adjacent lymph nodes, is the only chance for cure. However, two-thirds of patients present with advanced disease that is incurable by surgical excision alone. Controversy persists about what is considered an optimal surgical resection; opinion differs regarding the extent of resection necessary for cancers found in different parts of the stomach and the extent of lymph node dissection required in addition to resection of the tumor. Discussion of these issues is beyond the scope of this review. In practice, the extent of dissection is determined primarily by tumor location, preoperative staging, and the condition of the patient. Generally, proximal gastric tumors require more extensive resection than distal gastric tumors. Palliative rather than curative surgery may still be considered in certain circumstances, for example, when there is tumor obstruction, perforation, or bleeding.

Gastric carcinoma is relatively resistant to radiotherapy, which usually is administered only to palliate symptoms and not to improve survival. Chemotherapeutic regimens have shown only modest results, with a decrease in measurable tumor mass in about 15% of patients and only a minimal effect on prolonging survival.

OTHER GASTRIC TUMORS

Gastric Lymphoma

Primary gastric lymphoma is a rare malignant disease that accounts for less than 5% of all gastric malignancies, although after adenocarcinoma, lymphomas are the most common gastric malignancy. Of note, the incidence of primary gastric lymphoma appears to be increasing, especially among the elderly. The stomach is the most common extranodal site for the occurrence of lymphoma, and of the primary gastrointestinal lymphomas, nearly one-half originate in the stomach, occurring less frequently in the small intestine and colon.

Like adenocarcinoma, the clinical features of gastric lymphoma are nonspecific and include abdominal discomfort, dyspepsia, gastric outlet complaints due to obstruction or impairment of gastric motility, anorexia, weight loss, and anemia due to blood loss from ulceration; bleeding occurs in about 20% of patients.

Endoscopically, gastric lymphoma may be difficult to differentiate from adenocarcinoma. Lymphomatous involvement of the stomach may have various presentations, including large, firm rugal folds, eroded nodules, or exophytic ulcerated masses. The enlarged folds reflect the subepithelial infiltrative growth pattern seen with lymphomas, particularly MALTomas (see below), especially in early stages.

When the disease is suspected, conventional endoscopic biopsy specimens may not be revealing, especially with submucosal involvement only. Deeper biopsy or snare biopsy specimens from a polypoid mass or large rugal fold may be needed to make the diagnosis. If lymphoma is suspected, extra biopsy specimens should be obtained for immunoperoxidase staining or lymphoid markers, which increase diagnostic accuracy.

CT of the abdomen and chest is useful for determining if there is nodal involvement above or below the diaphragm (or both). EUS is highly accurate in determining the extent of gastric wall infiltration, thus providing additional information for treatment planning.

Most gastric lymphomas are B cell in origin. Non-Hodgkin's lymphoma, especially the diffuse histiocytic type, is the most common form of gastric lymphoma, whereas Hodgkin's disease of the stomach is uncommon. Stage I disease is limited to the stomach, and stage II disease implies localized involvement of abdominal lymph nodes. In stage III disease, both sides of the diaphragm are involved. Stage IV disease represents diffuse or disseminated involvement. The 5-year survival rate for all patients with gastric lymphoma is about 50%. However, patients with stage I or II tumors smaller than 5 cm in diameter have a 10-year survival rate greater than 80%.

Therapy for non-Hodgkin's gastric lymphomas depends primarily on tumor stage. Exploratory laparotomy and partial gastrectomy are indicated when stage I disease is suspected. For stage II, III, or IV disease, chemotherapy is the primary therapeutic modality. Radiotherapy is usually reserved for debulking large lesions or controlling localized disease.

MALTomas

An important gastric lymphoma subtype is MALToma. It is a low-grade B-cell lymphoma and is associated with chronic *H. pylori* infection in more than 90% of cases. It has been postulated that infection caused by *H. pylori* induces an increased number of plasma cells and lymphocytes, which may organize into lymphoid follicles. As these follicles become prominent, they develop B-cell monoclonal populations that appear to be induced and sustained by stimuli that come from *H. pylori*–sensitized T cells. As the B-cell monoclonal populations proliferate, they begin to spill into the gastric epithelium. These monoclonal B cells are part of the mucosal inflammatory reaction. In some instances, however, they gradually evolve into malignant lymphoma cells with autonomous and uncontrolled growth.

Even for an experienced endoscopist, the diagnosis of MALToma can be difficult because the mucosal surface may appear normal or there may be erosions, subtle nodularity, ulcerations, or a protruding mass lesion. Diagnosis depends on examination of gastric biopsy specimens (Fig. 3). Immunostaining of paraffin-embedded specimens for several B-cell surface receptors characteristically expressed in MALTomas is extremely useful in making the diagnosis. Examination of the involved portions of the gastric wall with EUS is the most reliable method for determining the infiltration depth of the MALToma and hence its tumor stage. Infiltration depth serves as a predictor of the response to therapy. Superficial MALTomas are more likely to have a favorable response to therapy than deeper or transmural tumors.

If *H. pylori* is eradicated, the lymphoma can regress. Several clinical studies have documented that complete remission occurs in approximately 50% to 90% of patients with low-grade MALToma detected at an early clinical stage and treated for *H. pylori* infection. If untreated, the T-cell dependence ultimately appears to fade and the lymphoid proliferation acquires the independent neoplastic nature that characterizes malignant lymphomas. This may explain why some low-grade MALTomas do not regress after *H. pylori* eradication. Most lymphomas of this type remain slow growing and well-differentiated. Rarely, some MALTomas differentiate and form large-cell, highly malignant neoplasms, which tend to follow a more aggressive natural history, spreading to local and distant lymph nodes and other organs.

The treatment of low-grade MALToma is eradication of *H. pylori* infection. As suggested above, patients with early-stage disease are more likely to have complete regression of MALToma after anti–*H. pylori* therapy, and antibiotic treatment should be considered first-line therapy for these patients. Frequent endoscopic follow-up is required after the initial therapy to verify treatment response. If no regression is seen, referral to an oncologist is recommended for consideration of other treatment modalities, including surgery, chemotherapy, and radiotherapy.

Gastric Carcinoid Tumors

Gastric carcinoid tumors tend to occur in the body of the stomach. They may be single or multiple (in approximately 14% of cases), and to the endoscopist, they may look like an ordinary ulcer, polyp, or tumor mass. They frequently are round and yellowish. Approximately 2% to 3% of all carcinoids are located in the stomach, but gastric carcinoids represent only 0.3% of all gastric tumors.

Gastric carcinoid tumors can produce an array of active substances, including 5-hydroxytryptamine, and thus are capable of producing the classic flushing symptoms associated with carcinoid syndrome. However, most of these tumors do not produce symptoms related to vasoactive peptides and usually are discovered incidentally, although they can cause epigastric pain and can present with bleeding.

Gastric carcinoid tumors occur more frequently in patients with pernicious anemia and atrophic gastritis, with resulting achlorhydria. They also appear to be more common in patients with Zollinger-Ellison syndrome. The link between these clinical situations appears to be hypergastrinemia; thus, any condition in which serum levels of gastrin are increased for a long period should heighten the clinician's awareness that gastric carcinoid tumors could develop.

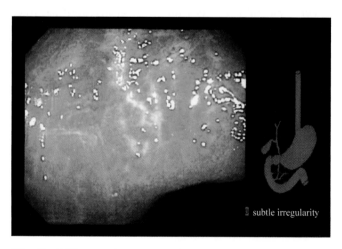

subtle irregularity

Fig. 3. Diffuse erythema and surface irregularity of the body of the stomach. Biopsy specimens revealed MALToma.

Because most gastric carcinoid tumors are slow growing and have low invasive or metastatic potential, the best treatment for all gastric carcinoids is controversial. If the tumor is large or responsible for symptoms, excision is usually recommended. Lesions smaller than 1 cm generally can be removed endoscopically. If the lesion is large, if more than five lesions occur in an area such as the antrum, if malignant cells are present, or if the lesion has recurred after being removed, then surgical resection, typically involving antrectomy, is indicated.

Gastrointestinal Stromal Tumors

Gastrointestinal stromal tumors (GISTs) are rare. They can arise throughout the gastrointestinal tract, although the most common site for malignant tumors is the stomach. Most, but not all, GISTs are thought to be of smooth muscle differentiation and include leiomyomas and leiomyosarcomas. They typically are asymptomatic and are found incidentally at endoscopy or surgery. Large GISTs (average size at the time of presentation, 4.5 cm) may present with gastrointestinal tract bleeding or abdominal pain. If the tumor is submucosal, routine endoscopic biopsy specimens usually are not diagnostic.

Leiomyosarcomas account for approximately 1% of malignant gastric tumors. They tend to be larger than leiomyomas at the time of discovery (average, 7.5 cm), although there is much overlap in size. Recently, the use of EUS has been helpful for determining 1) the submucosal nature of the tumor and 2) whether invasion through the gastric walls or extragastric extension is present (more suggestive of leiomyosarcoma). EUS-directed fine-needle aspiration biopsy can help to distinguish between a benign and a malignant smooth muscle tumor. Surgical resection of the tumor is the only treatment option, and curative resection generally can be attempted in one-third to one-half of patients.

Metastatic Tumors of the Stomach

When a patient presents with upper gastrointestinal tract symptoms and a history of a primary extragastric neoplasm, metastatic involvement of the stomach should be considered a possible explanation of the symptoms.

Malignant melanoma is one of the more frequently encountered metastatic lesions. At endoscopy, it usually presents as a slightly elevated black nodule. Cancer of the breast, lung, ovary, testis, liver, colon, or parotid gland has been shown to metastasize to the stomach. Kaposi's sarcoma can also involve the stomach, especially in patients with acquired immunodeficiency syndrome.

RECOMMENDED READING

Anonymous. Infection with *Helicobacter pylori*. IARC Monogr Eval Carcinog Risks Hum. 1994;61:177-240.

Blot WJ, Devesa SS, Kneller RW, Fraumeni JF Jr. Rising incidence of adenocarcinoma of esophagus and gastric cardia. JAMA. 1991;265:1287-9.

Botterweck AA, Schouten LJ, Volovics A, Dorant E, van Den Brandt PA. Trends in incidence of adenocarcinoma of the oesophagus and gastric cardia in ten European countries. Int J Epidemiol. 2000;29:645-54.

Correa P. Chronic gastritis: a clinico-pathological classification. Am J Gastroenterol. 1988;83:504-9.

Correa P. A human model of gastric carcinogenesis. Cancer Res. 1988;48:3554-60.

Fuchs CS, Mayer RJ. Gastric carcinoma. N Engl J Med. 1995;333:32-41.

Huang JQ, Sridhar S, Chen Y, Hunt RH. Meta-analysis of the relationship between *Helicobacter pylori* seropositivity and gastric cancer. Gastroenterology. 1998;114:1169-79.

Keller G, Rotter M, Vogelsang H, Bischoff P, Becker KF, Mueller J, et al. Microsatellite instability in adenocarcinomas of the upper gastrointestinal tract: relation to clinicopathological data and family history. Am J Pathol. 1995;147:593-600.

Laurén P. The two histological main types of gastric carcinoma: diffuse and so-called intestinal-type carcinoma: an attempt at a histo-clinical classification. Acta Pathol Microbiol Scand. 1965;64:31-49.

Morgner A, Bayerdorffer E, Neubauer A, Stolte M. Malignant tumors of the stomach: gastric mucosa-associated lymphoid tissue lymphoma and *Helicobacter pylori*. Gastroenterol Clin North Am. 2000;29:593-607.

Sipponen P, Marshall BJ: Gastritis and gastric cancer: Western countries. Gastroenterol Clin North Am. 2000;29:579-92.

Stalnikowicz R, Benbassat J. Risk of gastric cancer after gastric surgery for benign disorders. Arch Intern Med. 1990;150:2022-6.

Uemura N, Okamoto S, Yamamoto S, Matsumura N, Yamaguchi S, Yamakido M, et al. *Helicobacter pylori* infection and the development of gastric cancer. N Engl J Med. 2001;345:784-9.

CHAPTER 9

Gastrointestinal Motility Disorders

Michael Camilleri, M.D.

INTRODUCTION

Motility disorders result from impaired control of the neuromuscular apparatus of the gut. Associated symptoms include recurrent or chronic nausea, vomiting, bloating, and abdominal discomfort, constipation, or diarrhea, which occur in the absence of intestinal obstruction. Occasionally, gastroparesis and intestinal pseudo-obstruction are associated with generalized disease processes that affect other regions of the gastrointestinal tract and extraintestinal organs, including the urinary bladder. Other motility disorders affecting the stomach and small intestine are characterized by signs and symptoms of accelerated transit.

CONTROL OF GASTROINTESTINAL MOTOR FUNCTION

Motor function of the gastrointestinal tract depends on the contraction of smooth muscle cells and their integration and modulation by enteric and extrinsic nerves. Derangement of the mechanisms that regulate gastrointestinal motor function may lead to altered gut motility. Neurogenic modulators of gastrointestinal motility include the central nervous system (CNS), the autonomic nerves, and the enteric nervous system (ENS). Extrinsic neural control of gastrointestinal motor function consists of the cranial and sacral parasympathetic outflow (excitatory to nonsphincteric muscle) and the thoracolumbar sympathetic supply (excitatory to sphincters, inhibitory to nonsphincteric muscle). The cranial outflow is predominantly through the vagus nerve, which innervates the gastrointestinal tract from the stomach to the right colon and consists of preganglionic cholinergic fibers that synapse with the ENS. The supply of sympathetic fibers to the stomach and small bowel arises from levels

T5 to T10 of the intermediolateral column of the spinal cord. The prevertebral ganglia have an important role in the integration of afferent impulses between the gut and the CNS and reflex control of abdominal viscera.

The ENS is an independent nervous system consisting of approximately 100 million neurons organized into ganglionated plexuses. The larger myenteric (or Auerbach) plexus is situated between the longitudinal and circular muscle layers of the muscularis externa and contains neurons responsible for gastrointestinal motility. The submucosal (or Meissner) plexus controls absorption, secretion, and mucosal blood flow. The ENS also is important in visceral afferent function.

The ENS develops in utero by migration of neural crest cells to the developing alimentary canal. This migration and the sequence of innervation of different levels of the gut are regulated by specific signaling molecules, which include transcription factors (e.g., Mash1), neurotrophic factors (e.g., glial-derived neurotrophic factor), and the neuregulin signaling system. These facilitate the growth, differentiation, and persistence of the migrating nerve cells after they arrive in the gut. The receptors for neuregulin proteins are tyrosine kinases, which are important in cell signaling.

Myogenic factors regulate the electrical activity generated by gastrointestinal smooth muscle cells. The interstitial cells of Cajal, located at the interface of the circular and longitudinal muscle layers of the small intestine, form a non-neural pacemaker system and function as intermediaries between the neurogenic (ENS) and myogenic control systems. The interstitial cells of Cajal are in proximity to the gastrointestinal smooth muscle cells. Electrical control activity spreads through the contiguous segments of the gut through neurochemical activation by excitatory (e.g., acetylcholine, substance P) and inhibitory (e.g., nitric oxide, somatostatin, vasoactive intestinal peptide) transmitters.

GASTRIC AND SMALL-BOWEL MOTILITY

The motor functions of the stomach and small intestine are characterized by distinct manometric patterns of activity in the fasting and postprandial periods (Fig. 1). The fasting (or interdigestive) period is characterized by a cyclic motor phenomenon called the "interdigestive migrating motor complex." In healthy persons, one cycle of the interdigestive migrating motor complex is completed every 60 to 90 minutes. The interdigestive migrating motor complex has three phases: a period of quiescence (phase I), a period of intermittent pressure activity (phase II), and an activity front (phase III) during which the stomach and small intestine contract at highest frequency (3 per minute in the stomach and 12 per minute in the upper small intestine). Phase III migrates for a variable distance through the small intestine; there is a gradient in the frequency of contractions from ~12 per minute in the duodenum to ~8 per minute in the ileum. Another characteristic interdigestive motor pattern in the distal small intestine is the "giant migrating complex," or power contraction; it serves to empty residue from the ileum into the colon in bolus transfers.

In the postprandial period, the interdigestive migrating motor complex is replaced by an irregular pressure response pattern of variable amplitude and frequency, which enables mixing and absorption. This pattern is observed in the regions in contact with food. The maximal frequency of contractions is lower than that noted during phase III of the interdigestive migrating motor complex. The duration of the postprandial motor activity is proportional to the number of calories consumed during the meal: ~1 hour for every 200 kcal ingested. Segments of the small intestine that are not in contact with food continue to display interdigestive motor patterns.

The proximal stomach accommodates food through a decrease in its tone, facilitating the ingestion of food without an increase in pressure. This reflex is mediated by the vagus nerve and involves an intrinsic nitrergic neuron.

Liquids empty from the stomach in an exponential manner (Fig. 2). The half-emptying time for nonnutrient liquids in healthy persons is usually less than 20 minutes. Solids are selectively retained in the stomach until particles have been triturated to less than 2 mm in diameter. Therefore, gastric emptying of solids is characterized by an initial lag period followed by a linear post-lag emptying phase. The small intestine transports solids and liquids at approximately the same rate. Because of the lag phase for the transport of solids from the stomach, liquids typically arrive in the colon before solids. Chyme moves from the ileum to the colon intermittently in boluses (Fig. 2).

PATHOGENESIS OF MOTILITY DISORDERS

Gastrointestinal motility disturbances result from disorders of the extrinsic nervous system, interstitial cells of Cajal (or intestinal pacemakers), or smooth muscle (Table 1). Combined

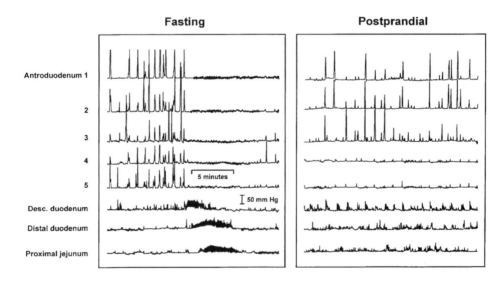

Fig. 1. Fasting and postprandial gastroduodenal manometric recordings in a healthy volunteer. A 535-kcal meal was ingested during the study. Note the cyclic interdigestive migrating motor complex (*left*) and the sustained, high-amplitude but irregular pressure activity after the meal (*right*). Desc., descending. (From Coulie B, Camilleri M. Intestinal pseudo-obstruction. Annu Rev Med. 1999;50:37-55. Used with permission.)

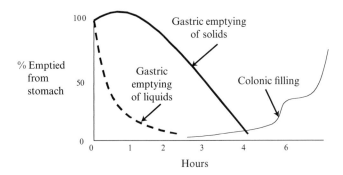

Fig. 2. Schematic representation of typical gastric emptying and colonic filling curves. Note the exponential emptying of liquids, in contrast to the initial retention of solids (lag phase), which is followed by a generally linear post-lag emptying rate. The colonic filling curve is characterized by intermittent bolus transfers.

disorders occur in systemic sclerosis, amyloidosis, and mitochondrial cytopathy and can present initially with neuropathic patterns; later, with disease progression, they can display myopathic characteristics. Motility disorders can be congenital (affecting the development of the motility apparatus) or acquired.

Embryologic Processes: Ontogeny of the Gut Neuromuscular Apparatus

Genetic defects in migration, differentiation, and survival of enteric neurons have been identified in several causes of gut dysmotility, including abnormalities of *cRET* (the gene that encodes for the tyrosine kinase receptor), the endothelin B system (which tends to retard development of neural elements, thereby facilitating colonization of the entire gut from the neural crest), Sox10 (a transcription factor that enhances maturation of neural precursors), and c-kit (a marker for the interstitial cells of Cajal). Disturbances in these mechanisms result in syndromic dysmotilities such as Hirschsprung's disease, Waardenburg-Shah syndrome (pigmentary defects, piebaldism, neural deafness, megacolon), and idiopathic hypertrophic pyloric stenosis.

Extrinsic Neuropathic Disorders

Extrinsic neuropathic processes include vagotomy, diabetes mellitus, trauma, Parkinson's disease, amyloidosis, and a paraneoplastic syndrome usually associated with small cell carcinoma of the lung. Another common "neuropathic" problem met in clinical practice results from the effect of medications such as α_2-adrenergic agonists and anticholinergic agents on neural control.

Damage to the autonomic nerves by trauma, infection, neuropathy, or neurodegeneration may lead to motor, secretory,

Table 1. Classification of Gastroparesis and Pseudo-obstruction

Type	Neuropathic	Myopathic
Infiltrative	Progressive systemic sclerosis	Progressive systemic sclerosis
	Amyloidosis	Amyloidosis
		Systemic lupus erythematosus
		Ehlers-Danlos syndrome
		Dermatomyositis
Familial	Familial visceral neuropathies	Familial visceral myopathies
		Metabolic myopathies
Idiopathic	Sporadic hollow visceral myopathy	Idiopathic intestinal pseudo-obstruction
Neurologic	Porphyria	Myotonia
	Heavy-metal poisoning	Other dystrophies
	Brainstem tumor	
	Parkinson's disease	
	Multiple sclerosis	
	Spinal cord transection	
Infectious	Chagas' disease	
	Cytomegalovirus	
	Norwalk virus	
	Epstein-Barr virus	
Drug-induced	Tricyclic antidepressants	
	Narcotic agents	
	Anticholinergic agents	
	Antihypertensives	
	Dopaminergic agents	
	Vincristine	
	Laxatives	
Paraneoplastic	Small cell lung cancer	
	Carcinoid syndrome	
Postoperative	Postvagotomy with or without pyloroplasty/ gastric resection	
Endocrine	Diabetes mellitus	
	Hypothyroidism/ hyperthyroidism	
	Hypoparathyroidism	

and sensory disturbances, most frequently resulting in constipation rather than upper gastrointestinal tract motility disorders. However, the latter may occur in patients with a high spinal cord injury or occur secondarily to constipation and fecal impaction. Parkinson's disease and multiple sclerosis are two neurologic diseases involving the extrinsic nervous system that are associated frequently with constipation. In Parkinson's disease, a decrease in the number of dopamine-containing neurons and the presence of Lewy bodies in myenteric plexus neurons have been described. Also, failure of the striated muscles of the pelvic floor to relax may be an extrapyramidal manifestation of Parkinson's disease. Multiple sclerosis is associated with slow colonic transit and absence of the postprandial motor contractile response in the colon. Gastroparesis and pseudo-obstruction are less frequent than constipation in these two diseases.

A broad spectrum of gastrointestinal motility disorders may be related to diabetes mellitus: gastroparesis, pylorospasm, intestinal pseudo-obstruction, diarrhea, constipation, and incontinence. All these manifestations may be caused by autonomic dysfunction (Table 2), although recent evidence points to the importance of acute changes in glycemia and, more importantly, to changes in the structure and function of the ENS. From a population perspective, constipation is the most important gastrointestinal symptom in patients with diabetes because it is the most prevalent symptom. Moreover, in a large group that had screening tests for autonomic neuropathy, the prevalence of constipation was 22% among the diabetic patients with neuropathy but only 9.2% among those without neuropathy, which was not significantly different from that of the healthy control group. In a questionnaire-based study of diabetic patients in the community, constipation was more prevalent in insulin-dependent diabetes mellitus than in noninsulin-dependent diabetes mellitus and was associated with symptoms of dysautonomia and use of constipating drugs, for example, calcium channel blockers. In hospital practice, gastroparesis is frequently encountered as a complication of diabetes. Apart from added attention needed for metabolic control, its management follows that of other causes of gastroparesis and pseudo-obstruction.

Enteric or Intrinsic Neuropathic Disorders

Disorders of the ENS are usually the result of a degenerative, immune, or inflammatory process. Only rarely can the cause be ascertained in these disturbances. Virally induced gastroparesis (e.g., rotavirus, Norwalk virus, cytomegalovirus, or Epstein-Barr virus) and pseudo-obstruction as well as degenerative disorders associated with infiltration of the myenteric plexus by inflammatory cells suggest that infection may be an important predisposing factor. In idiopathic chronic intestinal pseudo-obstruction, there is no disturbance of extrinsic neural control and no identified cause for ENS abnormality.

A full-thickness biopsy specimen from the intestine may be required to evaluate the myenteric plexus and interstitial cells of Cajal. The decision to perform a biopsy needs to be weighed against the risk of complications, including the subsequent formation of adhesions and, possibly, mechanical obstruction superimposed on episodes of pseudo-obstruction.

Smooth Muscle Disorders

Disturbances of smooth muscle may result in major disorders of gastric emptying and small-bowel and colonic transit. These disturbances include systemic sclerosis and amyloidosis. Dermatomyositis, dystrophia myotonica, and metabolic muscle disorders such as mitochondrial cytopathy are seen infrequently. In rare instances, there is a positive family history (e.g., hollow visceral myopathy may occur either sporadically or in families). Motility disturbances may be the result of metabolic disorders such as hypothyroidism or hyperparathyroidism, but these patients more commonly present with constipation.

Scleroderma may result in focal or general dilatation, diverticula (often wide-mouthed, especially in the colon), and delayed transit at the levels affected. The amplitude of contractions is

Table 2.   Gastrointestinal (GI) Manifestations of Diabetes Mellitus

GI manifestation of diabetes	Associated disease	Clinical presentation
↓ Gallbladder motility		Gallstones
Antral hypomotility pylorospasm	Exocrine pancreatic insufficiency	Gastric stasis Bezoars
↓ α_2-Adrenergic tone in enterocytes	Celiac sprue	Diarrhea, steatorrhea
SB dysmotility	SB bacterial overgrowth	Gastric or SB stasis or rapid SB transit
Colonic dysmotility	Bile acid malabsorption	Constipation or diarrhea
Anorectal dysfunction Sensory neuropathy IAS-sympathetic neuropathy EAS-pudendal neuropathy		Diarrhea or incontinence

EAS, external anal sphincter; IAS, internal anal sphincter; SB, small-bowel.
Modified from Camilleri M. Gastrointestinal problems in diabetes. Endocrinol Metab Clin N Am. 1996;25:361-78. Used with permission.

decreased (average < 30 mm Hg in the distal esophagus, < 40 mm Hg in the antrum, < 10 mm Hg in the small bowel) compared with that of controls. Bacterial overgrowth is common and may result in steatorrhea or pneumatosis intestinalis.

A mitochondrial disorder that affects the gut is called "mitochondrial neurogastrointestinal encephalomyopathy." It is referred to also as "oculogastrointestinal muscular dystrophy" or "familial visceral myopathy type II" and is an example of a spectrum of diseases that affect oxidative phosphorylation. It is an autosomal recessive condition with gastrointestinal and liver manifestations that may present at any age, typically with hepatomegaly or liver failure in the neonate, seizures or diarrhea in infancy, and liver failure or chronic intestinal pseudo-obstruction in children or adults.

Mitochondrial neurogastrointestinal encephalomyopathy is characterized also by external ophthalmoplegia, ptosis, periph-eral neuropathy, and leukoencephalopathy. The small intestine is dilated or has multiple diverticula, and the amplitude of contractions is low, typical of a myopathic disorder. Some patients have a combination of intestinal dysmotility or transfer dysphagia due to abnormal coordination and propagation of the swallow through the pharynx and the skeletal muscle portion of the esophagus. This becomes even more devastating when the smooth muscle portion of the esophagus is affected by the associated mitochondrial neurogastrointestinal encephalopathy.

MANAGEMENT OF GASTROPARESIS AND PSEUDO-OBSTRUCTION

Clinical Features

The clinical features of gastroparesis and chronic intestinal pseudo-obstruction are similar and include nausea, vomiting, early satiety, abdominal discomfort, distension, bloating, and anorexia. In patients in whom stasis and vomiting are important problems, there may be considerable weight loss and depletion of mineral and vitamin stores. The severity of the motility problem often manifests itself most clearly in the degree of nutritional and electrolyte depletion. Disturbances of bowel movements, such as diarrhea and constipation, indicate that the motility disorder is more extensive than gastroparesis. Severe vomiting may be complicated by aspiration pneumonia or Mallory-Weiss tears that may result in gastrointestinal tract hemorrhage. When patients have a more generalized motility disorder, they may also have symptoms referable to abnormal swallowing or delayed colonic transit.

A family history and medication history are essential for identifying underlying etiologic factors. A careful review of systems helps reveal an underlying collagen vascular disease (e.g., scleroderma) or disturbances of extrinsic neural control that also may be affecting the abdominal viscera. Such symptoms

include orthostatic dizziness, difficulties with erection or ejaculation, recurrent urinary tract infections, difficulty with visual accommodation in bright light, absence of sweating, and dry mouth, eyes, or vagina.

A succussion splash detected on physical examination is usually indicative of a region of stasis within the gastrointestinal tract, typically the stomach. The hands and mouth may show signs of Raynaud's phenomenon or scleroderma. Testing pupillary responses to light and accommodation, testing external ocular movement, and measuring blood pressure in the supine and standing positions and the general features of peripheral neuropathy can identify patients who have a neurologic disturbance or oculogastrointestinal dystrophy associated typically with mitochondrial cytopathy.

Conditions to be differentiated are mechanical obstruction (e.g., from peptic stricture or Crohn's disease in the small intestine), functional gastrointestinal disorders, and eating disorders such as anorexia nervosa and rumination syndrome. The degree of impairment of gastric emptying in eating disorders is relatively minor compared with that of diabetic or post-vagotomy gastric stasis.

A typical history of a person with rumination syndrome is early (0-30 minutes) postprandial, effortless regurgitation of undigested food that happens with virtually every meal. This condition occurs in mentally challenged children (e.g., Down's syndrome), but it increasingly is recognized among adolescents and adults of normal intelligence. It is treatable with behavioral modification.

Investigation

A motility disorder of the stomach or small bowel should be suspected whenever large volumes are aspirated from the stomach, particularly after an overnight fast or when undigested solid food or large volumes of liquids are observed during esophagogastroduodenoscopy. The following four questions should be considered in the management of each patient:

1. Are the symptoms acute or chronic?
2. Is the disease due to a neuropathy or myopathy?
3. What is the status of hydration and nutrition?
4. What regions of the digestive tract are affected?

The recommended sequence of investigations is as follows:

1. Suspect and exclude mechanical obstruction. In patients with pseudo-obstruction, plain radiographs of the abdomen taken at the time of symptoms typically show dilated loops of small bowel with associated air-fluid levels. Mechanical obstruction should be excluded by means of upper gastrointestinal endoscopy and barium studies, including a small-bowel follow-through series. Barium studies fortuitously may suggest the presence of a motor disorder, particularly if there is gross dilatation or dilution of barium or if solid food is retained within the stomach. However, these studies rarely identify the cause.

An exception is small-bowel systemic sclerosis, which is characterized by megaduodenum and packed valvulae conniventes in the small intestine.

2. Assess gastric and small-bowel motility. After mechanical obstruction and alternative diagnoses such as Crohn's disease have been excluded, a transit profile of the stomach or small bowel (or both) should be performed. Efficiency in the emptying of solids is the most sensitive measurement of upper gastrointestinal tract transit. Scans are typically performed at 0, 1, 2, 3, 4, and 6 hours after ingestion of a radiolabeled meal. If the cause of the motility disturbance is obvious, such as gastroparesis in a patient with long-standing diabetes mellitus, further diagnostic testing usually is not needed. If the cause is unclear, gastroduodenal manometry, using a multilumen tube with sensors in the distal stomach and proximal small intestine, can distinguish between neuropathic and myopathic processes (Fig. 3). Neuropathies are characterized by contractions of normal amplitude but abnormal patterns of contractility. In contrast, the predominant disturbance in myopathic disorders is the low amplitude of contractions in the segments affected (Fig. 3).

3. Identify the pathogenesis. Causes of gastroparesis and intestinal pseudo-obstruction are outlined in Table 1. In the absence of a cause for a neuropathic pattern of motor activity in the small intestine, it is necessary to pursue further investigations, including testing for autonomic dysfunction, type 1 antineuronal nuclear autoantibodies associated with paraneoplastic syndromes, and magnetic resonance imaging of the brain to exclude a brainstem lesion (Fig. 4). Autonomic testing includes evaluation for orthostatic hypotension, assessment of supine and standing serum norepinephrine levels, measurement of the heart rate interval change during deep breathing, and plasma pancreatic polypeptide response to modified sham feeding. This testing can identify sympathetic adrenergic or vagal neuropathy. Rarely, brain imaging is indicated for patients with vomiting. The identification of a myopathic disorder on initial testing should lead to a search for amyloidosis (immunoglobulin electrophoresis, fat aspirate, or rectal biopsy), systemic sclerosis (Scl-70, an autoantibody), and a family history of gastrointestinal motility disorders. Laboratory studies to consider include assessment of thyroid function and levels of antinuclear antibody, lactate, creatine phosphokinase, aldolase, and porphyrins and serologic study for Chagas' disease. In certain cases, a laparoscopically obtained full-thickness biopsy specimen from the small intestine may be required. Special staining techniques may be needed to identify metabolic muscle disorders, including mitochondrial myopathy. Genetic testing is available to assess for certain mitochondrial myopathies.

4. Identify complications of the motility disorder: bacterial overgrowth, dehydration, and malnutrition. In patients who present with diarrhea, it is important to assess nutritional status (essential element and vitamin levels) and to exclude bacterial

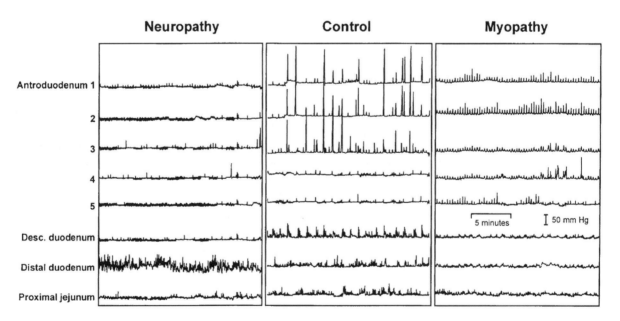

Fig. 3. Postprandial manometric profiles in small-bowel dysmotility due to neuropathy (diabetes mellitus, *left*) and myopathy (systemic sclerosis, *right*). Note the simultaneous, prolonged contractions of low amplitude during the fasting and postprandial periods in myopathy. Although the contraction amplitudes are normal in neuropathy, contractile activity is uncoordinated and contractile frequency is decreased. Desc., descending. (From Coulie B, Camilleri M. Intestinal pseudo-obstruction. Annu Rev Med. 1999;50:37-55. Used with permission.)

Abnormal Gastric or Small-Bowel Transit

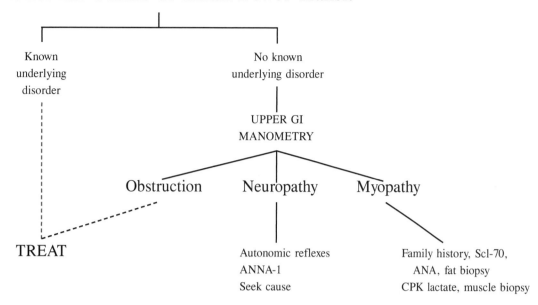

Fig. 4. Flow diagram outlining steps involved in diagnosing gastroparesis and intestinal pseudo-obstruction. ANA, antinuclear antibodies; ANNA-1, antineuronal nuclear antibodies type 1; CPK, creatine phosphokinase; GI, gastrointestinal. (Modified from Camilleri M, Prather CM. Gastric motor physiology and motor disorders. In: Feldman M, Sleisenger MH, Scharschmidt BF, editors. Sleisenger & Fordtran's gastrointestinal and liver disease: pathophysiology/diagnosis/management. Vol 1. 6th ed. Philadelphia: WB Saunders Company; 1998. p. 572-86. Used with permission.)

overgrowth by culture of small-bowel aspirates. Bacterial overgrowth is relatively uncommon in neuropathic disorders but is more common in myopathic conditions, such as scleroderma, that more often are associated with bowel dilatation or low-amplitude contractions. Bacterial overgrowth may be difficult to detect in cultures of small-bowel aspirates; however, breath hydrogen after a glucose or lactose load is a nonspecific test that should be interpreted with caution and in conjunction with small-bowel transit time because the early breath hydrogen peak may be due to bacterial metabolism of the substrate in the colon resulting from fast small-bowel transit. Often, an empiric trial of antibiotic therapy is used as a surrogate for formal testing.

TREATMENT OF GASTROPARESIS AND INTESTINAL PSEUDO-OBSTRUCTION

Treatment should be designed for each patient, depending on the findings of the investigation. The principal methods of management include correction of hydration and nutritional deficiencies, use of prokinetic and antiemetic medications, suppression of bacterial overgrowth, decompression, and surgical treatment.

Correction of Hydration and Nutritional Deficiencies

Rehydration, electrolyte repletion, and nutritional supplementation are particularly important during acute exacerbations of gastroparesis and chronic intestinal pseudo-obstruction. Restoration of nutrition can be achieved orally, enterally, or parenterally, depending on the severity of the clinical syndrome. Initial nutritional measures include low-fiber supplements with the addition of iron, folate, calcium, and vitamins D, K, and B_{12}. In patients with more severe symptoms, enteral or parenteral supplementation of nutrition may be required. If it is anticipated that enteral supplementation may be required for more than 3 months, it is usually best to provide feedings through a jejunostomy tube. Gastrostomy tubes should be avoided in gastroparesis except for venting purposes. Many patients who require long-term parenteral nutrition continue to tolerate some oral feeding.

Prokinetics and Medications

Increasingly, medications are being used to treat neuromuscular motility disorders. However, there is little evidence that they are effective in myopathic disturbances, except for the rare case of dystrophia myotonica affecting the stomach and for small-bowel systemic sclerosis.

Erythromycin, a macrolide antibiotic that stimulates motilin receptors at higher doses (e.g., 250-500 mg) and cholinergic mechanisms at lower doses (40-80 mg), results in the dumping of solids from the stomach. It has been shown to accelerate gastric emptying in gastroparesis; it also increases the amplitude of antral contractions and improves antroduodenal coordination. Erythromycin is most effective when it is given intravenously during acute exacerbations of gastroparesis or intestinal pseudo-obstruction. The usual dose of intravenous erythromycin lactobionate is 3 mg/kg every 8 hours. The effect of oral erythromycin appears to be restricted by tolerance and gastrointestinal side effects, which often prevent treatment for more than 1 month; sometimes a low dose of liquid formula erythromycin (e.g., 40-80 mg three times daily before meals) can be tolerated. The elixir formulation may improve absorption in the setting of dysmotility. Although initial studies demonstrated that 2 weeks of treatment was effective in patients with diabetic gastroparesis, there is little evidence that continued therapy produces long-term improvement in gastric emptying or associated symptoms.

Metoclopramide is a dopamine antagonist that has both prokinetic and antiemetic properties. Antiemetic effects are due partly to its anti-serotonergic$_3$-(5-HT$_3$) antagonist actions. Long-term use of metoclopramide is limited by the side effects of tremor and Parkinson-like symptoms, a consequence of antidopaminergic activity in the CNS. It is available in tablet or elixir form and is typically taken 30 minutes before meals and at bedtime. Usual doses range from 5 to 20 mg four times daily.

Serotonergic (5-HT) agents may prove to be beneficial in the treatment of gastroparesis and intestinal pseudo-obstruction. The combined 5-HT$_4$ agonist and 5-HT$_3$ antagonist, cisapride, was essentially the only medication for which there was evidence for efficacy in the medium- and long-term; the medication is no longer available for prescription because of the risks of cardiac dysrhythmias (torsades de pointes).

Octreotide, a cyclized analogue of somatostatin, has been shown to induce activity fronts in the small intestine that mimic phase III activity of the interdigestive migrating motor complex. Activity fronts in the small bowel are characterized by a simultaneous or very rapidly propagated activity front that is not well coordinated. The clinical effects of octreotide include an initial acceleration of gastric emptying, a decrease in postprandial gastric motility, and inhibition of small-bowel transit. Therefore, the therapeutic efficacy of octreotide in intestinal dysmotility associated with gastroparesis and pseudo-obstruction requires further assessment in clinical trials. Currently, octreotide appears to be more useful in the treatment of dumping syndromes associated with accelerated transit. However, it may be used at nighttime to induce interdigestive migrating motor complex activity and avoid bacterial overgrowth. If required during the daytime, octreotide is often given in combination with oral erythromycin to "normalize" the gastric emptying rate.

Antiemetics, including diphenhydramine, trifluoperazine, and metoclopramide, are important in the management of nausea and vomiting of patients with gastroparesis and intestinal pseudo-obstruction. The more expensive serotonin 5-HT$_3$ antagonists (e.g., ondansetron) have not proved to have greater benefit than the less expensive alternatives.

Antibiotic therapy is indicated for patients who have documented symptomatic bacterial overgrowth. Although formal clinical trials have not been conducted, it is common practice to use different antibiotics for 7 to 10 days each month in an attempt to avoid development of resistance. Common antibiotics include doxycycline (100 mg twice daily), metronidazole (500 mg three times daily), ciprofloxacin (500 mg twice daily), and double-strength trimethoprim-sulfamethoxazole (two tablets twice daily). Antibiotic therapy for patients with diarrhea and fat malabsorption due to bacterial overgrowth produces considerable symptomatic relief.

Decompression

Decompression is rarely necessary in patients with chronic pseudo-obstruction. However, venting enterostomy (jejunostomy) is effective in relieving abdominal distension and bloating. It has been shown to markedly decrease the frequency of nasogastric intubations and hospitalizations for acute exacerbations of severe intestinal pseudo-obstruction in patients requiring central parenteral nutrition. Access to the small intestine by enterostomy also provides a way to deliver nutrients enterally and should be considered for patients with intermittent symptoms. The currently available enteral tubes allow for aspiration and feeding by a single apparatus.

Surgical Treatment

Surgical treatment has a limited role for patients with gastroparesis and intestinal pseudo-obstruction. For patients who have had multiple abdominal operations, it becomes difficult to discern whether exacerbations of symptoms reflect an underlying disease or adhesions and mechanical obstruction. Surgical treatment should be considered whenever the motility disorder is localized to a resectable portion of the gut. Three instances in which to consider this approach include 1) duodenojejunostomy or duodenoplasty for patients with megaduodenum or duodenal atresia in children, 2) completion gastrectomy for patients with postgastric surgical stasis syndrome, and 3) colectomy with ileorectostomy for intractable constipation associated with chronic colonic pseudo-obstruction.

Novel Therapies

Preliminary data suggest that gastric pacing may improve gastric emptying and symptoms in patients with severe gastroparesis. In humans, gastric pacing has not been able to entrain gastric slow waves to normalize gastric dysrhythmias or to accelerate gastric emptying. Gastric electrical stimulation is an approved treatment, but data on efficacy are inconclusive and further controlled clinical trials are needed to assess the long-term benefits, complications, and optimal selection of patients for this treatment.

Currently, small-bowel transplantation is limited to patients with intestinal failure who have reversible total parenteral nutrition (TPN)-induced liver disease or life-threatening or recurrent catheter-related sepsis. Combined small-bowel and liver transplantation is being performed in patients with irreversible TPN-induced liver disease. Complications following small-bowel transplantation include infection, rejection, and lymphoproliferative disorders due to long-term immunosuppression and Epstein-Barr virus infection. Studies have suggested that small-bowel transplantation may improve quality of life and be more cost-effective than long-term TPN. In the future, improvements in immunosuppressive regimens, earlier detection of rejection, and treatment of cytomegalovirus infection based on polymerase chain reaction detection may enable small-bowel transplantation to become the definitive treatment for short-bowel syndrome or severe pseudo-obstruction uncontrolled by TPN. In the meantime, parenteral nutrition is the treatment of choice for most patients.

DUMPING SYNDROME AND ACCELERATED GASTRIC EMPTYING

Dumping syndrome and accelerated gastric emptying typically occur after truncal vagotomy and gastric drainage procedures. With the introduction of highly selective vagotomy and the advent of effective anti-acid secretory therapy, the prevalence of these problems is decreasing.

Rapid gastric emptying is thought to result from impaired gastric accommodation after the ingestion of a meal and the presence of the drainage procedure. A high caloric (usually carbohydrate) content of the liquid phase of the meal evokes a rapid insulin response, with secondary hypoglycemia. These patients also may have impaired antral contractility and gastric stasis of solids, which paradoxically may result in the clinical features of both gastroparesis (for solids) and dumping (for liquids). The most useful investigation is a dual-phase radioisotopic gastric emptying test.

The management of dumping syndrome includes dietary maneuvers (avoidance of high-nutrient liquid drinks and, possibly, addition of guar gum or pectin to retard gastric emptying of liquids). Rarely, pharmacologic treatment with octreotide (50-100 μg subcutaneously before meals) is needed. It retards intestinal transit and inhibits the hormonal responses that lead to hypoglycemia.

RAPID TRANSIT DYSMOTILITY OF THE SMALL BOWEL

Rapid transit of material through the small bowel may occur in postvagotomy diarrhea, short-bowel syndrome, diabetic diarrhea, carcinoid diarrhea, and irritable bowel syndrome. Except for irritable bowel syndrome, these conditions may cause severe diarrhea and result in substantial losses of fluids and electrolytes. Idiopathic bile acid catharsis may represent an inability of the distal ileum to reabsorb bile acids because of rapid transit and decreased contact time with ileal mucosa; this condition may induce colonic secretion and secondary diarrhea. Accelerated transit may be confirmed by scintigraphic studies.

Treatment

The objectives of treatment are to restore hydration and nutrition and to slow small-bowel transit.

Dietary Interventions

These include the avoidance of hyperosmolar drinks and replacement with iso-osmolar or hypo-osmolar oral rehydration solutions. The fat content in the diet should be reduced to approximately 50 g to avoid delivery of unabsorbed fat to the colon. All electrolyte and nutritional deficiencies of calcium, magnesium, potassium, and water- and fat-soluble vitamins should be corrected. In patients who have less than 1 m of residual small bowel, it may be impossible to maintain fluid and electrolyte homeostasis without parenteral support. In patients who have a longer residual segment, oral nutrition, pharmacotherapy, and supplements are almost always effective.

Drug Therapy

The opioid agent loperamide (4 mg 30 minutes before meals and at bedtime for a total dose of 16 mg/day) has been shown to suppress the motor response to feeding and to improve symptoms. Verapamil (40 mg twice daily) or clonidine (0.1 mg twice daily) (or both) may be given in addition to loperamide. Octreotide (50 μg subcutaneously three times daily before meals) may be given to patients in whom the oral agents are ineffective or poorly tolerated. The 5-HT$_3$ antagonists (e.g., ondansetron) may be effective in treating carcinoid diarrhea.

SUMMARY

Disorders of gastric and small-bowel motility may result in either stasis or accelerated transit. Understanding the mechanisms that control motility and pathophysiology in the patient is the key to optimal management. Simple, quantitative measures of transit and an algorithmic approach to identifying the underlying cause may lead to correction of abnormal function. Correcting dehydration and nutritional abnormalities and providing symptomatic relief are important steps in the management of these patients. Patient education is essential to avoid aggravation of symptoms caused by dietary indiscretions.

RECOMMENDED READING

Bytzer P, Talley NJ, Leemon M, Young LJ, Jones MP, Horowitz M. Prevalence of gastrointestinal symptoms associated with diabetes mellitus: a population-based survey of 15,000 adults. Arch Intern Med. 2001;161:1989-96.

Camilleri M. Enteric nervous system disorders: genetic and molecular insights for the neurogastroenterologist. Neurogastroenterol Motil. 2001;13:277-95.

Coulie B, Camilleri M. Intestinal pseudo-obstruction. Annu Rev Med. 1999;50:37-55.

Coulie B, Camilleri M. Gastrointestinal complications of diabetes mellitus. In: Leahy JL, Clark NG, Cefalu WT, editors. Medical management of diabetes mellitus. New York: Marcel Dekker; 2000. p. 387-406.

Di Lorenzo C. Pseudo-obstruction: current approaches. Gastroenterology. 1999;116:980-7.

Maleki D, Locke GR III, Camilleri M, Zinsmeister AR, Yawn BP, Leibson C, et al. Gastrointestinal tract symptoms among persons with diabetes mellitus in the community. Arch Intern Med. 2000;160:2808-16.

O'Brien MD, Bruce BK, Camilleri M. The rumination syndrome: clinical features rather than manometric diagnosis. Gastroenterology. 1995;108:1024-9.

Pachnis V, Durbec P, Taraviras S, Grigoriou M, Natarajan D. Role of the RET signal transduction pathway in development of the mammalian enteric nervous system. Am J Physiol. 1998;275:G183-6.

Parkman HP, Hasler WL, Fisher RS, American Gastroenterological Association. American Gastroenterological Association technical review on the diagnosis and treatment of gastroparesis. Gastroenterology. 2004;127:1592-622.

Rayner CK, Samsom M, Jones KL, Horowitz M. Relationships of upper gastrointestinal motor and sensory function with glycemic control. Diabetes Care. 2001;24:371-81.

von der Ohe MR, Camilleri M, Kvols LK, Thomforde GM. Motor dysfunction of the small bowel and colon in patients with the carcinoid syndrome and diarrhea. N Engl J Med. 1993;329:1073-8.

Wood JD, Alpers DH, Andrews PL. Fundamentals of neurogastroenterology. Gut. 1999;45 Suppl 2:II-6-16.

Stomach

Questions and Answers

QUESTIONS

Multiple Choice (choose the one best answer)

1. A 40-year-old migrant worker from Mexico presents to the emergency department with complaints of epigastric pain, melena, and nausea. Esophagogastroduodenoscopy shows a 2-cm duodenal ulcer, and antral biopsy specimens are positive for *Helicobacter pylori*. The primary reason to eradicate *H. pylori* infection in this patient is to:
   a. Reduce the risk of gastric cancer
   b. Heal the duodenal ulcer
   c. Heal the duodenal ulcer and decrease the risk of recurrent ulcer
   d. Prevent an inevitable MALToma
   e. Prevent transmission to his wife

2. On further questioning, the patient in question 1 recalls having a similar episode of gastrointestinal tract hemorrhage 5 years previously. Upon discharge, you tell the patient and his family that:
   a. A 14-day course of medication will solve the problem
   b. In addition to 14 days of triple therapy, he will need 6 weeks more of antiulcer medication
   c. His risk of reinfection from other infected family members who are positive for *H. pylori* is approximately 15%-20%
   d. In addition to proper medical therapy to eradicate *H. pylori* infection and to heal the ulcer, the patient will need a test to confirm that infection has been eradicated
   e. You now are concerned about a possible Zollinger-Ellison syndrome

3. An 82-year-old man who is active and in excellent health recently injured his back while riding a lawnmower. He began a course of ibuprofen therapy in addition to his usual 81 mg of aspirin. He complains of fatigue, shortness of breath, dizziness, and a pale appearance. He states that he has no abdominal pain, nausea, vomiting, or diarrhea. His stool is dark in color. However, he mentions that he recently took Pepto-Bismol for his "flulike symptoms." The patient is at increased risk for gastric ulcer complications because of:
   a. Age
   b. Recent gastrointestinal flu
   c. History of "stomachache" in high school
   d. His overall health status
   e. Pepto-Bismol

4. A 29-year-old woman complains of recurrent peptic ulcer disease. She has been hospitalized three times for bleeding duodenal ulcers. Currently, she is taking a proton pump inhibitor twice a day and complains of headache, diarrhea, and gastroesophageal reflux symptoms. The best initial test to diagnose her condition would be:
   a. Serum parathyroid hormone
   b. Serum prolactin
   c. Serum gastrin
   d. 24-hour 5-HIAA (5-hydroxyindoleacetic acid)
   e. *Giardia* stool antigen

5. The patient is found to have elevated levels of gastrin, parathyroid hormone, and prolactin. This clinical condition is known as:

a. Multiple endocrine neoplasia (MEN) type I

b. MEN type II

c. Zollinger-Ellison syndrome

d. Carcinoid syndrome

e. Mastocytosis

6. A 65-year-old woman with a past history of hypothyroidism who is receiving replacement therapy is referred to you for evaluation of gastrointestinal tract upset and a serum gastrin level of 1,200 pg/mL. She has been told she has Zollinger-Ellison syndrome. The initial test of choice to evaluate this patient should be:

a. Repeat serum gastrin level

b. Serum calcium level

c. Gastric analysis

d. Parathyroid hormone level

e. Thyroid-stimulating hormone level

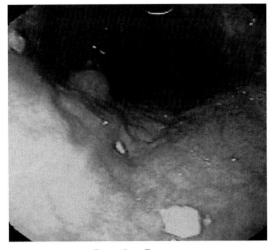

Question 7

7. A patient undergoes esophagogastroduodenoscopy and, at the time of gastric analysis, is noted to have multiple small nodules (2-3 mm) (Figure). Biopsy specimens from these nodules show carcinoid tumor. You recommend:

a. Subtotal gastrectomy

b. Somatostatin therapy

c. Proton pump inhibitor therapy to suppress gastrin level

d. Endoscopic resection of the nodules

e. Computed tomography of the abdomen to rule out metastatic disease

8. A 24-year-old alcoholic with chronic hepatitis C infection is admitted with hematemesis and melena. The endoscopic findings noted at esophagogastroduodenoscopy are shown (Figure). The diagnosis of the etiologic cause for his bleeding is:

a. Ectopic varices

b. Gastric antral vascular ectasia

c. Portal hypertensive gastropathy

d. Nonsteroidal anti-inflammatory drug (NSAID) gastropathy

e. Alcoholic gastritis

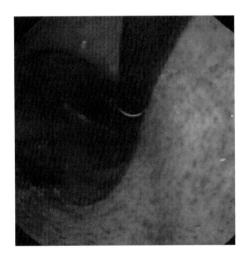

Question 8

9. A 75-year-old man presents with belching, vague abdominal pain, and a remote history of *Helicobacter pylori* infection treated 10 years earlier. The patient's father died of gastric cancer. The esophagogastroduodenoscopic findings (Figure) are of concern because of an association with:

a. Achlorhydria

b. Vitamin B_{12} deficiency

c. Risk for gastrointestinal tract hemorrhage

d. Risk for dysplasia

e. Nonulcer dyspepsia

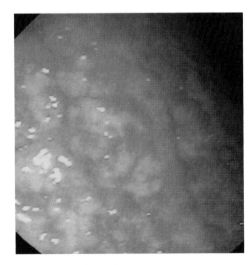

Question 9

10. A 24-year-old man complains of epigastric pain, flatulence, loose stool, and depression. He has been told he has irritable bowel syndrome. You order esophagogastroduodenoscopy, and a biopsy specimen from the endoscopic finding (Figure) shows an infiltration of lymphocytes. You recommend the following:
    a. *Helicobacter pylori* serologic study
    b. Serum tissue transglutaminase level
    c. Computed tomography with attention to the lymphatic system
    d. Serologic study for Whipple's disease
    e. Discontinue nonsteroidal anti-inflammatory drug therapy

11. A 72-year-old man presents with dysphagia, 25-lb weight loss, early satiety, aversion to meat, and melena. He has a great fear of gastric cancer because his father died of it at age 59. The esophagogastroduodenoscopic findings are shown in the Figure. You recommend to the patient:
    a. Imatinib mesylate to shrink the tumor
    b. Radiotherapy and chemotherapy
    c. Eradication of *Helicobacter pylori* to reverse the condition
    d. Surgical resection
    e. YAG laser therapy

12. The patient in question 11 states that he fears his sibiling and children are at risk for gastric cancer, and he asks if there is any way to prevent this disease from developing in them. You suggest:
    a. Genetic counseling for possible family cancer syndrome
    b. Folate, vitamin B_{12}, vitamin C, vitamin A, and vitamin E supplementation
    c. Screening for *Helicobacter pylori* infection
    d. Yearly endoscopic surveillance with biopsy
    e. No need for concern

13. The most frequent gastric tumor caused by *Helicobacter pylori* is:
    a. MALToma
    b. Gastrointestinal stromal tumor
    c. Adenocarcinoma
    d. Carcinoid tumor
    e. T-cell lymphoma

14. A 62-year-old woman with a past history of stage I adenocarcinoma of the breast presents with painless hematemesis and melena. Emergent esophagogastroduodenoscopy (EGD) was performed. The lesion shown in the Figure is most likely a:
    a. Gastrointestinal stromal tumor
    b. Leiomyoma
    c. Leiomysarcoma

d. Metastatic lesion from breast cancer
e. Kaposi's sarcoma

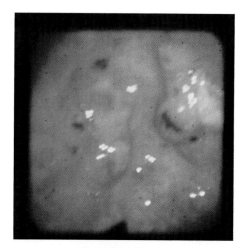

Question 10

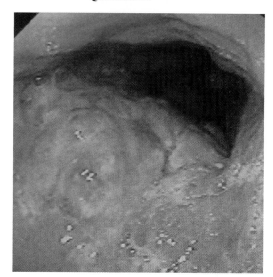

Question 11

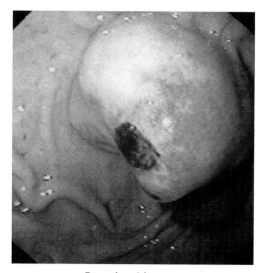

Question 14

15. The recommended treatment for the lesion in question 14 would be:
    a. Imatinib mesylate
    b. Endoscopic resection
    c. Surgical resection
    d. Local radiation
    e. Systemic chemotherapy

16. Which of the following is a *false* statement about metoclopramide (Reglan)?
    a. Metoclopramide is FDA-approved for the treatment of gastroesophageal reflux disease
    b. Metoclopramide is FDA-approved for the treatment of diabetic gastroparesis
    c. Metoclopramide is FDA-approved for the treatment of idiopathic gastroparesis
    d. Metoclopramide is pregnancy category B
    e. The dosing of metoclopramide is reduced in renal failure

17. Which of the following statements about upper gastrointestinal tract symptoms is *false*?
    a. Postprandial fullness severe enough to change usual activities is associated with delayed gastric emptying
    b. Early satiety is associated with impaired gastric accommodation
    c. A therapeutic response to a trial of metoclopramide is an effective way to diagnose gastroparesis
    d. Symptom patterns alone are unable to distinguish between functional dyspepsia and organic disease
    e. Postprandial fullness can be secondary to partial small-bowel obstruction

18. Which of the following statements about normal gastric function is *true*?
    a. In the postprandial period, the largest size food particle that can pass through the pylorus is 10 mm
    b. In the postprandial period, the largest size food particle that can pass through the pylorus is 6 mm
    c. In the postprandial period, the largest size food particle that can pass through the pylorus is 2 mm
    d. In the postprandial period, the largest size food particle that can pass through the pylorus is 1 mm
    e. The presence of phase III of the migrating motor complex (MMC) in the postprandial period ensures that the enteric nerves are working well

19. Gastroduodenal manometry (GDM) is a useful clinical test in which of the situations below?
    a. In the evaluation of a patient with scleroderma who has delayed gastric emptying
    b. In the evaluation of a patient with suspected rumination syndrome
    c. In a patient with unexplained obstructive symptoms and history of previous abdominal surgical procedures
    d. In the evaluation of a patient with severe upper gastrointestinal tract symptoms when all other tests are entirely normal
    e. In the evaluation of a patient with amyloidosis who has delayed gastric emptying

20. All the following statements about octreotide are *true* except:
    a. Octreotide is the treatment of choice for severe dumping syndrome refractory to diet
    b. The most common side effect of octreotide is constipation
    c. Octreotide induces phase III activity of the migrating motor complex
    d. Chronic use of octreotide is associated with the development of cholelithiasis
    e. Octreotide reduces portal pressure in patients with cirrhosis

21. A 52-year-old man who takes warfarin (Coumadin) and has an international normalized ratio (INR) of 2.3 presents with hematemesis and orthostasis. His INR is corrected with fresh frozen plasma to 1.2. He undergoes upper endoscopy after volume resuscitation within 8 hours after his original presentation. A 2-cm gastric ulcer was seen, with a nonbleeding, 1-mm, visible vessel on the greater curvature of the stomach in the antrum, and was treated with epinephrine injection and heater-probe therapy. The patient is prescribed an oral proton pump inhibitor twice daily. The patient's hemoglobin values are listed below:

Day	Hemoglobin, g/dL	INR
Admission	14.2	2.3
1	10.2	1.6
2	9.4	2.0
3	8.6	1.9

On day 2, he passes two formed black stools; on day 3, he passes one formed black stool. His vital signs are stable. Appropriate treatment on day 3 would be:
    a. Advance diet and observe
    b. Repeat esophagogastroduodenoscopy
    c. Infuse two more units of fresh frozen plasma
    d. Infuse two more units of fresh frozen plasma and repeat upper endoscopy

22. A 72-year-old woman had two episodes of red hematemesis associated with orthostasis over a 5-day period. She has three alcoholic drinks per day and uses ibuprofen daily. She had two upper endoscopy studies that were normal; both were performed about 5 hours after each episode. The most likely diagnosis is:
    a. Gastric varices
    b. Gastric Dieulafoy's lesion
    c. Gastric vascular ectasia
    d. Nonsteroidal anti-inflammatory drug (NSAID) gastric ulcer

23. A 62-year-old man with diabetes mellitus and chronic obstructive pulmonary disease has an upper gastro-intestinal tract hemorrhage requiring two units of packed red blood cells transfused for a 1-cm posterior duodenal ulcer that did not require endoscopic therapy. He was CLO (*Campylobacter*-like organism) test-negative and negative for *H. pylori* antibody. He takes no nonsteroidal anti-inflammatory drugs (NSAIDs) or aspirin and does not smoke. You see him in the clinic 5 days after discharge. The most appropriate treatment would be:
    a. Proton pump inhibitor twice daily for 8 weeks
    b. Proton pump inhibitor once a day for life
    c. Proton pump inhibitor once a day for 4 weeks
    d. Proton pump inhibitor once a day for 4 weeks with amoxicillin 1 g twice daily and clarithromycin 1 g twice daily for 2 weeks

24. A 28-year-old woman presents with necrotizing gallstone pancreatitis. She undergoes endoscopic sphincterotomy and stone extraction on day 2. Several extrapancreatic and one 8-cm intrapancreatic collections of fluid develop and are seen with computed tomography on day 10. On day 13, hematochezia and orthostasis develop, and she receives four units of packed erythrocytes. Upper endoscopy shows a maroon clot in the distal duodenum without evidence of active bleeding. The clot was washed, showing no evident underlying abnormality and no active bleeding. The ampulla seen with the side-viewing scope showed only a sphincterotomy site. The patient was hemodynamically stable for 12 hours and then tachycardia and hematochezia developed. The most likely successful therapeutic option would be:
    a. Esophagogastroduodenoscopy and epinephrine injection of the sphincterotomy site
    b. Diagnostic laparotomy
    c. Angiographic embolization
    d. Octreotide (Sandostatin) infusion

25. A 70-year-old woman presents with a 6-hour history of left-sided crampy abdominal pain. She passed several loose, watery stools and then three maroon stools. Her blood pressure is 130/70 mm Hg, pulse 92 without orthostatic change. Physical examination shows abdomen is soft, with moderate left-sided abdominal tenderness with some localized left-sided rebound tenderness. Hemoglobin is 12.8 g/dL. Leukocyte count is 13.4×10^9/L. The most likely diagnosis is:
    a. Diverticular hemorrhage
    b. *E. coli* O157:H7 colitis
    c. Colonic vascular ectasia
    d. Ischemic colitis

ANSWERS

1. Answer c

The primary reason to eradicate *H. pylori* infection in this patient is the need to heal the present duodenal ulcer and decrease the risk of recurrent ulceration in the future. Although 85% of gastric cancers are associated with *H. pylori*, the incidence of gastric cancer in the United States is 0.5%. Also, MALTomas are associated with *H. pylori* in 72% to 80% of patients with this tumor, but the risk of that lesion is certainly small and not inevitable. Infection with *H. pylori* occurs worldwide, and the overall prevalence of infection is strongly correlated with socioeconomic conditions. The prevalence among middle-aged adults is more than 80% in many developing countries such as Mexico. The infection is acquired by oral ingestion of the bacterium and is mainly transmitted within families during early childhood.

2. Answer d

Because the patient has had two episodes of gastrointestinal tract hemorrhage within 5 years, it is necessary to eradicate *H. pylori* and to confirm that it has been eradicated in order to prevent further recurrent ulcer with hemorrhage. A 14-day course of triple therapy would treat the *H. pylori* but would not be appropriate for eradicating the present ulcer. Risk of reinfection from other family members who are positive for *H. pylori* is small and reinfection rates are less than 3%.

3. Answer a

Risk factors for ulcer complications with nonsteroidal anti-inflammatory drug (NSAID) use include age older than 75 years, concomitant use of NSAIDs and anticoagulants, NSAIDs and corticosteroids, history of previous gastrointestinal tract bleeding, history of ulcer disease, and a comorbid history of heart disease.

4. Answer c

This patient presents with the clinical manifestations of Zollinger-Ellison syndrome. The initial test to diagnose her condition would be to determine the serum gastrin level. Although increased serum parathyroid hormone and prolactin levels may be associated with Zollinger-Ellison syndrome, they do not confirm the diagnosis. This patient does not manifest a carcinoid syndrome, and a 24-hour 5-HIAA would not be appropriate. Giardiasis can cause acid peptic symptoms and diarrhea; however, it should not be associated with bleeding duodenal ulcers, and a *Giardia* stool antigen test is not indicated.

5. Answer a

MEN type I is characterized by a gastrin-secreting tumor in the "gastrinoma triangle" associated with hypercalcemia, hyperparathyroidism, and pituitary tumors. MEN type II is associated with medullary carcinoma of the thyroid, pheochromocytomas, and hyperparathyroidism. These patients may present with a secretory diarrhea. Carcinoid syndrome is characterized by a watery secretory diarrhea associated with wheezing, flushing, cough, asthma, and skin rash caused by the secretion of serotonin, histamine, catecholamines, prostaglandins, and substance P.

6. Answer c

This patient does not have Zollinger-Ellison syndrome but has atrophic gastritis and pernicious anemia. The diagnostic test of choice is a gastric analysis to confirm achlorhydria.

7. Answer d

Multiple small carcinoid tumors are frequently associated with atrophic gastritis as a result of high levels of gastrin from the patient's achlorhydria. These lesions, for the most part, follow a benign course, and there are reports to support endoscopic resection of the nodules to prevent their growth and spread. There is no indication for subtotal gastrectomy or somatostatin treatment. Proton pump inhibitor therapy is to be avoided because it will increase the gastrin level and potentially stimulate further enterochromaffin cell–like growth.

8. Answer c

The endoscopic findings are those of portal hypertensive gastropathy associated with portal hypertension related to the patient's alcoholism, chronic hepatitis C, and presumed cirrhosis. The changes of portal hypertensive gastropathy primarily affect the proximal stomach. Gastric antral vascular ectasia involves the antrum and crosses the pylorus. NSAID gastropathy is very mild and nonspecific and usually presents with submucosal hemorrhage as opposed to the "mosaic" appearance of the proximal stomach in this case. Certainly, the patient could suffer from alcoholic gastritis, but this is more of a diffuse hemorrhagic type lesion and is not consistent with the endoscopic finding.

9. Answer d

The endoscopic findings shown are those of multifocal atrophic gastritis. This lesion is associated with dysplasia and a risk for gastric cancer. Because the patient has a first-degree relative with gastric cancer which places him at increased risk, this endoscopic finding is of concern. The patient has long-standing *H. pylori* infection; thus, he no doubt has an associated atrophic gastritis, which is associated with achlorhydria and vitamin B_{12} deficiency. This patient would benefit from vitamin B_{12} replacement.

10. Answer b

The endoscopic finding is characteristic of lymphocytic gastritis and is associated with celiac sprue as well as microscopic colitis. The test of choice would be to determine serum tissue transglutaminase level to evaluate for celiac sprue (gluten-sensitive enteropathy). Although *H. pylori* is associated with mucosa-associated lymphoid tissue lymphoma, the endoscopic findings are more consistent with lymphocytic gastritis. The pathologist may use special immunohistochemical staining to look for evidence of a monoclonal population of lymphocytes. The histopathologic features are not consistent with Whipple's disease, which is classically an infiltration of macrophages with the presence of characteristic bacilli.

11. Answer d

The endoscopic findings are those of adenocarcinoma of the stomach. The treatment of choice for this condition is surgical resection if there is no evidence of metastatic disease preoperatively. Imatinib mesylate has been used to shrink gastrointestinal stromal tumors before resection. Radiotherapy and chemotherapy may be warranted postoperatively if there is evidence of metastatic disease at the time of laparotomy. It has been recommended by the MAASTRICHT 2-2000 consensus report on treatment of *H. pylori* that patients who have had a resection for gastric carcinoma should have treatment to eradicate the bacillus. However, this will not reverse the condition.

12. Answer c

Gastric cancer is associated with *H. pylori* infection in 85% to 95% of all cases of adenocarcinoma of the stomach. Reports support that first-degree relatives of patients with gastric cancer have a higher incidence of *H. pylori* infection and also an increased risk of adenocarcinoma of the stomach. No data support supplementation with vitamins. Gastric cancer alone would not necessitate genetic counseling for a family cancer syndrome. No data support annual endoscopic surveillance with biopsies unless the patient lives in a country with a high risk for gastric cancers, for example, Japan or Chile.

13. Answer c

Studies by Uemura have reported that persons with *H. pylori* infection in developing countries have an incidence of gastric cancer of approximately 3% where gastric cancer did not develop in persons who are not infected. Gastric MALTomas have been associated also with *H. pylori* infection but are not as common as gastric adenocarcinomas. Gastrointestinal stromal tumors, carcinoid tumors, and T-cell lymphomas are not associated with *H. pylori* infection.

14. Answer a

The lesion seen on EGD is characteristic of gastrointestinal stromal tumors, which are submucosal tumors that often ulcerate in the center and have a high tendency to bleed. Historically, these lesions were thought to be either leiomyomas or leiomyosarcomas. However, current knowledge indicates that gastrointestinal stromal tumors have been misdiagnosed in the past and that leiomyomas and leiomyosarcomas are in fact rare lesions. One needs to keep in mind that breast cancer does metastasize to the stomach, and this certainly is in the differential diagnosis but unlikely with stage I disease. Kaposi's sarcoma is most often associated with profoundly immunosuppressed patients, such as those with human immunodeficiency virus infection and acquired immunodeficiency syndrome.

15. Answer c

The recommended treatment for gastrointestinal stromal tumors is surgical resection. Endoscopic resection has been performed on small lesions. However, it is imperative that the margins of resection be free of tumor, and it may necessitate the use of endoscopic ultrasonography in the endoscopic approach. Imatinib mesylate, which is a tyrosine kinase inhibitor, has been shown to shrink gastrointestinal stromal tumors, and treatment with it preoperatively may be indicated to make surgical excision easier. Imatinib mesylate has also been administered to patients with metastatic disease.

16. Answer c

There is no FDA-approved medication for the treatment of idiopathic gastroparesis.

17. Answer c

An empiric trial of a drug with a low therapeutic index for a condition that is not documented is poor practice.

18. Answer d

Choice e is false because the presence of the MMC in the postprandial period indicates failure of conversion to the fed pattern and is generally considered a sign of vagal dysfunction.

19. Answer c

Some manometric findings are reasonably specific for mechanical obstruction even when radiographic studies are negative. Patients who have a specific diagnosis that is associated with delayed gastric emptying, such as scleroderma, amyloidosis, or diabetes, do not need an additional diagnostic test. Rumination is diagnosed by history; manometric findings are less sensitive and specific. GDM testing is invasive and not always well tolerated, and it is unlikely to be helpful in a setting in which other assessments of gastrointestinal function (e.g., scintigraphy) are normal.

20. Answer b

Diarrhea occurs in 30% to 50% of patients treated for acromegaly, compared with 5% to 10% receiving placebo; constipation occurs in less than 10%.

21. Answer a

The slow decrease in hemoglobin concentration is consistent with reequilibration. There is no evidence of clinical bleeding and the one formed black stool is consistent with recent bleeding. No specific treatment is needed.

22. Answer b

All the choices are possible explanations, but Dieulafoy's lesion is the best answer. Gastric varices and the NSAID ulcer would likely be seen with endoscopy. The vascular ectasia could be difficult to visualize, but the red hematemesis and orthostasis are consistent with arterial bleeding, as seen with Dieulafoy's lesion. The majority of these occur in the upper stomach.

23. Answer b

Most duodenal ulcers will heal in 4 weeks with once-daily proton pump inhibitor therapy. A false-negative CLO test may be seen with upper gastrointestinal tract bleeding, but *H. pylori* serologic testing, although not completely sensitive, should remain positive. Anti-*H. pylori* therapy might still be supportable but is not the best answer. Patients with bleeding from peptic ulcer disease have a 5-year recurrent bleeding rate of about 30%. Patients without a correctable etiologic factor for peptic ulcer

disease (*H. pylori*, NSAIDs), especially those with comorbidities, should be receiving long-term proton pump inhibitor or full-dose histamine blocker prophylaxis.

24. Answer c

The most likely source of the major bleeding is a pseudo-aneurysm due to necrotic pancreatitis. This is difficult to operate on because of acute pancreatic necrosis, and it is best treated with angiographic embolization. Bleeding from the sphincterotomy site is possible but not the best answer. This would be less likely with the normal appearance of the sphincterotomy, and it is out more than a week after the procedure. Octreotide (Sandostatin) may be a temporizing measure for exsanguinating bleeding but is not the best answer.

25. Answer d

This is a classic description of ischemic colitis with pain, followed by nonbloody diarrhea and eventually hematochezia. *E. coli* O157:H7 can present with nonbloody diarrhea, followed by bloody diarrhea as well. Although pain may be present with *E. coli* infection, it generally is not the chief complaint; this would be a reasonable, but not the most likely, answer. Diverticular bleeding and vascular ectasia bleeding generally are painless.

SECTION III

Small Bowel and Nutrition

CHAPTER 10

Malabsorption

John A. Schaffner, M.D.

Malabsorption can be caused by various disordered physiologic processes that can be classified into three primary categories: luminal defects, mucosal defects, and delivery defects (Table 1). Although malabsorption frequently is synonymous with fat malabsorption, each class of nutrients (carbohydrate, protein, and fat) can have associated disorders that differ clinically.

The gastrointestinal and systemic consequences of malabsorption are listed in Table 2.

EVALUATION OF CARBOHYDRATE MALABSORPTION

Isolated carbohydrate malabsorption should be suspected in patients with symptoms of increased gas, distention, and possibly diarrhea. These symptoms usually are mild and not accompanied by weight loss. An extensive dietary history should be obtained to exclude obvious dietary causes, including high-fiber foods, fructose, and nonabsorbable carbohydrates (sorbitol, mannitol, lactulose). A history suggestive of a more global malabsorptive picture should preclude an evaluation of carbohydrate malabsorption.

A fecal pH less than 6 or the presence of reducing substances in the stool is evidence for carbohydrate malabsorption. Intestinal biopsy with quantitative analysis of mucosal enzyme activity is the most accurate method of assessing disaccharidase activity but is invasive and not widely available.

Oral tolerance tests with specific carbohydrates, particularly lactose, are done to determine whether the serum glucose level is increased. These tests generally have been replaced by more sensitive and easier hydrogen breath tests. An increase in breath hydrogen of 20 parts/million is indicative of colonic fermentation of the lactose by bacteria. False-positive results can occur in patients with bacterial overgrowth, and false-negative results can occur after antibiotic therapy or in patients who do not carry hydrogen-producing bacteria in their colon.

EVALUATION OF PROTEIN MALABSORPTION

Disorders of isolated protein malabsorption are rare. The evaluation generally looks for evidence of fat malabsorption. Protein losses can be measured in protein-losing enteropathies with α_1-antitrypsin clearance or, less commonly, radiolabeled macromolecules (most notably technetium Tc 99m-labeled albumin).

EVALUATION OF FAT MALABSORPTION

Measurement of fecal fat excretion remains the standard test for fat malabsorption. A 72-hour collection for fat quantitation usually is required, but shorter collections of 24 to 48 hours may be adequate if stool frequency is very great. A high fat intake of 100 g/day is necessary to ensure accurate results and must be started several days before the test. Normal fat excretion may vary slightly but should be between 6 and 8 g/24 hours. The qualitative stool fat test with Sudan staining is insensitive but may be valuable as a screening test in patients with fat excretion of more than 20 g/24 hours.

Carbon 14-triolein breath testing and other breath tests with labeled triglycerides are not widely available and are fraught with interpretation problems and lack of sensitivity in mild pancreatic insufficiency. No other test is yet available to replace stool fat collections.

Table 1.   Types of Malabsorption Syndromes

Category	Defect	Cause	Disease
Luminal defect	Defective hydrolysis of fat	Decreased lipase	Pancreatic insufficiency
		Decreased duodenal pH	Zollinger-Ellison syndrome
		Impaired mixing	Postgastrectomy
	Defective hydrolysis of protein	Decreased proteases (trypsin, chymotrypsin, elastase, carboxypeptidases)	Pancreatic insufficiency
		Absent enterokinase	Congenital enterokinase deficiency
	Impaired solubilization	Decreased micelle formation	Liver disease
			Biliary tract obstruction
			Altered enterohepatic circulation
			Poor mixing
			Drug effects (ETOH), neomycin, cholestyramine
		Deconjugation of bile salts	Bacterial overgrowth
Mucosal defect	Diffuse mucosal damage	Diminished surface area	Celiac disease, tropical sprue, Whipple's disease, Crohn's disease, infections, enteropathy (AIDS, GVHD), amyloid, drug effects, etc.
		Altered fluid absorption and secretion	
	Decreased brush border enzymes	Congenital deficiency	Lactase, sucrase-isomaltase, trehalase
		Acquired deficiency	
		Small bowel damage	
	Transport defects	Single enzyme congenital defects	Hartnup disease, cystinuria, B_{12} malabsorption
	Epithelial processing	Missing a transfer protein	Abetalipoproteinemia
Delivery defect	Lymphatic obstruction	Reduced chylomicron and lipoprotein absorption	Primary intestinal lymphangiectasia
			Lymphatic invasion by neoplasia

AIDS, acquired immunodeficiency syndrome; ETOH, ethyl alcohol; GVHD, graft-versus-host disease.
Data from Riley SA, Marsh MN. Maldigestion and malabsorption. In: Feldman M, Scharschmidt BF, Sleisenger MH, editors.
Sleisenger & Fordtran's gastrointestinal and liver disease: pathophysiology/diagnosis/management. Vol 2. 6th ed. Philadelphia: WB
Saunders Company; 1998. p. 1501-22.

Once steatorrhea is established, determination of the cause is the next step. In the absence of clinical clues, a D-xylose test is easy to perform, although there is considerable controversy about the value of this test. After ingestion of 25 g of D-xylose, a 1-hour serum specimen and a 5-hour urine collection are obtained. Often only the serum specimen is obtained, although this may not be as accurate as the urine specimen. Low values are indicative of small-bowel mucosal disease. Falsely low levels may occur with vomiting, gastric outlet obstruction, ascites, or poor urine collection. D-Xylose breath testing measuring hydrogen in expired air is another alternative to the serum and urine collections, although it is neither more sensitive nor specific than the urine and serum D-xylose tests.

For patients with an abnormal D-xylose result, the differential diagnosis is narrowed to small-bowel disease or bacterial overgrowth. For determination of small-bowel disease, the two available tests are small-bowel radiography and small-bowel biopsy. Which of these tests is ordered depends on the clinical circumstances. There is no correct first step.

Radiologic findings of malabsorption include flocculation and segmentation of barium, changes in mucosal fold pattern, and dilatation of intestinal loops. In addition, small-bowel studies are useful for determining the location of disease. Enteroclysis has a higher yield of abnormal findings in malabsorptive disorders than standard barium studies, although use of enteroclysis requires agreement of both the patient and the physician to have the test performed.

Small-bowel biopsy can be diagnostic in several cases in conjunction with the patient history and laboratory studies. The typical small-bowel diseases (celiac disease, Whipple's disease, tropical sprue, and infections) usually are diffuse processes, and biopsy of distal duodenum or proximal jejunum will provide an answer. Crohn's disease and lymphoma may be patchy, and obtaining adequate diagnostic tissue may be difficult.

Pancreatic insufficiency can be difficult to prove. Pancreatic calcifications may provide a clue but usually require severe pancreatic damage and are present in only 20% to 30% of patients with pancreatic insufficiency. Abdominal computed tomography, endoscopic retrograde cholangiopancreatography, and endoscopic ultrasonography also may show anatomical changes in chronic pancreatitis. The secretin test is difficult to perform and time-consuming, and because of a shortage of secretin it is rarely performed. During that test, bicarbonate and volume are measured in the duodenal aspirate. Cholecystokinin also can be administered and the pancreatic output of trypsin and lipase can be measured. This test is available in only a few centers. Empiric trials of pancreatic enzymes may be necessary for some patients.

Table 2. Consequences of Malabsorption

Signs and symptoms	Pathophysiologic mechanisms	Laboratory abnormalities
	Gastrointestinal	
Diarrhea	Malabsorption of nutrients	Stool weight >200 g
	Increased secretion due to crypt hyperplasia, inflammatory mediators, bile and fatty acids	Increased stool osmotic gap
Weight loss	Nutrient malabsorption, anorexia in mucosal diseases	Increased stool fat, decreased serum proteins
Flatulence, borborygmi, distention	Bacterial fermentation of carbohydrate and protein	Increased flatus
Bulky, greasy stools	Fat malabsorption	Increased stool fat, decreased carotene
Abdominal pain	If severe, due to chronic pancreatitis	
	If mild, distention of bowel	
	Hematopoietic	
Anemia	Iron, folate, vitamin B_{12}, pyridoxine	Microcytic, macrocytic, or dimorphic anemia
Coagulopathy	Vitamin K deficiency	Prolonged prothrombin time
	Musculoskeletal	
Bone pain (osteopenic bone disease)	Calcium, vitamin D, and protein malabsorption	Hypocalcemia, hypophosphatemia, increased alkaline phosphatase
Tetany	Calcium, magnesium, vitamin D malabsorption	Above plus hypomagnesemia
	Endocrine	
Amenorrhea, infertility, impotence	Malabsorption with protein-calorie malnutrition	Low serum protein; may have abnormal gonadotropin secretion
Secondary hyperparathyroidism	Probably vitamin D and calcium deficiency	Increased alkaline phosphatase, increased serum parathyroid hormone
	Skin and mucous membranes	
Cheilosis, glossitis, stomatitis	Iron, riboflavin, niacin, folate, vitamin B_{12} deficiency	Low serum iron, folate, vitamin B_{12}
Purpura	Vitamin K deficiency	Prolonged prothrombin time
Follicular hyperkeratosis	Vitamin A deficiency	Low serum carotene
Scaly dermatitis	Zinc and essential fatty acid deficiency	Low serum or urine zinc
Hyperpigmented dermatitis	Niacin deficiency	
Edema or ascites	Protein malabsorption	Low serum albumin
	Nervous system	
Xerophthalmia and night blindness	Vitamin A deficiency	Decreased serum carotene
Peripheral neuropathy	Vitamin B, thiamine deficiency	

CHAPTER 11

Small-Bowel Disease and Bacterial Overgrowth

John A. Schaffner, M.D.

SMALL-BOWEL DISEASE

Celiac Disease

Celiac disease is associated with many clinical presentations, although the majority of patients are asymptomatic. The disease is being detected with increased frequency, and in many screened populations the incidence may be higher than 1 in 250 persons.

The clinical features of the disease are often nonspecific and may manifest as symptoms outside the gastrointestinal tract. Nutritional deficiencies can include fat, protein, and carbohydrate malabsorption. Anemia may be due to iron, folate, or vitamin B_{12} deficiency. Deficiencies can include pyridoxine, vitamins A, C, D, E, and K, niacin, and pantothenic acid. Deficiencies of calcium, magnesium, zinc, and copper can occur.

Gastrointestinal complaints are those related to malabsorption, including diarrhea, bulky, foul-smelling stools, cramps, and weight loss. Patients may be anorectic or have a voracious appetite. Other complaints can include malaise, depression, weakness, menstrual problems, growth disturbance, or neurologic complaints.

Abnormalities on basic laboratory studies include a decreased hemoglobin concentration with an abnormal mean corpuscular volume, decreased calcium level, abnormal results on liver function tests, and increased fecal fat. Several disorders associated with celiac disease are listed in Table 1.

Celiac disease is a genetically inherited disease associated with the HLA locus found on the short arm of chromosome 6. Certain genes confer susceptibility. HLA-DQ2 (heterodimers DQA1*0501, DQB1*0201/0202) is present in 95% of patients with celiac disease, and HLA-DQ8 (DQA1*0301, DQB*0302) is present in the remainder of patients.

Absence of the *DQ* gene argues strongly against celiac disease. Because HLA-DQ2 and HLA-DQ8 are present in 20% to 30% of the general Western population, other factors must play a role. Further evidence of an environmental factor in the pathogenesis includes manifestation of the disease at virtually any age and presence of the disease in only about 70% of monozygotic twins.

Table 1. Disorders Associated With Celiac Disease

Endocrine disorders	Skin diseases
Diabetes	Dermatitis herpetiformis
Thyroid disease	Atopy
Addison's disease	Psoriasis
Connective tissue disorders	Down syndrome
Sjögren's syndrome	Osteopenia
Rheumatoid arthritis	Amenorrhea
Pulmonary disorders	Infertility
Asthma	Psychiatric disorders
Sarcoidosis	Liver disease
Renal disease	Malignancy
Neurologic disorders	Lymphoma
Seizures	Esophageal
Dementia	Oropharyngeal
Peripheral neuropathy	IgA deficiency
Inflammatory bowel disease	

Pathology

Figure 1 shows the histologic stages of celiac disease devised by Marsh. The preinfiltrative stage is indistinguishable from normal. Type 1 has an increase in γ/δ T-cell receptor intraepithelial lymphocytes. This lesion usually is not associated with gastrointestinal symptoms. Type 2 has enlarged crypts along with the intraepithelial lymphocytes. Type 3 is present in all symptomatic patients, but many patients with this lesion are asymptomatic. Type 4 is irreversible and is found in patients who do not respond to gluten withdrawal and in patients with lymphoma. There is not a good correlation between the severity of the lesion and the symptoms, although the sensitivity of the serologic markers may depend on the severity of the lesion.

The finding of flat mucosa is well recognized to occur in other diseases. These disorders include collagenous sprue, giardiasis, lymphoma, tropical sprue, cow's milk allergy, bacterial overgrowth, eosinophilic gastroenteritis, viral gastroenteritis, and Zollinger-Ellison syndrome.

The pathologic findings of celiac disease are shown in Figure 2.

Diagnosis

The ability to diagnose celiac disease requires a suspicion for the various presentations. Apart from the signs and symptoms and suggestive laboratory data, the endoscopic appearance of duodenal scalloping and reduced folds should prompt biopsy of the small bowel. The absence of endoscopic findings should not rule out biopsy. Biopsy of jejunal mucosa may be more accurate than duodenal biopsy.

Serologic screening, which in some studies has very high sensitivity, may not be accurate in all patients. Sensitivity varies considerably among laboratories and with the severity of the disease. If presence of the disease is to be proved, it is crucial that patients not be receiving a gluten-free diet. Gliadin antibody tests are not very specific and may lead to unnecessary testing. Antireticulin antibodies are another option but offer no

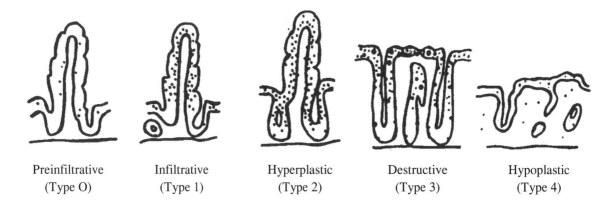

| Preinfiltrative (Type O) | Infiltrative (Type 1) | Hyperplastic (Type 2) | Destructive (Type 3) | Hypoplastic (Type 4) |

Fig. 1. Histologic stages of celiac disease. (From Mearin ML, Mulder CJ. Celiac disease [gluten-sensitive enteropathy]. In: Haubrich WS, Schaffner F, editors. Bockus gastroenterology. Vol 2. 5th edition. Philadelphia: WB Saunders; 1995. p. 1027-48. Used with permission.)

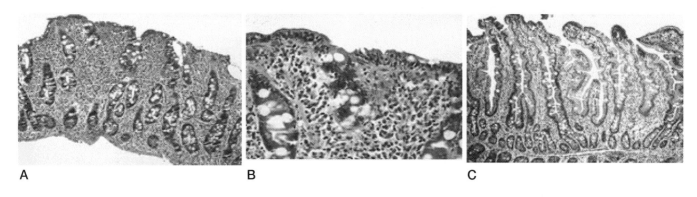

A   B   C

Fig. 2. *A*, Untreated celiac disease, showing a flat surface with severe enteritis, crypt hyperplasia, disarray of enterocytes, and extensive inflammatory infiltrate. *B*, In untreated celiac disease, the epithelial cells are cuboidal and vacuolated. There are numerous intraepithelial lymphocytes and plasma cells. *C*, Normal epithelium. (From Farrell RJ, Kelly CP. Celiac sprue. N Engl J Med. 2002;346:180-8. Used with permission.)

advantage over gliadin antibodies. Endomysial antibodies are not as sensitive as gliadin but are more specific. Tissue transglutaminase is the antigen against which endomysial antibody is directed. Although testing is easier to perform and less expensive, it is not yet clear that tissue transglutaminase has any diagnostic advantage over endomysial antibody.

A positive endomysial antibody test or tissue transglutaminase test has been indicative of celiac disease, but several studies have shown a small number of people who had positive serologic results but normal biopsy results. Likewise, a negative test result does not preclude presence of the disease. Therefore, biopsy should be performed in all patients who are suspected of having the disease regardless of serologic evidence.

A compatible biopsy with serologic confirmation indicates the need for treatment. Whether patients with serologic abnormalities and normal biopsy results should be treated remains controversial.

Treatment

The treatment of celiac disease is a gluten-restricted diet, including wheat, rye, and barley. Oats do not contain gluten, but they do contain the less toxic avenin. Studies have shown that small amounts of oats are well tolerated without inducing mucosal damage. A major issue regarding oats in the United States is contamination during processing. Recent investigations have shown that many pure oat products are contaminated with gluten. Thus, many physicians and American celiac societies advise against ingesting oats, particularly in the first months after diagnosis. Figure 3 shows the grain family tree.

Some patients do not respond to gluten withdrawal. All attempts should be made to ensure that there is no gluten in the diet before continuing symptoms are attributed to treatment failure. Occasional patients may require corticosteroid therapy and nutritional support. There are reports of using azathioprine and cyclosporine for refractory cases.

Patients who continue to have diarrhea despite gluten withdrawal should be examined for other causes of diarrhea. Microscopic colitis is relatively common among patients with celiac disease and responds to appropriate therapy. A considerable percentage of patients have pancreatic insufficiency and respond to enzyme replacement. Further investigations for lymphoma also should be undertaken in unresponsive patients.

Complications

The two major complications of celiac disease are refractory sprue and T-cell lymphoma. A diagnosis of refractory sprue is based on lack of response to a strict gluten-free diet and no other cause being found. In refractory sprue, severe complications can develop, including ulcerative jejunitis, collagenous sprue, and lymphoma. The lymphoma is associated with a high mortality rate. The risk for development of lymphoma can apparently be markedly reduced by strict adherence to a gluten-free diet, although the relative risk of this complication is unknown.

Patients with celiac disease also have an increased risk of esophageal cancer and oropharyngeal cancer and have an increase in autoimmune diseases. The risk of all these disorders seems to be reduced by dietary compliance.

Tropical Sprue

Tropical sprue is a distinctive illness that can manifest as an acute or chronic illness. The chronic disease, which usually requires 2 to 4 years of residence in a tropical area, occurs in three stages. Stage 1 is characterized by fatigue, malaise, abdominal cramps with or without diarrhea, and steatorrhea. Stage 2 has various gastrointestinal complaints, including dyspepsia, diarrhea, and manifestations of malabsorptive deficiencies. Stage 3 is characterized by macrocytic anemia and pancytopenia. Acute tropical sprue is not dependent on length of stay. The clinical stages are compressed, and onset is rapid.

The diagnosis of tropical sprue should be considered in any patient with signs of malabsorption and severe megaloblastic anemia who has been to a tropical climate. The differential diagnosis can include *Giardia lamblia*, *Strongyloides stercoralis*, *Isospora belli*, *Capillaria philippinensis*, and *Metagonimus yokogawai*.

The endoscopic finding of scalloping in the duodenum has been reported. Pathologically, the mucosa has shortening and broadening of villi with lengthening of crypts and an increase in chronic inflammatory cells. Fat staining shows accumulation of lipid droplets adjacent to the surface epithelium.

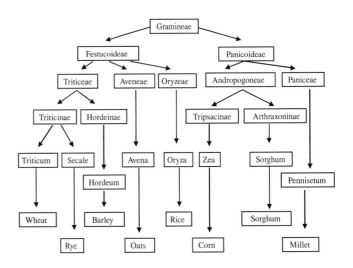

Fig. 3. Grain family tree, showing the distinction of wheat, rye, and barley.

The treatment of tropical sprue is folic acid 5 mg/day for 1 year, which usually results in a considerable response within days. Vitamin B_{12} may be given if symptoms have been present for more than 4 months.

Antibiotics usually result in a response within weeks. Reversal of anemia and glossitis, return of appetite, and weight gain are usually delayed. Tetracycline 250 mg four times a day is the recommended dosage for up to 6 months. An alternative is succinylsulfathiazole 4 g daily for 4 months followed by 2 g for 5 months. A combination of antibiotics and folic acid usually brings about a more rapid clinical response.

Whipple's Disease

Whipple's disease is a very rare infectious disease that has numerous potential manifestations. The patients are predominantly white males (male:female ratio, 9:1). The disease develops most often in the fourth or fifth decade of life.

There are various clinical presentations depending on the organ system involved. Table 2 illustrates the protean nature of the disease.

Whipple's disease is diagnosed on the basis of periodic acid-Schiff–positive macrophages in gut mucosa (Fig. 4). What

Table 2. Manifestations of Whipple's Disease

Organ system	Manifestations
Pulmonary	Chest pain, shortness of breath, cough
Renal	Focal embolic glomerulonephritis from endocarditis or direct bacillus involvement
Ocular	Central scotoma, papilledema, vitreous opacities, vitreous hemorrhage, ophthalmoplegia, keratitis, optic atrophy, nystagmus, gaze palsies, uveitis
Cardiac	>50%: congestive heart failure, pericarditis, valvular lesions
Neurologic	10%: dementia, headache, lethargy, coma, convulsions, sensory deficits, incoordination, polydipsia, cranial nerve problems
Rheumatologic	67% have joint symptoms, 30% >5 years, large and small joints affected, nondeforming
Gastrointestinal	Steatorrhea and diarrhea
Systemic signs and symptoms	Fever >50%, low-grade; lymphadenopathy is common
Other	Myopathies, ascites, inferior vena cava obstruction, thrombocytosis, pancytopenia

was once a pathognomonic biopsy of periodic acid-Schiff–positive macrophages now requires the tissue to be stained for acid-fast organisms. The finding of sickle-shaped particles in cells on electron microscopy is also definitive. Polymerase chain reaction for *Tropheryma whippelii* also can confirm the diagnosis. Periodic acid-Schiff–positive macrophages also have been found in *Mycobacterium avium-intracellulare*, *Rhodococcus equi*, histoplasmosis, macroglobulinemia, ceroid deposits, melanosis coli and rectal muciphages, EDTA therapy, and normal individuals.

The probable treatment of choice is trimethoprim-sulfamethoxazole because of penetration of the blood-brain barrier, although there are no conclusive studies of the disease, given its rarity. Other choices include penicillin, ceftriaxone, chloramphenicol, tetracycline, and penicillin plus streptomycin. Relapse has been reported with most antibiotic regimens. Treatment should be for at least 1 year.

Disaccharidase Deficiency

The clinical features of disaccharidase deficiency relate to the unabsorbed osmotic load and bacterial fermentation of the unabsorbed material. The symptoms of bloating and cramping usually have an onset of 1 to 2 hours after ingestion, although the symptoms may be delayed. Loose stools may occur depending on the amount of carbohydrate ingested. There are congenital and acquired deficiencies. Similar symptoms may occur after the ingestion of any nonabsorbed carbohydrate, although the amount of fiber contained in the carbohydrate could alter the symptom presentation.

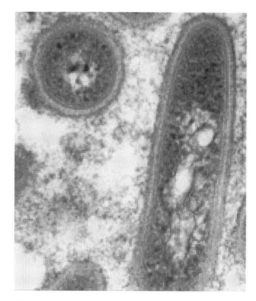

Fig. 4. Electron microscopy of bacillus in Whipple's disease. The plasma membrane is surrounded by a thin homogeneous wall, itself surrounded by a plasma-membrane–like structure. (From Dobbins WO III. The diagnosis of Whipple's disease. N Engl J Med. 1995;332:390-2. Used with permission.)

Lactase Deficiency

Three syndromes are associated with lactase deficiency. The congenital form, present from birth, is very rare and there appears to be evidence of an autosomal recessive inheritance. The primary form is genetically determined and is dependent on the population (Table 3). The onset is usually delayed. The secondary or acquired form of lactase deficiency occurs after intestinal injury.

Sucrase-isomaltase deficiency is rare, except in Greenland. It occurs in 5% of American Eskimos and Canadian Indians. It is inherited as an autosomal-recessive disorder. Some individuals may tolerate isomaltose.

Trehalase deficiency is very rare and related to trehalose, a sugar found in mushrooms and algae. Other types of carbohydrate malabsorption include glucose-galactose malabsorption, fructose malabsorption, and sorbitol, mannitol, and lactulose intolerance.

The diagnosis of a specific disaccharidase deficiency can be made with quantitative analysis of mucosal enzyme activities by biopsy. Lactase deficiency can be determined from the serum glucose response to an oral disaccharide load. The easiest and most reliable way of determining carbohydrate malabsorption is by measuring breath hydrogen response to an oral disaccharide load. This does require an adequate amount of fermenting colonic bacteria.

The treatment of carbohydrate intolerance is simple. For lactose intolerance, it is either avoidance of lactose or the use of lactase supplements. The treatment of sucrase-isomaltase deficiency is elimination of sucrose from the diet and limiting starch and possibly enzyme replacement therapy.

Table 3.   Population Distribution of Adult Hypolactasia

Population	Prevalence of hypolactasia, %
Northern European	5-15
Mediterranean and Near Eastern	60-85
Saharan and sub-Saharan Africa	85-100
East Asian and Pacific	90-100
Southern Asian	60-90
White American	10-25
Black American	45-80
Native American	50-95
Latin American	40-75

From Lloyd ML, Olsen WA. Disaccharide malabsorption. In: Haubrich WS, Schaffner F, editors. Bockus gastroenterology. Vol 2. 5th edition. Philadelphia: WB Saunders; 1995. p. 1087-1100. Used with permission.

Small-Bowel Neoplasia

Fortunately, malignant neoplasia of the small bowel is rare.

Adenocarcinoma

Adenocarcinoma is the most common malignancy of the small bowel. The proximal small bowel and duodenum are the most likely sites in which this malignancy arises. Possible reasons why the small bowel is relatively protected from adenocarcinoma are rapid transit through the small bowel, decreased concentration of carcinogens, enzyme systems that may detoxify carcinogens, an active gut immune system, rapidly proliferating cells, and low bacterial flora.

Disease associations with an increased risk of small-bowel adenocarcinoma include Crohn's disease, celiac disease, Peutz-Jeghers syndrome, and familial polyposis.

The most common presentation of small-bowel carcinoma is obstruction.

Lymphoma

Several types of lymphoma affect the small intestine as the primary organ. The Western type arises in normal small intestine and occurs primarily in the ileum. The Mediterranean type is associated with immunoproliferative small-bowel disease or α-chain disease. This disorder is characterized by the loss of normal mucosa and an increase in B-lymphoid cells. The lymphoma associated with celiac disease is a T-cell lymphoma and has been called enteropathy-associated T-cell lymphoma. Unlike adenocarcinoma, lymphoma rarely affects the duodenum. The most common presentation of lymphoma is obstructive symptoms.

Other Tumors

Other small-bowel tumors include stromal tumors (leiomyoma and leiomyosarcoma), carcinoid, and metastases (carcinomatosis, lymphoma, breast, melanoma).

Intestinal Lymphangiectasia

Intestinal lymphangiectasia occurs as a primary or secondary disorder. The primary disorder is rare and presents with hypoproteinemia, edema, and lymphocytopenia. The disease usually is diagnosed in childhood and may be associated with other lymphatic disorders, including lymphedema, chylothorax, or chylous ascites. Symptoms include diarrhea (93%), nausea or vomiting (6%-60%), abdominal pain (<10%), and growth retardation when presentation is earlier than age 10 years. Several other diseases have been associated with intestinal lymphangiectasia, including Noonan's syndrome, peliosis, Charcot-Marie-Tooth disease, Turner's syndrome, and hypobetalipoproteinemia.

The secondary form of intestinal lymphangiectasia can be due to congestive heart failure, neoplasia, and an assortment of inflammatory disorders (tuberculosis, sarcoid, retroperitoneal fibrosis).

Diagnosis depends on a decrease in all plasma proteins (albumin, globulins, fibrinogen, ceruloplasmin, lipoproteins, transferrin, and α_1-antitrypsin). Lymphocytopenia is present and affects mainly T lymphocytes.

Measuring the clearance of α_1-antitrypsin is the best method of proving a protein-losing enteropathy. The test is invalidated by severe α_1-antitrypsin deficiency, in neonates younger than 1 week, in Zollinger-Ellison syndrome, and with gastrointestinal bleeding. Technetium Tc 99m-labeled albumin and indium In 111-labeled transferrin are rarely used.

The disorder is treated with medium-chain triglycerides. Rarely, a localized resection may benefit the patient. For the secondary type, the underlying disorder is treated.

Eosinophilic Gastroenteritis

The disease is different depending on the tissue affected. Most forms have peripheral eosinophilia, although it does not have to be present. The sedimentation rate may be low. Less than 50% of cases have an identifiable precipitant. Mucosal disease is characterized by diarrhea, malabsorption, and protein-losing enteropathy. The submucosal pattern presents with obstructive symptoms. The serosal pattern is characterized by eosinophilic ascites and peritonitis. Diet has had a limited role in treatment. Corticosteroids usually bring about a prompt response. There are a few reports of the successful use of sodium cromoglycate.

Other Disorders With Malabsorption

Several diseases and conditions are associated with malabsorption (Table 4).

BACTERIAL OVERGROWTH

Cause

Bacterial overgrowth results from proliferation of bacteria caused by interference with the normal protective mechanisms. Gastric acid and a functioning ileocecal valve can play a role in reducing proliferation of intestinal flora. Stasis of intestinal contents as a result of impaired gastrointestinal motility, mechanical obstruction, or lack of intestinal continuity is the primary cause of the syndrome of bacterial overgrowth. Potential causes of bacterial overgrowth are listed in Table 5.

Manifestations

Bacterial overgrowth can result in malabsorption of fat, protein, and carbohydrate. Fat malabsorption can occur for several reasons. Deconjugation of conjugated bile salts by bacteria within the gut lumen is an important factor, although not the

Table 4. Diseases and Conditions Associated With Malabsorption

Infections
  Giardia lamblia
  Cryptosporidium
  Isospora belli
  Kala-azar
  Acute *Plasmodium falciparum*
  Strongyloides
  Capillaria philippinensis
Drugs
  Alcohol
  Neomycin
  Cholestyramine
  p-Aminosalicylic acid
  Aluminum hydroxide
  Colchicine
  Methotrexate
  Tetracycline
  Methyldopa
  Laxatives
Genetic disorders
  Cronkhite-Canada syndrome: severe malabsorption and
    protein-losing enteropathy
  Abetalipoproteinemia: autosomal recessive, causing a
    defect in synthesis of apolipoprotein B. Biopsy shows
    excess fat droplets in mucosal cells
  Familial enteropathy
  Specific absorption abnormalities
    Juvenile multiple carboxylase deficiency
    Iron malabsorption
    Hypophosphatemic rickets
    Familial vitamin B_{12} malabsorption (Imerslund-
      Grasbeck syndrome)
Miscellaneous disorders
  Immunoproliferative small intestinal disease (α-chain
    disease): thickened jejunum with infiltration of the
    lamina propria and submucosa; a benign disease that
    progresses to malignancy; abnormal heavy chains can
    be found in serum
  Collagen vascular diseases: scleroderma, systemic
    lupus erythematosus, rheumatoid arthritis
  Amyloidosis: most malabsorption due to bacterial
    overgrowth
  Mastocytosis: flushing, headache, tachycardia, and
    pruritus (urticaria pigmentosa). Pathogenesis of
    malabsorption in this disease is unclear. Biopsy shows
    intact villi with some edema and clubbing with
    infiltration of eosinophils and increase in mast cells.
    Patients may respond to sodium cromoglycate
Endocrine disorders
  Diabetes mellitus: autonomic dysfunction and bacterial
    overgrowth
  Hypoparathyroidism
  Thyrotoxicosis
  Hypothyroidism

Table 5. Disorders Associated With Bacterial Overgrowth of the Small Intestine

Gastric proliferation
Hypochlorhydria or achlorhydria
Gastric atony or outlet obstruction
Small intestinal stagnation
    Anatomical
        Afferent loop of gastrojejunostomy
        Duodenal or jejunal diverticulosis
        Surgical blind loop with end-to-side
          enteroenterostomy
        Obstruction (stricture, adhesion, cancer)
    Motor
        Scleroderma
        Intestinal pseudo-obstruction
        Diabetic autonomic neuropathy
        Derangements of interdigestive motor complex
    Abnormal communication between upper and lower
      gastrointestinal tracts
        Gastrocolic or jejunocolic fistula
        Resection of ileocecal valve
Miscellaneous
    Chronic pancreatitis
    Immunodeficiency syndrome
    Cirrhosis

From Toskes PP. Bacterial overgrowth syndromes. In: Haubrich WS, Schaffner F, editors. Bockus gastroenterology. Vol 2. 5th edition. Philadelphia: WB Saunders; 1995. p. 1174-82. Used with permission.

only mechanism. The deconjugation of bile salts may lead to a decrease in the concentration needed to form micelles. Deconjugated bile salts may inhibit uptake and esterification of fatty acids. Mucosal damage may impair uptake of fat and may even cause a "fat-losing enteropathy." Mucosal injury can occur as a result of metabolic products of bacterial digestion or by bacteria or bacterial toxins.

Several factors may lead to carbohydrate malabsorption, including bacterial fermentation, a decrease in brush-border enzymes enhancing carbohydrate intolerance due to mucosal damage, and destruction of mucosal disaccharidases by bacterial proteases.

Protein absorption also may be affected in overgrowth syndromes. Mechanisms include bacterial metabolism of protein-producing ammonia and fatty acids making less protein available, bacterial overgrowth causing diminished brush-border peptidase levels and decreased uptake of amino acids, and decreased enterokinase levels impairing pancreatic proteases.

Overgrowth may cause excess fluid and electrolyte losses by secretagogues (including hydroxy fatty acids and deconjugated

bile) and altered motility. Vitamin B_{12} absorption is affected primarily by anaerobic bacteria that use B_{12} even when complexed to intrinsic factor, whereas aerobic bacteria do not substantially affect the vitamin B_{12}–intrinsic factor complex. The folate value is either normal or high as a result of bacterial production and release of folate. Other vitamin or mineral deficiencies are uncommon in overgrowth syndromes.

Diagnosis

Direct aspiration of aerobes and anaerobes from small bowel is the standard for diagnosis. An abnormal result is more than 10^5 organisms/mL, although even a finding of more than 10^3 may indicate overgrowth.

Alternative methods include labeled carbon dioxide and hydrogen breath tests. Carbon 14- or 13-labeled substrates, such as ^{14}C-cholylglycine, have a sensitivity of approximately 65% and are seldom used. Simultaneous fecal bile salt analysis helps distinguish overgrowth from other causes of ileal malabsorption. Diagnostic tests for bacterial overgrowth are listed in Table 6.

[^{14}C]D-Xylose (1-g dose) is more sensitive and more specific. Sensitivities more than 95% are reported, and such tests are better than a jejunal culture. [^{13}C]D-Xylose tests do not appear to have the same sensitivity and specificity of the ^{14}C compounds.

Hydrogen breath testing can be used, although it has a reported sensitivity less than 70% with lactulose. Approximately a third of patients with overgrowth may have a high fasting breath hydrogen result.

Treatment

If the cause of overgrowth is not correctable, treatment with antibiotics can be undertaken. Numerous antibiotics have been used for treatment, and there is no obvious or proven benefit of one regimen over another. Generally, a course of therapy is given for 7 to 10 days and usually needs to be repeated when

Table 6. Diagnostic Tests for Bacterial Overgrowth

Culture of proximal small bowel contents
Urinary indican
Jejunal aspirate for fatty acids or bile acids
Breath tests
    Fasting hydrogen breath test
    [^{14}C]Bile acid breath test
    Glucose-hydrogen breath test
    [^{14}C]Xylose breath test
    [^{13}C]Xylose breath test
    Lactulose-hydrogen breath test
White cell scintigraphy (?)
Schilling test

symptoms recur. Rarely, longer courses of therapy may be necessary. Antibiotic choices include metronidazole 250 mg twice a day, tetracycline 250 mg four times a day, amoxicillin-clavulanic acid 250 to 500 mg four times a day, cephalosporins, fluoroquinolones, or chloramphenicol.

Additional measures that may help include the use of medium-chain triglycerides with restriction of dietary long-chain triglycerides, lactose-free diet or lactase supplementation, and vitamin replacement, including B_{12}.

Promotility agents also may be useful in some individuals with underlying motility disorders. Octreotide stimulates intestinal motor activity and can lead to clearance of bacteria and improvement in symptoms. Data on other agents are not available.

CHAPTER 12

Vitamins and Minerals

Stephen C. Hauser, M.D.

Vitamins and minerals are critical to normal health because of the vast assortment of metabolic functions for which they are essential. This chapter focuses on selected important vitamins and minerals and their relationships to gastrointestinal disorders.

WATER-SOLUBLE VITAMINS

Vitamin B_{12}

Dietary intake of vitamin B_{12} (cobalamin) requires the ingestion of animal products (meat, dairy, fish, and shellfish). Because cobalamin is bound to animal proteins, it must be released. Gastric contractions, gastric acid, and gastric pepsins accomplish this function. Free vitamin B_{12} then binds to salivary and gastric R proteins (haptocorrins), a process that is facilitated by the acid pH in the stomach. Gastric parietal cell production and secretion of intrinsic factor (IF) are critical for the transfer of cobalamin from haptocorrins to IF, which occurs in the duodenum and is facilitated by pancreatic proteases (degradation of haptocorrins) and the more neutral pH of the duodenum. Finally, in the terminal ileum, the cobalamin-IF complex is bound to specific receptors, and vitamin B_{12} is absorbed into the circulation bound to transcobalamin II. About half of the circulating vitamin B_{12} in cobalamin-transcobalamin II is secreted into bile, half of which recycles and half of which is excreted in stool. Cobalamin in bile is bound to a biliary haptocorrin, and this binding protein is then degraded by pancreatic proteases in the duodenum, once again liberating vitamin B_{12} for its binding to IF.

Deficiency of vitamin B_{12} results in megaloblastic anemia and hyperhomocystinemia, identical to that in folic acid deficiency.

In contrast to folate deficiency, vitamin B_{12} deficiency can cause neuropsychiatric abnormalities, including dementia and subacute combined degeneration of the posterior columns of the spinal cord (loss of lower extremity vibration and sometimes position sensation), and loss of taste, anorexia, and diarrhea. Serum methylmalonic acid levels (normal in folate deficiency) may be increased (abnormal) before vitamin B_{12} levels are subnormal. Because large amounts of cobalamin are stored in the body, especially in the liver, lack of adequate dietary vitamin B_{12} (e.g., in a person who decides to be a true vegan, without supplements) may take years to result in cobalamin deficiency. Achlorhydria is a not uncommon cause of vitamin B_{12} deficiency in the elderly. Pernicious anemia is another not uncommon cause of vitamin B_{12} deficiency due to lack of IF and acid. In contrast to achlorhydria, hyperacidity, such as that in Zollinger-Ellison syndrome, can disrupt the duodenal phase of absorption (lack of more neutral pH and inactivation of pancreatic proteases) of cobalamin and result in cobalamin deficiency. Vitamin B_{12} deficiency rarely occurs with pancreatic insufficiency itself or with the use of acid-suppressive medications. Bacterial overgrowth, infestation with *Diphyllobothrium latum*, and ileal disease or resection also can result in deficiency of vitamin B_{12}. Finally, gastric bypass surgery often is complicated by subsequent cobalamin deficiency (lack of IF, acid, and gastric grinding function). Pitfalls of the Schilling test include the use of crystalline (not food-bound) cobalamin, which bypasses the first step in vitamin B_{12} absorption (release of cobalamin from its food-bound state, such as in elderly persons with achlorhydria), false-normal values, and abnormal ileal absorption due to ileal macrocytosis (ongoing uncorrected cobalamin deficiency).

Folic Acid

There are many dietary sources of folate, including green leafy vegetables, grains, orange juice, and organ meats. Hydrolysis of dietary folylpolyglutamates is followed by active transport of folylmonoglutamates, principally in the duodenum and upper jejunum. Megaloblastic anemia, diarrhea (macrocytic enterocytes), glossitis, neural tube defects in newborns (maternal folate deficiency in the first 2 weeks of pregnancy), and increased risk of colorectal cancer and cardiovascular disease may occur as a result of folate deficiency. Persons with dietary deficiency of folate (body stores may last for up to 4 months), intestinal malabsorption states (small-bowel diseases, drugs such as sulfasalazine, methotrexate, and alcohol), pregnancy, and chronic liver disease are at increased risk of folate deficiency.

Other Water-soluble Vitamins

Vitamin C deficiency results in scurvy, which may include perifollicular hyperkeratotic papules and petechiae; swollen, red, bleeding gums; or anemia. Persons with severe malabsorptive disease and chronic alcoholics are at increased risk for vitamin C deficiency. Vitamin C supplementation can increase the risk of adverse cardiovascular events in persons with advanced iron storage disease (hemochromatosis). Thiamine (vitamin B_1) deficiency can result in beriberi with cardiac (cardiomyopathy, high-output failure) or neurologic (peripheral neuropathy, cerebellar dysfunction, gaze pareses, Wernicke-Korsakoff syndrome) disorders, which may be exacerbated by glucose administration to thiamine-deficient patients. Chronic alcoholism, pregnancy, and chronic malnutrition all are risk factors for thiamine deficiency. Riboflavin (vitamin B_2) deficiency can cause angular stomatitis, cheilosis, glossitis, a seborrheic dermatitis, and visual impairment. Persons with chronic alcoholism and malabsorptive disorders are at risk. Niacin (vitamin B_3) deficiency due to malabsorptive syndromes, chronic alcoholism, carcinoid syndrome, and isoniazid therapy can result in pellagra (diarrhea, dermatitis, and dementia), glossitis, and angular stomatitis. Pyridoxine (vitamin B_6) deficiency can occur in patients treated with isoniazid, hydralazine, oral contraceptives, dopamine, and D-penicillamine. Malabsorptive syndromes and chronic alcoholism also are risk factors. Glossitis, cheilosis, angular stomatitis, a seborrheic dermatitis, sideroblastic anemia, and peripheral neuropathy may supervene. Vitamin B_6 deficiency may be responsible for both the only modest increase of the aminotransferase values and the increased ratio of aspartate aminotransferase to alanine aminotransferase in alcoholic hepatitis.

FAT-SOLUBLE VITAMINS

Vitamin A

Like the other fat-soluble vitamins, absorption of vitamin A requires luminal bile salts and pancreatic esterases, assembly into chylomicrons, and lymphatic transport. Lack of vitamin A can result in night blindness, xerophthalmia, a follicular hyperkeratotic rash, abnormal taste and smell, and increased risk of infections. Liver disease may be accompanied by vitamin A deficiency, especially alcoholic liver disease. However, persons with alcoholic liver disease and vitamin A deficiency who are given supplements of vitamin A are at risk of hepatotoxicity. Similar to other fat-soluble vitamins, excess vitamin A can cause toxicity (liver failure, increased cerebrospinal fluid pressure, desquamating rash, vitamin D, alopecia, hypercalcemia).

Vitamin D

Diet, dietary supplementation, and sunlight result in adequate vitamin D levels. Liver disease and kidney disease, as well as malabsorptive conditions, are the major risk factors for vitamin D deficiency. Excess vitamin D can result in anorexia, nausea, vomiting, constipation and abdominal pain (hypercalcemia), and polyuria and kidney stones (hypercalciuria).

Vitamin E

Malabsorptive disorders and, in particular, chronic cholestasis in children are major risk factors for vitamin E deficiency. Manifestations of vitamin E deficiency include neurologic symptoms (posterior column disease, peripheral neuropathy, brainstem and cranial nerve damage), retinal disease, and hemolysis. High doses of vitamin E may cause coagulation disorders.

Vitamin K

Vitamin K is acquired from exogenous dietary sources (green leafy vegetables) and endogenous (intestinal bacteria) sources. Malabsorptive syndromes, dietary inadequacy, and antibiotic administration are risk factors for vitamin K deficiency. Factor VII usually is the rate-limiting factor for a normal prothrombin time (or international normalized ratio).

MINERALS

Iron

Loss of endogenous iron from the gastrointestinal tract, urinary tract, and skin and menstrual loss in women need to be matched by iron absorption from the duodenum and upper jejunum. Iron contained in the form of heme from meat is much more readily absorbed (up to 25%) than inorganic ferric iron salts (3%-10%). Gastric grinding, gastric acid, and gastric ascorbate help make ferric iron compounds more soluble. Ferric reductase (duodenal cytochrome B), as well as ascorbate, reduce inorganic iron from the ferric to the ferrous form. An iron transporter, divalent metal transporter 1, facilitates absorption of ferrous iron. Ferroportin 1 with the ferroxidase hephaestin transports iron into the circulation, oxidizes it to the ferric form, and allows it to bind to transferrin. Normally, with adequate total body iron stores, up to about 10% of dietary inorganic iron can be absorbed. With iron deficiency, this may increase to 30%.

Iron deficiency can result in microcytic hypochromic anemia, angular stomatitis, koilonychia, and atrophic lingual papillae. Lack of dietary iron, increased gastrointestinal loss of iron (bleeding), poor absorption of iron (upper small bowel mucosal dysfunction, such as that in celiac disease), bypass of the upper small bowel (gastrojejunal bypass surgery), gastric resection and achlorhydria, and persistent ingestion of iron-binding compounds (soil, laundry starch) all can contribute to iron deficiency. Iron overload is discussed in Chapter 34, Metabolic Liver Disease.

Zinc

Zinc is required as a cofactor for many enzymes (e.g., alkaline phosphatase), and its deficiency impairs growth, development, and reproductive and immune functions. Chronic diarrhea, short-bowel syndrome, cystic fibrosis, pancreatic insufficiency, cirrhosis, alcoholism, chronic renal failure, anorexia nervosa, pregnancy, sickle cell anemia, and use of the drug D-penicillamine are risk factors for zinc deficiency. A scaly red rash involving the face, groin, and hands may occur with zinc deficiency itself or as a result of the autosomal recessive disorder of zinc metabolism, acrodermatitis enteropathica. Alopecia, loss of taste, growth retardation, poor wound healing, hypogonadism, diarrhea, and night blindness also may occur as a result of zinc deficiency. Excess zinc intake (e.g., supplements, such as those used in the treatment of Wilson's disease) can result in copper deficiency.

Copper

Copper deficiency can result in a microcytic hypochromic anemia, leukopenia, neutropenia, diarrhea, and bony changes. Clinical conditions in adults predisposing to copper deficiency include total parenteral nutrition without copper supplementation, malabsorptive syndromes, and chronic biliary fistulas. Toxicity from excess administration of oral copper includes acute hemorrhagic gastritis.

Miscellaneous Minerals

Deficiencies of selenium (cardiomyopathy, myositis), chromium (hyperglycemia, neurologic symptoms), or manganese (night blindness, tachycardia, tachypnea, headache, vomiting) may develop in patients receiving long-term total parenteral nutrition or tube feeding.

RECOMMENDED READING

Annibale B, Capurso G, Delle Fave G. The stomach and iron deficiency anaemia: a forgotten link. Dig Liver Dis. 2003;35:288-95.

Basu TK, Donaldson D. Intestinal absorption in health and disease: micronutrients. Best Pract Res Clin Gastroenterol. 2003;17:957-79.

Klein S. A primer of nutritional support for gastroenterologists. Gastroenterology. 2002;122:1677-87.

Leslie WD, Bernstein CN, Leboff MS, American Gastroenterological Association Clinical Practice Committee. AGA technical review on osteoporosis in hepatic disorders. Gastroenterology. 2003;125:941-66.

Miret S, Simpson RJ, McKie AT. Physiology and molecular biology of dietary iron absorption. Annu Rev Nutr. 2003;23:283-301. Epub 2003 Feb 26.

Scott EM, Gaywood I, Scott BB, British Society of Gastroenterology. Guidelines for osteoporosis in coeliac disease and inflammatory bowel disease. Gut. 2000;46 Suppl 1:1-8.

CHAPTER 13

Nutrition Disorders and Parenteral and Enteral Nutrition

Darlene G. Kelly, M.D., Ph.D.

Nutrition is closely related to gastroenterology. Many gastrointestinal diseases have a major impact on nutrition status, and nutrition therapy has an impact on many gastrointestinal diseases.

WHEN IS NUTRITION SUPPORT BENEFICIAL?
Nutrition support with enteral or parenteral nutrition should be considered for normally nourished patients expected to be without oral intake for more than 7 to 10 days. For patients who are malnourished, the time to starting nutrition support is adjusted depending on the degree of malnutrition, the estimated metabolic stress, and the expected duration of lack of oral intake.

WHAT IS THE BEST INDICATOR OF MALNUTRITION?
The only criterion of malnutrition that has proved to offer predictive value is unintentional weight loss during the prior 3 months. Patients who have lost more than 20% of baseline weight have severe protein-calorie malnutrition. Those who have lost 10% to 20% of body weight in that period have moderate protein-calorie malnutrition. A weight loss of less than 10% of body weight in 3 months is considered to be mild protein-calorie malnutrition.

WHEN SHOULD NUTRITION SUPPORT BE STARTED IN MALNOURISHED PATIENTS?
For patients who are severely malnourished, nutrition support should be started immediately if oral intake is not possible. In those who are mildly malnourished, nutrition support should be started within 3 to 5 days. For those who are not malnourished, a period of 7 to 10 days without oral intake is generally well tolerated as long as fluids and electrolytes are maintained.

SHOULD NUTRITION SUPPORT BE ENTERAL (TUBE FEEDING) OR PARENTERAL?
The basic guideline for source of nutrition is "If the gut works, use it." If there is a delivery problem, such as inability to swallow, gastroparesis, or unwillingness to eat, the enteral route is indicated. However, if there is a problem with digestion or absorption, parenteral nutrition is appropriate.

SHOULD THE PATIENT DECIDE THE ROUTE OF NUTRITION?
A recent publication indicated that the patient should decide the route of nutrition, but risks, benefits, and costs must be considered. Enteral nutrition is associated with fewer risks to the patient's health and survival. The cost of enteral nutrition is a fraction of the cost of parenteral nutrition.

WHAT ARE THE TYPES OF FORMULA USED FOR ENTERAL NUTRITION?
Standard tube feeding formulas, in general, are least expensive, providing about 1 kcal/mL. Typically, they are lactose-free and gluten-free. They contain variable amounts of long- and medium-chain triglycerides, as well as intact protein; they are usually isotonic; and they provide complete nutrition at intakes of 1,500 to 2,000 kcal.

Calorically dense formulas contain 1.5 to 2 kcal/mL. They are hypertonic. Because they do not provide adequate water, additional water usually must be given by tube flushes to avoid dehydration.

Nutrition-dense formulas provide extra amounts of protein or lipid. Many contain added special nutrients. Examples are immunomodulating formulas that include ω-3 fatty acids, RNA, and arginine; glutamine-containing formulas; and fiber-containing formulas. Many of these are more expensive than standard formulas.

Elemental formulas contain free amino acids; thus, they are hypertonic with osmolalities as high as 700 mOsm/kg. Semi-elemental formulas contain partially hydrolyzed proteins yielding small peptides. Some are isotonic. These formulas also are more expensive than the basic formulas.

Disease-specific formulas are designed for diabetes, pulmonary disease, renal disease, and hepatic disease. In general, there are no data to support the use of these expensive formulas.

WHAT ARE THE CHOICES FOR LOCATIONS OF FEEDING AND FOR TUBES?

Nasogastric tubes, percutaneous endoscopic gastrostomy tubes, or surgical G tubes all can be used for intragastric feedings. These use normal gastric emptying and sometimes have been considered to be more physiologic. This route allows bolus feedings and infusing feedings by gravity without requiring infusion pumps. When these feedings are given in the hospital, infusion rates typically are monitored by checking residual volumes within the stomach. This approach is intended to minimize the risk of aspiration. Institutions' guidelines vary, but, usually, if the residual volume exceeds 200 mL or more than half the hourly infusion rate, feeding should be held and the residual volume rechecked in 1 hour. Persistently high residual volumes may indicate that jejunal feedings should be used.

Nasoenteric tubes, percutaneous endoscopic jejunostomies, percutaneous endoscopic gastrostomy with a jejunal extension tube, or surgical J tubes have been purported to decrease aspiration. Infusion pumps are required in most cases.

WHAT ARE THE CONTRAINDICATIONS TO ENTERAL NUTRITION?

The following are general contraindications to enteral feedings: inability to establish enteral access, bowel obstruction, severe intestinal dysmotility (pseudo-obstruction), high-output fistula (unless tubes can be placed beyond the fistula origin), intractable vomiting, intractable severe diarrhea, bowel ischemia, severe malabsorption, and patient refusal.

WHAT ARE THE MOST COMMON COMPLICATIONS OF ENTERAL NUTRITION?

Problems with tube placement are among the most serious complications. These can result in infusion of the formula into the lungs. Consequently, confirmation of the tube site is essential *before* the tube is used.

Diarrhea rarely results from the formula itself. The risk of diarrhea occurring from a formula can be minimized by using an isotonic formula and slowly increasing the infusion rate. More commonly, the diarrhea is related to other issues. In the evaluation of diarrhea during tube feeding, one should determine whether the patient is receiving sorbitol-containing medications, magnesium-containing antacids, and hypertonic oral preparations such as potassium. Another explanation is gut atrophy after a period of time without enteral feedings. This reverses quickly with resumption of oral nutrients. Additionally, many patients have received antibiotics, and these may have altered gut flora and caused diarrhea, even in the absence of *Clostridium difficile*.

Tube discomfort can be decreased by polyurethane feeding tubes. Furthermore, the smallest possible tube should be used. Esophageal strictures can be avoided by using a standard feeding tube rather than a large nasogastric tube.

Some medications may interact with formula components. For example, phenytoin is bound by feeding formula, and vitamin K alters anticoagulation by warfarin.

Tube clogging is a common complication in patients receiving enteral nutrition. This can be minimized by using a tube of adequate caliber. Care must be taken to use water flushes after administration of medications and during infusion of the feeding.

Aspiration of feeding formula can be avoided by elevating the head of the bed to 30°. The use of postpyloric feeding tubes to prevent aspiration is not well supported by the literature.

WHAT ARE THE COMPONENTS OF A PARENTERAL NUTRITION FORMULA?

Formulas vary with institutional guidelines. In general, calories usually are provided at about basal needs (basal metabolic rate) for patients in an intensive care unit, and at a level to provide basal needs +20% for ambulatory patients. For long-term home parenteral nutrition (HPN), calories are adjusted as needed to support weight gain or to maintain weight.

Macronutrients include amino acids (1-1.5 g/kg body weight) that provide 4 kcal/g, dextrose that provides 3.4 kcal/g (hydrated formula is less calorically dense than free carbohydrate), and lipid formulations (primarily linoleic acid, soybean-based, available in the United States) that provide 1.1 kcal/mL of 10% and 2 kcal/mL of 20% lipid. New lipid formulations using medium-chain lipid are being studied, and olive oil-based formulas are being used in Europe.

Multivitamin formulas for parenteral use, as mandated by the Food and Drug Administration, contain 13 water-soluble and fat-soluble vitamins, now including 150 µg of vitamin K per dose and very high amounts of vitamin C.

Minerals include calcium, phosphorus, and magnesium, which are added individually. Calcium phosphate can precipitate and cause emboli, a lethal complication, so amounts of calcium and phosphorus are monitored closely to prevent this complication. Trace elements are available as combinations of four, five, six, and seven elements. The formulas containing only zinc, copper, chromium, and manganese (MTE4) must not be used for long-term total parenteral nutrition (TPN) because they are devoid of selenium and have been associated with many cases of deficiency of this trace element. For long-term use, MTE5 (also contains selenium) is *essential*.

WHAT ARE THE MOST COMMON COMPLICATIONS OF PARENTERAL NUTRITION?

Mechanical complications include pneumothorax (~4% of line placements), which is most common in emaciated patients; malposition of the catheter tip; and, rarely, hydropneumothorax, hemothorax, arterial insertion, or brachial plexus injury. Normal wear and tear of long-term lines can be repaired with the line in situ.

Catheter infections are the most common complication. For inpatients, catheters usually are removed without attempts at treatment. For stable outpatients with long-term central lines, attempts should be made to treat most infections with the catheter in situ. Infections present as bacteremias and fungemias, exit site infections, and tract infections involving the tunneled portion of the catheter. Catheter tract infections cannot be treated effectively and do require catheter removal.

Central venous thrombosis is clinically evident in 1% to 4% of central lines and is radiologically evident in 20% to 45%. Pulmonary emboli are unusual in the setting of central venous thrombosis due to central lines.

Nutrient excess or deficiency is not uncommon. There is recent evidence for manganese deposition in the basal ganglia of humans receiving HPN, and neurologic manifestations have been reported in experimental animals. Aluminum toxicity due to contamination of TPN components may cause deposition in bone, increasing the fracture potential. Copper and manganese excesses can occur in patients with cholestatic liver disease related to HPN. Chromium deficiency has been reported to cause weight loss, peripheral neuropathy, and glucose intolerance in patients receiving HPN. Selenium deficiency occurs in patients on HPN who are not receiving selenium; severe cardiomyopathy, muscle pain and tenderness, white nail beds, and macrocytosis are possible sequelae. Iron deficiency anemia occurs in some patients

receiving HPN. Normally iron is not a component of TPN, although iron dextran can be added to TPN bags not containing lipid if the patient has had a test dose without reaction.

Metabolic bone disease has been reported in patients receiving HPN. Whether long-term TPN is an independent risk factor for osteomalacia and osteoporosis is not certain. Many patients who receive TPN are already at risk for metabolic bone disease because of prolonged malabsorption, malnutrition, and corticosteroid use. Many have osteomalacia at the time TPN is initiated. Factors that may predispose consumers of HPN to bone disease include large sodium and amino acid loads, hyperinsulinemia from large dextrose loads, cycling TPN, aluminum contamination, high phosphate loads, and heparin added to TPN bags.

TPN-related hepatobiliary disease may take the form of temporarily increased liver enzyme values, cholestasis, sludge and gallstones, and hepatocellular disease. Particularly in neonates, a very aggressive cholestatic process is common, although this progressive liver disease now is more common in adults than previously. Factors that may predispose to liver disease in association with HPN include use of large amounts of lipids, systemic infusion of nutrients (compared with portal route with first-pass hepatic clearance for oral nutrients), sepsis, small intestinal bacterial overgrowth with increased lithocholic acid production, decreased enterohepatic circulation, and various nutrient excesses and deficiencies.

WHAT ARE THE RISKS ASSOCIATED WITH AGGRESSIVE THERAPY OF MALNUTRITION?

Refeeding syndrome can occur in the severely malnourished patient in whom high-glucose, high-volume feedings are started abruptly. It presents as a result of electrolyte (notably potassium, magnesium, phosphate) shifts from the extracellular space to the intracellular space which leave the patient profoundly hypokalemic, hypomagnesemic, and hypophosphatemic. There is altered glucose metabolism. Increased reabsorption of sodium and water in the kidney occurs rapidly with initiation of feeding. Sequelae include rapid expansion of the extracellular fluid space, anasarca, congestive heart failure, respiratory depression, respiratory acidosis, ketoacidosis, neuromuscular dysfunction, increased erythrocyte affinity for oxygen resulting in tissue hypoxia, osmotic diuresis, prerenal azotemia, hypotension, and hyperosmolar nonketotic coma. Sudden death can result. Although refeeding syndrome occurs most commonly with TPN, it also can occur with enteral nutrition.

Refeeding syndrome can be avoided by the use of parenteral thiamine (100 mg/day for 3 days), slow initiation of feeding with liberal amounts of potassium, magnesium, and phosphate, conservative use of dextrose (100-150 g initially), sodium and volume adjustment as indicated by clinical examination (attention to evolving edema), and attention to intake and output records and laboratory results.

Persons at risk include those with protein-calorie malnutrition due to underfeeding or malabsorption, chronic alcoholics, the morbidly obese with massive weight loss, those who receive no oral intake for 7 to 10 days with evidence of stress and nutritional depletion, and those who have had prolonged intravenous hydration or fasting.

WHAT ARE THE SEQUELAE OF VITAMIN AND MINERAL DEFICIENCY?

Table 1 lists the consequences of deficiencies.

RECOMMENDED READING

Buchman AL, editor. Clinical Nutrition in Gastrointestinal Disease. Therofare, NJ: Slack (in press).

Jacobs DO, editor. Proceedings of the Home Parenteral and Enteral Workshop. JPEN J Parenter Enteral Nutr. 2002 Suppl:26:S1-75.

Table 1. Sequelae of Vitamin and Mineral Deficiencies

Vitamin or mineral	Sequelae of deficiency
Vitamin A	Night blindness, Bitot's spots, conjunctival xerosis
Vitamin D	Nausea, vomiting, weakness, fatigue, diarrhea, anorexia, confusion, psychosis, headache, hypercalciuria
Vitamin E	Increased platelet aggregation, decreased erythrocyte survival, hemolytic anemia, neuronal degeneration, decreased deep tendon reflexes
Vitamin K	Excess bruising, bleeding
Vitamin C	Bleeding gums, petechiae, impaired wound healing, fatigue, depression, anorexia, muscle pain, increased susceptibility to stress and infections
Thiamine	Paresthesias, anesthesia, weakness (especially lower extremities), cardiac failure, hepatomegaly, tachycardia, oliguria, Wernicke's encephalopathy
Riboflavin	Cheilosis, angular stomatitis, glossitis, seborrheic dermatitis (face and scrotum), photophobia, corneal vascularization, normochromic/normocytic anemia
Niacin	Dermatitis, diarrhea, dementia, apathy, depression, vomiting, headache, fatigue
Pyridoxine, vitamin B_6	Seborrheic dermatitis, microcytic anemia, convulsions, confusion, angular stomatitis, glossitis, cheilosis
Vitamin B_{12}	Megaloblastic anemia, macrocytosis, hypersegmented neutrophils, leukopenia, thrombocytopenia, neurologic symptoms
Folic acid	Megaloblastic/macrocytic anemia
Pantothenic acid	(Only with metabolic antagonists or synthetic diet free of pathothenic acid) Listlessness, fatigue, irritability, restlessness, malaise, nausea, abdominal cramps, vomiting, diarrhea, muscle cramps, staggering gait
Choline	Fatty liver
Biotin	Anorexia, pallor, glossitis, nausea, vomiting, hair loss, lethargy, depression
Iron	Microcytic, hypochromic anemia
Calcium	Metabolic bone disease
Magnesium	Neuromuscular hyperexcitability, weakness
Copper	Microcytic anemia (conditioned iron deficiency), Menkes (kinky hair) syndrome
Zinc	Growth arrest, hypogonadism, suppressed cellular immunity, poor wound healing, slowed hair growth, decreased plasma proteins
Selenium	Dilated cardiomyopathy, muscular weakness
Manganese	Abnormal collagen growth, altered prothrombin levels
Molybdenum	Low uric acid level, increased oxypurines, neurologic abnormalities, coma
Iodine	Hypothyroidism, goiter
Chromium	Glucose intolerance

Small Bowel and Nutrition

Questions and Answers

QUESTIONS

Multiple Choice (choose the one best answer)

1. A 24-year-old woman presents with a 3-month history of diarrhea with a 20-lb weight loss. She has no family history, no travel history, no alcohol use, and no other associated symptoms. Laboratory studies indicate mild iron deficiency anemia. A fecal fat study shows 28 g of fat/24 h. Results of D-xylose study are abnormal. Small-bowel radiography is normal. The endomysial antibody value is increased. What should be done next?
   a. Pancreatic function testing
   b. Quantitative small-bowel culture
   c. Small-bowel biopsy
   d. Tissue transglutaminase assay
   e. Treatment with a gluten-free diet

2. In the patient described in question 1, celiac disease is diagnosed and a gluten-free diet is started. Instructions for dietary compliance would allow for which of the following grains in a gluten-free diet?
   a. Rye
   b. Wheat
   c. Millet
   d. Oats
   e. Barley

3. Scenario 1: While following a strict gluten-free diet, the woman described in questions 1 and 2 responds well but diarrhea recurs after about 6 months. She denies any other symptoms. Her stool frequency is 5 or 6 times a day. Review of her diet shows strict compliance, and the endomysial antibody value is now normal. Stool studies show only 6 g of fat/24 h. What is the next step?
   a. Repeat the small-bowel biopsy
   b. Small-bowel follow-through
   c. Abdominal computed tomography
   d. Colonoscopy with biopsies
   e. Bacterial aspirate of small-bowel contents

4. Scenario 2: While following a strict gluten-free diet, the woman described in questions 1 and 2 responds well but diarrhea recurs after about 6 months. She denies any other symptoms. Her stool frequency is 5 or 6 times a day. Review of her diet shows strict compliance, and the endomysial antibody value is now normal. Stool studies show 36 g of fat/24 h. What would *not* be included in the evaluation?
   a. Repeated small-bowel biopsy
   b. Abdominal computed tomography
   c. Small-bowel follow-through
   d. Pancreatic function testing
   e. Colonoscopy with biopsies

5. The patient described in questions 1 and 2 has several family members who are asymptomatic. What is an appropriate screening recommendation for her siblings?
   a. HLA typing
   b. Small-bowel biopsy
   c. Intestinal permeability studies
   d. Serologic testing
   e. Nothing until symptoms develop

6. The 28-year-old sister of the patient described in questions 1 and 2 had started following a gluten-free diet more than a year ago because of some information she had found on the Internet. She now wants to know whether she has celiac disease. She is asymptomatic. What should you recommend?
   a. HLA typing
   b. Small-bowel biopsy
   c. Intestinal permeability studies
   d. Serologic testing
   e. Nothing until symptoms develop

7. A 55-year-old man presents to his physician with complaints of diarrhea and weight loss. He had operation for refractory ulcer disease 10 years earlier. He thinks part of his stomach was removed. He has had intermittent diarrhea for many years, particularly when he eats sweets, but it has worsened during the past 6 months. He has lost about 25 lb. The patient has macrocytosis without any history of alcohol intake. The hemoglobin value is 11.6 g/dL, and the mean corpuscular volume is 102 fL. His reticulocyte count is normal. Stool studies show 18 g of fat/24 h and a volume of 350 mL/day. What is the next study?
   a. Colonoscopy
   b. Esophagogastroduodenoscopy with duodenal aspirate
   c. Computed tomography
   d. Upper gastrointestinal series and small-bowel follow-through
   e. Stool electrolyte test

8. What should be the treatment for bacterial overgrowth?
   a. Metronidazole
   b. Ciprofloxacin
   c. Tetracycline
   d. Amoxicillin/clavulanate potassium
   e. Any of the above

9. For the patient described in question 7, which of the following scenarios is likely to be present with the macrocytic anemia if the cause of his problem is bacterial overgrowth?
   a. Low vitamin B_{12}, low folate values
   b. Normal vitamin B_{12}, low folate values
   c. Low vitamin B_{12}, high folate values
   d. Normal vitamin B_{12}, normal folate values
   e. None of the above

10. The patient described in question 7 responds to a course of antibiotics but his symptoms recur in about 6 weeks. He again responds to a course of therapy. However, the symptoms return after a month. What do you recommend?
    a. Daily low-dose antibiotics
    b. *Lactobacillus*

c. Tegaserod
d. Surgical consultation to shorten the limb
e. A monthly course of antibiotics

11. A 63-year-old woman presents with anorexia, weight loss, hair loss, and diarrhea. She complains that her food "tastes bad." Twenty-five years ago, she underwent a vagotomy and antrectomy for peptic ulcer disease. Recently, she was questioned by the police for putting garbage bags onto neighbors' cars. On physical examination, the tongue is erythematous with atrophic lingual papillae. Which of the following is most likely?
    a. She is hypothyroid
    b. She has pancreatic insufficiency
    c. A serum methylmalonic acid level is increased
    d. A serum homocysteine level is decreased
    e. Her basal acid output is 12 mmol/h

12. A 53-year-old woman is admitted to the medical intensive care unit with a history of recent-onset confusion. Her family notes that "she drinks a lot, eats poorly, and bumps into things." She has had chronic diarrhea and substantial weight loss. On admission, she is alert, disoriented, confused, and weak. She has tachycardia and slightly diminished blood pressure and temperature. The blood glucose value is slightly low, and she has a mild metabolic acidosis. Which of the following is more important to administer intravenously?
    a. Glucose
    b. Bicarbonate
    c. Phosphorus
    d. Thiamine
    e. Thyroid hormone

13. A 38-year-old man presents with anorexia, hair loss, diarrhea, and a rash. He says his food "tastes bad." He drives a beer truck and recently has had to stop driving at night. On physical examination he has a scaly, red rash on the palms of his hands and around the corners of his mouth and nasolabial folds. Which of the following is most likely?
    a. Diminished serum vitamin A level
    b. Increased serum vitamin A level
    c. Diminished plasma zinc level
    d. Syphilis
    e. Hyperthyroidism

14. In a 23-year-old woman, anemia develops 3 years after successful Roux-en-Y gastrojejunal bypass. Her weight decreased from 310 lb preoperatively to 250 lb 2 years later, and her current weight is 185 lb. Her blood smear shows hypochromic microcytic red blood cells. Her physical

examination is unremarkable. A stool sample is guaiac-negative. Which of the following is the next best course of action?

a. Iron supplementation
b. Colonoscopy
c. Capsule enteroscopy
d. Vitamin B$_{12}$ supplementation
e. Chromium supplementation

15. A 49-year-old man with a long history of alcoholism and diarrhea had recent development of a scaly, hyperpigmented rash involving his face, neck, and the tops of his hands. Two months ago he had positive results of the purified protein derivative test and isoniazid therapy was begun. His skin findings, given the history, are most consistent with which of the following?

a. Riboflavin deficiency
b. Carcinoid syndrome
c. Cutaneous tuberculosis
d. Pyridoxine deficiency
e. Niacin deficiency

16. A 71-year-old man is admitted, intubated, to the intensive care unit after a car accident. His wife says that he has lost 25 lb during the past 3 months. You are consulted regarding a feeding program for this patient. What would you recommend?

a. Immediate total parenteral nutrition because of the ventilator
b. Enteral feedings through a percutaneous endoscopic gastrostomy tube after 5 days
c. Immediate enteral feedings through a nasogastric tube
d. D5W, normal saline with 20 mEq/L potassium chloride until the ventilator is no longer being used
e. Enteral feedings through a percutaneous endoscopic jejunostomy tube after 5 days

17. A 66-year-old woman with a long history of diabetes presents with nausea, vomiting, and postprandial abdominal discomfort. She has lost 15 lb in the last 3 months. She has had peripheral neuropathy for several years and has an increased creatinine level. She has recently undergone laser coagulation of retinal hemorrhages. What approach to long-term nutrition support would you consider?

a. Home total parenteral nutrition
b. A pureed oral diet
c. Enteral feedings through a percutaneous endoscopic gastrostomy tube
d. Enteral feedings through a laparoscopically placed jejunostomy tube
e. A low-fat diet

18. A 49-year-old alcoholic patient is admitted with a weight loss of 20 kg during the past 6 months; his current weight is 50 kg. His body mass index is 13.2. He has been actively drinking during the past 6 months. On admission, the house officer decided to "beef him up" and started total parenteral nutrition, 2 L daily consisting of 100 g of amino acids, 250 mL 10% lipid, and 400 g of dextrose, a multivitamin dose, and "standard" electrolytes and trace elements. You are consulted on day 3 because of severe edema, dyspnea, and lethargy. What is the most likely issue related to his nutrition?

a. The patient is thiamine-deficient and has altered glucose metabolism (remember the Krebs cycle?)
b. He is hypophosphatemic and probably has respiratory muscle weakness
c. He has congestive heart failure related to overfeeding
d. He has refeeding syndrome and total body depletion of magnesium, potassium, and phosphorus
e. All of the above

19. A 55-year-old woman is referred to you because she complains of fatigue. She has been receiving total parenteral nutrition at home for 4 years because of short-bowel syndrome resulting from multiple intestinal resections for radiation enteritis. On examination, she has marked tenderness of the calves. A chest radiograph shows an enlarged cardiac silhouette. What would you consider doing next?

a. Check the selenium level
b. Check the creatinine kinase level
c. Check the albumin level
d. Measure folate levels
e. Check the chromium level

20. You are asked to see a 30-year-old man in the hospital who has an aspartate aminotransferase value of 2 times the upper limit of normal. He has severe Crohn's disease with extensive stricturing. Total parenteral nutrition was started 10 days ago because he has lost weight and the surgeons want to delay surgical intervention. The man has had no known history of liver disease and does not drink significant amounts of alcohol. Which of the following considerations should be made in evaluating the abnormal liver enzyme value?

a. Check for any medications that cause aminotransferase increases
b. Determine whether he has any risks for hepatitis
c. Review the total parenteral nutrition formula to ensure that overfeeding is not an issue
d. If other test results are negative, be assured that aminotransferase values are often increased after 1 to 2 weeks of total parenteral nutrition and usually improve during the subsequent 2 to 4 weeks
e. All of the above

ANSWERS

1. Answer c

The steatorrhea and abnormal D-xylose result indicate small-bowel disease. The increased endomysial antibody value is highly suggestive of celiac disease. A tissue transglutaminase test would not add anything at this point. In cases of suspected celiac disease, a small-bowel biopsy is always indicated. Treatment should never be started without a firm diagnosis because of the difficulty of proving the diagnosis when the patient is receiving a gluten-free diet. Pancreatic function testing and quantitative small-bowel culture would not be performed at this point given the high probability of celiac disease.

2. Answer c

Wheat, rye, and barley are all prohibited in a gluten-free diet. Oats are permitted in Europe but generally are not allowed in the United States because of contamination in processing. There is considerable debate on the issue of allowing oats.

3. Answer d

In this scenario, the patient responded to a gluten-free diet but has recurrence of diarrhea. However, this time she does not have steatorrhea. One of the most common causes of recurrent diarrhea in patients with treated celiac disease is microscopic colitis detected on random colonic biopsy specimens from normal-appearing mucosa.

4. Answer e

In this scenario, the recurrent steatorrhea but negative serologic results indicate dietary compliance. However, refractory sprue or lymphoma may be developing and thus a small-bowel biopsy, small-bowel follow-through, and computed tomography are needed. Patients with celiac disease also have a higher incidence of pancreatic insufficiency and may require pancreatic function testing. Colonoscopy would not be indicated for steatorrhea.

5. Answer d

In asymptomatic individuals, serologic tissue transglutaminase or endomysial antibody testing is adequate. If celiac disease is highly suspected, a biopsy is indicated even with negative serologic results.

6. Answer a

The diagnosis of celiac disease is very difficult in asymptomatic individuals following a gluten-free diet because serologic and biopsy results may be negative. HLA typing will at least establish whether the person is at risk with the DQ2 focus. Very few individuals with celiac disease are DQ2-negative.

7. Answer b

The patient has mild steatorrhea with previous operation, possibly a Billroth II procedure. The previous diarrhea is indicative of dumping, but something has changed. One possibility is stenosis of the afferent limb causing bacterial overgrowth. The diagnosis would best be determined with aspiration of the afferent limb for bacteria. A small-bowel follow-through might give a clue to the anatomy but will not confirm the diagnosis. Stool electrolyte studies are unnecessary in documented steatorrhea. There is no reason to start with computed tomography for evaluating steatorrhea unless pancreatic cancer is suspected.

8. Answer e

All of these antibiotics have proved effective for treating bacterial overgrowth. There are no studies showing superiority of one over another.

9. Answer c

Bacterial overgrowth results in consumption of ingested vitamin B_{12} but production of bacterial folate. Diminished B_{12} levels and B_{12} deficiency will not occur for at least 4 years after stopping vitamin B_{12} ingestion.

10. Answer e

The best therapy is a monthly course of antibiotics with rotating antibiotics to diminish resistant strains. Daily antibiotic therapy is rarely needed. There are no convincing data that a blind loop can be repopulated with *Lactobacillus*. There also is no proof that prokinetic agents help blind loops empty better. Operation would be indicated only with an obstructed or very long loop.

11. Answer c

This patient most likely has vitamin B_{12} deficiency with anorexia, abnormal taste, diarrhea (macrocytosis of intestinal lining cells), neuropsychiatric abnormalities, and glossitis. Her previous operation and her age could be responsible (gastric atrophy, loss of parietal cells). The most sensitive test result for vitamin B_{12} deficiency is an increased serum methylmalonic acid. Serum homocysteine levels also would be increased (not decreased). She could be hypothyroid (association with autoimmune pernicious anemia), but there is no evidence for pancreatic insufficiency. Although pancreatic insufficiency decreases vitamin B_{12} absorption, it rarely causes clinical vitamin B_{12} deficiency. After a vagotomy, she should not have an increased basal acid output.

12. Answer d

The best answer is thiamine. This alcohol-ingesting patient is chronically ill with diarrhea, and her weakness, confusion, bumping into things (ataxia), tachycardia (high-output heart failure), and acidosis (lactic acidosis) most likely represent features of thiamine deficiency with Wernicke's syndrome. Although her glucose value is slightly low, administration of glucose before that of thiamine could be disastrous. Likewise, administration of thyroid hormone (slightly low temperature) could be dangerous if she has hypothyroidism due to pituitary disease (hence, hypoadrenalism as well). Bicarbonate for the mild acidosis and phosphorus repletion (refeeding syndrome) might be needed later, but they are not as important as administration of thiamine before glucose.

13. Answer c

This patient's rash and the alopecia, loss of taste, diarrhea, and night blindness fit best with zinc deficiency, which is associated with alcoholism. Vitamin A deficiency, which also occurs in alcoholics, can cause night blindness, but the rash is follicular hyperkeratotic. Vitamin A toxicity can cause alopecia and a desquamating rash. Syphilis can include red rashes on the palms. Hyperthyroidism can cause fast-transit diarrhea.

14. Answer a

This patient most likely is iron-deficient as a result of decreased intake (her operation, small gastric pouch), lack of gastric grinding activity, lack of gastric acid production, and bypass of the duodenum, hence the development of a hypochromic microcytic anemia. Colonoscopy and capsule enteroscopy to look for a bleeding source are not indicated in this 23-year-old patient with guaiac-negative stool. Vitamin B_{12} supplementation is required in patients who have had a bypass, but not for the anemia described. Chromium deficiency does not cause a hypochromic microcytic anemia (copper deficiency can, rarely).

15. Answer e

The rash in sun-exposed areas is most consistent with pellagra (niacin deficiency), which is a complication of alcoholism. Isoniazid administration without pyridoxine supplementation can worsen niacin deficiency (decreased tryptophan to niacin conversion). Nothing in the history suggests cutaneous tuberculosis or carcinoid syndrome (depletion of the niacin precursor tryptophan by conversion to serotonin). Riboflavin deficiency and pyridoxine deficiency cause a seborrheic dermatitis.

16. Answer c

The patient has moderate-to-severe malnutrition on the basis of the weight loss. Enteral feedings are commonly used in the intensive care unit for intubated patients.

17. Answer d

The patient most likely has gastroparesis as a result of diabetic autonomic neuropathy. She needs postpyloric feedings for long-term nutrition.

18. Answer e

This patient has refeeding syndrome and all of the complications listed.

19. Answer a

Selenium deficiency is characterized by dilated cardiomyopathy and muscle disease. Many companies provide MTE4 as the trace element source, but this product is devoid of selenium.

20. Answer e

All of the considerations should be made. If no other explanation is found for the aminotransferase increase, it is true that transient increases occur early in the course of total parenteral nutrition. These usually resolve but should be monitored periodically.

SECTION IV

Miscellaneous Disorders

CHAPTER 14

Gastrointestinal Manifestations of Human Immunodeficiency Virus Infection

Stephen C. Hauser, M.D.

Nearly 40 million people worldwide are infected with human immunodeficiency virus (HIV) type 1. Highly active antiretroviral therapies (HAARTs) with multiple drugs—now widely used in the United States and highly effective—have greatly diminished the incidence of opportunistic infections in patients infected with HIV. Suppression of viral load to less than 50 copies/mL and maintenance of adequate CD4 lymphocyte counts ($>500/\mu L$) are crucial. Opportunistic infections and malignancies are uncommon in HIV-infected patients with plasma HIV viral loads less than 10,000 copies/mL and CD4 counts greater than 200 to $500/\mu L$. However, not all patients with HIV receive adequate therapy because of cost, compliance, lack of availability of treatment in certain parts of the world, drug resistance, drug toxicity, and drug-drug and drug-alternative substance interactions. In immunosuppressed HIV-infected patients, multiple simultaneous infections often occur. Presentations may be typical or atypical, and there is great overlap in clinical signs and symptoms between infections and malignancies. In patients with successfully treated HIV, gastrointestinal disorders are more likely to be similar to those in non–HIV-infected, otherwise healthy persons (e.g., dysphagia due to gastroesophageal reflux disease rather than an opportunistic infection).

Side effects of antiretroviral therapy involving the gastrointestinal tract (and liver) are common and need to be considered in patients with common complaints and disorders such as anorexia, nausea, vomiting, oral ulcers, abdominal pain, diarrhea, pancreatitis, or liver function test abnormalities (Table 1).

Table 1. **Antiretroviral Therapy Toxicity and the Gastrointestinal Tract and Liver**

Drug class	Drug	Selected toxicities
Nucleoside reverse transcriptase inhibitors	All (e.g., zidovudine, abacavir, emtricitabine, tenofovir)	Nausea/vomiting, diarrhea, hepatic steatosis, lactic acidosis
	Didanosine, zalcitabine, stavudine, lamivadine	Pancreatitis
Nonnucleoside reverse transcriptase inhibitors	All (e.g., nevirapine, most liver-toxic, and delaviridine)	Nausea/vomiting, diarrhea, abnormal liver function tests
	Efavirenz	Pancreatitis
Protease inhibitors	All (saquinavir, ritonavir, most GI side effects, indinavir, nelfinavir, amprenavir, lopinavir, atazanavir, fosamprenavir)	Nausea/vomiting, diarrhea, abnormal liver function tests, pancreatitis; more GI bleeding in hemophiliacs

GI, gastrointestinal.

- Successful antiretroviral drug therapy has greatly diminished the incidence of opportunistic infections in patients infected with HIV.
- Multiple simultaneous infections often occur in immunosuppressed HIV-infected patients.
- Side effects of antiretroviral drug therapy involving the gastrointestinal tract are common.

ORAL CAVITY

Oral lesions are common in HIV-infected patients (up to 80%) and may be the first symptom in up to 10% of patients (Table 2).

ESOPHAGUS

Case—A 27-year-old man who has HIV infection presents with new dysphagia to solids. He is an injection drug user and has been noncompliant with antiretroviral drug therapy. Thrush is found on physical examination. The CD4 count is $110/\mu L$, and his plasma HIV viral load is more than 30,000 copies/mL.

The clinical presentation of this patient strongly suggests an opportunistic infection of the esophagus with *Candida*, and initial treatment should focus on the HIV infection and empiric administration of fluconazole.

Common symptoms of esophageal disorders include dysphagia, odynophagia, and chest pain unrelated to swallowing. With successful antiretroviral treatment of HIV, common disorders such as gastroesophageal reflux disease and pill esophagitis are more likely to occur than infectious esophagitis. Of the opportunistic infections involving the esophagus, *Candida* is the most common fungal infection and cytomegalovirus (CMV) is the most common viral infection; herpes simplex virus (HSV) infection is less common. *Candida* often causes dysphagia, whereas CMV, HSV, and idiopathic esophageal ulceration (IEU) often cause odynophagia. Two-thirds of patients with *Candida* esophagitis have oral thrush, hence the role of empiric therapy, but nearly 25% have a second cause for their symptoms (multiple coexistent pathogens). CMV and IEU are unusual if the CD4 lymphocyte count is more than $100/\mu L$.

Empiric treatment with fluconazole is recommended for patients with mild to moderate symptoms (dysphagia, odynophagia) who have thrush. About 75% have a response in 3 to 5 days to a 200-mg loading dose on the first day, followed by 100 mg/day for 14 to 28 days. Endoscopy is indicated for patients who do not have a response to treatment or who are severely symptomatic. Barium studies are not useful. At endoscopy, brush cytology is more sensitive than biopsy to diagnose *Candida* esophagitis, although the typical appearance (multiple plaquelike, often linear or confluent creamy-white lesions, with bleeding points when removed) is very specific. *Candida* often (up to 50% of cases) is an oral commensal and usually (up to 90% of cases) is found in stool specimens. Finally, *Candida* esophagitis can be asymptomatic. Treatment may be topical for mild cases. Ketoconazole and itraconazole absorption are dependent on acid in the stomach. Only rare cases with frequent, severe recurrences merit fluconazole (100-200 mg/day) secondary prophylaxis. Primary prevention is not recommended.

CMV infection often produces large, but sometimes small, shallow or deep, focal or serpiginous, usually painful (odynophagia, chest pain) ulcers in the middle to distal third of the esophagus. Erosions, strictures, fistulas, perforations, or mass lesions are less frequent. Up to 15% of persons with CMV esophagitis have concomitant retinitis. The diagnosis requires endoscopy, with biopsy specimens taken from the base of the ulcer (CMV involves the vessels and endothelium, whereas HSV affects epithelial cells at the edge of ulcers) to look for cytopathic (intranuclear inclusions, perinuclear halo, and cytoplasmic inclusions) effects. Serologic (most patients are already positive) and culture (contamination with blood) studies are less specific. Immunohistochemistry and in situ hybridization can improve sensitivity. Treatment with ganciclovir usually helps (foscarnet for resistant cases, more expensive), and lifelong secondary prophylaxis often is recommended (Table 2). Primary ganciclovir prophylaxis can be considered in HIV, CMV-positive patients with CD4 counts less than $50/\mu L$.

HSV esophagitis often presents with multiple small, superficial ulcers ("volcano" ulcers) or erosive esophagitis (Fig. 1). Strictures and fistulas are rare. Vesicles rarely are visualized. Biopsy specimens from the edge of ulcerations should show cytopathic changes (ground-glass nuclei, eosinophilic Cowdry type A intranuclear inclusions, multinucleate cells). Treatment with acyclovir usually is successful (Table 2). Primary prophylaxis is not recommended. Some patients with frequent, severe recurrences require secondary prophylaxis.

Idiopathic esophageal ulcers may be single or multiple, and they often occur in the distal esophagus. By definition, all diagnostic studies (biopsy, brush, cultures, special studies) are negative. Pain is the norm, and fistulas may occur. Treatment includes corticosteroids or thalidomide (Table 2).

Other unusual causes of esophageal lesions include infections with papillomavirus, Epstein-Barr virus, papovavirus, *Histoplasma*, *Aspergillus*, Mucorales, *Cryptococcus*, *Actinomyces*, *Nocardia*, bacillary angiomatosis, *Leishmania*, *Cryptosporidium*, *Pneumocystis*, *Mycobacterium tuberculosis*, and *Mycobacterium avium-intracellulare*, as well as lymphomatoid granulomatosis, non-Hodgkin's lymphoma, and Kaposi's sarcoma.

Table 2. Oral Lesions in HIV-Infected Persons

Condition	Features	Treatment	Secondary prophylaxis
Candidiasis (usually *albicans*; non-*albicans* strains may be azole-resistant)	With/without pain: pseudo-membranous (thrush), erythematous (atrophic), hyperplastic (painless, white, does not rub off) Culture, KOH, Gram stain, rarely biopsy	Topical nystatin, clotrimazole, amphotericin suspension vs. systemic fluconazole, itraconazole, amphotericin	Not recommended
Cryptococcus, histoplasmosis, geotrichosis, *Penicillium marneffei* (Asia), *Leishmania*	Painful, nodular, ulcerated: rare	Antifungals	No
Oral hairy leukoplakia (Epstein-Barr virus)	Painless, often on tongue, not red, does not peel off Biopsy, viral studies	If symptomatic, high-dose acyclovir or ganciclovir	No
Herpes simplex virus	Biopsy, Tzanck preparation	Acyclovir, famciclovir, valacyclovir If resistance, foscarnet or cidofovir	Not recommended
Herpes zoster	Rare	Antivirals	
Cytomegalovirus	Rare	Ganciclovir or foscarnet	Usually recommended
Oral condylomata	Human papillomavirus		
Aphthous ulcers	Painful; no organisms in biopsy specimen HIV-induced (?)	Topical anesthetics, dexamethasone, systemic corticosteroids, thalidomide	
Bacillary angiomatosis	*Bartonella henselae* or *quintana*, papules or ulcers Biopsy		
Syphilis	Rare		
Lymphomatoid granulomatosis	Rare		
Granuloma annulare	Rare		
Mycobacterium avium-intracellulare	Rare		
Non-Hodgkin's lymphoma			
Kaposi's sarcoma			
Squamous cell carcinoma			
Necrotizing gingivitis and periodontitis			

HIV, human immunodeficiency virus.

- *Candida* and CMV are the most common opportunistic infections of the esophagus.
- Cytopathic changes diagnostic of CMV or HSV ulceration involving the esophagus most often are found in biopsy specimens from the base or edge of the ulceration, respectively.

STOMACH

Gastric disorders related to immunosuppression in persons infected with HIV are uncommon. Epigastric discomfort may be due to CMV involving the stomach or, more likely, gastroesophageal reflux disease, distal esophageal ulceration (due to CMV, IEU, or herpes simplex), peptic ulcer disease, or dyspepsia. Gastric lymphoma can present with anorexia, nausea, vomiting, pain, or bleeding, whereas Kaposi's sarcoma involving the stomach is more likely to be asymptomatic. Whether "AIDS gastropathy" (achlorhydria or hypochlorhydria with gastric atrophy and antiparietal cell antibodies) exists is unclear. Rare infections of the stomach include cryptosporidiosis, histoplasmosis, bacillary angiomatosis, herpes zoster, and infection with

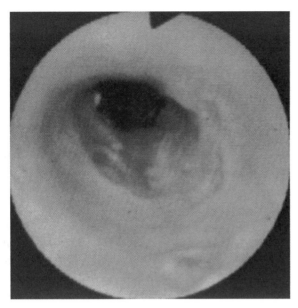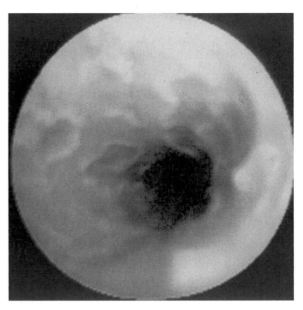

Fig. 1. Endoscopic photograph of herpes simplex esophagitis showing multiple superficial ulcers. (From Treadwell TL, Peppercorn MA, Koff RS. The gastroenterology teaching project, unit 6—gastrointestinal infections and AIDS. Used with permission.)

M. avium-intracellulare. Idiopathic aphthous ulcers also have been identified in the stomach.

SMALL BOWEL

Case—A 35-year-old woman with HIV infection successfully treated with antiretroviral drugs presents with voluminous watery diarrhea after a trip to Haiti. She complains of nausea, cramps, and a recent 5-lb weight loss, but she states that she does not have fever or gastrointestinal tract bleeding. Fecal leukocytes and occult blood are not observed on stool examination. Standard stool cultures for bacteria are negative. Mild eosinophilia is apparent on a peripheral blood smear.

The clinical presentation of this patient is consistent with *Isospora belli* infection of the small bowel, which is endemic in Haiti. This should respond promptly to antibiotic treatment with trimethoprim-sulfamethoxazole. Because antiretroviral drug therapy has been successful in this patient, recurrent infection is not likely.

The principal presentation of small-bowel disease in HIV-infected patients is enteritis, with diarrhea that is often high-volume, watery, and fecal-leukocyte–negative and sometimes with nausea, vomiting, bloating, periumbilical cramps, weight loss, or malabsorption. Diarrhea of colonic origin is more likely to be small-volume, with frequent, urgent, loose stools, lower abdominal pain, and often fecal-leukocyte–positive, with or without blood. Opportunistic infections are more likely to

occur in persons with CD4 lymphocyte counts less than 100 to 200/µL. Medications used to treat HIV infection commonly are implicated (Table 1). In diarrhea thought to be due to infection, a pathogen is identified in only 50% to 85% of cases, and, in up to 25% of cases, more than one pathogen may be discovered.

The initial diagnostic approach to chronic diarrhea in HIV-infected patients should include the following: 1) freshly collected stools for bacterial culture (including *Salmonella*, *Campylobacter*, *Shigella*), ova and parasites, fecal leukocytes, and *Clostridium difficile* toxin; 2) special studies (monoclonal antibodies, modified acid-fast and trichrome stains) for *Giardia*, *Cryptosporidium*, and Microsporida; and 3) blood cultures for enteric pathogens and *M. avium-intracellulare* (especially if the patient is febrile). If these studies are negative, especially in sicker and more immunosuppressed patients, endoscopic evaluation is indicated. Persons who are less ill and have a CD4 lymphocyte count greater than 200/µL and no pronounced weight loss usually do not have an opportunistic infection and can be given an empiric trial of antidiarrheal medications. Endoscopy with small bowel (preferably distal duodenum or proximal jejunum) biopsy and aspiration for parasites can be performed when a small-bowel source for the diarrhea is suspected. Colonoscopy with ileoscopy and biopsy can be helpful in the detection of selected small-bowel infections (*Cryptosporidium*).

Small-bowel infections often include the following: *Cryptosporidium*—This parasite is ubiquitous and transmitted as a zoonosis (humans, cats, dogs, calves, lambs, and other animals, especially newborn pets), by fecal-oral transmission, and, worldwide, through food (raw oysters, unpasteurized juices) and water (including recreational) contamination, by as little as 10 to 100 oocysts. It usually infects small-bowel epithelial cells (apical, small [2-8 μm], extracytoplasmic but intracellular sporozoites [Fig. 2]), with variable degrees of villous atrophy, but it also can involve the esophagus, stomach, colon, biliary tree, or lung. Diagnosis can be made by examining the stool for oocysts (modified acid-fast stain, enzyme-linked immunosorbent assay) or performing biopsy of the small bowel (biopsy of the terminal ileum may be more sensitive than biopsy of the proximal small bowel). Severe high-volume diarrhea with wasting (malabsorption, lactose intolerance, vitamin B_{12} deficiency) is most common when CD4 counts are less than 50/μL. Specific therapy is investigational. Antiretroviral therapy has the best chance of improving the diarrhea.

Microsporida—Two species of this parasite, *Enterocytozoon bieneusi* and *Encephalitozoon* (Septata) *intestinalis*, can be transmitted as a zoonosis or by fecal-oral transmission. *E. bieneusi* involves small-bowel epithelium (small-bowel biopsy, intracellular, 1-2-mm meronts and spores [Fig. 3]) or the hepatobiliary tree. *E. intestinalis* involves intestinal and often extraintestinal sites (kidney, lung). Currently, the diagnosis usually can be made with stool examination (modified trichrome stain, chemofluorescent agents, monoclonal antibody testing) or with small-bowel biopsy (villous atrophy may be seen) or aspiration. The clinical presentation of immunosuppressed HIV-infected patients is similar to that of patients infected with *Cryptosporidium*. No specific therapy is available for *E. bieneusi*. The less common *E. intestinalis* infection can be treated with albendazole. *E. intestinalis* may be identified in the lamina propria of the small intestine and in urine sediment.

Isospora—*I. belli* is another protozoan that is transmitted among humans by fecal-oral routes and contaminated water. It is endemic in developing countries (Haiti, Africa). Multiple large intracellular forms (schizonts, merozoites, gametocytes), mild villous atrophy, and infiltrating eosinophils can be identified in small-bowel biopsy specimens, and stool examination (modified acid-fast stain) may show large oocysts and Charcot-Leyden crystals. Eosinophilia can be observed in peripheral blood smears. Infection with this parasite is treated with trimethoprim-sulfamethoxazole, although recurrences are common and may require repeat courses of therapy or secondary prophylaxis.

Cyclospora—This parasite is larger than *Cryptosporidium* but smaller than *Isospora*, and the species that infects humans, *Cyclospora cayetanensis*, is transmitted through fecal-oral routes and contaminated water and fruit. Diagnosis can be made with stool examination (acid-fast stains) or small-bowel biopsy (variable degrees of villous atrophy are seen in biopsy specimens). As for *Isospora* infection, trimethoprim-sulfamethoxazole therapy is effective, but relapse may be frequent and require re-treatment or secondary prophylaxis.

Giardia—*Giardia lamblia* infections are not more common, severe, or prolonged in HIV-infected patients than in non–HIV-infected patients; however, infections are more common in those who practice oral-anal sex. Stool examination (for cysts and trophozoites), duodenal aspirates, and stool antigen tests are used to make the diagnosis. Treatment is with metronidazole.

Cytomegalovirus—Infection with CMV can occur throughout the gastrointestinal tract but is most common in the esophagus and colon.

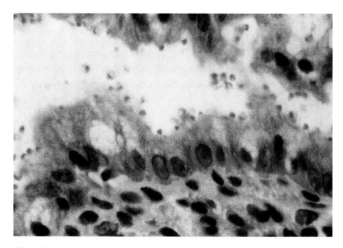

Fig. 2. Jejunal biopsy specimen has apical sporozoites of *Cryptosporidium parvum*. (Hematoxylin-eosin; original magnification, x400.) (From Goodgame RW. Understanding intestinal spore-forming protozoa: *Cryptosporidia, Microsporidia, Isospora,* and *Cyclospora.* Ann Intern Med. 1996;124:429-41. Used with permission.)

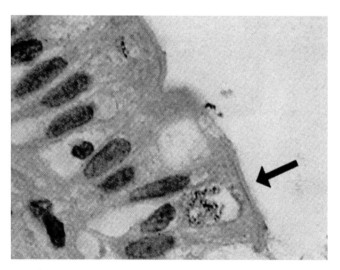

Fig. 3. Small intestinal biopsy specimen has a cluster of microsporidial spores within apical cytoplasm (*arrow*). (Hematoxylin-eosin; original magnification, x350.) (From Case Records of the Massachusetts General Hospital [Case 51-1993]. N Engl J Med. 1993;329:1946-54. Used with permission.)

Mycobacterium—M. avium-intracellulare can involve the small bowel. At endoscopy, patchy areas of edema, erythema, friability, erosions, nodularity, a frosted appearance, or yellowish plaques may be found. Patients with this infection usually have low CD4 lymphocyte counts (< 100/μL) and often have fever, weight loss, diarrhea, abdominal pain, anemia, and malabsorption. Small bowel biopsy specimens typically show macrophages stuffed with many acid-fast organisms. Stool and blood cultures also may be diagnostic. Differentiation from *M. tuberculosis* requires culture results. Patients with mycobacterial infections may have extensive and bulky mesenteric or retroperitoneal adenopathy, with areas of central necrosis seen on computed tomography (Fig. 4). Multidrug therapeutic regimens improve symptoms, and secondary prophylaxis usually is recommended until a sustained (longer than 6 months) increase in the CD4 count greater than 100/mL occurs in response to HAART (and at least 1 year of therapy for *M. avium-intracellulare* and no signs or symptoms of the infection). Primary prophylaxis is recommended for patients with CD4 lymphocyte counts less than 50/μL, and discontinuation of primary prophylaxis may be considered for patients whose CD4 counts increase to more than 100/μL for at least 3 months.

Other, more uncommon infections that may involve the small intestine include leishmaniasis, toxoplasmosis, histoplasmosis, candidiasis, coccidioidomycosis, aspergillosis, cryptococcosis, mucormycosis, and strongyloidiasis. Intestinal involvement with Kaposi's sarcoma, often related to human herpesvirus 8 (purplish red submucosal lesions, frequently difficult to diagnose with endoscopic biopsy), is usually asymptomatic, but some of the lesions can hemorrhage. Recent reports suggest that saliva is an infectious source. Non-Hodgkin's lymphoma often involves the small intestine and frequently is associated with fever, weight loss, abdominal pain, mass lesions, bleeding, and diarrhea. Most of these are of B-cell origin.

- Small-bowel disease often can be distinguished from large-bowel disease on the basis of clinical presentation.
- Medications used to treat HIV infection commonly cause gastrointestinal symptoms.
- Patients who are less ill, have CD4 counts greater than 200/mL, and do not have pronounced weight loss usually do not have opportunistic infections and can be given an empiric trial of antidiarrheal medications.

COLON

Case—A 32-year-old man who recently was found to be infected with HIV comes to the emergency department with new fever, abdominal pain, and bloody diarrhea. He recently bought his daughter a puppy at the local mall. The puppy has had nonbloody diarrhea.

The clinical presentation of this patient is consistent with colitis due to *Campylobacter* infection acquired from the infected young dog and emphasizes the importance of preventing exposure in HIV-infected persons.

Diarrhea due to colon disease is extremely common in HIV-infected patients. Immunosuppressed patients are more likely to have enteric infections from *Salmonella*, *Shigella*, or *Campylobacter*. These infections, some of which also can involve the small bowel, tend to be more common, more persistent, and more likely to recur or relapse. Some persons with recurrent enteric infections and *Salmonella* sepsis may benefit from secondary prophylaxis. Blood cultures and stool examination for fecal leukocytes often are positive. Other bacterial infections include *Yersinia*; *Aeromonas*; enteroadherent, enteroinvasive, and enteropathogenic *Escherichia coli*; *Vibrio vulnificus* (raw shellfish); and *Listeria*. Exposure to the following should be avoided: reptiles (*Salmonella*); young or sick pets (*Salmonella*, *Campylobacter*, *Cryptosporidium*); raw or undercooked eggs; meat and shellfish (*Salmonella*, noncholera vibrios, *E. coli* O157:H7); unpasteurized dairy products, poorly washed produce, soft cheeses, ready-to-eat cold cuts or hot dogs (*Listeria*, *Salmonella*); raw seed sprouts, refrigerated meat spreads, deli foods that cannot be reheated, and unpasteurized apple cider (*E. coli* O157:H7). *Streptococcus bovis* sepsis and endocarditis may be associated with gastrointestinal abnormalities, such as colon cancer. Empiric treatment with

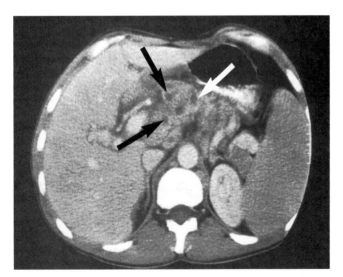

Fig. 4. Abdominal computed tomogram showing punctate areas of central necrosis within enlarged celiac and peripancreatic lymph nodes (*arrows*). (From Jeffrey RB Jr. Abdominal imaging in AIDS. Curr Probl Diagn Radiol. 1988;17:109-17. Used with permission.)

ciprofloxacin or trimethoprim-sulfamethoxazole may be useful for presumed bacterial infections before the agent is identified. Thus, HIV-infected patients should avoid the following: human and animal feces, contaminated water (drinking and recreational), newborn and very young pets, calves, lambs, reptiles, stray pets, contaminated soil, raw meat, raw fish, raw shellfish, travel to parts of the world with probable exposure to unsafe food or water, unpasteurized juices, raw seed sprouts, questionable cold cuts, unclean produce, soft cheeses (e.g., Brie, Camembert, feta, and blue-veined and Mexican-style cheese such as queso fresco), refrigerated pâtes, refrigerated meat spreads, poorly cooked eggs, poorly cooked and reheated leftovers, many deli foods, and food from street vendors.

CMV often affects the colon, with diarrhea, abdominal pain, bleeding, ulceration (Fig. 5), mass lesion, perforation, fistula, and weight loss as clinical manifestations. The CD4 lymphocyte counts usually are low (< 50 to 100/µL). Infection may be asymptomatic. Diagnosis requires tissue biopsy specimens showing cytopathic changes; biopsy specimens from even normal-appearing areas can be diagnostic and should be taken. Up to 18% of cases may involve the right colon alone and would not be diagnosed with flexible sigmoidoscopy.

Clostridium difficile colitis is common, but it is not more severe, persistent, or recurrent in immunosuppressed than in nonimmunosuppressed persons. Other less common infections are due to *M. avium-intracellulare*, *M. tuberculosis*, *Bartonella henselae* (bacillary angiomatosis), *Cryptosporidium*, *Entamoeba histolytica* (symptomatic colitis is rare), *Cryptococcus*, *Toxoplasma*, *Pneumocystis*, *Leishmania*, *Penicillium marneffei* (Southeast Asia), and *Candida*. Histoplasmosis and schistosomiasis are also less common than *C. difficile* infections.

Several organisms found in stool samples are of uncertain clinical significance, including non-*histolytica Entamoeba*, *Balantidium coli*, spirochetosis, *Blastocystis hominis*, adenovirus, *Rotavirus*, *Astrovirus*, coronavirus, picobirnavirus, and *Calicivirus*.

Other processes may occur, including lymphoma, Kaposi's sarcoma, toxic megacolon (bacterial infections, CMV, *C. difficile*, *Cryptosporidium*, and Kaposi's sarcoma-related), typhlitis (sometimes without neutropenia), pneumatosis intestinalis (often associated with infections such as CMV, *C. difficile*, *Cryptosporidium*, and *M. avium-intracellulare*), idiopathic colonic ulcer, and intussusception (due to infections, neoplasms, lymphoid hyperplasia). Anorectal disease is common with herpes simplex (chronic cutaneous perianal ulcers, pain, tenesmus, mucopurulent discharge, inguinal lymphadenopathy, dysuria, and saddle paresthesias), CMV, gonorrhea, syphilis, idiopathic ulcer, condylomata (human papillomavirus), molluscum contagiosum, anal squamous cell carcinoma, and *Chlamydia*,

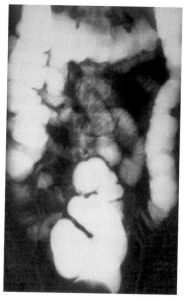

Fig. 5. Barium enema shows cytomegalovirus colitis. Note mucosal edema, ulcerations, and narrowing of the transverse colon. These findings are nonspecific and can occur in other infections as well as in ischemic colitis. (From Treadwell TL, Peppercorn MA, Koff RS. The gastroenterology teaching project, unit 6—gastrointestinal infections and AIDS. Used with permission.)

as well as *Actinomyces*, Kaposi's sarcoma, lymphoma, and *Leishmania*.

- Many infections in immunocompromised HIV-infected patients can be prevented.
- Enteric infections may be diagnosed with blood culture and stool studies.
- Noninfectious causes of diarrhea in HIV-infected, antiretroviral medication-treated patients have become more common.

PANCREAS

Pancreatic involvement in immunosuppressed HIV-infected patients often results from medications and infections (pancreatitis) and less often from malignancy. Hyperamylasemia, pancreatic in origin or due to renal failure or macroamylasemia, may occur in asymptomatic persons. Medications often implicated in pancreatitis include dideoxycytidine, dideoxyinosine, pentamidine, dapsone, and trimethoprim-sulfamethoxazole. Infections reported to involve the pancreas are protean and include CMV, *Toxoplasma*, *Pneumocystis*, *Candida*, *Cryptococcus*, histoplasmosis, aspergillosis, *M. avium-intracellulare*, and *M. tuberculosis*. Kaposi's sarcoma and lymphoma also may affect the pancreas.

RECOMMENDED READING

Call SA, Heudebert G, Saag M, Wilcox CM. The changing etiology of chronic diarrhea in HIV-infected patients with CD4 cell counts less than 200 cells/mm^3. Am J Gastroenterol. 2000;95:3142-6.

Cappell MS. The pancreas in AIDS. Gastroenterol Clin North Am. 1997;26:337-65.

Clayton F, Clayton CH. Gastrointestinal pathology in HIV-infected patients. Gastroenterol Clin North Am. 1997;26:191-240.

Datta D, Gazzard B, Stebbing J. The diagnostic yield of stool analysis in 525 HIV-1-infected individuals. AIDS. 2003;17:1711-3.

Department of Health and Human Services/NIH AIDS treatment and information service [cited 2005 Mar 21]. Available from: http://www.aidsinfo.nih.gov.

Horvath KD, Whelan RL. Intestinal tuberculosis: return of an old disease. Am J Gastroenterol. 1998;93:692-6.

Lew EA, Poles MA, Dieterich DT. Diarrheal diseases associated with HIV infection. Gastroenterol Clin North Am. 1997;26:259-90.

Mönkemüller KE, Call SA, Lazenby AJ, Wilcox CM. Declining prevalence of opportunistic gastrointestinal disease in the era of combination antiretroviral therapy. Am J Gastroenterol. 2000;95:457-62.

Noyer CM, Simon D. Oral and esophageal disorders. Gastroenterol Clin North Am. 1997;26:241-57.

Pare AA, Gottesman L. Anorectal diseases. Gastroenterol Clin North Am. 1997;26:367-76.

Wei SC, Hung C-C, Chen M-Y, Wang CY, Chuang CY, Wong JM. Endoscopy in acquired immunodeficiency syndrome patients with diarrhea and negative stool studies. Gastrointest Endosc. 2000;51:427-32.

Wilcox CM. Current concepts of gastrointestinal disease associated with human immunodeficiency virus infection. Clin Perspect Gastroenterol. 2000;3:9-17.

CHAPTER 15

Gastrointestinal Infections and Diverticulitis

Darrell S. Pardi, M.D.

Infections are a common cause of gastrointestinal disease. This chapter focuses on the more common infectious causes of diarrhea, food poisoning, and diverticulitis. It does not review *Helicobacter pylori*, bacterial overgrowth, or infections in human immunodeficiency virus (HIV)-positive patients, which are considered in other chapters.

Worldwide, an estimated 1 billion cases of infectious diarrhea occur annually, and death rates are second only to cardiovascular disease. It is estimated that infectious diarrhea causes the death of one child younger than 5 years every 10 seconds worldwide. Thus, in some areas, diarrheal diseases are responsible for more years of life lost than all other causes combined. Infectious diarrhea is more common in children and in developing countries than in adults in developed countries. In developed countries, the infections are usually mild and self-limited, and thus antibiotic therapy is unnecessary. In some specific cases, antibiotics are not effective (Table 1). The clinical features of infectious diarrhea vary, depending on whether the organism is invasive and whether the infection occurs in the small bowel or colon (Table 2).

VIRUSES

In the United States, most gastroenteritis is viral and is typically brief and self-limited (Table 3). Viral gastroenteritis typically is characterized by diarrhea of brief duration, often with nausea and vomiting, but absence of high fever, severe abdominal pain, and bloody diarrhea. Therapy is symptomatic with antiemetics, antipyretics, and attention to adequate hydration.

Table 1. Effectiveness of Antibiotic Therapy for Infectious Diarrhea

Antibiotics are effective and indicated
  Salmonella enterocolitis in an immunocompromised host
  Salmonella typhoid fever
  Shigella
  Clostridium difficile
  Yersinia sepsis or systemic infection
  Moderate-to-severe traveler's diarrhea
  Campylobacter dysentery or sepsis
  Vibrio cholerae
  Giardia
  Amebiasis
Antibiotics are possibly effective
  Enteroinvasive *Escherichia coli*
  Enteropathogenic *Escherichia coli*
  Campylobacter enteritis
  Vibrio parahaemolyticus
Antibiotics probably are not effective
  Enterohemorrhagic *Escherichia coli* (including O157:H7)
  Salmonella enterocolitis
  Yersinia enteritis without sepsis
  Mild-to-moderate traveler's diarrhea

Modified from Banerjee S, LaMont JT. Treatment of gastrointestinal infections. Gastroenterology. 2000;118 Suppl 1:S48-S67. Used with permission.

Table 2. Clinical Features of Infectious Diarrhea

Feature	Location	
	Small bowel	**Large bowel**
Pathogens	*Salmonella*	*Campylobacter*
	Vibrio cholerae	*Salmonella*
	Escherichia coli	*Shigella*
	(ETEC, EPEC)	*Yersinia*
	Yersinia	*Escherichia coli*
	Rotavirus	(EIEC, EHEC)
	Norwalk virus	*Clostridium difficile*
	Adenovirus	*Entamoeba*
	Giardia	*histolytica*
	Cryptosporidium	Cytomegalovirus
Location of pain	Mid abdomen or	Lower abdomen,
	diffuse	rectum
Volume of stool	Large	Small
Type of stool	Watery	Mucoid, blood
Fecal leukocytes	Rare	Common
Other	Dehydration,	Tenesmus if
	malabsorption	proctitis

EIEC, enteroinvasive serogroups; EHEC, enterohemorrhagic groups; EPEC, enteropathogenic strains; ETEC, enterotoxigenic strains.
Modified from Hamer DH, Gorbach SL. Infectious diarrhea and bacterial food poisoning. In: Feldman M, Sleisenger MH, Scharschmidt BF, editors. Sleisenger and Fordtran's gastrointestinal and liver disease: pathophysiology, diagnosis, management. Vol 2. 6th ed. Philadelphia: WB Saunders Company; 1998. p. 1594-632. Used with permission.

Rotavirus

Rotavirus is the most common cause of diarrhea in young children worldwide. Adult infection often occurs after contact with a sick child or as part of an institutional epidemic. In tropical climates, rotavirus infection occurs year-round; in temperate climates, it is more common in the winter. Spread is by the fecal-oral route, facilitated by prolonged survival in the environment and resistance to many disinfectants. Symptoms occur within 72 hours after exposure, last up to 5 days, and include mild fever, diarrhea, and vomiting. Most adults are mildly symptomatic or asymptomatic, but the disease can be severe in persons who are immunocompromised, malnourished, or chronically ill. Death can occur from dehydration and acidosis, usually in the very young or elderly. Symptoms may be prolonged because of transient disaccharidase deficiency caused by severe small-bowel infection. Treatment focuses on dehydration. Oral rehydration is optimal, because oral nutrition stimulates mucosal repair, leading to shorter duration and less severe diarrhea. Protective immunity may not develop

Table 3. Summary of Viral Diarrhea

Virus	Incubation, days	Duration, days
Rotavirus	1-3	4-5
Norwalk virus	1-2	2-3
Adenovirus	8-10	7-14
Astrovirus	2-4	3-5

Modified from Czachor JS, Herchline TE. Infectious diarrhea in immunocompetent hosts. Part 1. Bacteria, viruses and parasites. Hosp Physician. 1996;8:10-7. Used with permission.

after natural infections, although reinfection tends to be less severe. An effective vaccine was developed but was withdrawn because of an association with intussusception.

Caliciviruses

Caliciviruses, also known as small round-structured viruses, are the most important cause of viral gastroenteritis in adults, and they cause many outbreaks in young children and adults. The most common caliciviruses are the Norwalk-like viruses. Outbreaks are associated with contaminated food (e.g., shellfish), water, or person-to-person spread. Caliciviruses are common in the environment and are resistant to disinfectants and chlorination. The incubation period is less than 48 hours, followed by illness lasting up to 3 days. Infection occurs in the proximal small bowel. Diarrhea, nausea, vomiting, abdominal pain, fever, headache, and malaise are common but typically mild. Postinfectious immunity is not permanent or fully protective against reinfection.

Astrovirus

Astrovirus is an important cause of diarrhea in infants and children, particularly in developing countries. Nausea and vomiting are common, although usually less severe than with rotavirus. The incubation period is 2 to 4 days. Illness is mild and lasts up to 5 days.

Enteric Adenovirus

Most adenoviruses cause respiratory infection, although some strains cause diarrhea. Respiratory symptoms may precede gastrointestinal manifestations. A long incubation period (up to 10 days) and diarrhea of long duration (1-2 weeks) are characteristic.

BACTERIA

Bacteria are relatively uncommon causes of acute diarrhea, and the indiscriminate culturing of stool from patients with acute diarrhea results in few positive findings, with an unacceptably high cost per positive culture. However, stool cultures are appropriate for patients with bloody diarrhea, high fever or pain, fecal leukocytes, immunocompromise, or diarrhea persisting longer than a few days. In most laboratories, routine stool cultures detect *Salmonella*, *Shigella*, and *Campylobacter*. *Escherichia coli* O157:H7, *Yersinia*, *Vibrio*, and others often require a special request.

Many bacterial causes of diarrhea do not require antibiotic therapy in healthy adults. However, in those presenting with bloody stools or high fever or those with a chronic illness, including immunocompromise, empiric antibiotic therapy is often given while the results of stool culture are pending. Quinolones are usually given for empiric coverage in adults. The more common causes of bacterial diarrhea are summarized in Table 4.

Campylobacter

Campylobacter is the most commonly identified bacterial cause of diarrhea in the United States and is twice as common as *Salmonella* and sevenfold more common than *Shigella*. Most infections are due to *C. jejuni* and typically are acquired from contaminated poultry (up to 90% of chickens may be colonized) or unpasteurized milk in the summer or early autumn. Infection is most common in very young children, teens, and young adults.

Fevers, myalgias, malaise, abdominal pain, and headache follow an incubation period of 1 to 4 days. Diarrhea begins later and ranges from profuse watery to bloody, lasting up to 1 week. Prolonged carriage can occur for several months, and recurrent infection can occur in up to 25% of patients. A chronic carrier state is rare. Hemolytic uremic syndrome (HUS), reactive arthritis (HLA-B27), and Guillain-Barré syndrome can occur.

In most healthy patients, symptoms are mild to moderate, and by the time the slow-growing *Campylobacter* is identified, the patient's condition has begun to improve. For these patients, antibiotic therapy is unnecessary. Antibiotics are recommended for prolonged (> 1 week) or worsening symptoms, dysentery, high fever, bacteremia, pregnant women, and persons at risk for complications (extremes of age, immunocompromise, cirrhosis). Quinolones and erythromycin are effective therapy. Erythromycin is less expensive, with less resistance, but treatment must be started early (within the first 3 days of symptoms). Treatment with quinolones can be started later in the illness, but high rates of resistance have been reported.

Salmonella

Infection with *Salmonella* causes a spectrum of diseases ranging from gastroenteritis to typhoid fever (Table 5). Infection can be complicated by bacteremia resulting in disseminated infection. *S. typhi* and *S. paratyphi* cause typhoid fever. The remaining serotypes (~ 2,000 described) cause nontyphoidal salmonellosis. *S. enteritidis* and *S. typhimurium* are the two most commonly isolated serotypes in the United States.

Outbreaks typically occur in the summer or autumn and are associated with contaminated food (undercooked or raw chicken or eggs, meat, or dairy products), reflecting the high colonization rates of *Salmonella* in poultry and livestock. Pets, including turtles, reptiles, cats, and dogs, can carry and transmit the organism. Person-to-person spread is also important in outbreaks and in developing countries. Because typhoidal *Salmonella* exists only in humans, a new case of typhoid fever indicates exposure to a carrier. Attack rates are highest among

Table 4. Summary of Bacterial Diarrhea

Bacteria	Incubation, days	Duration, days	Dysentery (blood/mucus)*	Source
Salmonella				Chicken, eggs, meat, dairy
Gastroenteritis	1-2	3-7	0	
Colitis	1-2	14-21	+ to + +	
Typhoid fever	7-14	28	+	
Shigella	1-2	3-5	+ + +	P-P, egg salad, dairy
Campylobacter	1-4	5-10	+ +	Poultry, milk
Escherichia coli O157:H7	2-7	3-8	+ + +	Hamburger, salami
Vibrio parahaemolyticus	1-2	2-7	0 to + +	Shellfish
Vibrio cholerae	1-3	4-7	0	Water, shellfish
Yersinia	4-7	7-21	0 to +	Pork, milk

Scale: 0 = no to + + + = common.
P-P, person-to-person.
Modified from Czachor JS, Herchline TE. Infectious diarrhea in immunocompetent hosts. Part 1. Bacteria, viruses and parasites. Hosp Physician. 1996;8:10-7. Used with permission.

Table 5.   Clinical Syndromes of *Salmonella* Infection

Syndrome	Incidence, %
Gastroenteritis	75
Varies from mild to severe (dysentery)	
Bacteremia	5-10
With or without gastroenteritis	
Consider AIDS	
Typhoid (enteric) fever	5-10
With or without gastroenteritis	
Systemic infection	5
Osteomyelitis, arthritis, meningitis,	
cholecystitis, abscess	
Carrier state >1 year	<1

AIDS, acquired immunodeficiency syndrome.
Modified from Hamer DH, Gorbach SL. Infectious diarrhea and bacterial food poisoning. In: Feldman M, Sleisenger MH, Scharschmidt BF, editors. Sleisenger and Fordtran's gastrointestinal and liver disease: pathophysiology, diagnosis, management. Vol 2. 6th ed. Philadelphia: WB Saunders Company; 1998. p. 1594-632. Used with permission.

infants, the elderly, and persons with decreased stomach acid. Conditions predisposing to *Salmonella*, in addition to eating raw or undercooked eggs and poultry, are listed in Table 6.

Gastroenteritis occurs in 75% of infections and typically begins within 48 hours after exposure, with nausea and vomiting, followed by diarrhea and cramps. Diarrhea may range from mild to severe and from watery to bloody. Fever and abdominal pain are common. Localized tenderness can simulate an acute abdomen and is often localized to the right lower quadrant, reflecting the ileal location of most infections. Gastroenteritis typically lasts for 7 or fewer days, although in unusual cases primarily with colitis, symptoms can last for weeks. Bacteremia occurs in 5% to 10% of infections, often resulting in distant infections (e.g., central nervous system infections, endocarditis, osteomyelitis). Recurrent or persistent bacteremia can occur in patients with acquired immunodeficiency syndrome (AIDS).

Typhoid fever (enteric fever) is a systemic infection characterized by a longer incubation period of 1 to 2 weeks, followed by systemic symptoms that include fevers, malaise, arthralgia, myalgia, headache, and delirium. Gastrointestinal symptoms are often delayed and include abdominal pain and constipation more than diarrhea. Delayed bowel perforation and bleeding can occur. Physical findings include bradycardia relative to fever, hepatosplenomegaly, lymphadenopathy, and a macular rash (rose spots). Typhoid fever is associated with recurrent or sustained bacteremia, resulting in metastatic infections. Symptoms typically last 4 weeks, although antibiotic therapy can hasten recovery. Recurrent infection, occurring 7 to 10 days after apparent recovery, is not uncommon. The incidence of typhoid fever is decreasing in the United States.

Prolonged asymptomatic fecal shedding of *Salmonella* is common (average, ~5 weeks), although most patients clear the organism within 3 months. Chronic carriage (> 1 year) occurs in fewer than 1% of patients with gastroenteritis and in up to 3% with typhoid fever. Risk factors include extremes of age and cholelithiasis (associated with chronic gallbladder infection).

Therapy in uncomplicated gastroenteritis includes hydration and avoidance of antimotility agents. Antibiotics may prolong the carrier state, select resistant organisms, do not improve outcomes, and are not indicated for healthy subjects with uncomplicated gastroenteritis. Antibiotics (e.g., quinolones, amoxicillin, trimethoprim-sulfamethoxazole [TMP-SMX]) are indicated for colitis, for patients with or at risk for bacteremia (extremes of age, immunocompromise [HIV, medications, malignancy], valvular heart disease, hemoglobinopathy, orthopedic implants), for severe disease, or for chronic carriers. Multidrug resistance is becoming a problem; therapy should be guided by sensitivity testing. Prolonged therapy is necessary for metastatic infections.

Table 6.   Conditions Predisposing to *Salmonella* Infection

Hemolytic anemia
    Sickle cell disease
Malignancy
    Lymphoma
    Leukemia
    Disseminated carcinoma
Immunosuppression
    AIDS
    Corticosteroids
    Chemotherapy/radiation
Achlorhydria
    Gastric surgery
    Proton pump inhibitors
    Idiopathic
Ulcerative colitis
Schistosomiasis

AIDS, acquired immunodeficiency syndrome.
Modified from Hamer DH, Gorbach SL. Infectious diarrhea and bacterial food poisoning. In: Feldman M, Sleisenger MH, Scharschmidt BF, editors. Sleisenger and Fordtran's gastrointestinal and liver disease: pathophysiology, diagnosis, management. Vol 2. 6th ed. Philadelphia: WB Saunders Company; 1998. p. 1594-632. Used with permission.

For typhoid fever, therapy is recommended. Quinolones or third-generation cephalosporins are typically given as empiric therapy while sensitivity data are pending. Resistance to chloramphenicol, TMP-SMX, and ampicillin makes these drugs inappropriate for empiric therapy. Corticosteroids also may be beneficial in patients with severe disease. In chronic carriers, therapy with a quinolone (e.g., norfloxacin, 400 mg twice daily for 4 weeks) may lead to clearance. If not, cholecystectomy may be needed to remove the nidus of chronic infection.

Shigella

Shigella has 40 serotypes in four species (*S. dysenteriae*, *S. flexneri*, *S. boydii*, and *S. sonnei*). Spread is typically person-to-person, facilitated by a low infective dose because of resistance to stomach acid. Outbreaks are related to contaminated food and water. *S. sonnei* produces the mildest disease and is the most common type in the United States. Symptoms typically begin within 48 hours after ingestion and include fever, malaise, abdominal pain, and watery diarrhea. Rectal pain or burning can be prominent. Respiratory complaints are common, and children may have neurologic manifestations, including seizures. The diarrhea may decrease and become bloody with mucus and pus (i.e., dysentery). This classic progression occurs in a small proportion of cases and is least common for *S. sonnei* infections.

The initial watery diarrhea is thought to be due to the Shiga toxin, whereas dysentery is due to mucosal invasion, which occurs primarily in the colon. Bacteremia is uncommon. Predictors of severity include extremes of age, malnutrition, immunocompromise, and infection with *S. dysenteriae*. *S. dysenteriae* is most likely to cause complications such as HUS (see below), dysentery, and toxic megacolon. Shigellosis typically lasts for 1 to 3 days in children and 5 to 7 days in adults. Although chronic carriage is unusual, prolonged infections can occur and be difficult to differentiate from ulcerative colitis. A delayed asymmetric large-joint arthritis can occur, usually in those with HLA-B27.

Treatment focuses on hydration and perhaps avoidance of antimotility agents. Healthy patients whose condition improves spontaneously may not require therapy. However, antibiotics have been shown to decrease disease duration and mortality. Therefore, for most patients, particularly those with chronic illnesses (including malnutrition and HIV), the elderly, day care or health care workers, or food handlers, antibiotic therapy (quinolones, TMP-SMX, ampicillin) is indicated for 1 to 5 days, depending on severity of the infection. Resistance to multiple antibiotics has been reported, and if therapy is begun before sensitivity data are available, quinolones are recommended (in adults). For all patients, handwashing and other hygienic practices are necessary to decrease person-to-person spread and to limit outbreaks.

Escherichia coli

Enterohemorrhagic *E. coli* (e.g., *E. coli* O157:H7)

Enterohemorrhagic *E. coli* (EHEC) produces Shiga toxin and causes colitis after an incubation period of 3 to 5 days. *E. coli* O157:H7 accounts for more than 90% of EHEC cases in the United States; 100 other serotypes have been identified. Although several outbreaks have attracted considerable media attention, most cases of EHEC are sporadic. It has been estimated that 50% of cattle and 90% of hamburger lots are contaminated with EHEC. Thus, EHEC is associated with the ingestion of undercooked hamburger but also of salami, sprouts, and unpasteurized milk or juice. Although the infectious dose is low, EHEC is effectively killed at temperatures higher than 156°F. A pink center in a hamburger is associated with lower temperatures and an increased risk of infection. Irradiation of hamburger also effectively kills EHEC, but whether the public embraces irradiated foods remains to be seen.

EHEC typically produces watery diarrhea that progresses to bloody diarrhea after a few hours to a few days. One study suggested that EHEC is the most common cause of bloody diarrhea in the United States. Systemic symptoms (fatigue, myalgias, headache), severe abdominal pain, nausea, and vomiting are common, but fever is not. Illness typically lasts 5 to 10 days. In the elderly, EHEC may be misdiagnosed as ischemic colitis.

EHEC can lead to HUS/thrombotic thrombocytopenic purpura (TTP) in 5% of patients, resulting in hemolytic anemia and renal failure with or without central nervous system symptoms. The pathophysiologic mechanism of EHEC appears to be vascular endothelial damage that leads to platelet aggregation and initiation of the coagulation cascade. This, in turn, leads to ischemia of the colon and results in hemorrhagic colitis. In fact, some cases of "ischemic colitis" probably represent misdiagnosed cases of EHEC. Similar thrombi and ischemia in the kidney may be the cause of renal insufficiency in HUS. HUS/TTP can have high morbidity and mortality, particularly in the very young and very old.

In some laboratories, specific testing for *E. coli* O157:H7 (sorbitol-MacConkey agar or a newer stool toxin assay that may be more sensitive) must be requested; thus, the condition can be underdiagnosed. In several large series reported from North America, *E. coli* O157:H7 was the second to fourth most commonly identified bacterium in acute diarrheal illnesses. Antibiotics do not appear to be beneficial and may increase toxin production or release (or both). This, in turn, may increase the risk of HUS/TTP and, perhaps, death. Also, antimotility agents, including narcotics, may increase the risk of HUS. Thus, antibiotics and antimotility agents should be avoided if EHEC infection is suspected clinically (e.g., absence of fever in a patient with bloody diarrhea of suspected infectious origin).

Patients with EHEC should be placed in contact isolation, and any personal contacts with gastrointestinal symptoms should be tested for EHEC. It has been recommended that children, food handlers, and health care workers delay their return to school or work until they are asymptomatic and have had several stool cultures negative for EHEC.

Enterotoxigenic *E. coli*

Enterotoxigenic *E. coli* (ETEC) is a common cause of diarrhea in travelers and in children in developing countries. The organism attaches to the small bowel and causes diarrhea through enterotoxins. The disease ranges from mild to severe watery diarrhea often associated with mild upper gastrointestinal tract symptoms that last for 2 to 5 days. Rehydration is the mainstay of therapy. Antibiotics (quinolones, TMP-SMX, tetracycline) often are given empirically for moderate-to-severe traveler's diarrhea. As for most gastrointestinal infections, multiple-drug antibiotic resistance has been reported with ETEC, although resistance to quinolones does not appear to be a major problem yet.

Enteropathogenic *E. coli*

Enteropathogenic *E. coli* (EPEC) is primarily a problem in infants. It caused several epidemics with high mortality in neonatal nurseries in the early 1900s. Currently, it most often occurs in developing countries. EPEC attaches to the small-bowel mucosa and causes watery mucoid diarrhea by producing structural changes in the microvilli. Antibiotics are effective therapy, although resistance to TMP-SMX is emerging.

Enteroinvasive *E. coli*

Enteroinvasive *E. coli* (EIEC) is a rare cause of diarrhea associated with fever and abdominal pain. The diarrhea is usually watery, but it can be accompanied by fever and leukocytes (i.e., dysentery). EIEC is similar to *Shigella* in its ability to invade the colonic mucosa and produce a Shiga-like toxin. Resistance to TMP-SMX is common, but not to quinolones.

Enteroaggregative *E. coli*

Enteroaggregative *E. coli* (EAEC) is primarily a problem in infants in developing countries and in HIV-infected adults, although it also can cause traveler's diarrhea. EAEC causes persistent diarrhea that can be watery or bloody. Specific tests for EAEC are not available clinically. Quinolones are effective therapy, suggesting that empiric treatment with these agents may be reasonable in patients with HIV who have diarrhea and negative findings on evaluation.

The different types of *E. coli* are summarized in Table 7.

Vibrio

Vibrio species are halophilic and are associated with consumption of raw or undercooked saltwater fish or shellfish (oysters, crabs, mussels) or contamination of food with seawater.

V. parahaemolyticus is a common cause of diarrhea in the coastal United States and Japan, particularly during warm months. Several toxins can be produced, resulting in various clinical presentations. The incubation period is less than 1 to 2 days, and the primary symptom is watery diarrhea. Abdominal pain, vomiting, and headaches are also common. *V. parahaemolyticus*

Table 7.   Types of *Escherichia coli* Causing Infectious Diarrhea

Type	Patients affected	Pathophysiology	Clinical feature
Enteropathogenic (EPEC)	Infants in developing countries, some travelers	Attachment alters brush border	Watery diarrhea
Enterotoxigenic (ETEC)	Children in developing countries, travelers	Enterotoxin-mediated secretion	Watery diarrhea
Enteroinvasive (EIEC)	Rare Food and water outbreak	Direct invasion	Usually watery diarrhea, 10% have dysentery
Enterohemorrhagic (EHEC, e.g., O157:H7)	Food (hamburger), sporadic or outbreak	Shiga-like cytotoxins	Watery then bloody diarrhea, HUS/TTP
Enteroaggregative (EAEC)	Infants in developing countries, HIV-positive	Adherence, toxins	Prolonged watery diarrhea

HIV, human immunodeficiency virus; HUS, hemolytic uremic syndrome; TTP, thrombotic thrombocytopenic purpura.
Modified from Hamer DH, Gorbach SL. Infectious diarrhea and bacterial food poisoning. In: Feldman M, Sleisenger MH, Scharschmidt BF, editors. Sleisenger and Fordtran's gastrointestinal and liver disease: pathophysiology, diagnosis, management. Vol 2. 6th ed. Philadelphia: WB Saunders Company; 1998. p. 1594-632. Used with permission.

may uncommonly cause frank dysentery and mucosal ulceration. Illness typically lasts 2 to 5 days, and antibiotics usually are not necessary. The role of antibiotics is uncertain, even for patients with severe or prolonged symptoms. If antibiotics are administered, a reasonable choice is quinolones, doxycycline, or tetracyline.

V. cholerae infection is not common in the United States, although sporadic cases occur along the Gulf Coast and in travelers returning from endemic areas (Latin America, Africa, Asia). The infectious dose is large, although hypochlorhydria decreases it. Cholera toxin can cause profound dehydration from profuse diarrhea (up to 1 L/h or more) and vomiting. However, milder cases (and asymptomatic carriage) are possible. In severe cases, stools are described as "rice water" because of the watery consistency with flecks of mucus. Hypotension, renal failure, and hypokalemic acidosis occur in severe cases, often leading to death without aggressive rehydration. Oral rehydration solution can be life-saving, but severe cases typically require intravenous fluids, with attention to potassium and bicarbonate replacement. Infection can be treated with various antibiotics, including tetracycline, doxycycline, TMP-SMX, or erythromycin, and even a single dose of quinolones can be effective.

V. vulnificus also can cause diarrhea. It can be acquired through wound contamination by infected seawater or by direct consumption, particularly in the summer months. In immunocompromised patients or those with chronic liver disease, systemic infection with sepsis is a risk, with high mortality. These patients should be instructed not to eat or to handle raw seafood, particularly oysters.

Yersinia

Yersinia enterocolitica is less common in the United States than in northern Europe. *Yersinia* is typically acquired in cold months from contaminated food, milk, or water and has an incubation period of 4 to 7 days. Many animals can harbor the organism and be a source of infection, which occurs primarily in the terminal ileum. Symptoms range from mild (fever, diarrhea, nausea, cramps) to severe (reflecting invasion). Uncommonly, *Yersinia* causes bacteremia with sepsis or distant infection. Arthralgias and rash are more common in adults than in children. Postinfectious arthritis also can occur (HLA-B27).

In healthy patients, symptoms typically last 1 to 3 weeks. Antibiotic therapy has not been shown to be of benefit in uncomplicated disease. Patients at risk for sepsis (cirrhosis, iron overload, immunocompromise) and those with severe or prolonged symptoms, bacteremia, or distant infections may benefit from antibiotic therapy (tetracycline, quinolones, TMP-SMX with or without aminoglycosides). *Yersinia* ileocolitis can simulate Crohn's disease (including extraintestinal manifestations: aphthous ulcers, arthralgias, erythema nodosum), and

right-lower-quadrant tenderness with mesenteric lymphadenitis can simulate appendicitis.

PARASITES

Stool evaluation for ova and parasites is particularly helpful in immunocompromised patients and those with an appropriate exposure or travel history. Most parasites are shed intermittently, and a single stool evaluation is relatively insensitive. To increase sensitivity, three or more separate stools should be analyzed.

Giardia lamblia

Giardia, the most common parasitic infection in the United States, is acquired by the ingestion of water or food contaminated with cysts or by person-to-person spread (day care, nursing home). Cysts can survive for months in the environment and are resistant to chlorination. In the United States, the peak incidence occurs in the summer and early autumn. Excystation occurs in the small bowel where the trophozoites attach to and damage the mucosa. High-risk groups are travelers to endemic areas, children in day care, patients with immunoglobulin deficiencies, and homosexual men. Symptoms, including watery diarrhea, cramps, nausea, bloating, and flatulence, occur 1 to 2 weeks after ingestion. Patients may present with acute disease, although diarrhea may be intermittent, leading to a delay in seeking medical attention. Chronic symptoms also may occur and can be associated with malabsorption. Some persons become asymptomatic carriers with chronic cyst passage.

Examination of multiple stools for trophozoites or cysts is reasonably sensitive in acute watery diarrhea. With chronic symptoms or less watery stools, this examination is insensitive and duodenal aspirate and biopsy (organisms or lack of plasma cells) or fecal analysis for *Giardia* antigen may be better. Metronidazole (250 mg 3 times daily for 5 to 7 days) is usually effective therapy. Treatment of asymptomatic carriers provides no benefit for the individual but may help prevent outbreaks, for example, in day care or health care workers.

Cryptosporidium parvum

Although *Cryptosporidium* has been increasingly recognized as a pathogen during the AIDS epidemic, it also can cause diarrhea in immunocompetent hosts. Infection is commonly acquired from contaminated water or person-to-person spread. It can resist chlorination, resulting in outbreaks even in industrialized areas. Several U.S. outbreaks have been attributed to contaminated water sources. *Cryptosporidium* invades the small-bowel mucosa and causes inflammation, villous blunting, and malabsorption. In most healthy patients, disease is mild and self-limited, with watery diarrhea, nausea, cramps, and flatulence developing 7 to 10 days after ingestion. Stools may be intermittent and mucoid but should not contain much blood or pus.

Diarrhea can last 6 weeks or longer. Headaches, fevers, or myalgias are common. The diagnosis can be made by stool analysis (immunoassays are more sensitive than microscopy) or small-bowel biopsy. In healthy patients, treatment usually is not necessary. Cryptosporidiosis in patients with AIDS is discussed in Chapter 14, Gastrointestinal Manifestations of Human Immunodeficiency Virus Infection.

Entamoeba histolytica

Amebiasis is the most common parasitic diarrhea in the world, although it is less common in the United States. Most cases in the United States occur in travelers or immigrants from endemic areas (Latin America, Africa, India) and in homosexual men. Infection is acquired through the ingestion of contaminated food or water. Amebic cysts excyst in the small bowel and infect the colon. Symptoms begin 7 to 21 days after ingestion and include bloody diarrhea, abdominal pain, fever, and tenesmus, consistent with invasive colitis. Amebic colitis can vary from mild to fulminant, with severe bleeding or perforation. Because the risk of perforation is increased by corticosteroid use, it is important to differentiate amebic colitis from ulcerative colitis. Amebic ulcers are caused by mucosal invasion by trophozoites. The ulcers vary from mild to severe, with the classic description being that of undermined edges leading to a flask-shaped ulcer. Amebae can penetrate the bowel wall, enter the portal circulation, and cause liver or splenic abscesses. Patients with liver abscesses tend to be males, and they may not have a discernible history of colitis. Distant infection (peritonitis, empyema, central nervous system infection) also can occur. A localized infection surrounded by granulation tissue or a dense fibrous coat (ameboma) can resemble colon cancer.

Diagnosis is made by stool examination. Three or more samples may be needed to make the diagnosis by microscopy, although stool antigen testing and polymerase chain reaction for *Entamoeba histolytica* DNA are more sensitive. Metronidazole (750 mg 3 times daily for 7 to 10 days) is the drug of choice for treating colitis or liver abscesses. Patients with severe colitis or abscesses may require intravenous therapy. Cysts are relatively resistant to metronidazole and require a second agent such as diloxanide furoate, paromomycin, or iodoquinol. Drainage of liver abscesses is not recommended unless rupture is imminent or medical therapy is ineffective.

Numerous nonpathologic amebae can inhabit the human colon, including *Entamoeba coli*, *Entamoeba hartmanni*, and *Endolimax nana*. Distinguishing between these organisms and *E. histolytica* can be difficult by routine microscopy, even for experienced examiners, although serologic testing and stool polymerase chain reaction should help.

Blastocystis hominis

Blastocystis is found occasionally on routine "ova and parasite" stool examinations. Its pathogenicity is uncertain, particularly in immunocompetent hosts. However, if no other cause for a patient's symptoms is found, a trial of metronidazole can be considered.

TRAVELER'S DIARRHEA

Infectious diarrhea affects 10% to 50% of travelers to high-risk areas of Southeast Asia, the Middle East, India, Africa, and Latin America. The incidence of diarrhea varies depending on the specific area visited (e.g., urban or rural), the traveler's age, time of year, and local conditions such as flooding or a cholera outbreak. Bacteria cause 80% to 90% of cases of traveler's diarrhea, and the other 10% to 20% are due to parasites, viruses, or toxins. ETEC is a common cause. The unusual case of prolonged traveler's diarrhea is more likely to be caused by a parasite such as *Giardia* or *Cyclospora cayetanensis*. The risk of infection can be decreased by avoiding uncooked foods, local water (including ice), and unpasteurized drinks.

Symptoms typically begin several days after the person arrives in the area and last for 3 to 5 days. Watery diarrhea, bloating, fatigue, and cramps are common. Bloody diarrhea and high fever are uncommon; their presence suggests an invasive organism and should prompt an evaluation for a specific organism. For most travelers, antibiotic prophylaxis is not recommended. However, patients with immunocompromise, severe chronic illness, hypochlorhydria, or proton pump inhibitor therapy may benefit from prophylaxis (e.g., ciprofloxacin, 500 mg daily). Bismuth subsalicylate (2 tablets 4 times daily) is an alternative prophylaxis.

Mild cases of traveler's diarrhea can be treated with rehydration and antidiarrheals or bismuth (if no fever, severe pain, or bloody diarrhea) for 1 to 3 days. For moderate-to-severe diarrhea, a quinolone is recommended, often together with an antidiarrheal. Ampicillin and TMP-SMX are not recommended because of the high rates of resistance in some areas.

FOOD POISONING

From 1988 to 1992 in the United States, 2,423 food-borne outbreaks affected more than 77,000 people. Because of underreporting, the true burden of disease may be 10 to 100 times higher. Most cases of bacterial diarrhea, as indicated in Table 4, are acquired from food and can be considered forms of "food poisoning." Also, some bacteria cause acute gastrointestinal symptoms due to preformed toxins that are ingested with contaminated foods. Common symptoms of food poisoning and typical offending agents are listed in Table 8.

Staphylococcus aureus toxin causes 1 to 2 days of severe vomiting, cramps, and diarrhea that begin 2 to 6 hours after ingestion (cream-filled pastries, meat, potato or egg salad). Severe infection can cause dehydration.

Table 8. Food Poisoning Syndromes

Symptoms	Incubation period, h	Possible agents
Acute nausea, vomiting	6	Preformed toxins of *Staphylococcus aureus*, *Bacillus cereus*
Watery diarrhea	6-72	*Clostridium perfringens*, *B. cereus*, ETEC, *Vibrio cholerae*, *Giardia*
Inflammatory ileocolitis ("dysentery")	16-72	*Salmonella*, *Shigella*, *Campylobacter*, EIEC, EHEC (O157:H7), *V. parahaemolyticus*, *Yersinia*

EHEC, enterohemorrhagic Escherichia coli; EIEC, enteroinvasive E. coli; ETEC, enterotoxigenic E. coli.
Modified from Guerrant RL, Bobak DA: Bacterial and protozoal gastroenteritis. N Engl J Med. 1991;325:327-40. Used with permission.

Clostridium perfringens toxin results in 1 to 2 days of abdominal pain and watery diarrhea that begin 8 to 24 hours after ingestion of foods typically prepared in advance and left to sit unrefrigerated (beef, poultry, gravy). An uncommon strain of *C. perfringens* produces the potentially fatal enteritis necroticans or pigbel, a condition that occurs primarily in poor tropical regions.

Bacillus cereus toxin causes nausea and vomiting that occur within 2 to 6 hours after ingestion (pork, creams or sauces, or fried rice) and last 6 to 10 hours. Diarrhea may occur later, probably from a toxin formed in vivo. In healthy hosts, antibiotic therapy is not necessary for these acute forms of food poisoning due to preformed enterotoxins.

Listeria monocytogenes can be found in many foods (hot dogs, lunch meat, cheeses), and its growth is not substantially inhibited by refrigeration. It can cause gastroenteritis, often with fever, that is typically mild and self-limited, lasting 1 to 2 days. However, in chronically ill or immunosuppressed patients and in the very young, the elderly, and pregnant women, *Listeria* also can produce severe disease with bacteremia and disseminated infection associated with a high mortality rate. Therapy, usually with ampicillin and gentamicin, is indicated.

DIVERTICULITIS

In Western societies, colonic diverticulosis affects 5% to 10% of the population older than 45 years and 80% of those over 85 years. Uninflamed and nonbleeding diverticula are asymptomatic. Approximately 20% of patients with diverticula have an episode of symptomatic diverticulitis. Diverticular hemorrhage is the second most common cause of colonic bleeding after vascular lesions.

Pathophysiology

Diverticulosis predominantly affects the sigmoid colon but may involve the entire colon. High luminal pressure is believed to cause mucosal protrusion through weak areas where the vasa recta penetrate the bowel wall, resulting in diverticula. There is an association between diverticulosis and a Western diet,

high in refined carbohydrates and low in dietary fiber; whether this represents cause and effect is unproved. If the neck of a diverticulum is obstructed, it may distend and lead to bacterial overgrowth and invasion, often with perforation, which is generally walled off by the adjacent mesocolon or appendices epiploicae.

Classification

Stage I diverticulitis is characterized by small confined pericolonic abscesses, and stage II disease includes larger confined pericolonic collections. Stage III involves generalized suppurative peritonitis ("perforated diverticulitis"); because the diverticular neck is generally obstructed by a fecolith, peritoneal contamination by feces may not occur. Stage IV indicates fecal peritonitis.

- Colonic diverticula are common but do not cause symptoms unless they are infected or bleeding.
- Diverticula form predominantly in the sigmoid colon by mucosal protrusion through weak spots in the bowel wall.
- Virtually all patients with diverticulitis have a microperforation.
- Stage I, small confined abscess; stage II, large confined abscess; stage III, suppurative peritonitis; stage IV, fecal peritonitis.

Clinical Features

Symptoms of diverticulitis include lower abdominal pain, fever, and altered bowel habits (typically diarrhea). The stool may contain trace blood, but profuse bleeding is very uncommon. Dysuria, urinary frequency, and urgency reflect bladder irritation, whereas pneumaturia, fecaluria, or recurrent urinary tract infection suggests a colovesical fistula. Physical findings include fever, left lower quadrant tenderness, or a mass.

Complications

Rupture of a peridiverticular abscess or uninflamed diverticulum causes peritonitis, occurs more commonly in elderly and immunosuppressed persons, and is associated with a high mortality rate. Repeated episodes of acute diverticulitis may lead to colonic obstruction. Jaundice or hepatic abscesses suggest pylephlebitis. A massively dilated (> 10 cm) cecum, signs of cecal necrosis (i.e., air in the bowel wall), or marked tenderness mandates immediate surgical consultation. Colovesical and, less frequently, colovaginal and colocutaneous fistulas may occur.

Diagnostic Studies

A contrast enema shows diverticula but not diverticular inflammation. Moreover, contrast studies may cause a perforation. If the clinical features are highly suggestive of diverticulitis, imaging studies are unnecessary. If the diagnosis is uncertain, or if an abscess is suspected, computed tomography is preferred, although the results may be false-negative in up to 20% of cases. Ultrasonography also may show diverticular inflammation, but it is more operator-dependent than computed tomography and abdominal tenderness may preclude application of sufficient external pressure. Flexible sigmoidoscopy is necessary only if carcinoma or colitis is a concern.

- A contrast enema shows diverticula but not inflammation.
- Indications for computed tomography: uncertain diagnosis, concern for abscess.
- Sigmoidoscopy is necessary only to exclude carcinoma or colitis.

Treatment

Therapy is influenced by severity, ability to tolerate oral intake, prior history of diverticulitis or bleeding, and complications.

- Mild first attack, tolerate oral intake: Outpatient therapy with a liquid diet and oral broad-spectrum antibiotics (e.g., ciprofloxacin and metronidazole). After the acute attack has resolved, a high-fiber diet and colonoscopy (to exclude cancer) are advisable. Approximately 5% to 10% of patients will have a second attack within 2 years.
- Severe pain, inability to tolerate oral intake, persistent symptoms despite adequate outpatient therapy: Hospitalization, nothing by mouth, and broad-spectrum intravenous antibiotics. Computed tomography to exclude abscess or perforation. Consider computed tomography-guided percutaneous drainage of an abscess to control systemic sepsis, permitting a single-stage surgical procedure, if necessary, at a later stage.
- Surgery: Emergency operation is indicated for peritonitis, uncontrolled sepsis, perforation, and clinical deterioration. Indications for elective surgery include fistula formation, stricture, and recurrent diverticulitis.

If operation can be deferred until acute inflammation heals, then a single-stage primary resection and reanastomosis, perhaps laparoscopically, can be accomplished with minimal morbidity and mortality. For emergency indications, the first stage of a two-stage procedure involves resection of the diseased segment and creation of an end colostomy with oversewing of the distal colonic or rectal stump (Hartmann's procedure). Colonic continuity may be reestablished in a second operation.

RECOMMENDED READING

Banerjee S, LaMont JT. Treatment of gastrointestinal infections. Gastroenterology. 2000;118 Suppl 1:S48-S67.

Casburn-Jones AC, Farthing MJ. Management of infectious diarrhoea. Gut. 2004;53:296-305.

DuPont HL. Guidelines on acute infectious diarrhea in adults: the Practice Parameters Committee of the American College of Gastroenterology. Am J Gastroenterol. 1997;92:1962-75.

Hamer DH, Gorbach SL. Infectious diarrhea and bacterial food poisoning. In: Feldman M, Friedman LS, Sleisenger MH, editors. Sleisenger & Fordtran's gastrointestinal and liver disease: pathophysiology/diagnosis/management. Vol 2. 7th ed. Philadelphia: Saunders; 2002. p. 1864-913.

Oldfield EC III. Emerging foodborne pathogens: keeping your patients and your families safe. Rev Gastroenterol Disord. 2001;1:177-86.

Surawicz CM, editor. Infectious diarrhea. Gastroenterol Clin N Am. 2001;30:599-861.

Tytgat GNJ, editor. Best Pract Res Clin Gastroenterol. 2002;16(4):527-662.

CHAPTER 16

Gastrointestinal Endocrine Tumors

Thomas R. Viggiano, M.D.

Gastrointestinal endocrine tumors comprise a diverse group of tumors. They are classified as "functional" or "nonfunctional" depending on whether the clinical syndrome is due to hormone release. Advances in knowledge and technology have improved our understanding of these tumors and enhanced our ability to diagnose and treat the resulting clinical syndromes. This chapter summarizes the clinical syndromes associated with the important functional gastrointestinal endocrine tumors (Table 1).

Gastrointestinal endocrine tumors are uncommon. Of these tumors, carcinoid tumors are the most common, occurring in 15 per 1,000,000 population annually. All other gastrointestinal endocrine tumors combined have a prevalence of 10 per 1,000,000 population annually. Gastrinomas and insulinomas are the next most common and occur with an approximately equal prevalence of 0.5 to 2.0 per 1,000,000 population annually. VIPomas (VIP, vasoactive intestinal polypeptide) are rare tumors, but the prevalence has not been well defined. Rarer still are glucagonomas, with fewer than 200 cases reported. Somatostatinomas are the most rare, with only approximately 50 cases reported. Nonfunctional gastrointestinal endocrine tumors are commonly reported as incidental findings at surgery or autopsy. However, the exact prevalence of nonfunctional tumors is unknown.

Originally, gastrointestinal endocrine tumors were thought to arise from ectodermal tissue from the neural crest, but now it is thought that they arise from endodermal stem cells of the neuroendocrine system. These tumors have been called "APUDomas" (APUD, amine precursor uptake and decarboxylation) because they share cytochemical properties in the production of peptides. Histologically, the tumors consist of innocuous-appearing cells that have uniform nuclei and cytoplasm; mitotic figures are rare. With light microscopy, pathologists are not able to distinguish different tumors of this neuroendocrine family. These tumors are slow growing, and pathologists may not be able to tell histologically whether a tumor is benign or malignant. Electron microscopy can demonstrate secretory granules, and immunocytochemical staining may help identify secretory products. It is important for clinicians to understand that malignancy of these slow-growing tumors often can be determined only by the clinical evidence of metastasis or invasion.

Previously, the pancreas was thought to be the most common location of noncarcinoid gastrointestinal endocrine tumors. However, with advances in tumor localization, intestinal and extraintestinal locations are known to be more common than previously recognized. In a small percentage of patients with a functional endocrine syndrome, no tumor is found at surgery, and hyperplasia of the pancreatic islets is the cause of the syndrome. The ability of the standard imaging studies such as computed tomography (CT), ultrasonography, and magnetic resonance imaging (MRI) to localize a gastrointestinal endocrine tumor depends on the size of the tumor or the presence of metastases. If tumor size is less than 1 cm, the detection rate by conventional imaging studies is less than 10%. If tumor size is more than 3 cm, the localization rate is 50%. Insulinomas and gastrinomas are the more common tumors and tend to present when the tumor is small. Overall, CT, ultrasonography, and MRI localize fewer than 40% of these tumors.

More than 90% of gastrinomas, VIPomas, glucagonomas, and somatostatinomas and more than 75% of carcinoid tumors have somatostatin receptors. A radiolabeled somatostatin analogue, octreotide, can be given to localize both tumors and

Table 1.   Gastrointestinal Endocrine Tumors

Tumor	Annual incidence (per million population)	Common symptoms	Initial study to localize tumor	Rate of malignancy	Management consideration (see text)
Gastrinoma	0.5-2.0	Abdominal pain Ulcer, dyspepsia Diarrhea	Somatostatin receptor scintigraphy	>60%	Surgery if no MEN syndrome and no metastases Octreotide Acid antagonists ?Chemotherapy
Insulinoma	0.5-2.0	Hypoglycemia Neuropsychiatric	Endoscopic ultrasonography	<10%	Surgery if no metastases Diazoxide
VIPoma	0.05-0.2	Diarrhea	Abdominal computed tomography	>75%	Surgery if no metastases Octreotide ?Chemotherapy
Glucagonoma	0.01-0.1	Diabetes Dermatitis Weight loss Diarrhea	Abdominal computed tomography	>75%	Nutritional support Insulin Octreotide ?Chemotherapy
Somatostatinoma	Rare	Diarrhea	Abdominal computed tomography	>85%	?Octreotide ?Chemotherapy

MEN, multiple endocrine neoplasia; VIP, vasoactive intestinal peptide.

metastases and is the basis for somatostatin receptor scintigraphy or octreotide scanning. Except for insulinomas, octreotide scanning is the most sensitive and effective imaging method for gastrointestinal endocrine tumors. Currently, octreotide scanning is recommended as the initial test for localizing these elusive tumors.

Endoscopic ultrasonography is particularly sensitive for identifying endocrine tumors within the pancreas. However, it is less effective for imaging extrapancreatic tumors and metastatic disease. Endoscopic ultrasonography requires considerable expertise, whereas octreotide scanning is performed well in most radiology departments. Both endoscopic ultrasonography and octreotide scanning frequently fail to localize small extrapancreatic gastrointestinal endocrine tumors.

The development of treatments directed at somatostatin receptors has improved our ability to alleviate symptoms and slow tumor growth. In cases of most tumors with somatostatin receptors, octreotide therapy usually produces symptomatic improvement. Preliminary evidence indicates that octreotide may also inhibit tumor growth and either stabilize or decrease tumor size.

Gastrointestinal endocrine tumors are hypervascular. Previously, selective abdominal angiography was the most

sensitive method for localizing primary tumors, and it identified approximately 60% of tumors, including some small ones. The hypervascularity of the tumors also provides an opportunity for treatment. For example, the liver derives only 20% to 25% of its blood supply from the hepatic artery. In patients who have diffuse metastatic disease of the liver with minimal or no other metastases and whose hormone symptoms cannot be controlled with chemotherapy or octreotide, hepatic artery embolization is helpful.

Gastrointestinal endocrine tumors may occur in a sporadic (nonfamilial) form or as part of an autosomal-dominant inherited multiple endocrine neoplasia (MEN) syndrome. All gastrointestinal endocrine tumors can be associated with MEN type 1 (MEN 1). MEN 1, or Wermer's syndrome, is characterized by pituitary, parathyroid, and pancreatic hyperplasia or tumors. Most commonly, MEN presents with 1) hypercalcemia from hyperparathyroidism, 2) a functional or nonfunctional pancreatic endocrine tumor, and 3) a silent pituitary tumor. Recognition of MEN 1 is important because there are differences in the clinical presentation, in clinical and diagnostic approaches to the tumors, and in options for treatment.

Nonfunctional gastrointestinal endocrine tumors include tumors that release peptides but do not cause a distinct clinical syndrome. Pancreatic polypeptide and neurotensin do not produce a syndrome. Ironically, most gastrointestinal endocrine tumors produce multiple hormones; however, it is not understood why such tumors are usually associated with one or no clinical syndrome. Gastrointestinal endocrine tumors also produce substances other than peptides, for example, chromogranins, which can be localized with immunochemical studies. Nonfunctional gastrointestinal endocrine tumors may be malignant. Human chorionic gonadotropin is a chromogranin that has been proposed as an indicator for malignant tumors. However, the presence of human chorionic gonadotropin has not been established as a marker for malignancy.

Gastrointestinal endocrine tumors share many properties that affect diagnosis and treatment. Identifying these tumors, however, depends on recognizing the distinct syndromes that result from hormone release.

CARCINOID TUMORS AND CARCINOID SYNDROME
Carcinoid tumors, the most common gastrointestinal endocrine tumors, are slow growing and may occur anywhere in the gut. The clinical presentation varies from an asymptomatic incidental finding to symptomatic tumors, including a classic syndrome resulting from release of biogenic amines.

Etiology and Pathogenesis
Carcinoid tumors arise from neuroendocrine intestinal cells, also known as "enterochromaffin cells" or "Kulchitsky cells." The tumors occur most commonly in the appendix, ileum, rectum, and stomach, but they also may occur in the bronchus, biliary duct, thymus, breast, and ovary.

Approximately half of intestinal carcinoids are appendiceal tumors, which are asymptomatic and are found incidentally at appendectomy. Appendiceal carcinoids are usually smaller than 1 cm, solitary, and benign. They are found in 0.3% to 0.5% of appendectomy specimens. Local invasion of appendiceal carcinoids is common, but metastatic spread is rare.

Rectal carcinoid tumors are also usually asymptomatic and are found incidentally during proctosigmoidoscopic examinations. More than 90% of these tumors occur in a zone from 4 to 13 cm above the anal verge and can be recognized as a small gray-yellow nodule. Although these tumors have been reported only in middle-aged persons, it is this population that undergoes sigmoidoscopic examination for screening purposes.

Gastric carcinoid tumors may arise from histamine-secreting enterochromaffin-like cells in patients with chronic atrophic gastritis and achlorhydria associated with *Helicobacter pylori* infection or pernicious anemia. The combination of chronic inflammation and hypergastrinemia associated with atrophic gastritis is believed to be responsible for the development of this tumor.

Small intestinal carcinoid tumors are the most important clinically because they are more likely to present with intestinal symptoms and carcinoid syndrome. Most small intestinal carcinoids occur in the ileum within 2 ft of the ileocecal valve. Ileal carcinoids tend to be larger than other small intestinal carcinoids at the time of diagnosis but most are smaller than 2 cm. Ileal carcinoids may also be multicentric and have a higher likelihood of metastatic spread to regional lymph nodes and the liver, resulting in carcinoid syndrome. Small intestinal carcinoids may invade through the mesentery and cause a characteristic fibroblastic reaction that may produce intestinal obstruction and periodic abdominal pain.

Clinical Features
Carcinoid tumors are slow growing, originate deep in the mucosal layer, and are usually small when diagnosed. Thus, many of them may be asymptomatic. Appendiceal, rectal, and many gastric carcinoids are asymptomatic incidental findings at the time of diagnosis. Small intestinal carcinoids may present with intestinal symptoms of obstruction, abdominal pain, or, rarely, intestinal bleeding, but the most common clinical presentation is abdominal pain caused by intermittent bowel obstruction. The median duration of symptoms before diagnosis is more than 2 years.

Carcinoid syndrome occurs when the tumor releases biogenic amines into the systemic circulation, which nearly always means that liver metastases are present. The most common symptoms are diarrhea and facial flushing, and the most common physical finding is hepatomegaly. Wheezing from bronchospasm and right-sided valvular heart disease from endocardial fibrosis also may be present. Carcinoid syndrome is not associated with hypertension but may be associated with paroxysmal hypotension. Small intestinal carcinoids arise from mid-gut neuroendocrine tissue. However, carcinoid tumors that cause carcinoid syndrome may arise from foregut tissue and may occur in the bronchus, stomach, or duodenum.

Diagnosis
Carcinoid tumors usually are asymptomatic and are discovered incidentally. Symptoms due to the direct effects of a tumor in the intestinal tract include abdominal pain, intestinal obstruction, nausea, weight loss, or intestinal bleeding. Carcinoid syndrome usually occurs in patients with liver metastases.

Intestinal carcinoids may be found with esophagogastroduodenoscopy, flexible sigmoidoscopy or colonoscopy, radiographic contrast studies of the intestine, or CT of the abdomen. Urinary 5-hydroxyindoleacetic acid secretion should be measured in patients with carcinoid syndrome. Because foregut carcinoid tumors lack aromatic L-amino acid decarboxylase, urinary 5-hydroxytryptamine levels are increased. Octreotide scanning identifies the site of primary tumors and metastatic disease in more than 75% of patients. MRI and selective angiography are also sensitive for detecting metastases to the liver. Echocardiography is useful for evaluating patients with suspected cardiac valvular disease.

Treatment

Appendiceal carcinoids usually are found incidentally at appendectomy. Of these tumors, 98% are smaller than 1 cm and have no evidence of metastasis. Appendectomy is considered curative for all appendiceal carcinoids smaller than 2 cm. For tumors larger than 2 cm, right hemicolectomy is recommended.

Eighty percent of rectal carcinoids are smaller than 1 cm, and wide local excision usually is adequate treatment. Only 5% of rectal carcinoids are larger than 2 cm, and these larger tumors have a higher risk of metastasizing. Rectal ultrasonography should be performed to examine for invasion or lymph node involvement. If invasion is found on preoperative testing or at the time of wide local excision, a more radical cancer operation is recommended, depending on the patient's age, operative risk, and acceptance of a permanent colostomy.

Small gastric carcinoids and polypoid gastric carcinoids may be removed endoscopically. Larger or invasive gastric carcinoids require surgical treatment.

Many patients with intestinal carcinoid tumors live comfortably for many years, even after advanced spread of disease. The best treatment in the early stage for many patients may be no treatment at all. Surgery may be effective palliative treatment for patients with intestinal symptoms.

Carcinoid syndrome almost always means that liver metastases are present. Diarrhea may be controlled with hypomotility agents. If patients have had ileal resection, diarrhea may respond to cholestyramine. Octreotide inhibits hormone secretion by carcinoid cells and provides effective control of diarrhea, flushing, and wheezing in more than 75% of patients. Corticosteroids may be helpful for relieving wheezing due to bronchospasms.

Surgery may be useful for palliation of intestinal obstruction. Although resection of liver metastases has produced some symptomatic improvement, it has not improved survival. Carcinoid tumors generally are radioresistant, and radiation is helpful only for relieving pain caused by bone metastases. Arterial embolization of liver metastases provides relief from symptoms for up to 1 year in 90% of patients. Chemotherapy is reserved for patients with debilitating symptoms that cannot be controlled with octreotide or for patients with impaired liver function or carcinoid cardiac involvement. Combination therapy with streptozotocin and doxorubicin is associated with a small but significant increase in survival. Interferon alfa improves symptoms but not survival. Overall, the 5-year survival rate for patients with local carcinoid tumors is 95%; for those with regional lymph node involvement, 65%; and for those with liver metastases, 20%. The median duration of survival for patients with carcinoid syndrome is 2.5 years after the first episode of flushing.

GASTRINOMA (ZOLLINGER-ELLISON SYNDROME)

Gastrinomas produce the classic triad of symptoms called "Zollinger-Ellison syndrome." This syndrome consists of peptic ulcer disease, gastric acid hypersecretion, and a gastrin-producing tumor. Gastrinomas are rare and occur in fewer than 1% of patients who have peptic ulcer disease. Gastrinomas frequently are associated with MEN 1.

Etiology and Pathogenesis

The majority of gastrinomas were thought to be non-β islet cell tumors of the pancreas. With advances in technology, it has been learned that extrapancreatic gastrinomas are common. As many as 50% of gastrinomas occur in the duodenal wall; the pancreas is the second most common site. However, more than 90% of gastrinomas occur in an anatomical area called the "gastrinoma triangle."

Gastrinomas are slow growing, and it is difficult to differentiate benign tumors from malignant ones. Approximately two-thirds of gastrinomas are malignant. The best indicator of malignancy is the presence of metastases, which are usually in regional lymph nodes or the liver. It is important to determine whether liver metastases are present. If they are, the patient is not a candidate for surgical treatment.

Approximately a third of gastrinomas are associated with MEN 1. In addition to gastrinomas, tumors or hyperplasia of the pituitary and parathyroid glands may be present. Surgical resection of tumors or hyperplasia in MEN 1 is nearly impossible because the tumors are multicentric.

Clinical Features

Peptic ulcer disease is the most common sign of gastrinoma and occurs in more than 90% of patients. Although the ulcer disease associated with gastrinomas was thought to be more refractory to medical treatment or to present in an unusual way (e.g., multiple large duodenal ulcers or postbulbar duodenal ulcers), the most common type of ulcer associated with gastrinoma is an ordinary ulcer located in the duodenal bulb.

Diarrhea occurs in 30% to 50% of patients with gastrinoma. Multiple factors contribute to the development of diarrhea, including the volume of acid hypersecretion, morphologic small-bowel changes from acid hypersecretion and inflammation, and decreased water and sodium absorption because of hypergastrinemia. Also, the low pH may inactivate pancreatic lipase and cause bile salts to precipitate, resulting in fat malabsorption or steatorrhea.

Now, esophageal symptoms are widely recognized to occur with gastrinomas. Severe gastroesophageal reflux disease occurs in as many as 50% to 70% of patients and is often refractory to conventional treatments for reflux. Gastrin has no important effect in decreasing lower esophageal sphincter pressure.

From 20% to 30% of patients with gastrinoma have coexisting MEN 1. This syndrome has been referred to as the "three Ps" (pituitary, parathyroid, pancreas). Both parathyroid tumors and hyperplasia most commonly present with hypercalcemia, and both are usually clinically silent.

Several clinical presentations should raise suspicion that gastrinoma may be present. Gastrinoma should be considered in all patients who have a duodenal ulcer that is not caused by *H. pylori* infection or aspirin or nonsteroidal anti-inflammatory drugs. Patients with duodenal ulcer disease and diarrhea may have a gastrinoma. Patients with refractory peptic ulcer disease or severe refractory gastroesophageal reflux disease and those whose ulcer disease presents with a complication may have a gastrinoma. If patients have a duodenal ulcer associated with hypercalcemia or a family history of peptic ulcer disease, MEN 1 should be suspected. Also, gastrinoma should be considered in patients who have recurrent ulcers after surgery for peptic ulcer disease. If gastrinoma is suspected, the serum concentration of gastrin should be measured.

Diagnostic Tests

The criteria to establish the diagnosis of gastrinoma, or Zollinger-Ellison syndrome, include the following: 1) a compatible clinical presentation (peptic ulcer disease, diarrhea, and so forth); 2) gastric acid hypersecretion, which is defined as more than 15 mEq of HCl per hour secretion in patients who have not had gastric surgery or more than 5 mEq of HCl per hour secretion in those who have had gastric surgery; and 3) hypergastrinemia.

The first screening test is usually measurement of the serum level of gastrin. If the gastrin level is increased, the next step is to determine whether there is gastric acid hypersecretion. Some laboratories still perform gastric analysis. A screening test is to suction gastric fluid and determine the pH. A pH greater than 2.5 usually is not consistent with a hypersecretory state.

A serum level of gastrin more than 1,000 pg/mL strongly suggests the presence of a gastrinoma. A level less than 1,000 pg/mL may be consistent with several conditions that cause hypergastrinemia. The most common cause of hypergastrinemia is hypochlorhydria. Thus, hypergastrinemia with acid hyposecretion is seen most commonly in chronic atrophic gastritis, gastric ulcer, or gastric carcinoma or in patients who have had vagotomy or who are currently taking proton pump inhibitors. Gastrinoma is not the only cause of hypergastrinemia with normal or increased acid secretion. Duodenal ulcer disease, gastric outlet obstruction, a retained gastric antrum in patients with previous gastric surgery, or a rare condition called "antral G-cell hyperplasia" or hyperfunction also may cause hypergastrinemia with increased acid secretion.

If a patient has pronounced hypergastrinemia and acid hypersecretion but the serum gastrin level is less than 1,000 pg/mL, an intravenous secretin injection test is indicated. After secretin is injected intravenously, the serum level of gastrin increases at least 200 pg/mL over the basal gastrin level in patients with Zollinger-Ellison syndrome. For other causes of hypergastrinemic hyperchlorhydria, only a slight or no increase occurs in the serum level of gastrin.

Recent technologic advances have improved our ability to localize gastrinomas. Most gastrinomas have somatostatin receptors. Radiolabeled octreotide localizes 85% of tumors and detects more than 80% of metastases. Thus, octreotide scanning currently is the initial test of choice. Endoscopic ultrasonography is also sensitive and helps localize approximately 80% of gastrinomas. CT of the abdomen detects approximately 50% of tumors and may be useful for directing biopsy of liver metastases, if present. Selective angiography localizes only 33% of gastrinomas, and portal venous catheterization is rarely needed to localize tumors. Exploratory laparotomy by an experienced surgeon with intraoperative endoscopy may help localize tumors at the time of surgery.

Treatment

The two objectives of treatment of Zollinger-Ellison syndrome are to control gastric acid hypersecretion and to treat the malignant neoplasm, if present.

Medical treatment to decrease gastric acid hypersecretion includes proton pump inhibitors at higher doses than for treating routine peptic ulcer disease. The aim is to keep the basal acid output at less than 10 mEq of HCl per hour before the next dose of medication. Somatostatin is a gastric acid secretory inhibitor, and octreotide may be useful in the treatment of acid hypersecretion.

Surgical treatment is recommended to patients who are good surgical risks and in whom curative resection may be possible. Patients with liver metastases or MEN 1 are not candidates for surgical treatment. Currently, surgery cures approximately 30% of patients with gastrinoma.

Tumor excision is the surgical treatment of choice. Some also advocate a highly selective or parietal cell vagotomy so that the medication requirement to control symptoms will be reduced. Previously, total gastrectomy was performed; however, it is not recommended because of the associated morbidity and mortality. Also, total pancreatectomy is not recommended because it is associated with high morbidity and mortality and may not be curative.

INSULINOMA

Insulinomas are insulin-secreting tumors that nearly always originate in the pancreas and cause symptoms of hypoglycemia. Insulinomas are one of the more common pancreatic endocrine tumors.

Etiology and Pathogenesis

Insulinomas are β-cell tumors and almost all arise in or adjacent to the pancreas. They are usually solitary, but approximately 2% may be multiple, and multiple insulinomas should raise suspicion of the presence of MEN 1. Solitary insulinomas usually are distributed evenly in the head, body, and tail of the pancreas, but because they are small, localization can be difficult. Although malignant insulinomas occur in only 5% to 10% of patients, many malignant tumors have metastasized to the liver and regional lymph nodes at the time of diagnosis.

Clinical Features

Insulinomas usually occur in persons 20 to 75 years old, and 60% occur in females. Most patients present with neurologic manifestations of hypoglycemia, referred to as "neuroglycopenic symptoms." The more common of these symptoms are altered consciousness or loss of consciousness, confusion, dizziness, and visual symptoms (diplopia, blurred vision). Symptoms can also result from catecholamine release caused by hypoglycemia. Catecholamine-mediated symptoms include anxiety, weakness, fatigue, headache, palpitations, tremor, and sweating. The symptoms produced by insulinomas are nonspecific and may be vague, and the key to diagnosis of these tumors is an awareness by the physician that an insulinoma may be present. Typically, symptoms occur with fasting, when a meal is delayed or missed, or during exercise. Patients may learn to avoid symptoms by eating frequently, and 40% of patients have a history of weight gain from increased eating. The average duration of symptoms may be long; for 25% of patients, it is more than 3 years.

Diagnosis

For many years, it was thought that the Whipple triad—hypoglycemic symptoms, fasting blood glucose level less than 50 mg/dL, and relief of hypoglycemic symptoms with glucose ingestion—was specific for the diagnosis of insulinoma. However, this triad is not specific for insulinoma.

No absolute glucose level defines hypoglycemia; thus, the presence of an insulinoma is best determined by the combination of a low fasting blood glucose level and an inappropriately increased plasma insulin level. However, this combination is identified in only 65% of patients with insulinoma. The next step is to begin a 72-hour fast, with blood glucose and insulin levels determined at regular intervals and when the patient becomes symptomatic. With this fasting test, symptoms develop in 75% of patients within 24 hours, in 92% to 98% by 48 hours, and in virtually 100% within 72 hours.

Other causes of fasting hypoglycemia must be excluded, including exogenous insulin administration, sulfonylurea ingestion, tumors that release insulin-like growth factors, and autoantibodies to insulin or insulin receptors. Plasma sulfonylurea levels, antibodies to insulin, and C-peptide and plasma proinsulin levels may distinguish among these conditions. Plasma proinsulin accounts for more than 20% of circulating insulin in 80% to 90% of patients with insulinoma. Because commercial insulin contains no C-peptide, patients with insulinomas tend to have increased or normal plasma concentrations of C-peptide, whereas those with surreptitious insulin use have increased plasma insulin and low C-peptide levels. C-peptide does not differentiate surreptitious use of oral hypoglycemic agents from insulinoma, but plasma sulfonylurea levels may be helpful.

Localization of insulinomas may be difficult. Because most tumors are small, CT of the abdomen detects only 50% of them. A major advance has been endoscopic ultrasonography, which detects 80% to 90% of insulinomas. Angiography with selective venous sampling for insulin levels is also sensitive (80%). Because insulinomas have somatostatin receptors less commonly than other gastrointestinal endocrine tumors, octreotide scans localize only 50% of these tumors. In addition to localizing the tumor, it is important to determine whether it has metastasized to regional lymph nodes or the liver because patients with metastatic disease are not candidates for surgery. The sensitivity of MRI for detecting liver metastases is 80%.

Treatment

After the diagnosis of insulinoma has been established, initial treatment is to reverse the hypoglycemic symptoms. Diazoxide directly inhibits insulin release and enhances glycogenolysis and is effective in 60% of patients. Also, octreotide frequently inhibits insulin secretion by these tumors and may be effective for acute management.

Definitive treatment is surgical removal of the tumor, and this is indicated for any patient in whom metastatic disease has not been identified. If the tumor is not localized preoperatively, careful surgical exploration by an experienced surgeon is indicated. If no tumor is found, a stepwise distal pancreatectomy is performed until frozen section pathologic analysis indicates that all tumor has been removed. If still no tumor is found, a 70% to 80% pancreatectomy is performed, preserving both endocrine and exocrine pancreatic function. According to most reports, 70% to 95% of all patients treated surgically are cured.

Patients with metastatic disease and those whose insulinomas have not been removed by partial pancreatectomy can be managed with hyperglycemic agents such as diazoxide and octreotide. Patients with metastatic insulinoma also may be given chemotherapy. The most effective combination chemotherapy is streptozocin and doxorubicin.

VIPOMA

VIPoma syndrome is caused by a neuroendocrine tumor that is usually located in the pancreas and produces VIP. The syndrome is characterized by severe watery diarrhea, hypokalemia, and achlorhydria and is known as the "WDHA syndrome" (watery diarrhea, hypokalemia, achlorhydria) or "Verner-Morrison syndrome."

Etiology and Pathogenesis

Approximately 90% of VIPomas are in the pancreas. Although other tumors, including intestinal carcinoids, pheochromocytomas, and bronchogenic carcinomas, may produce VIP, they rarely cause this syndrome. A VIPoma is usually a solitary non-β pancreatic islet cell tumor, and more than 75% of them occur in the body or tail of the pancreas. Although these tumors are slow growing, they frequently reach a large size before diagnosis. Approximately 75% of VIPomas are malignant, and 50% have metastasized at the time of diagnosis. VIPomas cannot be differentiated from other pancreatic endocrine tumors by conventional histologic or electron microscopic examination. However, the demonstration of immunoreactive VIP in the tumor and plasma establishes the diagnosis. VIP induces intestinal water and chloride secretion and inhibits gastric acid secretion.

Clinical Features

The clinical features of VIPomas include severe secretory diarrhea, hypokalemia, achlorhydria, and dehydration. Stool volume exceeds 3 L per day in 75% of patients and is greater than 1 L per day in all patients. The watery diarrhea resembles that of cholera, hence the term "pancreatic cholera." A useful clinical observation with secretory diarrhea syndromes is that diarrhea persists despite fasting.

Hypokalemia, with potassium levels often less than 2.5 mEq/L, occurs in more than 90% of patients. More than 90% of patients have dehydration, and almost all patients report weight loss that cannot be accounted for by dehydration alone. Erythematous flushing of the head and trunk may be seen in 20% of patients. In approximately 30% of patients, hyperglycemia develops because of VIP- and hypokalemia-induced glycogenolysis in the liver. VIPomas may release other peptide hormones, including peptide histidine-methionine, somatostatin, and neurotensin, which may contribute to some clinical features in individual patients.

Diagnosis

VIPoma syndrome should be suspected in patients who present with high-volume watery diarrhea that persists despite fasting and is associated with hypokalemia and dehydration. The diagnosis is confirmed by the finding of an increased plasma concentration of VIP. Because these tumors are large, frequently malignant, and metastatic, CT of the abdomen should be performed to localize and determine the extent of tumor involvement. MRI is also effective for localizing the tumor and demonstrating metastatic disease. Other imaging studies may not be necessary. Preliminary data indicate that somatostatin receptor scanning and endoscopic ultrasonography are effective for imaging these tumors.

Treatment

The first priority of treatment is to correct dehydration and electrolyte abnormalities. Patients may require 5 L or more of fluid per day, with aggressive potassium replacement. Renal insufficiency and renal failure have been reported in this syndrome.

Long-acting somatostatin analogues such as octreotide control the diarrhea in 85% to 90% of patients with VIPomas, and these agents are considered the initial treatment of choice. For patients who do not have a response to somatostatin analogues, concomitant administration of glucocorticoids should be tried.

After imaging studies have localized and determined the extent of tumor involvement, surgery should be considered for all patients without evidence of metastatic disease. Surgical resection of a pancreatic VIPoma relieves all symptoms and is curative in approximately 30% of patients. Surgery also may be indicated to relieve local effects produced by the large size of the tumor.

For patients with metastatic disease, the most effective treatment options are chemotherapy and hepatic artery embolization. Streptozotocin and doxorubicin or streptozotocin and fluorouracil are the most effective chemotherapy regimens and achieve partial remission in up to 90% of patients. Long-term treatment with octreotide may be necessary to control symptoms.

GLUCAGONOMA

Glucagonomas produce a rare syndrome of dermatitis, glucose intolerance, weight loss, and anemia associated with a pancreatic islet cell tumor.

Etiology and Pathogenesis

Glucagonomas are usually solitary large tumors that have an average size of 5 to 6 cm at the time of diagnosis. Sixty-five percent of the tumors are located in the head of the pancreas, and the rest occur equally in the body and tail. More than 75% of the tumors are metastatic at the time of diagnosis, most commonly with metastases to the liver, bone, and mesentery. Glucagon stimulates glycogenolysis, gluconeogenesis, lipolysis, ketogenesis, and insulin secretion and inhibits pancreatic and gastric secretion and intestinal motility.

Clinical Features

Glucagonomas occur in persons 45 to 70 years old. The characteristic presentation is that of a distinct dermatitis called "necrolytic migratory erythema," which usually develops a mean of 7 years before the onset of other symptoms. This rash starts as an erythematous area, typically in an intertriginous area such as the groin, buttocks, thighs, or perineum or it may start in periorificial areas. The erythematous lesions spread laterally and then become raised, with a superficial central blistering or bullous formation. When the bullae rupture, crusting occurs and the lesions begin to heal in the center. Healing is associated with hyperpigmentation. The entire sequence usually takes 1 to 2 weeks and presents as a mixed pattern of erythema, bullous formation, epidermal separation, crusting, and hyperpigmentation, which wax and wane. Glossitis, angular stomatitis, dystrophic nails, and hair thinning are other clinical findings.

Most patients have some glucose intolerance and some may have frank diabetes mellitus. The glucose intolerance is a result of liver glycogenolysis and gluconeogenesis. Most patients with glucagonoma also have noticeable weight loss, even if the tumor is found incidentally and is small. It is believed that glucagon exerts a catabolic effect. Some patients also may have anorexia.

Most patients with glucagonoma also have hypoaminoacidemia, which may be responsible for the rash. Treatment with amino acids and nutrition results in improvement of the rash. Patients with glucagonoma may have hypocholesterolemia. Approximately 25% of patients have an increased risk of thromboembolic disease and 15% have clinically important diarrhea.

Diagnosis

Glucagonoma should be suspected when a patient has a refractory rash consistent with necrolytic migratory erythema. The patients also usually have weight loss and glucose intolerance. The diagnosis can be confirmed by the finding of an increase in plasma glucagon concentration more than 1,000 pg/mL. Hyperglucagonemia may occur in other conditions, including chronic renal insufficiency, hepatic insufficiency, septicemia, diabetic ketoacidosis, severe stress, severe burns, prolonged starvation, acromegaly, or acute pancreatitis, but the glucagon level usually does not exceed 500 pg/mL. CT or ultrasonography of the abdomen or angiography usually localizes the tumor because glucagonomas tend to be large and occur in the pancreas.

Treatment

The initial objective of treatment is to control the symptoms and hyperglycemia and to restore nutritional status. The surgical risk of these patients usually is increased because of the catabolic effects of glucagon, glucose intolerance, and hypoaminoacidemia. Patients should receive nutritional support, and the hyperglycemia should be corrected. The rash may improve with correction of the hypoaminoacidemia. If anemia is pronounced, transfusion may be needed.

Octreotide is useful for controlling symptoms, and it improves the dermatitis, weight loss, diarrhea, and abdominal pain but not diabetes mellitus.

Surgery is offered to all patients who are acceptable surgical risks and who do not have evidence of metastatic spread of the tumor, but it is curative in only 20% of them. Surgical debulking reportedly may be of benefit even in patients who have metastatic disease. Hepatic artery embolization of the tumor may produce clinical improvement. Because affected patients are at increased risk for thromboembolic events, surgical patients should receive precautions to prevent postoperative thromboembolic complications.

In patients with metastatic disease, it is important to remember that the tumors are slow growing and survival is good even for those who do not receive chemotherapy. There is no clear evidence that chemotherapy has any important effect on these tumors. The most commonly used chemotherapeutic agents are streptozotocin, fluorouracil, and doxorubicin.

SOMATOSTATINOMAS

Somatostatinomas are the least common of gastrointestinal endocrine tumors. They produce a distinct syndrome of diabetes mellitus, gallbladder disease, and steatorrhea.

Etiology and Pathogenesis

Somatostatinomas are neuroendocrine tumors that occur in the pancreas and intestine: 60% of them are located in the pancreas and 40% in the duodenum or jejunum. Because pancreatic tumors tend to have higher levels of somatostatin, they are more likely to produce symptoms. Somatostatinomas are usually solitary and large, and 85% have metastasized at the time of diagnosis. Somatostatin inhibits insulin release, gallbladder motility, and the secretion of pancreatic enzymes and bicarbonate. Somatostatinomas are not associated with MEN 1. However, somatostatinomas have been found in patients with pheochromocytoma, café au lait spots, and neurofibromatosis, suggesting a possible association with MEN 2B. Other tumors such as small cell lung cancer, medullary thyroid carcinoma, pheochromocytomas, and paragangliomas may secrete somatostatin.

Clinical Features

Somatostatinomas usually occur in patients 40 to 60 years old. All the symptoms and findings of somatostatinoma syndrome are more common in patients with pancreatic tumors than in those with intestinal tumors. Diabetes mellitus occurs in half of the patients. Gallbladder disease occurs in 65% of patients and usually is manifested as cholelithiasis, acalculous cholecystitis, or obstructive jaundice from local tumor invasion. Steatorrhea occurs in 35% of patients and is more common with pancreatic than intestinal tumors.

Diagnosis

Most somatostatinomas are found incidentally when laparotomy is performed for gallbladder disease. The diagnosis is established by the finding of somatostatin-containing D cells in the resected tumor and an increased plasma concentration of somatostatin-like immunoreactive material. Tumors are localized with CT or ultrasonography of the abdomen.

Treatment

Because patients may be malnourished, initial treatment involves correction of nutritional deficiencies. Diabetes mellitus is usually mild and responds to oral hypoglycemic agents or low doses of insulin. No specific medical treatment exists. Octreotide may be helpful in treatment. However, somatostatinomas are rare and more reports are needed to determine the efficacy of octreotide.

Surgical excision is the treatment of choice; however, 85% of patients present with metastatic disease. If imaging studies show a possibly resectable tumor, surgical resection may be beneficial. Cytotoxic chemotherapy is offered to patients with evidence of metastatic disease, but there is no clear evidence that this treatment is effective.

RECOMMENDED READING

Anthony T, Kim L. Gastrointestinal carcinoid tumors and the carcinoid syndrome. In: Feldman M, Friedman LS, Sleisenger MH, editors. Sleisenger & Fordtran's gastrointestinal and liver disease: pathophysiology/diagnosis/management. Vol 2. 7th ed. Philadelphia: Saunders; 2002. p. 2151-68.

Jensen RT. Endocrine neoplasms of the pancreas. In: Yamada T, editor. Textbook of gastroenterology. Vol 2. 4th ed. Philadelphia: Williams & Wilkins; 2003. p. 2108-46.

Jensen RT, Norton JA. Pancreatic endocrine tumors. In: Feldman M, Friedman LS, Sleisenger MH, editors. Sleisenger & Fordtran's gastrointestinal and liver disease: pathophysiology/diagnosis/management. Vol 1. 7th ed. Philadelphia: Saunders; 2002. p. 988-1016.

Pisegna JR. Zollinger-Ellison syndrome and other hypersecretory states. In: Feldman M, Friedman LS, Sleisenger MH, editors. Sleisenger & Fordtran's gastrointestinal and liver disease: pathophysiology/diagnosis/management. Vol 1. 7th ed. Philadelphia: Saunders; 2002. p. 782-92.

CHAPTER 17

Nonvariceal Gastrointestinal Tract Bleeding

Jeffrey A. Alexander, M.D.

UPPER GASTROINTESTINAL TRACT BLEEDING

Upper gastrointestinal tract (UGI) bleeding constitutes 75% to 80% of all acute gastrointestinal tract bleeding. The mortality rate from acute UGI bleeding is low, ranging from 5% to 10%, but it has not changed appreciably in the past 50 years. This lack of change in mortality rate likely is related to the increased age of patients presenting with UGI bleeding and the increase in associated comorbid conditions. Peptic ulcers are the most common source of UGI bleeding, accounting for about 40% of cases. Gastric erosions (15%-25%), bleeding varices (5%-30%), and Mallory-Weiss tears (5%-15%) are the other major causes of UGI bleeding. Aspirin or nonsteroidal anti-inflammatory drug (NSAID) use is prevalent in 45% to 60% of all patients with acute bleeding. Moreover, the risk of UGI bleeding is increased in patients taking as little as one baby aspirin a day.

Initial Approach to the Patient

The initial evaluation of a patient with UGI bleeding should focus on 1) hemodynamic assessment and 2) assessment of comorbid conditions.

Melena can result when as little as 100 mL of blood is instilled into the UGI tract, whereas instillation of 1,000 mL or more initially leads to hematochezia. Hematochezia from UGI bleeding is a sign of considerable bleeding and, if associated with a red nasogastric aspirate, has a mortality rate near 30%. Patients still bleed whole blood; therefore, the hematocrit value may not drop immediately with acute bleeding. Extravascular fluid enters the vascular space to restore volume for up to 72 hours, thereby leading to a subsequent decrease in hematocrit. Similarly, the hematocrit value may continue to decrease for a few days after bleeding has stopped, and a decrease in the hematocrit value without clinical evidence of blood loss is not diagnostic of recurrent bleeding. Adequate intravenous access should not be overlooked. Volume and blood resuscitation as well as stabilization of any other comorbid active medical conditions should take place before endoscopy. Rarely, there is massive bleeding that cannot be adequately stabilized before endoscopy. Intubation for airway protection should be considered in patients with ongoing hematemesis or those with suspected active bleeding and decreased consciousness or loss of gag reflex. There is no evidence that nasogastric lavage helps stop bleeding, although it may be helpful for cleansing the stomach before endoscopy. Intravenous administration of erythromycin before endoscopy improves the quality of the examination.

Prognostic Factors

Clinical

Age older than 70 years is a risk factor for mortality. Comorbid conditions that increase mortality include pulmonary disease (acute respiratory failure, pneumonia, symptomatic chronic obstructive pulmonary disease), malignancy, hepatic disorders (cirrhosis, alcoholic hepatitis), neurologic disorders (delirium, recent stroke), sepsis, the postoperative state, and possibly cardiac disease (congestive heart failure, ischemic heart disease, dysrhythmia) and renal disorders (acute renal failure, creatinine > 4 mg/dL, dialysis). Signs of large-volume bleeding include fresh hematemesis or bright red nasogastric aspirate and shock, the two most predictive risk factors for mortality. Tachycardia (heart rate > 100 beats/min), orthostasis, and hypotension (systolic blood pressure < 100 mm Hg) are predictive of rebleeding. Coffee-ground emesis has no prognostic value. A transfusion requirement of 4 units of blood or more per resuscitative event is predictive of rebleeding, and a transfusion requirement of 6 units or more is predictive of mortality. Laboratory factors of note include thrombocytopenia, leukocytosis, and abnormal coagulation profile, all of which increase mortality. Corticosteroid use increases mortality, and anticoagulant use increases the risk of rebleeding.

Endoscopic

Only the finding of varices or gastric cancer clearly have been shown to be predictors of mortality. Active arterial spurting has been associated inconsistently with increased mortality. Endoscopic findings, however, have clear prognostic value for assessing rebleeding rates. Endoscopy should be performed within 24 hours of presentation for reliable prognostication of rebleeding. Nearly 94% of rebleeding occurs by 72 hours and 98%, within 96 hours. The three endoscopic observations that are independent predictors of rebleeding regardless of the type of lesion are arterial spurting (rebleeding, 70%-90%), visible vessel or pigmented protuberance (40%-50%), and adherent clot resistant to washing (10%-35%). Ulcers larger than 2 cm and posterior duodenal bulb ulcers also are predictive of rebleeding.

Specific Lesions

Peptic Ulcers

The approach to the patient who has bled from peptic ulcer disease is determined at endoscopy. There are many options for endoscopic therapy. Thermal-coaptive coagulation involves the placement of the coagulating probe directly on the bleeding vessel. This is uniformly effective for vessels up to 2 mm in diameter with the heater probe (typical peptic ulcer disease setting of 30 J) or bipolar electrocoagulation (14-16 W). Injection therapy results in short-term tamponade and vasospasm and can be induced with the liberal use of epinephrine (1:10,000). Vasodestruction is long-term and can be induced by sclerosants or alcohol (not to exceed a total injection volume of 2 mL). Ligation therapy with endoscopically placed clips has appeal for use in patients with coagulation disorders or in those in whom further coaptive coagulation may not be desirable. Endoscopic therapy is indicated for patients with active arterial bleeding and those with a nonbleeding visible vessel or pigmented protuberance. An adherent clot is a predictor of rebleeding; the role of endoscopy in the management of clots has been controversial, but recent evidence favors clot removal and treatment.

All three endoscopic treatment options have relatively similar efficacy; however, many endoscopists favor a more permanent treatment option (coagulation, vasodestruction) after control of ulcer bleeding with epinephrine injection. Patients with a clean ulcer base (rebleeding rates < 5%) and a flat pigmented spot (rebleeding rates 5%-10%) do not require endoscopic therapy and likely could be dismissed soon after endoscopy. Deep ulcers may tend to expose larger vessels that may not be amenable to endoscopic coagulation. Deep ulcers in the stomach, particularly those in the upper body on the lesser curvature (left gastric artery), or posterior duodenal bulb (gastroduodenal artery) with nonbleeding visible vessels larger than 2 to 3 mm in diameter should not be treated. Rebleeding after endoscopic therapy occurs in 20% to 30% of cases. Retreatment for recurrent bleeding maintains long-term hemostasis in more than 70% of cases.

If endoscopic therapy fails, angiographic embolization of the bleeding vessel is an option in a patient who is a poor operative risk. No available data support the use of histamine$_2$ blockers or antacids for peptic ulcer bleeding. Several recent studies suggest that omeprazole is of benefit in patients with peptic ulcer bleeding and high-risk stigmata, both with and without endoscopic therapy. Presumably, the benefit is related to clot stabilization occurring in a nonacid environment. In vitro studies suggest that a pH of more than 6.0 is required for platelet aggregation and fibrin formation, whereas a pH of less than 5.0 is associated with clot lysis. It is unclear whether this increase in pH can be obtained in patients receiving oral proton pump inhibitor therapy. In torrential bleeding, octreotide may be of some benefit as a temporizing measure because of its effects on decreasing splanchnic blood flow.

Patients with UGI bleeding and *Helicobacter pylori* infection should be treated, and *H. pylori* eradication should be proved. Patients taking NSAIDs should avoid them, if possible. Patients without a reversible cause of peptic ulcer disease should receive long-term ulcer prophylaxis with either full-dose histamine$_2$ blocker (ranitidine, 300 mg/d) or proton pump inhibitor. Without treatment, ulcer bleeding will recur in approximately one-third of these patients in 3 to 5 years. This rate can be decreased to less than 10% with full-dose histamine$_2$-blocker prophylaxis. Limited data suggest that ulcer rebleeding is uncommon in patients with proven *H. pylori* eradication who avoid the use of NSAIDs. However, ulcer prophylaxis may be reasonable in patients with *H. pylori* who have a serious comorbid condition, especially if they are using NSAIDs continuously or intermittently.

Mucosal Erosive Disease

Endoscopic esophagitis, gastritis, and duodenitis are defined by the endoscopic finding of hemorrhage, erythema, or erosions. These lesions rarely are associated with major UGI bleeding. Large hiatal hernias can be associated with chronic blood loss related to Cameron lesions, which are linear erosions along the crests of gastric folds at or near the diaphragmatic hiatus (Fig. 1).

Gastric erosive disease usually is related to NSAID use, alcohol intake, or stress gastritis. Bleeding usually is minor unless ulceration develops. Prophylaxis of NSAID injury with misoprostol or omeprazole or therapy with cyclooxygenase-2–specific NSAIDs decreases the risk of ulcer development. Stress gastritis leads to clinically significant UGI bleeding in less than 3% of patients in intensive care units. At higher risk are patients who receive mechanical ventilation for more than 48 hours, those with coagulopathy, and those with head injury or extensive burn injuries. Prophylactic therapy with histamine$_2$-receptor antagonists or sucralfate should be reserved for these groups. Although not universally agreed on, histamine$_2$-receptor antagonists may be slightly more effective than sucralfate, although they may be associated with a greater incidence of pneumonia and, possibly, mortality. Data are limited on proton pump inhibitor therapy for stress ulcer prophylaxis, but it appears to be beneficial.

Mallory-Weiss Tear

Mallory-Weiss tears occur at the gastroesophageal junction and often are present with a classic history of recurrent retching, often in an alcoholic patient, before the development of hematemesis. Most tears occur on the gastric side of the gastroesophageal junction, but 10% to 20% may involve the esophagus. Bleeding stops spontaneously in 80% to 90% of patients and rebleeding occurs in 2% to 5%. Endoscopic therapy with thermal coagulation or injection therapy is of benefit for active bleeding. Angiographic therapy with intra-arterial vasopressin or embolization also can be effective, as can oversewing the lesion intraoperatively.

Portal Hypertensive Gastropathy

This lesion is more frequent in the proximal than the distal stomach and gives the gastric mucosa a mosaic or snakeskin appearance, with or without red spots. Severe portal hypertensive gastropathy has the mosaic pattern as well as diffuse red spots. Portal hypertensive gastropathy can be associated with chronic as well as acute gastrointestinal bleeding. Bleeding usually is not massive, and therapy is directed at lowering portal pressure. Rebleeding can be decreased with nonselective β-adrenergic blocker therapy.

Aortoenteric Fistula

Fistulas can occur between any major vascular structure and the gastrointestinal tract. Aortoesophageal fistulas are caused by thoracic aortic aneurysms, esophageal foreign bodies, or neoplasms. Up to 75% of aortoenteric fistulas communicate with the duodenum, usually in the third portion. They may develop from an aortic aneurysm, but more commonly they are related to an abdominal aortic (graft) reconstructive procedure. Infection seems to play a major pathogenic role in the

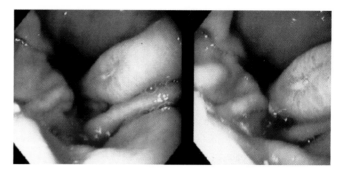

Fig. 1. Cameron lesion.

development of these fistulas, which usually develop off the origin of the graft, often with pseudoaneurysm formation. The classic "herald bleed," in which bleeding stops spontaneously hours to months before a massive bleed, occurs in about half of patients.

Evaluation should begin with extended upper endoscopy to look for evidence of distal duodenal bleeding (positive in <40% of cases) and to exclude other sources of bleeding. In a patient with an aortic graft, severe bleeding, and negative endoscopy findings, explorative surgery is indicated. Angiography rarely is helpful and may delay appropriate treatment. Computed tomography or magnetic resonance imaging may be helpful for demonstrating air surrounding the graft in proximity to the duodenum or an absence of a tissue plane between the graft and the duodenum, suggesting the diagnosis. A correct diagnosis is established preoperatively in as few as one-third of patients.

Hemobilia and Hemosuccus Pancreaticus

Hemobilia presents classically as UGI bleeding accompanied by biliary colic and jaundice. The diagnosis is made endoscopically by seeing blood coming from the ampulla. The most common cause of hemobilia is trauma to the liver or biliary tree, including liver biopsy. Extrahepatic or intrahepatic artery aneurysms often are caused by trauma and may communicate with the bile ducts. Bleeding also can be caused by gallstones, hepatic or bile duct tumors, and cholecystitis.

Hemosuccus pancreaticus usually indicates bleeding from peripancreatic blood vessels into the pancreatic duct. This usually is due to rupture of true aneurysms or pseudoaneurysms often associated with pancreatitis and pseudocysts. Angiography is used to locate the bleeding site, and transcatheter embolization is the treatment of choice. Surgery may be required for embolization failures.

Neoplasms

Bleeding can occur from primary (adenocarcinoma, stromal tumors, lymphomas, or neuroendocrine tumors) and occasionally metastatic UGI tumors (melanoma, breast). Leiomyomas, leiomyosarcomas, and lipomas often appear as a submucosal mass with central ulceration and are not an infrequent cause of severe UGI bleeding. Effective therapy generally is surgical.

Vascular Anomalies

Anomalies With Skin Lesions

Vascular lesions can be seen throughout the gastrointestinal tract in several systemic syndromes such as Osler-Weber-Rendu or hereditary hemorrhagic telangiectasias, the elastic tissue disorders of pseudoxanthoma elasticum and Ehlers-Danlos syndrome, CREST syndrome (calcinosis cutis, Raynaud's phenomenon, esophageal dysfunction, sclerodactyly, and telangiectasia), and blue rubber bleb nevus syndrome. Endoscopic coagulation is the treatment of choice. Therapy with high-dose estrogen-progesterone is of debatable value, but it has been reported to decrease bleeding in patients with hereditary hemorrhagic telangiectasia not amenable to complete endoscopic therapy.

Anomalies Without Skin Lesions

Vascular ectasias can occur anywhere in the UGI tract, but they are more common in the duodenum and stomach, particularly in older patients and those who have chronic renal failure or have had radiation therapy. These lesions are cherry red and often fernlike. Histologically, dilated, ectatic, or tortuous submucosal blood vessels are seen, the pathogenesis of which is unknown. These lesions may be diffuse or localized. Vascular ectasias are treated with endoscopic thermal coagulation. Estrogen-progesterone therapy occasionally is effective and can be tried if endoscopy fails.

Gastric antral vascular ectasia, or "watermelon stomach," is a specific type of localized ectasia often seen in elderly women presenting with iron deficiency anemia and evidence of mild UGI blood loss (Fig. 2). This lesion is associated with several other disease processes, most notably connective tissue disorders, atrophic gastritis, pernicious anemia, and portal hypertension. Red streaks traverse the gastric antrum and converge at the pylorus, resembling the stripes on a watermelon. Histologically, large blood vessels with intravascular fibrin thrombi and fibromuscular hyperplasia are seen, but the diagnosis usually is made by the classic endoscopic appearance. If iron replacement is inadequate to maintain a normal hemoglobin concentration, endoscopic thermal therapy often is helpful. Argon plasma coagulation is the preferred thermal treatment in gastric antral vascular ectasia because a large area usually requires therapy. Occasionally, antrectomy is necessary.

A Dieulafoy lesion is an abnormally large submucosal artery that can rupture and bleed (Fig. 3 and 4). The bleeding is arterial and usually moderate to severe. The majority of these lesions are within 6 cm of the esophageal junction, although they can occur in the duodenum and jejunum as well as esophagus, colon, rectum, and biliary tree. After the bleeding has stopped, the lesion can be difficult to diagnose, and several endoscopic examinations may be needed to identify it. After the lesion is identified, endoscopic tattooing often is helpful, especially if surgical therapy is planned. A Dieulafoy lesion appears as a small protruding vessel surrounded by normal mucosa or a minute mucosal defect. It is amenable to conventional endoscopic therapy as well as band ligation and endoscopic clipping. Rebleeding rates after endoscopic therapy are low. A visible nonbleeding vessel should be treated. Angiographic embolization can be effective in high-risk surgical patients.

LOWER GASTROINTESTINAL TRACT BLEEDING

Blood loss through the rectum which is not originating from the upper gastrointestinal tract is considered lower gastrointestinal tract bleeding. By convention, upper gastrointestinal tract sources are defined as those occurring proximal to the ligament of Treitz, and they are a common cause of hematochezia. Only 3% to 5% of gastrointestinal tract bleeding originates from the small intestine between the ligament of Treitz and the ileocecal valve.

Depending on the transit time, which is determined by the volume of bleeding, patients may present with melena, hematochezia, or occult bleeding. Sufficient time for bacterial metabolism is required for melena to be generated from fresh blood.

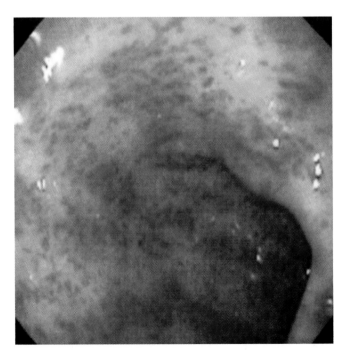

Fig. 2. Gastric antral vascular ectasia.

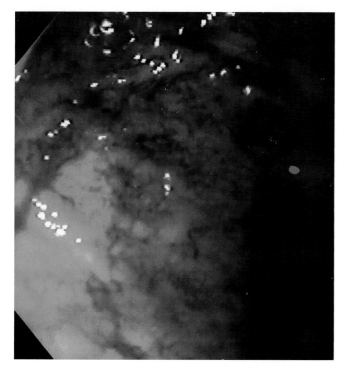

Fig. 3. Proximal stomach in patient with nonvisible Dieulafoy lesion.

Hematochezia most commonly indicates bleeding from a colonic source. However, a more proximal source is present in 5% to 10% of patients. Hematochezia from a proximal gastrointestinal tract source without hemodynamic evidence of bleeding is uncommon.

Hematochezia, particularly if limited to the toilet paper or surface of formed stool, is most suggestive of perianal bleeding (e.g., hemorrhoids, fissures). Tenesmus suggests a rectal origin (e.g., proctitis). The possibility of neoplasia must be considered in all patients.

Specific Lesions

Diverticular bleeding typically presents with acute blood loss, as manifested by maroon-colored stools or hematochezia. Minor or occult bleeding is not characteristic of diverticular bleeding. Diverticular bleeding and diverticulitis are two distinct entities that rarely, if ever, overlap. Diverticular bleeding is painless except for the cramping that may occur with the cathartic effect of blood within the colon.

Diverticular bleeding is thought to originate more commonly from the right colon, where ostia tend to be wider and the colon wall is thinner. Diverticular bleeding will develop in 3% to 5% of patients with diverticulosis. Bleeding most commonly occurs in the sixth and seventh decades of life and stops spontaneously in more than 75% of patients. Rebleeding occurs in approximately 25% of patients after a first bleed and in 50% of patients after a second bleed.

In patients who have ongoing or recurrent bleeding, angiography often is performed with hopes of identifying an actively bleeding vessel. If such a vessel is identified, transcatheter embolization can be attempted, although colonic infarction in some series has been as high as 20%. Transcatheter vasopressin can control bleeding in 90% of cases, but rebleeding rates are high. Endoscopic therapy has been reported to be safe and effective, although finding the actual bleeding lesion may be difficult.

Vascular ectasias are typically less than 5 mm in size and found in 3% to 6% of patients undergoing colonoscopy; they are most often found in the right colon but may be found anywhere in the gastrointestinal tract. These lesions are most commonly angiodysplasias, which are often multiple and believed to be related to the aging process. Less than 10% of patients with angiodysplasia eventually have bleeding. Not uncommonly, anticoagulation or platelet dysfunction is associated with clinically evident bleeding from these lesions. These lesions may lead to acute overt as well as occult gastrointestinal tract bleeding.

Many patients can be sufficiently managed with iron repletion therapy alone. Endoscopic therapy is effective but is associated with a high rebleeding rate. Angiographic embolization can be used in an acute setting. Estrogen-progesterone therapy may be of benefit in some patients, particularly those with hereditary hemorrhagic telangiectasia, but the data are mixed.

Neoplasms of the colon and small bowel may present with either acute or occult lower gastrointestinal tract bleeding. Tumors of the small intestine may be a relatively common cause of obscure lower gastrointestinal tract bleeding in patients younger than 50 years. Gastrointestinal stromal tumors,

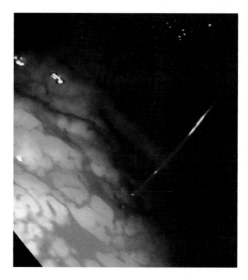

Fig. 4. Same stomach as in Figure 3, with active bleeding from the Dieulafoy lesion.

leiomyomas, and leiomyosarcomas cause more than half of bleeding neoplasms of the small intestine.

Ischemic colitis often presents with pain and low-volume hematochezia. It may occur in patients who have had abdominal vascular operation and patients with vasculitis, clotting disorders, or estrogen use. However, in most cases, no etiologic factor is identified. Large vessel disease is rare, and angiography generally is not indicated. There is no specific therapy, and recovery is usually complete in several days, although a colonic stricture occasionally develops.

Meckel's diverticulum is a remnant of the vitelline duct, usually located 100 cm proximal to the ileocecal valve. Autopsy series suggest a prevalence of 0.3% to 3%. Approximately 50% contain gastric mucosa and may present with bleeding, typically in a child or young adult.

Inflammatory bowel disease may present with gross, bloody diarrhea, which is the classic presentation for ulcerative colitis. Major hemorrhage is uncommon but can occur.

Benign recto-anal disease often presents with hematochezia. Painless hematochezia with blood on the toilet paper or the surface of formed stool is most suggestive of hemorrhoidal bleeding. Painful outlet bleeding is typical for an anal fissure.

Stercoral ulcers are associated with constipation and most commonly occur in the rectosigmoid area or occasionally the more proximal colon. They often manifest after disimpaction. Solitary rectal ulcer syndrome often is associated with excessive straining. The ulcer usually is located on the anterior wall, 6 to 10 cm above the anal verge. Both of these lesions may present with considerable bleeding.

Radiation proctitis may present months to years after radiation to the prostate or pelvic organs. Sigmoidoscopy reveals characteristic mucosal telangiectasias. The bleeding is rarely severe, and endoscopic argon plasma coagulation is the treatment of choice.

Infections may be associated with lower gastrointestinal tract bleeding. Obvious clues include a travel history and evidence of systemic toxicity such as fevers, rashes, arthralgias, eosinophilia, or diarrhea. In patients with human immunodeficiency virus, common causes for lower gastrointestinal tract bleeding are cytomegalovirus colitis and lymphoma.

NSAID enteropathy and colopathy is increasingly being recognized as an explanation for lower gastrointestinal tract bleeding. Autopsy studies have documented small intestine ulcers in 8% of patients who had taken NSAIDs within the preceding 6 months. Diaphragmatic strictures are strongly suggestive of NSAID-induced inflammation. NSAIDs also are known to reactivate inflammatory bowel disease.

Approach

The evaluation and management of patients presenting with lower gastrointestinal tract bleeding is largely determined by the clinical presentation of the patient and the differential diagnosis that has been generated. Key points to keep in mind are as follows:

1. Patients who are undergoing evaluation for positive results of fecal occult blood testing require colonic imaging. In the absence of signs or symptoms of upper tract disease or iron deficiency, the value of upper endoscopy is debatable.

2. In general, the yield of a small bowel follow-through in patients with obscure gastrointestinal bleedings is less than 5%. This rate increases to 5% to 10% with enteroclysis.

3. Technetium Tc-99m–tagged red blood cell radionuclide scanning can detect bleeding rates as low as 0.1 mL/min. The test may be repeated during a 12- to 24-hour period in an attempt to capture intermittent bleeding. Radionuclide scanning generally is not useful for identifying a specific site of bleeding. It is more sensitive for bleeding and less invasive than angiography and often is used to determine the best timing for angiography.

4. Mesenteric angiography is more accurate then radionuclide scanning but requires a faster bleeding rate (>0.5 mL/min). Angiographic yields are much greater during active gastrointestinal bleeding (60%-70%) than after bleeding has ceased (<20%). Angiographic therapy with transcatheter vasopressin infusion or embolization has been effective but is associated with a substantial risk of bowel infarction.

5. Capsule endoscopy clearly is the best method to evaluate the entire small bowel in cases of obscure bleeding, yielding an abnormal finding about 70% of the time. However, capsule retention requiring operation remains an issue.

6. Push enteroscopy has been reported to identify probable bleeding sites in 50% of patients with obscure gastrointestinal bleeding. This procedure can be done with an adult or pediatric colonoscope, but the depth of insertion is greater with a dedicated enteroscope (length, 200-250 cm) and use of an overtube. Curiously, about 25% of the lesions identified with push enteroscopy are within the reach of a standard endoscope.

7. Intraoperative enteroscopy has been reported to detect abnormalities in about 70% of patients. However, recurrent bleeding is not uncommon, and only 40% to 50% of patients are free of bleeding at 2 years.

RECOMMENDED READING

Nonvariceal Upper Gastrointestinal Tract Bleeding

Barkun A, Bardou M, Marshall JK, Nonvariceal Upper GI Bleeding Consensus Conference Group. Consensus recommendations for managing patients with nonvariceal upper gastrointestinal bleeding. Ann Intern Med. 2003;139:843-57.

British Society of Gastroenterology Endoscopy Committee. Non-variceal upper gastrointestinal haemorrhage. Guidelines. Gut. 2002;51 Suppl IV:1-6.

Cook DJ, Reeve BK, Guyatt GH, Heyland DK, Griffith LE, Buckingham L, et al. Stress ulcer prophylaxis in critically ill patients: resolving discordant meta-analyses. JAMA. 1996;275:308-14.

Jensen DM. Long term prevention of recurrent ulcer hemorrhage: issues and insights. Curr Viewpoints Dig Health. 1995;2:1-14.

Jensen DM. Current diagnosis and treatment of severe ulcer hemorrhage. ASGE Clin Update. 1999;6:1-4.

Laine L. Management of ulcers with adherent clots. Gastroenterology. 2002;123:632-6.

Laine L, Peterson WL. Bleeding peptic ulcer. N Engl J Med. 1994;331:717-27.

McCarthy DM. Prevention and treatment of gastrointestinal symptoms and complications due to NSAIDs. Best Pract Res Clin Gastroenterol. 2001;15:755-73.

Mueller X, Rothenbuehler JM, Amery A, Harder F. Factors predisposing to further hemorrhage and mortality after peptic ulcer bleeding. J Am Coll Surg. 1994;179:457-61.

Peterson WL, Cook DJ. Antisecretory therapy for bleeding peptic ulcer. JAMA. 1998;280:877-88.

Rockall TA, Logan RF, Devlin HB, Northfield TC. Incidence of and mortality from acute upper gastrointestinal haemorrhage in the United Kingdom. Steering Committee and members of the National Audit of Acute Upper Gastrointestinal Haemorrhage. BMJ. 1995;311:222-6.

Rockall TA, Logan RF, Devlin HB, Northfield TC. Risk assessment after acute upper gastrointestinal haemorrhage. Gut. 1996;38:316-21.

Yavorski RT, Wong RK, Maydonovitch C, Battin LS, Furnia A, Amundson DE. Analysis of 3,294 cases of upper gastrointestinal bleeding in military medical facilities. Am J Gastroenterol. 1995;90:568-73.

Zimmerman J, Siguencia J, Tsvang E, Beeri R, Arnon R. Predictors of mortality in patients admitted to hospital for acute upper gastrointestinal hemorrhage. Scand J Gastroenterol. 1995;30:327-31.

Lower Gastrointestinal Tract Bleeding

Davies NM. Toxicity of nonsteroidal anti-inflammatory drugs in the large intestine. Dis Colon Rectum. 1995;38:1311-21.

Gostout CJ. The role of endoscopy in managing acute lower gastrointestinal bleeding. N Engl J Med. 2000;342:125-7.

Lewis BS. Small intestinal bleeding. Gastroenterol Clin North Am. 2000;29:67-95.

Van Cutsem E, Piessevaux H. Pharmacologic therapy of arteriovenous malformations. Gastrointest Endosc Clin N Am. 1996;6:819-32.

Zuckerman GR, Prakash C. Acute lower intestinal bleeding. Part II. Etiology, therapy, and outcomes. Gastrointest Endosc. 1999;49:228-38.

Obscure/Occult Gastrointestinal Bleeding

Barkin JS, Ross BS. Medical therapy for chronic gastrointestinal bleeding of obscure origin. Am J Gastroenterol. 1998;93:1250-4.

Rockey DC. Occult gastrointestinal bleeding. N Engl J Med. 1999;341:38-46.

Zuckerman GR, Prakash C, Askin MP, Lewis BS. AGA technical review on the evaluation and management of occult and obscure gastrointestinal bleeding. Gastroenterology. 2000;118:201-21.

CHAPTER 18

Vascular Disorders of the Gastrointestinal Tract

Stephen C. Hauser, M.D.

Mesenteric ischemia can occur from any of a myriad of conditions that decrease intestinal blood flow. Cappell divided these conditions into 1) secondary mesenteric ischemia due to extrinsic vascular compression or trauma (Table 1) and 2) primary mesenteric ischemia (mesenteric ischemic vasculopathy) resulting from arterial emboli, arterial or venous thrombi, low-flow states, or vasculitis. The esophagus receives its principal blood supply segmentally from small vessels from the aorta, right intercostal artery, bronchial arteries, inferior thyroid artery, left gastric artery, short gastric artery, and left phrenic artery. Vascular disease of the esophagus is extremely rare, except after surgical resection and in rare cases of vasculitis (Behçet's syndrome). The stomach has numerous arterial inputs with rich collateralization, and vascular disease of the stomach also is extremely rare except for the reasons mentioned above for the esophagus.

The principal arterial supply to the gut distal to the esophagus is from the celiac (CA), superior mesenteric (SMA), and inferior mesenteric (IMA) arteries. Embolic disease most frequently affects the SMA because of its large diameter and narrow angle of take-off from the abdominal aorta. Collaterals, which may include the meandering mesenteric artery or arc of Riolan at the base of the mesentery (connects SMA and IMA), the marginal artery of Drummond along the mesenteric border (connects SMA and IMA), the pancreaticoduodenal arcade (connects CA and SMA), the arc of Barkow (CA and SMA), and the arc of Buhler (connects CA and SMA), rapidly enlarge in response to localized mesenteric ischemia. The inferior mesenteric vein joins the splenic vein, which in turn joins the superior mesenteric vein to form the portal vein.

PATIENT HISTORY AND EXAMINATION

Primary mesenteric ischemia is responsible for about 1 per 1,000 hospital admissions. Risks include age (older than 50 years) and conditions that predispose to stasis, thrombosis, inflammation, or embolism of the mesenteric vasculature (Table 2). Symptoms may be acute (sudden, hours), subacute (days), chronic (intermittent), or a combination (usually acute and chronic). Abdominal pain often is severe, persistent (lasting hours), and poorly localized. The pain typically is more severe than the findings on abdominal palpation (i.e., pain is much greater than tenderness). Prompt evaluation is critical. Other nonspecific complaints can include fever, nausea, vomiting, abdominal distention, and diarrhea. Physical findings can

Table 1. Conditions Predisposing to Secondary Mesenteric Ischemia

Adhesions
Herniation
Volvulus
Intussusception
Median arcuate ligament syndrome
Mesenteric fibrosis
Retroperitoneal fibrosis
Carcinoid syndrome
Amyloidosis
Malignancy (peritoneal, mesenteric, colonic)
Neurofibromatosis
Trauma

Table 2. Conditions Predisposing to Primary Mesenteric Ischemia

Atherosclerosis or fibromuscular dysplasia
Cholesterol atheromatous embolism
Hypercoagulable or hyperviscosity states
Vasculitis (Fabry's disease, Behçet's syndrome, thromboangiitis obliterans, giant cell arteritis, Takayasu's arteritis, Buerger's disease, Crohn's disease, systemic lupus erythematosus, polyarteritis nodosa, rheumatoid arthritis, syphilis, Henoch-Schönlein purpura, dermatomyositis, Köhlmeier-Degos syndrome, Churg-Strauss syndrome, Wegener's granulomatosis, cryoglobulinemia, hypersensitivity vasculitis, Cogan's syndrome, Kawasaki disease, lymphocytic phlebitis, mesenteric phlebosclerosis)
Cardiac arrhythmias, valvular disease, subacute bacterial endocarditis, myxoma
Cardiomegaly, myocardial dyskinesia, intracardiac thrombosis
Cardiac catheterization, myocardial infarction
Aortic or mesenteric artery aneurysm or dissection
Low-flow states, systemic hypotension
Vasoconstrictive agents (digitalis, ergot, cocaine, amphetamines, sumatriptan, vasopressin, pseudoephedrine)
Abdominal trauma
Radiation

include abdominal distention, diminished or increased bowel sounds, and nonspecific diffuse abdominal tenderness. Localized abdominal tenderness, rebound, rigidity, altered mental status, and visible gastrointestinal tract bleeding usually are late manifestations of more severe ischemic gut damage (gastrointestinal bleeding is ominous in small-bowel ischemia and less ominous in ischemic colitis). Occult gastrointestinal bleeding can be an early finding. Leukocytosis with left shift, hemoconcentration, and an increase in amylase, aspartate aminotransferase, lactate, creatine kinase, lactate dehydrogenase, or phosphate levels may occur. Attention to predisposing conditions, their extraintestinal manifestations (congestive heart failure, hypotension, sepsis, arrhythmias, splanchnic vasoconstrictors such as digoxin and cocaine), and their initial management are critical in resuscitation of the patient (volume replacement, enhancing cardiac output, diminishing splanchnic vasoconstriction, administration of broad-spectrum antibiotics).

INITIAL DIAGNOSTIC EVALUATION

In an acutely ill patient, plain abdominal radiographs are important to rule out secondary causes of mesenteric ischemia and other causes of acute abdominal pain, principally obstruction and perforation. "Thumbprinting" may be seen. Pneumatosis intestinalis or portal venous gas are late findings that suggest transmural necrosis of the intestine (gangrene). Contrast-enhanced abdominal-pelvic computed tomography (CT) may help exclude other causes of acute intra-abdominal pain and has been recommended to diagnose acute (or acute on chronic) mesenteric venous thrombosis in patients with a history of deep venous thrombosis or thrombophlebitis or a family history of

a hypercoagulable state. The CT scan may be normal in acute mesenteric ischemia or may show nonspecific changes such as bowel wall thickening, submucosal hemorrhage, mesenteric stranding, and pneumatosis. CT should not defer resuscitation or arteriography in very ill patients with suspected acute mesenteric ischemia. Patients with subacute or chronic pain syndromes benefit from a more complete evaluation, including CT and duplex ultrasonography (see below).

Acutely ill patients require prompt diagnosis and treatment, for which selective mesenteric arteriography is the standard. If angiography is not readily available or transmural intestinal necrosis (gangrene) is suspected, laparotomy is indicated. Resuscitation and administration of broad-spectrum antibiotics constitute initial therapy for all patients.

SUPERIOR MESENTERIC ARTERY EMBOLUS

SMA embolus is common, accounting for 5% of peripheral emboli and 50% of cases of primary mesenteric ischemia. The emboli usually are from the heart; an aortic origin is less common. Arrhythmias, cardioversion, cardiac catheterization, myocardial infarction or dyskinesia, previous embolism, and age older than 50 are major risk factors. Peritonitis requires laparotomy, with or without resection and with or without embolectomy. Otherwise, embolectomy, usually surgical, is indicated (Fig. 1). Patients with acute onset of partial or small SMA branch occlusion may be candidates for thrombolytic therapy, intra-arterial papaverine, or anticoagulation. Generalized SMA vasoconstriction occurs from occlusion of a single SMA branch and often persists after embolectomy. Hence, many experts recommend intra-arterial papaverine

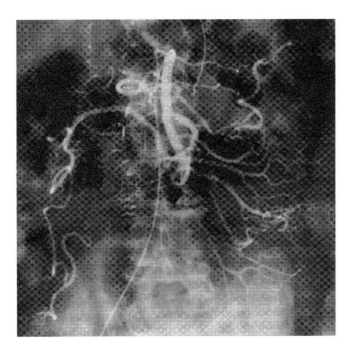

Fig. 1. Anteroposterior view of the aorta showing embolic occlusion of the proximal superior mesenteric artery. Note the normal-appearing proximal jejunal arterial branches and abrupt cutoff of the superior mesenteric artery. (From McKinsey JF, Gewertz BL. Acute mesenteric ischemia. Surg Clin North Am. 1997;77:307-18. Used with permission.)

before and for 24 hours after embolectomy or until a second-look operation (if indicated) is performed. Prophylaxis against further embolization (heparinization) usually is indicated.

SUPERIOR MESENTERIC ARTERY THROMBUS
SMA thrombus accounts for about 15% of cases of primary mesenteric ischemia. Risk factors for SMA thrombus include old age, low-flow states (arrhythmia, hypotension, sepsis, myocardial infarction, dyskinesia, congestive heart failure), atherosclerosis (acute on chronic ischemia, hypertension, diabetes mellitus, vasculopathy), hypercoagulable states, vasculitis, and aortic or mesenteric artery aneurysm. Up to one-third of patients have a history of chronic mesenteric ischemia (see below). Therapy usually involves intra-arterial papaverine and surgical thrombectomy or surgical bypass grafting, bowel resection, or some combination of these.

NONOCCLUSIVE MESENTERIC ISCHEMIA
Nonocclusive mesenteric ischemia accounts for 20% of cases of acute mesenteric ischemia. Risks for low-flow state include decreased cardiac output (myocardial infarction or dyskinesia, arrhythmia, shock, sepsis, pancreatitis, burns, multiple organ failure, congestive heart failure, hemorrhage), vasospasm

(digoxin, α-adrenergic agonists, cocaine), and preexisting atherosclerotic disease (hypertension, diabetes mellitus, hyperlipidemia, vasculopathy). Angiography can be diagnostic (lack of thrombus or embolus, alternating spasm and dilatation ["string-of-sausages" sign], pruning, and spasm of mesenteric arcades) (Fig. 2). Treatment involves optimization of cardiac output, avoiding vasospastic medications, and prolonged (up to several days) selective intra-arterial infusion of vasodilators such as papaverine, tolazoline, nitroglycerin, or glucagon. Laparotomy with or without resection and warm saline lavage may be needed in selected cases. Anticoagulation generally is not used. Broad-spectrum antibiotics should be administered.

MESENTERIC VENOUS THROMBOSIS
Mesenteric venous thrombosis, usually (up to 95%) SMV thrombosis, accounts for about 5% to 10% of cases of acute mesenteric ischemia. Risk factors include a personal or family history of hypercoagulopathy and a history of deep venous thrombosis. Causes include hypercoagulable states, hyperviscosity syndromes, intra-abdominal infections (pyelophlebitis) or inflammation, malignant obstruction, portal hypertension, and trauma (Table 3). Symptoms may be acute (hours) or subacute-chronic (days to months) and include abdominal pain (severe, out of proportion to physical findings, or less severe and vague), anorexia, nausea, vomiting, diarrhea, constipation, abdominal distention, and gastrointestinal bleeding. Patients may present with bacteremia (especially *Bacteroides*). Because the differential diagnosis is broad and includes obstruction, perforation, and other causes of acute abdominal pain and acute mesenteric ischemia, the initial evaluation usually includes plain abdominal radiography and contrast-enhanced CT; the latter usually is diagnostic of mesenteric venous thrombosis with or without portal vein or splenic vein thrombosis (Fig. 3). Although angiography is less reliable for the diagnosis of mesenteric venous thrombosis, it allows intra-arterial infusion of vasodilators. Therapy involves laparotomy with or without bowel resection when infarction is suspected, fluid resuscitation, broad-spectrum antibiotics, avoidance of vasoconstrictors, a nasogastric tube if there is distention, and anticoagulation (in the absence of bleeding). Selected patients with acute onset of mesenteric venous thrombosis may be candidates for thrombolytic therapy, followed by anticoagulation. Underlying conditions such as hypercoagulable states, hyperviscosity syndromes, intra-abdominal infections, and malignancy require concomitant diagnosis and treatment.

Mesenteric venous thrombosis may present as a subacute or chronic illness, with vague abdominal pain and distention or no symptoms. It may be an incidental CT finding in patients with portal hypertension, chronic pancreatitis, or malignancy. Long-term anticoagulation should be considered except for

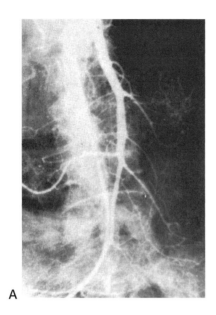

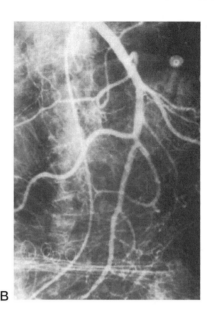

Fig. 2. Patient with nonocclusive mesenteric ischemia before, *A*, and after, *B*, treatment with papaverine. *A*, Angiogram showing spasm of main superior mesenteric artery, origins of its branches, and the intestinal arcades. *B*, Angiogram after 36 hours of papaverine infusion showing resolution of the arteriospasm. The abdominal symptoms and signs had resolved. (From Boley SJ, Brandt LJ, Veith FJ. Ischemic disorders of the intestines. Curr Probl Surg. 1978;15[4]:1-85. Used with permission.)

higher-risk patients such as the elderly or those with portal hypertension and prominent varices or portal hypertensive gastropathy.

CHRONIC MESENTERIC ISCHEMIA

Patients with classic chronic mesenteric ischemia present with episodic ischemic abdominal pain that typically is postprandial, lasts 1 to 3 hours, and becomes worse with time. Thus, patients lose weight because of fear of eating (sitophobia). Atherosclerotic stenosis of the origin of at least two of the three major visceral arteries usually is found on arteriography. However, this is a common angiographic finding in otherwise healthy age-matched controls. Rarely, vasculitis or aortic aneurysm can present as chronic mesenteric ischemia. A history of previous vascular disease, hypertension, diabetes mellitus, renal insufficiency, and smoking is common. Nausea, vomiting, diarrhea, constipation, and bloating may occur in addition to abdominal pain and weight loss. Some patients may have malabsorption, otherwise unexplained gastroduodenal ulcerations, and small-bowel biopsy findings of nonspecific surface cell flattening, chronic inflammation, and villous atrophy. More than one-half of the patients have a bruit on abdominal examination.

Doppler ultrasonography—if able to visualize the CA and SMA (each about 80%)—may show increased flow velocities, consistent with marked stenosis. However, thinking of the diagnosis, excluding other causes of abdominal pain and other

symptoms (i.e., pancreatic cancer, gastric cancer, gastroparesis, small-bowel bacterial overgrowth states, partial small-bowel obstruction, biliary disease, gastric volvulus, or paraesophageal hernias), and obtaining arteriographic results consistent with the clinical findings are crucial. Surgical reconstruction and, in selected cases, angioplasty with or without stents can be therapeutic.

ISCHEMIC COLITIS

Ischemic colitis represents nearly one-half of all cases of mesenteric ischemia. Atherosclerotic or thrombotic occlusion of the IMA or its branches and nonocclusive low-flow states are not uncommon causes of ischemic colitis (with associated vasospasm). Less common causes include embolus, vasculitis, hypercoagulable states, iatrogenic IMA ligation (aortic surgery), and colonic obstruction (colon cancer, diverticulitis, strictures). Other unusual associations include long-distance running, intra-abdominal infections or inflammatory disease, and use of birth control pills, danazol, alosetron, digitalis, vasopressin, gold, pseudoephedrine, psychotropic drugs, ergot, amphetamines, cocaine, or sumatriptan. Not uncommonly, there is no recognizable cause. Some gastrointestinal infections, such as cytomegalovirus, *Escherichia coli* O157:H7, and *Clostridium difficile* infections, and chronic inflammatory bowel disease can mimic ischemic colitis clinically and histologically. Ischemic colitis due to low-flow states often affects watershed areas such as the splenic flexure, descending colon, and rectosigmoid

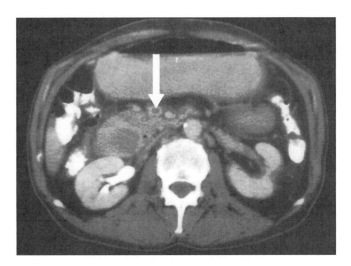

Fig. 3. Abdominal computed tomogram of a patient with acute mesenteric venous thrombosis. *Arrow*, thrombus in the superior mesenteric vein. (From Rhee RY, Gloviczki P. Mesenteric venous thrombosis. Surg Clin North Am. 1997;77:327-38. Used with permission.)

Table 3. Risk Factors for Mesenteric Venous Thrombosis

Hypercoagulable and hyperviscosity states
Protein S deficiency
Primary myeloproliferative disorder
G20210A factor II gene mutation
C677T *MTHFR* gene mutation
Antiphospholipid syndrome
G1691 factor V gene mutation
Antithrombin deficiency
Protein C deficiency
Hyperfibrinogenemia
Thrombocytosis
Sickle cell disease
Estrogen or progesterone
Intra-abdominal infections and inflammation
Appendicitis
Diverticulitis
Abscess
Crohn's disease
Pancreatitis
Cholecystitis
Neonatal omphalitis
Portal hypertension
Cirrhosis
Sclerotherapy of varices
Malignant obstruction
Trauma
Vasculitis

junction and the right colon. Often, but not always, the rectum is spared in ischemic colitis.

The clinical symptoms of ischemic colitis vary but often include acute abdominal pain (in two-thirds of patients, usually the left lower quadrant), urgency, diarrhea, distention, anorexia, nausea, vomiting, or bright red blood or maroon material per rectum (variable amounts), or some combination of these. Physical findings often include one or more of the following: abdominal tenderness over the affected bowel, distention, fever, and tachycardia. Laboratory findings range from normal in patients with less severe ischemic colitis to those found in persons with severe ischemic necrosis (see above). Plain radiographs of the abdomen may show evidence of submucosal edema and hemorrhage ("thumbprinting"), or the findings may be nonspecific. Colonoscopy often provides endoscopic and histologic findings consistent with ischemic colitis (segmental, patchy ulceration, edema, erythema, submucosal hemorrhagic or purple nodules) and helps exclude other causes of abdominal pain and gastrointestinal bleeding. CT may help exclude other disorders, especially in more symptomatic, sicker patients. Gastrointestinal infections (acute bacterial colitis, *C. difficile* infection, parasitic infections), inflammatory bowel disease, diverticulitis, pancreatitis, and other causes of acute abdominal pain (pelvic disorders in women) need to be excluded. Typically, angiography is not required, but it may be for patients with more severe ischemic colitis or with right-sided involvement (which may include the small bowel).

As for all types of mesenteric ischemia, treatment depends on the cause and includes supportive treatment (volume replacement, correction of low-flow states, broad-spectrum antibiotics, transfusions, avoiding vasoconstrictive medications) and, in selected cases, surgery (signs and symptoms of transmural necrosis, perforation, massive bleeding, recurrent sepsis, failure to improve over time, stricture formation). In most patients, ischemic colitis resolves promptly with supportive therapy alone. Younger patients should be evaluated for thrombophilic states. Recent studies lend support to the usefulness of thrombophilic screening in older patients with idiopathic ischemic colitis.

MISCELLANEOUS SYNDROMES

Celiac Artery Compression

CA compression, also called "median arcuate ligament syndrome," is a rare syndrome with abdominal pain, which most likely is caused by extrinsic compression of the celiac axis (neural structures, the wall of the CA) by the arcuate ligament. Rarely, the SMA also may be involved. Ischemia to the gut is unlikely to cause the pain (because only one vessel is involved and collateral vessels are well developed). Celiac artery compression usually occurs in young women, often with upper abdominal pain, especially after eating (increased blood flow through the CA), often with weight loss, and with a loud systolic bruit in the epigastric area on physical examination. Lateral aortography should demonstrate a typical concave defect over the superior aspect of the CA near its take-off from the aorta, with respiratory variability. Collaterals may be seen. Surgical release of the compression of the CA or reconstruction of the CA (or both) may be curative. Preoperatively, other possible causes of the symptoms must be excluded.

Vasculitis

Many vasculitic syndromes can involve the gastrointestinal tract. Buerger's disease can cause multiple distal occlusions of the mesenteric arterial circulation. Polyarteritis nodosa typically involves medium-sized vessels, resulting in segmental microaneurysms. Many affected patients have fever, an increased erythrocyte sedimentation rate, hypertension, and multiple organ involvement. Nearly half are infected with hepatitis B virus. Also, the gallbladder and spleen may be involved. The gastrointestinal tract often is involved in Churg-Strauss syndrome and Henoch-Schönlein purpura (sometimes with *E. coli* O157:H7 or *Campylobacter jejuni* infection); with Henoch-Schönlein purpura, IgA is deposited in multiple organs, including the walls of blood vessels. Patients with severe rheumatoid arthritis, high titers of rheumatoid factor, nodules, cryoglobulinemia, low serum levels of complement, and extra-articular manifestations also may have vascular lesions involving the gut, pancreas, gallbladder, spleen, and appendix, as may patients with systemic lupus erythematosus (especially those with antiphospholipid or cardiolipin antibodies). Vasculitis with bowel involvement is less common in patients with Behçet's syndrome or Wegener's granulomatosis. Mesenteric venous involvement can occur with Churg-Strauss syndrome, systemic lupus erythematosus, Behçet's syndrome, lymphocytic phlebitis, and idiopathic mesenteric phlebosclerosis.

Bowel as well as large-vessel rupture can be a life-threatening complication of Ehlers-Danlos syndrome type IV, with thin fragile skin, easy bruisability, hyperextensible distal interphalangeal joints, and splanchnic artery aneurysms due to a defect in type III collagen. Similar vascular catastrophes with gastrointestinal bleeding can occur in patients with pseudoxanthoma elasticum type I, which is often accompanied by peau d'orange skin and choroiditis. Occasionally, mesenteric vasculitis is found in patients with carcinoid syndrome. Splanchnic artery aneurysms include splenic artery aneurysms (due to atherosclerosis, fibrodysplasia of the media, portal hypertension, pregnancy, pancreatitis, vasculitis, or trauma), hepatic artery aneurysms (often due to trauma, including liver biopsy), mesenteric aneurysms (often due to atherosclerosis), and aneurysms of the arterial supply to the pancreas (often due to pancreatitis and pseudocysts)—all of which may present with gastrointestinal or intraperitoneal hemorrhage.

RECOMMENDED READING

American Gastroenterological Association Medical Position Statement. Guidelines on intestinal ischemia. Gastroenterology. 2000;118:951-3.

Amitrano L, Brancaccio V, Guardascione MA, Margaglione M, Iannaccone L, Dandrea G, et al. High prevalence of thrombophilic genotypes in patients with acute mesenteric vein thrombosis. Am J Gastroenterol. 2001;96:146-9.

Bassiouny HS. Nonocclusive mesenteric ischemia. Surg Clin North Am. 1997;77:319-26.

Bech FR. Celiac artery compression syndromes. Surg Clin North Am. 1997;77:409-24.

Brandt LJ, Boley SJ. AGA technical review on intestinal ischemia. Gastroenterology. 2000;118:954-68.

Cappell MS. Intestinal (mesenteric) vasculopathy. I. Acute superior mesenteric arteriopathy and venopathy. Gastroenterol Clin North Am. 1998;27:783-825.

Cappell MS. Intestinal (mesenteric) vasculopathy. II. Ischemic colitis and chronic mesenteric ischemia. Gastroenterol Clin North Am. 1998;27:827-60.

Hackworth CA, Leef JA. Percutaneous transluminal mesenteric angioplasty. Surg Clin North Am. 1997;77:371-80.

Koutroubakis IE, Sfiridaki A, Theodoropoulou A, Kouroumalis EA. Role of acquired and hereditary thrombotic risk factors in colon ischemia of ambulatory patients. Gastroenterology. 2001;121:561-5.

Krupski WC, Selzman CH, Whitehill TA. Unusual causes of mesenteric ischemia. Surg Clin North Am. 1997;77:471-502.

Kumar S, Sarr MG, Kamath PS. Mesenteric venous thrombosis. N Engl J Med. 2001;345:1683-8.

McKinsey JF, Gewertz BL. Acute mesenteric ischemia. Surg Clin North Am. 1997;77:307-18.

Midian-Singh R, Polen A, Durishin C, Crock RD, Whittier FC, Fahmy N. Ischemic colitis revisited: a prospective study identifying hypercoagulability as a risk factor. South Med J. 2004;97:120-3.

Moawad J, Gewertz BL. Chronic mesenteric ischemia: clinical presentation and diagnosis. Surg Clin North Am. 1997;77:357-69.

Nicoloff AD, Williamson WK, Moneta GL, Taylor LM, Porter JM. Duplex ultrasonography in evaluation of splanchnic artery stenosis. Surg Clin North Am. 1997;77:339-55.

Noyer CM, Brandt LJ. Colon ischemia: unusual aspects. Clin Perspect Gastroenterol. 2000;36:315-26.

Rosenblum JD, Boyle CM, Schwartz LB. The mesenteric circulation: anatomy and physiology. Surg Clin North Am. 1997;77:289-306.

Segatto E, Mortele KJ, Ji H, Wiesner W, Ros PR. Acute small bowel ischemia: CT imaging findings. Semin Ultrasound CT MR. 2003;24:364-76.

CHAPTER 19

Gastrointestinal Manifestations of Systemic Disease

Stephen C. Hauser, M.D.

Many systemic disorders can have gastrointestinal manifestations. This chapter is an overview of these diseases as they affect the gastrointestinal tract and liver, emphasizing disorders that are not considered elsewhere in this book.

SYMPTOMS AND SIGNS

Eating Disorders and Weight

Obesity can have adverse effects on the gastrointestinal tract, including an increased risk of symptomatic gastroesophageal reflux disease, a possible increased risk of esophageal, gallbladder, and colonic adenocarcinoma, increased gallstone formation in women, fatty liver and nonalcoholic steatohepatitis, and complications in obese patients with pancreatitis (gallstones, hypertriglyceridemia). Hypothyroidism, Cushing's syndrome, hypothalamic disorders, Stein-Leventhal syndrome, and drugs (especially antipsychotic agents, tricyclic antidepressants, monoamine oxidase inhibitors, lithium, and glucocorticoids) should be considered in the differential diagnosis of obesity. Crash *diets* with rapid weight loss can result in gallstones (increased cholesterol saturation of bile, decreased gallbladder motility), nausea, vomiting, diarrhea, or severe constipation. Patients with *eating disorders* (e.g., bulimia, anorexia nervosa) may present with a wide variety of gastrointestinal problems: nausea, vomiting, gas, abdominal pain, diarrhea, dysphagia, gastroesophageal reflux disease, rumination, Mallory-Weiss tear, gastroparesis, constipation, superior mesenteric artery syndrome, cholelithiasis, pancreatitis, increased values on liver function tests, and abnormal gastrointestinal motility.

Nausea and Vomiting

The differential diagnosis is protean and includes drugs (especially narcotics, dopamine agonists, digitalis, chemotherapy, nonsteroidal anti-inflammatory drugs), toxins (alcohol, hypervitaminosis A, poisoning), vestibular diseases, central nervous system diseases, pregnancy (see below), metabolic disorders (e.g., Reye's syndrome, Jamaican vomiting illness, uremia, parathyroid disease, diabetic ketoacidosis, hyperthyroidism, sepsis, Addison's disease), myocardial infarction (congestive heart failure), and radiation.

Diarrhea

On occasion, diarrhea can be caused by systemic disorders such as hyperthyroidism, Addison's disease, hypoparathyroidism, collagen vascular diseases, vasculitis, malignancies (e.g., carcinoid, gastrinoma, pheochromocytoma, VIPoma [vasoactive intestinal polypeptide], medullary carcinoma of the thyroid, glucagonoma, mastocytosis, other neuroendocrine tumors), immunologic disorders (see below), amyloidosis (see below), autonomic nervous system disease, diabetes mellitus (see below), and, more commonly, drugs and toxins, including alcohol and radiation.

Constipation

The differential diagnosis should include drugs and toxins, metabolic disorders (hypothyroidism, hypercalcemia, hypokalemia, hypopituitarism, diabetes mellitus, pheochromocytoma, glucagonoma), central, peripheral, or autonomic neurologic disorders, myopathies, collagen vascular disease, amyloidosis, porphyria, and pregnancy.

Abdominal Pain

Extra-abdominal causes of acute or intermittent abdominal pain include thoracic disorders (e.g., myocardial infarction, pulmonary embolus, pneumonia, pericarditis), metabolic disorders (diabetic ketoacidosis, pheochromocytoma, Addison's disease, uremia, hyperlipidemia, porphyria, angioedema [see below], hyperparathyroidism), hematologic disorders (sickle cell crisis, hemolysis, acute leukemia), neurologic diseases (herpes zoster, tabes dorsalis, abdominal epilepsy, abdominal migraine), drugs, toxins, narcotic withdrawal, and heat stroke.

Jaundice and Abnormal Results of Liver Function Tests

Unconjugated hyperbilirubinemia in the newborn can be caused by hypothyroidism. In adults, *congestive heart failure* is one of the most common causes of mild abnormal results of liver function tests, including mild unconjugated hyperbilirubinemia, mild increases of alanine aminotransferase and aspartate aminotransferase, and, less often, a mild increase of alkaline phosphatase. Many connective tissue diseases (see below) can be associated with abnormal liver function test results. *Hodgkin's disease* without involvement of the liver or biliary tree, like many infections and sepsis, can be associated with increased alkaline phosphatase levels and even jaundice.

SYSTEMIC DISORDERS

Dermatologic

Many dermatologic disorders can be associated with gastrointestinal vascular bleeding lesions. Hereditary hemorrhagic telangiectasia is an autosomal dominant disorder; telangiectasias can involve any part of the bowel and the lips, tongue, mouth, extremities, chest, nose, liver, central nervous system, retina, and lung. Endoscopically, these mucosal telangiectasias are indistinguishable from angiodysplastic lesions. Lesions may involve all histologic layers (mucosa to serosa) of the bowel wall. *Blue rubber bleb nevus syndrome*, sometimes autosomal dominant, consists of intestinal and cutaneous cavernous hemangiomas with a bluish, rubbery consistency. Other internal organs also may be involved. Intestinal lesions can result in intussusception. Similar hemangiomas may occur in the sporadic disorder Klippel-Trénaunay-Weber syndrome, involving gut and skin and hemihypertrophy of a limb and varicose veins. Malignant atrophic papulosis (Degos' syndrome) consists of painless skin papules with cigarette-paper–like white centers and a telangiectatic periphery and gastrointestinal and central nervous system involvement. All of these disorders can cause bleeding and require therapeutic endoscopic or surgical intervention.

Several bullous skin disorders can manifest with involvement of the gastrointestinal tract, including *epidermolysis bullosa* (trauma-induced blisters, oral cavity, esophagus, and anal area, with bullae, webs, strictures, dysphagia, bleeding, and constipation), *pemphigus vulgaris* (oral involvement, esophagus less common, occasionally the lower gastrointestinal tract with bleeding), and *bullous pemphigoid* (oral, less often esophageal or anal involvement). Dilatation (trauma) of strictures in epidermolysis bullosa may lead to more stricturing, and soft diets and corticosteroids may be helpful. Topical or systemic corticosteroids may be useful in bullous pemphigoid and pemphigus vulgaris.

Finally, *lichen planus* can affect the mouth and esophagus (strictures, pain, dysphagia; also, an association with hepatitis C virus infection), *psoriasis* can affect the skin and esophagus (webs, dysphagia), and *tylosis* (autosomal dominant) can affect the skin (palmoplantar keratoderma) and esophagus (squamous cell carcinoma, family screening and surveillance endoscopy are indicated).

Immunologic

A host of immunologic disorders have gastrointestinal manifestations. *X-linked (Burton's) hypogammaglobulinemia*, a maturational hereditary defect in B cells, results in gastrointestinal infections (*Campylobacter*, *Giardia*, rotavirus), small bowel bacterial overgrowth, and perirectal abscesses. Plasma cells typically are absent on rectal biopsy. *Selective IgA deficiency* occurs in about 1 in 500 persons; it is usually sporadic but is sometimes familial, and it is associated with a lack of secretory immunoglobulin A1 and A2. Most persons are well, and gastrointestinal infections (*Giardia*) are not common. Persons with celiac disease have an increased prevalence of immunoglobulin A deficiency (1:50). Other gastrointestinal associations include pernicious anemia, bacterial overgrowth with vitamin B_{12} deficiency, Crohn's disease, and nodular lymphoid hyperplasia. *Common variable (late-onset, acquired) hypogammaglobulinemia*, often sporadic, again involves abnormal maturation of B cells, gastrointestinal tract infections (*Giardia* and other parasites, small bowel bacterial overgrowth, rotavirus, bacterial diarrhea), malabsorption, pancreatic insufficiency, sprue-like disorders, pernicious anemia, gastric cancer, nodular lymphoid hyperplasia, cholelithiasis, autoimmune chronic hepatitis, sclerosing cholangitis, and biliary parasitosis (cryptosporidiosis). Carcinoma or lymphoma of the small and large bowel also may occur.

Chronic mucocutaneous candidiasis is a heterogeneous group of disorders with defective T-cell function, oropharyngeal or esophageal candidiasis, skin and nail lesions, and various autoimmune (pernicious anemia) and endocrine (hypoadrenal, hypothyroid, hypoparathyroid, diabetes mellitus) deficiencies. *Hereditary angioedema* is an autosomal dominant (chromosome 11q11-13) disorder with a quantitative or qualitative deficiency of C1 esterase inhibitor, resulting in attacks of nonpitting, painless, nonpruritic angioedema that can involve the skin, mouth, larynx, or gastrointestinal tract. Gastrointestinal tract involvement includes attacks of pain, sometimes with diarrhea, vomiting, intussusception, or transient ascites. Imaging may reveal edematous bowel. Similar presentations may be due to acquired C1 esterase inhibitor deficiency (collagen vascular diseases, lymphoproliferative disorders). Diagnostic testing includes C1 esterase inhibitor levels (low in 85%), C1 esterase function (low in the 15% with normal or increased inhibitor levels), and C4 levels (absent during attacks, reduced between attacks). C1 levels are normal. Danazol can prevent attacks, and C1 esterase inhibitor concentrate or fresh frozen plasma can be used during attacks. Angiotensin-converting enzyme inhibitors also can cause angioedema of the intestine, independent of diminished complement or C1 esterase inhibitor levels. Angiotensin II receptor antagonists also have been implicated. An estrogen-dependent inherited form of angioedema, also independent of diminished complement or C1 esterase inhibitor levels, has been reported during pregnancy or with the administration of exogenous estrogens.

Cardiovascular

Congestive heart failure can present with hepatic involvement (hepatomegaly, right upper quadrant pain, mild abnormal results of liver function tests, ascites with an increased serum to ascites albumin gradient) and gastrointestinal involvement (anorexia, nausea, bloating, abdominal pain, diarrhea, malabsorption, protein-losing enteropathy, low-flow mesenteric ischemia). It is now thought that valvular aortic stenosis might be associated with gastrointestinal angiodysplasia, perhaps on the basis of abnormal von Willebrand multimers. *Cardiac transplantation* may be complicated by an increased risk of bowel perforation, pancreatitis, and gallstone-related disease.

Pulmonary

α_1-*Antitrypsin deficiency* can be thought of as either a pulmonary disease with liver manifestations or a liver disorder with pulmonary consequences. Liver disease, including cirrhosis and hepatocellular carcinoma, is due to the inability of the liver to export an abnormal gene product (usually the ZZ protease inhibitor type, with low serum α_1-antitrypsin levels) and does not occur in the null-null phenotype (no gene product). Patients with *chronic obstructive pulmonary disease* are at increased risk for peptic ulcer disease. Chronic obstructive pulmonary disease and asthma can facilitate gastroesophageal reflux. *Sarcoidosis* is a systemic granulomatous disorder that commonly involves the liver (often asymptomatic, with or without mild increases of alanine aminotransferase, bilirubin, or alkaline phosphatase; occasionally progressive hepatic fibrosis resulting in cirrhosis; some patients with severe cholestasis with ductopenia). Less often, sarcoidosis affects the gastrointestinal tract (esophageal

involvement with dysphagia, dysmotility or stricture rare, often due to hilar or mediastinal lymph node involvement; stomach, with antral ulceration or pyloric stenosis or gastric outlet obstruction, occurs more often; small bowel disease, with malabsorption or protein-losing enteropathy, rare; colonic involvement very rare). *Lung transplantation* may be complicated by postoperative colonic perforation and vagal injury with esophageal and gastric dysmotility.

Renal

Chronic renal failure can be complicated by dysgeusia, anorexia, nausea, vomiting, esophagitis, gastritis, angiodysplasias of the gastrointestinal tract, peptic ulcer disease, duodenitis, duodenal pseudomelanosis (asymptomatic), abdominal pain, constipation, pseudo-obstruction, perforated colonic diverticula, small bowel and colonic ulceration, intussusception, gastrointestinal bleeding, amyloidosis, diarrhea, fecal impaction, and bacterial overgrowth. In patients undergoing *hemodialysis*, a refractory exudative ascites of unclear pathogenesis can develop, and this resolves with renal transplantation. In patients who have had *renal transplantation*, infections and ulcerative complications of the gastrointestinal tract, diverticulitis, and perforated colonic diverticula often develop. The adult form of *polycystic kidney disease* is associated with hepatic cysts, congenital hepatic fibrosis, and Caroli's disease. (There are rare reports of hyperammonemia and hepatic encephalopathy in patients with severe urease-producing *Proteus* or *Escherichia coli* bacterial infections, without previous liver disease.)

Endocrine

Endocrine disorders commonly affect the gastrointestinal tract and liver. *Diabetes mellitus* can be complicated by disorders of the esophagus (dysmotility, candidiasis), stomach (dysmotility, gastroparesis, bezoars, pernicious anemia), small bowel (dysmotility, bacterial overgrowth, celiac disease association), colon (dysmotility, constipation, fecal incontinence, diarrhea), biliary tree (cholelithiasis), and liver (fatty liver, nonalcoholic steatohepatitis). Diabetic neuropathy and ketoacidosis can present as abdominal pain, and diabetes mellitus is a risk factor for several forms of primary mesenteric ischemia. *Acromegaly* is associated with an enlarged tongue, an increased risk of colonic adenomas (colonoscopic screening, at least by age 50 years), and, perhaps, colon and stomach cancer. Gallstones are a risk in patients receiving octreotide treatment. *Addison's disease* may present with anorexia, nausea, vomiting, weight loss, malabsorption, abdominal pain, and diarrhea and may be associated with atrophic gastritis and pernicious anemia. Serum aminotransferase levels also may be increased. *Hypercortisolism* may be associated with gastric ulceration and increased aminotransferase levels. *Hyperthyroidism* may manifest as hyperphagia, weight loss, mild diarrhea, steatorrhea, abdominal pain, concomitant atrophic gastritis, dysphagia, ascites, and non-specific mild abnormalities in results of liver function tests. Autoimmune chronic hepatitis and primary biliary cirrhosis also may be associated disorders. *Hypothyroidism* often results in anorexia, weight gain, constipation, dysphagia, heartburn, and, less often, intestinal pseudo-obstruction, achlorhydria, and ascites (high protein). Associated gastrointestinal diseases include pernicious anemia, ulcerative colitis, primary biliary cirrhosis, autoimmune chronic hepatitis, and celiac disease. *Hyperparathyroidism*, with hypercalcemia, classically produces anorexia, nausea, vomiting, constipation, and abdominal pain; rarely, peptic ulcer disease and pancreatitis develop. *Hypoparathyroidism* can present with diarrhea, steatorrhea, abdominal pain, pseudo-obstruction, protein-losing enteropathy, and lymphangiectasia.

Hematologic

Sickle cell anemia often results in severe abdominal pain with sickle cell crisis. The liver also may be affected, with pain (congestion, infarction), fever, and increased values on liver function tests. As in other hemolytic states, cholelithiasis (black pigment stones) is common. *Hemolytic uremic syndrome* and *thrombotic thrombocytopenic purpura* can be complicated by gastrointestinal tract bleeding, ulceration, perforation, toxic megacolon, cholecystitis, and pancreatitis, and often they are associated with gram-negative infections, such as those caused by *E. coli* O157:H7, *Shigella*, *Salmonella*, *Yersinia*, and *Campylobacter*. A host of *hypercoagulable states*, some caused by hematologic malignancies, have been implicated in cases of Budd-Chiari syndrome, portal venous thrombosis, and primary mesenteric (venous and arterial) ischemic states. *Hypocoagulable states*, such as hemophilia, and platelet abnormalities often result in gastrointestinal bleeding, obstruction, intramural hematomas, or intussusception.

Four of the *porphyrias* can present with acute abdominal crises (abdominal pain, vomiting, constipation, and hyponatremia are common). These four are acute intermittent porphyria, variegate porphyria, hereditary coproporphyria, and aminolevulinic acid (ALA) dehydratase deficiency. The first three are autosomal dominant. *Acute intermittent porphyria* is the most common acute porphyria. It is associated with increased levels of ALA and porphobilinogen; there are no skin findings. *Variegate porphyria* is characterized by increases in urine coproporphyrin and stool protoporphyrin and coproporphyrin; patients can have skin disease, with or without an abdominal attack. In *hereditary coproporphyria*, stool and urine coproporphyrin levels are increased; skin disease can be present, usually with an abdominal attack. In the very rare *ALA dehydratase deficiency*, only ALA is increased; there are no skin findings, and the condition is autosomal recessive. Abdominal crises may be precipitated by fasting, medications,

alcohol, intercurrent illnesses, and menstruation. Urine ALA and porphobilinogen levels (ALA only with ALA dehydratase) are always increased during an acute abdominal crisis. In acute intermittent porphyria, urinary ALA and porphobilinogen values are usually increased between attacks also. *Porphyria cutanea tarda* affects only the skin and is associated with alcohol abuse or alcoholic liver disease, mild iron overload or hemochromatosis, and hepatitis B or C virus infection. *Erythropoietic protoporphyria*, with skin manifestations, can result in cirrhosis and liver failure due to hepatic deposition of protoporphyrin.

Mastocytosis is a systemic infiltrative disorder of bone marrow, skin, bone, spleen, the central nervous system, the gastrointestinal tract, and the liver. Periodic flushing (precipitated by alcohol, stress, heat, or medications), hypotension, urticaria pigmentosa, Darier's sign (urticaria after scratching), chest pain, dyspnea, abdominal pain, vomiting, diarrhea, and paresthesias may occur. Malabsorption, peptic ulcer disease (gastric acid hypersecretion), complicated gastroesophageal reflux disease, hepatomegaly, splenomegaly, increased serum alkaline phosphatase value, and, rarely, portal hypertension and hepatic fibrosis may occur.

Oncologic

Leukemias and *lymphomas* commonly involve the gastrointestinal tract and liver. Unusual tumors affecting the gut include α *heavy-chain disease* (Mediterranean lymphoma), which diffusely infiltrates the small bowel and adjacent lymph nodes (B cells, α heavy chains produced in excess); *mantle cell lymphomas*, which mimic a multiple polyposis syndrome; *multiple myeloma* or *amyloidosis*, with focal plasmacytomas (mass, ulceration, bleeding, or obstruction), gastrointestinal mucosal infiltration with malabsorption, or hyperviscosity syndrome (ischemia); *Waldenström's macroglobulinemia*, with gastrointestinal and hepatosplenic infiltration and malabsorption; and *small cell carcinoma of the lung*, with paraneoplastic pseudo-obstruction.

Bone marrow transplantation often is complicated by *graft-versus-host disease*. Acute graft-versus-host disease with rashes, small and large intestinal mucosal involvement (diarrhea, protein-losing enteropathy, malabsorption, pain, bleeding, apoptotic bodies on biopsy, even in endoscopically normal-appearing areas), and cholestatic liver disease usually occurs in the first 100 days after transplantation. Chronic graft-versus-host disease with cholestatic liver disease (vanishing bile ducts), esophageal disease (dysphagia, strictures, webs), skin disease, and polyserositis usually occurs after 100 days. *Veno-occlusive disease of the liver*, with bland, nonthrombotic obliteration of small hepatic veins and venules due to conditioning (radiation, chemotherapy) therapy, usually occurs 8 to 23 days after transplantation.

Neuromuscular

Many neurologic and muscular disorders affect the gastrointestinal tract. *Acute head injury* with intracranial hypertension, like many other serious illnesses, can result in stress gastritis. However, deep ulceration, sometimes with perforation, can occur in this setting, apparently as a result of vagal stimulation of gastrin and gastric acid production. Similar ulceration can occur after body burns with a large surface area. Abdominal pain, nausea, and vomiting rarely are attributed to *migraine* or temporal lobe *epilepsy*, the latter often including central nervous system symptoms. Cyclic vomiting may present with recurrent attacks of abdominal pain, nausea, and vomiting. *Cerebrovascular disease* and *cerebral palsy* commonly result in oropharyngeal dysphagia due to dysmotility. *Multiple sclerosis* frequently affects the gastrointestinal tract with oropharyngeal dysphagia, gastroparesis, constipation, or disorders of defecation or fecal incontinence. Patients with *Parkinson's disease* often have oropharyngeal dysphagia, gastroesophageal reflux disease, esophageal dysphagia, constipation, and fecal incontinence. *Amyotrophic lateral sclerosis* and *myasthenia gravis* both can cause oropharyngeal dysphagia. More diffuse gastrointestinal tract dysmotility syndromes occur with poliomyelitis, Huntington's chorea, dysautonomia syndromes, *Shy-Drager syndrome, Chagas' disease*, and *spinal cord injuries*. Patients with *dementia* may be at risk for aspiration because of oropharyngeal dysphagia, and they may have weight loss due to decreased intake, poor diet, and pica.

Muscular dystrophies such as *oculopharyngeal muscular dystrophy* (third nerve palsy, often French-Canadian ancestry) and *Duchenne's muscular dystrophy* can be complicated by oropharyngeal dysphagia. Duchenne's muscular dystrophy is associated with more widespread gastrointestinal tract dysmotility.

Rheumatologic

Involvement of the gastrointestinal tract in *scleroderma*, a common effect, is due to smooth muscle atrophy, fibrosis, small vessel involvement, and neural damage. Typically, the esophagus is affected (decreased motility, weak lower esophageal sphincter, gastroesophageal reflux disease, Barrett's esophagus, adenocarcinoma, pill esophagitis). However, the stomach (gastroparesis), small bowel (bacterial overgrowth, pseudo-obstruction), and colon and rectum (decreased motility, megacolon, fecal incontinence and impaction, rectal prolapse, anorectal sphincter dysfunction) also may be affected. Telangiectasias and diverticula may be found throughout the gastrointestinal tract, including gastric antral vascular ectasia, which is associated with connective tissue disease in general. Mild increases of the aminotransferases, autoimmune liver disease, and primary biliary cirrhosis may be associated with scleroderma, as in other connective tissue diseases.

Gastrointestinal tract manifestations may occur in other connective tissue disorders such as *rheumatoid arthritis* (esophageal dysmotility, vasculitis, amyloidosis), *systemic lupus erythematosus* (esophageal dysmotility, vasculitis, serositis, pancreatitis), *polymyositis* (oropharyngeal dysmotility, gut smooth muscle dysfunction, vasculitis), *dermatomyositis* (malignancies, including pancreatic, stomach, and colorectal), and *Sjögren's syndrome* (esophageal webs, pancreatic insufficiency). Rheumatoid arthritis may be part of *Felty's syndrome* (splenomegaly, neutropenia) with nodular regenerative hyperplasia and portal hypertension. *Nodular regenerative hyperplasia* itself also occurs with scleroderma, polymyalgia rheumatica, vasculitis, and lymphoproliferative or myeloproliferative syndromes. Rheumatoid arthritis also is associated with liver disease due to autoimmune chronic hepatitis, primary biliary cirrhosis, and amyloidosis (see below). *Sjögren's syndrome* is associated with autoimmune chronic hepatitis and primary biliary cirrhosis.

Patients with *seronegative spondyloarthropathies* may have ileocolonic inflammation similar to that of Crohn's disease. *Systemic vasculitides*, including *Behçet's disease* (oral and genital ulcers, gastrointestinal involvement similar to that of Crohn's disease, Budd-Chiari syndrome), *polyarteritis nodosa* (gallbladder, pancreas, appendix, gastrointestinal tract), *Wegener's granulomatosis* (gastrointestinal tract), and *Churg-Strauss syndrome* (gallbladder, gastrointestinal tract), can present with diverse gastrointestinal and hepatic manifestations.

Pregnancy and Gynecologic Conditions

Pregnancy has many effects on the gastrointestinal tract. Nausea and vomiting are extremely common during the first trimester of pregnancy. When these effects become protracted and severe (*hyperemesis gravidarum*), dehydration, weight loss, malnutrition, and liver function test abnormalities may occur (see Chapter 38, Liver Disease and Pregnancy). Risk factors include young age, obesity, multiparity, multiple births, first and molar pregnancies, and previous hyperemesis gravidarum. Hyperthyroidism must be excluded. Treatment is supportive, and symptoms usually resolve by week 20 of pregnancy.

Gastroesophageal reflux disease also is common during pregnancy because of the combined relaxing effects of estrogens and progestins on the smooth muscle of the body of the esophagus and the lower esophageal sphincter. Once symptoms occur during a pregnancy, they often persist until term and recur with subsequent pregnancies. Antacids (avoiding magnesium-containing antacids near term) and sucralfate appear safe, and cimetidine, ranitidine, and famotidine often are used. Nizatidine and all proton-pump inhibitors are best avoided during pregnancy. Endoscopy rarely is indicated during pregnancy; if used, it is usually for substantial bleeding, intractable emesis, or persistent, severe upper abdominal pain. Lidocaine spray and meperidine (50 mg) are preferred as medications, although many use midazolam or diazepam. Fetal monitoring should be performed during endoscopic procedures, certainly after week 23. Pregnancy appears to decrease the frequency, severity, and risk of complications with *peptic ulcer disease*.

Constipation is another common gastrointestinal tract manifestation in pregnancy. Altered motility (hormonal), altered diet, constipating medications (iron), compression of the sigmoid colon by an enlarged uterus, and decreased activity all contribute. Treatment should include dietary advice, liquids, activity, fiber, and, if necessary, docusate- and magnesium-containing cathartics (except close to term). Castor oil (premature labor), mineral oil (maternal malabsorption of fat-soluble vitamins, severe aspiration pneumonia), and anthraquinones (possible malformations) should be avoided. Pregnancy is unlikely to cause *diarrhea*. Fiber, pectin, kaolin, and loperamide can be used, but diphenoxylate with atropine (Lomotil) and any bismuth-containing compound (Pepto-Bismol) should not be used. Colonoscopy should be avoided during pregnancy. Flexible sigmoidoscopy is thought by many to be safe. *Small-bowel obstruction* during pregnancy (about 1:1,500) most often is due to adhesions; *volvulus* is the second most common cause, especially in the third trimester, when incarcerated hernias are less common. *Appendicitis* is not more common during pregnancy (about 1:1,500), but the diagnosis often is delayed, with increased maternal (up to 11%) and fetal (up to 37%) mortality, especially late in pregnancy, when the enlarged uterus pushes the appendix and cecum up into the right upper quadrant, resulting in atypical signs and symptoms.

Endometriosis, if severe, often affects the gut; the sigmoid colon is most often involved. It sometimes results in obstruction (adhesions), perforation, bleeding, diarrhea, and, more often, abdominal pain or constipation. These gastrointestinal tract symptoms may or may not be cyclical. Associated gynecologic symptoms, such as pain with intercourse, are common. Estrogen administration after menopause may be associated with symptoms. *Meigs' syndrome* presents with ascites and, often, pleural effusion in association with benign ovarian neoplasms.

Miscellaneous

Systemic amyloidosis includes AL amyloidosis (primary, myeloma, plasma cell-related), AA amyloidosis (secondary, chronic infections, inflammation), familial forms, dialysis-associated amyloidosis, and senile amyloidosis. Systemic forms can infiltrate the gastrointestinal tract, resulting in macroglossia (usually primary AL amyloidosis), esophageal dysphagia or dysmotility, gastroesophageal reflux disease, gastroparesis, gastric ulceration, tumors, bleeding, or obstruction, small and large bowel dysmotility or pseudo-obstruction, diarrhea, malabsorption, bacterial overgrowth, bleeding, ischemia, ulceration, constipation, and fecal incontinence. Liver involvement also is frequent, with hepatomegaly, increased alkaline phosphatase level, and, rarely, severe intrahepatic cholestasis (usually primary AL amyloidosis) or liver failure. Pancreatic exocrine insufficiency also has been described. Rectal, stomach, and liver (rare reports of rupture) biopsies often are diagnostic. Chemotherapy may be useful in primary AL amyloidosis, and colchicine may be useful in AA amyloidosis due to familial Mediterranean fever (fever, serositis, arthritis, vasculitis, chest or abdominal pain, family history, recessive, chromosome 16p13.3) and inflammatory bowel disease. Liver transplantation may be helpful for certain familial forms (autosomal dominant, mutant transthyretin protein) with symptoms, but not after severe irreversible (especially neurologic) damage has occurred.

Ehlers-Danlos syndrome type IV, usually autosomal dominant, often is associated with bowel perforation, vascular aneurysms, arteriovenous fistulas, and rupture. *Paraneoplastic syndromes* with diffuse gastrointestinal tract motor dysfunction most often occur with small cell lung carcinoma, often with autonomic neuropathy, cerebellar degeneration, peripheral neuropathy, seizures, or syndrome of inappropriate secretion of antidiuretic hormone. Antineuronal nuclear antibodies, type 1, usually are detectable.

RECOMMENDED READING

Chial HJ, McAlpine DE, Camilleri M. Anorexia nervosa: manifestations and management for the gastroenterologist. Am J Gastroenterol. 2002;97:255-69.

Elder GH, Hift RJ, Meissner PN. The acute porphyrias. Lancet. 1997;349:1613-7.

Falk RH, Comenzo RL, Skinner M. The systemic amyloidoses. N Engl J Med. 1997;337:898-909.

Golkar L, Bernhard JD. Mastocytosis. Lancet. 1997;349:1379-85.

Hasler WL, Chey WD. Nausea and vomiting. Gastroenterology. 2003;125:1860-7.

Iqbal N, Salzman D, Lazenby AJ, Wilcox CM. Diagnosis of gastrointestinal graft-versus-host disease. Am J Gastroenterol. 2000;95:3034-8.

Nzeako UC, Frigas E, Tremaine WJ. Hereditary angioedema: a broad review for clinicians. Arch Intern Med. 2001;161:2417-29.

Rose S, Young MA, Reynolds JC. Gastrointestinal manifestations of scleroderma. Gastroenterol Clin North Am. 1998;27:563-94.

Solomon JA, Abrams L, Lichtenstein GR. GI manifestations of Ehlers-Danlos syndrome. Am J Gastroenterol. 1996;91:2282-8.

Verne GN, Sninsky CA. Diabetes and the gastrointestinal tract. Gastroenterol Clin North Am. 1998;27:861-74.

Wald A. Constipation, diarrhea, and symptomatic hemorrhoids during pregnancy. Gastroenterol Clin North Am. 2003;32:309-22.

Yanovski SZ, Yanovski JA. Obesity. N Engl J Med. 2002;346:591-602.

Miscellaneous Disorders

Questions and Answers

QUESTIONS

Multiple Choice (choose the one best answer)

1. A 46-year-old man is referred to you for a treatment recommendation. Six weeks ago, he underwent an exploratory laparotomy for evaluation of chronic abdominal pain, postprandial abdominal bloating, and irregular bowel movements. The laparotomy was normal, and a cholecystectomy and appendectomy were performed. Pathologic analysis of the gallbladder was normal, but the appendix had a 1-cm carcinoid tumor and no inflammation. Preoperatively, computed tomography of the abdomen and pelvis was normal. Postoperatively, the patient's symptoms improved, and a colonoscopy showed a normal colon and terminal ileum. What is the most appropriate treatment recommendation?
   a. Exploratory laparotomy
   b. Laparoscopy
   c. Right hemicolectomy
   d. Octreotide
   e. Observation

2. A 39-year-old woman comes to your office with recurrent epigastric pain. She has had documented duodenal ulcers in the past and *Helicobacter pylori* studies have been negative. She denies use of alcohol, aspirin, and nonsteroidal anti-inflammatory drugs. Her weight has been stable. Laboratory results include a hemoglobin value of 10.0 g/dL, gastrin 1,243 pg/mL, and negative *H. pylori* serology. Esophagogastroduodenoscopy shows a duodenal bulb ulcer. Which of the following is the most appropriate next step in evaluation of this patient?

   a. Computed tomography of the abdomen
   b. Magnetic resonance imaging of the abdomen
   c. Octreotide scanning
   d. Endoscopic ultrasonography
   e. Angiography

3. A 50-year-old woman is admitted to the hospital with anxiety, palpitations, and episodic confusion of 2 years in duration. The fasting glucose level is low. A 72-hour fast test shows inappropriate glucose and insulin levels consistent with an insulinoma. Which of the following is the most appropriate next step in the evaluation of this patient?
   a. Computed tomography of the abdomen
   b. Magnetic resonance imaging
   c. Octreotide scanning
   d. Endoscopic ultrasonography
   e. Angiography with venous sampling

4. A 45-year-old man has had watery diarrhea for 6 months. Stool studies for fat and enteric pathogens have been negative, and upper and lower gastrointestinal endoscopy results have been normal. A vasoactive intestinal polypeptide level is increased, and computed tomography of the abdomen shows a 5-cm mass in the tail of the pancreas and multiple defects in the liver. Which of the following is the most appropriate treatment recommendation?
   a. Total pancreatectomy and octreotide
   b. Total pancreatectomy and chemotherapy
   c. Total pancreatectomy and radiation
   d. Total pancreatectomy and hepatic artery embolization
   e. Octreotide

5. You are asked to see a 39-year-old woman with peptic ulcer disease. She has had documented duodenal ulcers for 15 years. She denies use of alcohol, aspirin, and non-steroidal anti-inflammatory drugs. Multiple studies for *Helicobacter pylori* have been negative. She was treated empirically with antibiotics 2 years ago and her chronic diarrhea worsened. Laboratory values include hemoglobin 9.6 g/dL, calcium 11.4 mg/dL, and serum gastrin 1,114 pg/mL. Octreotide scanning shows activity in the body of the pancreas. Bone scanning is negative. What is the most appropriate next step in the management of this patient?
   a. Total pancreatectomy
   b. Partial pancreatectomy
   c. Partial pancreatectomy and octreotide
   d. Partial pancreatectomy and chemotherapy
   e. Octreotide

6. A 64-year-old man with a history of hypertension and diabetes mellitus is admitted to the coronary care unit with acute onset of chest pain and dyspnea, lasting 1 hour, relieved with the administration of morphine sulfate. He is comfortable and hemodynamically stable, and electrocardiography is normal. Before the myocardial enzymes are known, acute, severe periumbilical pain develops, and blood pressure is 115/80 mm Hg and the pulse rate is regular at 108 beats/min. Which of the following is most likely?
   a. He is having an inferior wall myocardial infarction presenting as abdominal pain
   b. He has nonocclusive mesenteric ischemia due to a recent myocardial infarction
   c. He has had a recent myocardial infarction now complicated by mesenteric arterial embolization
   d. He has diffuse atherosclerotic vascular disease now complicated by mesenteric arterial thrombosis
   e. He has Marfan's syndrome in combination with a thoracoabdominal dissecting aortic aneurysm

7. Acute cholecystitis develops in a 75-year-old woman and she undergoes laparoscopic cholecystectomy that is successful. After the procedure, nausea and abdominal distention develop. Results of laboratory tests and hepatoiminodiacetic acid scanning are normal. Abdominal-pelvic computed tomography shows nonspecific dilatation of multiple small bowel loops with increased gas and fluid, without a transition point. The patient's condition improves with a nasogastric tube, but worsening nausea, discomfort, and distention develop over several days whenever the tube is clamped. She has never had an abdominal or pelvic operation. She has a history of diabetes mellitus and hypertension, smokes cigarettes, but does not have a history of cardiac disease.

Which of the following is most likely?
   a. Endoscopic retrograde cholangiopancreatography shows choledocholithiasis
   b. She has had a perioperative myocardial infarction
   c. At mesenteric arteriography, pruning of arterial vessels is seen and is relieved by intra-arterial papaverine
   d. Small-bowel barium study shows a mid jejunal malignant gastrointestinal stromal tumor
   e. A high-grade thrombolic occlusion of the superior mesenteric artery and total atherosclerotic occlusion of the celiac artery are found

8. A 22-year-old woman completes her fifth marathon, after which she passes a loose stool with "about a cup" of bright red blood. She is otherwise healthy. Emergency colonoscopy shows three shallow ulcers in the cecum, without stigmata. Some old blood material and clot are seen here and there in the colon. Which of the following is most likely?
   a. The ulcers will be gone in 48 hours and are unlikely to recur
   b. The paient snorted cocaine before the marathon
   c. The patient takes tegaserod maleate for constipation
   d. The findings are the initial clinical manifestations of Crohn's colitis
   e. She should have a human immunodeficiency virus test performed

9. An 82-year-old woman with ischemic cardiomyopathy, severe congestive heart failure, and moderate hypotension is admitted to an intensive care unit. She also has severe chronic obstructive pulmonary disease. While she is in the intensive care unit, persistent, moderately severe periumbilical pain, nausea, and distention develop. Abdominal radiography shows mild distention of multiple loops of small bowel. Computed tomography without intravenous contrast (creatinine value is 1.5 mg/dL) shows similar findings. Which of the following is the best course of action?
   a. Blood cultures and intravenous antibiotics
   b. Surgical exploration to rule out partial small-bowel obstruction
   c. Anticoagulation
   d. Visceral arteriography
   e. Doppler ultrasonography of visceral arteries

10. A 28-year-old woman presents with acute, severe, constant periumbilical pain. She had her appendix removed at laparotomy 10 years ago and had postoperative right lower extremity deep venous thrombosis. She has no children but has had two miscarriages. She does not smoke and has otherwise been well. Her mother had some kind of

vasculitis. A pregnancy test is negative. There is no tenderness on examination of her abdomen, and bowel sounds are active. An abdominal radiograph, complete blood count, and sedimentation rate are normal. Which of the following should be done next?

a. Doppler ultrasonography of the portal, splenic, and superior mesenteric veins
b. Visceral arteriography
c. Exploration laparotomy
d. Abdominal-pelvic computed tomography
e. Doppler ultrasonography of the celiac, superior mesenteric, and inferior mesenteric arteries

11. A 60-year-old man presents with progressive fatigue, weight loss, diarrhea, and edema. Findings on physical examination are mild postural hypotension, mild hepatomegaly, and peripheral edema. Laboratory tests are remarkable for anemia and hypoalbuminemia, and liver function and creatinine values are normal. Stool studies are negative for pathogens and fecal leukocytes. Endoscopy and colonoscopy are planned, but on pre-procedure airway assessment his uvula is not visible (see Figure). Which of the following is most likely given these findings?

a. Urinalysis shows significant proteinuria
b. Findings at endoscopy and colonoscopy after anesthesia consultation are consistent with Crohn's ileocolitis
c. The 24-hour urine 5-hydroxyindoleacetic acid value is increased
d. Abdominal-pelvic computed tomography shows a cecal mass and multiple low-attenuation lesions in the liver consistent with advanced metastatic colon cancer
e. Results of serologic tests are consistent with celiac disease

12. A 21-year-old man presents with a 4-month history of colicky abdominal pain and diarrhea and a 2-year history of severe, recurrent episodes of oral ulceration. Physical examination is remarkable for right lower quadrant tenderness, erythematous, warm, and tender nodules on his shins, a swollen and painful left knee and right elbow, and an ulceration on the shaft of his penis. Multiple aphthous and punched-out ulcers in the terminal ileum and cecum are found at colonoscopy. Biopsies of these lesions are nonspecific but consistent with an active chronic colitis. Which of the following is most likely?

a. The patient is positive for HLA-B27 and had *Salmonella* gastroenteritis recently
b. The patient is from Sweden and had *Yersinia* enterocolitis recently
c. The patient is from Japan and had abnormal results on an eye examination recently

d. The patient's brother has ulcerative colitis and pyoderma gangrenosum
e. Bihilar adenopathy is found on chest radiography

13. A 32-year-old woman is seen in the emergency department with acute mid abdominal pain. She has had several previous episodes during the past year requiring emergency consultation. She has no history of medical or surgical illness and never has been pregnant. She has been referred to a psychiatric pain clinic. On physical examination, her abdomen is soft and relatively nontender despite her severe "10 out of 10" pain. A complete blood count and standard chemistry tests show mild hyponatremia. Which of the following is most likely?

a. Abdominal-pelvic computed tomography is consistent with early small-bowel obstruction
b. Doppler ultrasonography shows a respiratory-dependent indentation of the celiac artery near its origin
c. Hepatobiliary iminodiacetic acid scanning is abnormal
d. Sphincter of Oddi dysfunction is found on biliary manometry
e. The patient drinks alcohol, and her menstrual period started yesterday

14. A 33-year-old woman is sent to a gastroenterologist with several months of intermittent, crampy left lower quadrant pain, constipation, and small amounts of bright red blood on the stool. She denies diarrhea, weight loss, fever, or flushing. As a child, she had an appendectomy complicated by perforation. She has not been pregnant. As a pre-teenager, she was sexually abused. She is worried and notes recent dyspareunia. Her menstrual periods are

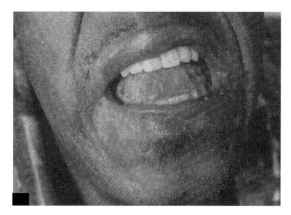

Question 11

From Gertz MA, Kyle RA. Primary systemic amyloidosis: a diagnostic primer. Mayo Clin Proc. 1989;64:1505-19. By permission of Mayo Foundation for Medical Education and Research.

unremarkable. On physical examination, there is mild left lower quadrant tenderness. At sigmoidoscopy, a biopsy specimen is obtained from a small, focal polypoid area in the distal sigmoid (see Figure). Which of the following is the most likely diagnosis?

a. Juvenile polyp
b. Endometriosis
c. Carcinoid tumor
d. Colonic adenocarcinoma
e. Metastatic ovarian carcinoma

15. A 35-year-old woman presents with a 2-week history of fever, dyspnea, weakness, jaundice, and confusion. She was well until the past 8 months, during which she has progressively lost weight and has had worsening diarrhea, abdominal distention, and lower extremity edema. On physical examination, she appears chronically ill, is confused and lethargic, and has tachypnea and tachycardia. Jaundice, hair loss, muscle wasting, a mildly increased jugular venous pressure, ascites, and edema are apparent. Her leukocyte count is 30×10^9/L, hemoglobin 8.0 g/dL, international normalized ratio 5.2, partial thromboplastin time 70 seconds, alkaline phosphatase 625 U/L, total bilirubin 34 mg/dL, and creatinine 4.2 mg/dL. Her platelet count, alanine aminotransferase, aspartate aminotransferase, and drug-toxin screens are unremarkable. Paracentesis of the ascites shows a protein value of 2.5,

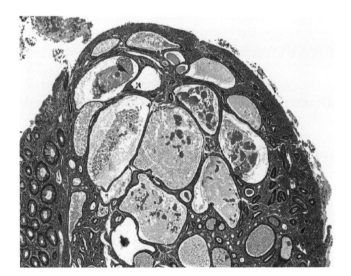

Question 14

From Emory TS, Carpenter HA, Gostout CJ, Sobin LH, editors. Atlas of gastrointestinal endoscopy & endoscopic biopsies. Washington, DC: Armed Forces Institute of Pathology; 2000. p. 361.

serum-to-ascites albumen gradient of 1.6, and a leukocyte count of 2.4×10^9/L with 78% polymorphonuclear leukocytes. Which of the following best explains this patient's history and examination and initial laboratory findings?

a. Cirrhosis with spontaneous bacterial peritonitis
b. Perforated cecal adenocarcinoma
c. Human immunodeficiency virus type 1 infection with sepsis
d. Adrenal insufficiency with sepsis
e. Thyroid storm with sepsis

16. A 26-year-old man with a long history of intravenous drug abuse and multiple sex partners (men and women) presents with an episode of hematemesis. He is known to be positive for human immunodeficiency virus, but has been noncompliant with therapy. He has previously been treated for *Candida* esophagitis, cytomegalovirus colitis, and multifocal *Mycobacterium avium-intracellulare*. He is hemodynamically stable, and at endoscopy three purplish nodules are found in his stomach. Biopsies are unremarkable. Which of the following is most likely to explain these lesions?

a. Non-Hodgkin's lymphoma, B-cell lineage
b. Kaposi's sarcoma
c. Cytomegalovirus gastritis
d. *Mycobacterium avium-intracellulare*
e. Gastrointestinal stromal tumor

17. A 28-year-old woman with a recent diagnosis of human immunodeficiency virus type 1 who has not yet started drug therapy is seen for a several-day history of watery diarrhea. There is no history of fever, chills, nausea, vomiting, abdominal pain, medications, travel, or exposure. Stool examinations for bacterial culture, ova and parasites, fecal leukocytes, occult blood, and *Clostridium difficile* are negative. Her symptoms improve rapidly with ciprofloxacin. Which of the following infections is most likely to explain all of this?

a. Enterotoxigenic *Escherichia coli*
b. Enteroadherent *E. coli*
c. Enterohemorrhagic *E. coli*
d. Enteroinvasive *E. coli*
e. Enteropathogenic *E. coli*

18. A 57-year-old African-American woman has had intermittent dysphagia to solids during the past 6 months. She has a history of human immunodeficiency virus type 1, successfully treated with medications. She also has mild attacks of asthma, particularly after she goes to bed, which have been less frequent since she started using a corticosteroid inhaler a few weeks ago. Unfortunately, she was

found to have oral thrush 10 days ago and is receiving treatment with oral fluconazole. Which of the following is most likely to be found at endoscopy?

a. *Candida* esophagitis
b. Cytomegalovirus esophagitis
c. Distal esophagitis, Los Angeles grade B
d. Esophageal adenocarcinoma with Barrett's esophagus
e. Pill esophagitis

19. A 22-year-old man with recently diagnosed asymptomatic human immunodeficiency virus type 1 receiving medical therapy has had moderately severe upper abdominal pain lasting for more than 24 hours. Which of the following is most likely to be the cause of this acute pain?

a. Choledocholithiasis
b. Trimethoprim-sulfamethoxazole–induced pancreatitis
c. Retroperitoneal B-cell lymphoma
d. Acquired immunodeficiency syndrome cholangiopathy due to *Cryptosporidium* infection
e. Idiopathic esophageal ulcer

20. A 76-year-old man previously infected with human immunodeficiency virus (HIV) type 1 takes a trip to California. Recently, he has felt well. He is receiving multiple medications for the HIV and is trying to figure out the new Medicare guidelines for obtaining these medications at less cost. While in California, he eats lunch at a "New Health, New Life" spa, including an organic vegetarian sandwich on whole-grain bread with iced tea. The next day, fever, chills, cramps, and watery diarrhea develop. Which of the following is most likely?

a. His stool will be positive for enterohemorrhagic *Escherichia coli*
b. Mayonnaise on his sandwich was infected with *Staphylococcus aureus*
c. Sprouts in his sandwich were contaminated with *Salmonella*
d. The ice cubes in the iced tea were contaminated with *Giardia*
e. His symptoms are due to his antiretroviral drug therapy

ANSWERS

1. Answer e

Carcinoid tumors are the most common gastrointestinal endocrine tumor, and the most common intestinal carcinoid tumors are located in the appendix. Appendiceal carcinoids are usually asymptomatic and found incidentally at operation. Ninety-eight percent of appendiceal carcinoids are solitary, benign, and less than 1 cm in size. Appendectomy is considered curative for all appendiceal carcinoids less than 2 cm in size. If an appendiceal carcinoid is larger than 2 cm or if there is evidence of malignancy and possible invasion, a right hemicolectomy is recommended.

2. Answer c

This woman has a history of chronic recurrent epigastric pain and previously documented duodenal ulcers. Consideration should be given to a hypersecretory syndrome when duodenal ulcers are not caused by nonsteroidal anti-inflammatory drugs or *H. pylori*. Under the circumstances described, a serum gastrin test should be ordered. In this patient, the gastrin level is clearly increased to a point that suggests a gastrinoma. Most gastrinomas have somatostatin receptors, and octreotide scanning localizes 85% of gastrinomas and detects more than 80% of metastases. Octreotide scanning currently is considered the initial test of choice to localize a gastrinoma.

3. Answer d

Insulinomas are common pancreatic endocrine tumors. Most patients present with neuroglycopenic symptoms caused by catecholamine release, which is due to hypoglycemia. The most common neuroglycopenic symptoms include altered consciousness, confusion, dizziness, diplopia, blurred vision, anxiety, weakness, fatigue, headache, palpitations, tremor, and sweating. The average duration of symptoms before detection of an insulinoma is longer than 3 years in 25% of patients. The diagnosis of insulinoma is not suggested by a fasting glucose level but is confirmed by a 72-hour fast test that shows inappropriate glucose and insulin levels. Localization of insulinomas may be difficult, and computed tomography of the abdomen and octreotide scanning localize only 50% of the tumors. Endoscopic ultrasonography detects 80% to 90% of insulinomas and is considered the initial test of choice.

4. Answer e

The VIPoma (vasoactive intestinal polypeptide tumor) syndrome is characterized by severe watery diarrhea, hypokalemia, and achlorhydria, and it is caused by a neuroendocrine tumor that produces vasoactive intestinal polypeptide. Ninety percent of VIPomas are located in the pancreas, approximately 75% are malignant, and 50% have metastases at the time of diagnosis.

Operation should be considered in patients with no evidence of metastatic disease or to relieve local effects produced by the large size of these tumors. In this patient, the tumor is located in the tail of the pancreas and there are no apparent local effects produced by this tumor. Total pancreatectomy is not indicated. Partial pancreatectomy may help in relieving symptoms but would not be curative in this patient because of the hepatic metastases. Octreotide controls diarrhea in 80% to 90% of patients and is considered the initial treatment of choice.

5. Answer e

This young woman has a 15-year history of duodenal ulcers that have not been caused by *Helicobacter pylori* or use of nonsteroidal anti-inflammatory drugs. She also has had diarrhea for at least 2 years. In these circumstances, a gastrinoma should be considered, and the serum gastrin level is increased to a point that suggests gastrinoma. The presence of hypercalcemia suggests multiple endocrine neoplasia syndrome; this syndrome presents with hypercalcemia from hyperparathyroidism, a functional or nonfunctional pancreatic endocrine tumor, and a silent pituitary tumor. Patients with gastrinoma who have multiple endocrine neoplasia syndrome or liver metastases are not candidates for surgical treatment. Somatostatin is a gastric acid secretory inhibitor and is useful in the treatment of acid hypersecretion.

6. Answer c

This 64-year-old man with a history of hypertension and diabetes mellitus is at high risk for silent and symptomatic atherosclerotic vascular disease. He likely has had an ischemic event, perhaps in the setting of previous coronary artery disease and myocardial dysfunction, both putting him at great risk for mesenteric arterial embolization. An inferior myocardial infarction can present with abdominal discomfort, but usually it is upper abdominal or epigastric in location. Nonocclusive ischemia (low-flow state) is unlikely given his blood pressure, and, although he is at risk for mesenteric arterial thrombosis, there is no particular reason why this should occur at this time. Marfan's syndrome with a dissecting aneurysm affecting both coronary and mesenteric arteries would be much less common.

7. Answer e

The clinical history of several days of small-bowel ileus and normal laboratory test results argue against choledocholithiasis as a good explanation. A perioperative myocardial infarction or nonocclusive mesenteric ischemia with pruning of the arterial vasculature could explain the patient's symptoms, but no supportive evidence (e.g., low-flow state, hypotension, sepsis) is provided for these diagnoses. The lack of a transition point or mass on computed tomography make a malignant, hence large, gastrointestinal stromal tumor unlikely.

Superior mesenteric artery thrombosis in a patient at risk for underlying chronic mesenteric atherosclerotic arterial disease, perhaps exacerbated by the acute cholecystitis, makes answer e the best choice. Surgical therapy or angioplasty could be beneficial.

8. Answer a

The most likely scenario for this clinical presentation in this previously healthy patient is ischemic colitis due to long-distance running. She obviously has run long distances before, and it is unlikely that this will happen again. Tegaserod maleate, unlike alosetron hydrochloride, has not been associated with ischemic colitis. There is nothing offered in the history to suggest Crohn's disease, cocaine use, or human immunodeficiency virus (cytomegalovirus colitis) exposure.

9. Answer d

Obtaining blood cultures and administration of intravenous antibiotics are both correct, but answer a is not the best answer. This patient is not a surgical candidate given her severe cardiopulmonary disease, and there is nothing to indicate anticoagulation or small-bowel obstruction. Doppler ultrasonography will not detect acute arterial thrombosis or embolism, both of which can best be diagnosed with visceral arteriography. The most likely diagnosis is nonocclusive mesenteric ischemia, best diagnosed and treated in this very ill patient with visceral arteriography with administration of an intra-arterial vasodilator.

10. Answer d

The clinical presentation is most suggestive of mesenteric ischemia. Early small-bowel obstruction also could present in this manner. Computed tomography is the best approach to detect early obstruction and to help exclude internal herniation, intussusception, or perforation (more sensitive than abdominal radiography). Her previous history of deep venous thrombosis and miscarriages suggests a hypercoagulable state, and computed tomography is the best test to evaluate her for mesenteric venous thrombosis. Because nothing in the history suggests arterial thrombosis or embolization, visceral arteriography and Doppler ultrasonography of the visceral arteries are not the best answers. Doppler ultrasonography of the visceral veins might show mesenteric venous thrombosis, but computed tomography can best determine whether this is intrinsic to the vein(s) involved or due to extrinsic compression (e.g., herniation, volvulus, pancreatic carcinoma) or disease (intra-abdominal abscess or inflammation, chronic liver disease). Laparotomy would not be the best choice at this time. If computed tomography were negative (normal), other testing then would be indicated (e.g., visceral arteriography to evaluate for arterial thrombus, arterial embolus, or vasculitis).

11. Answer a

The enlargement of the tongue, which does not allow visualization of the uvula, as well as the dental indentations on the tongue and the diarrhea, hepatomegaly, and postural hypotension are most consistent with systemic amyloidosis. Primary amyloidosis often includes proteinuria (answer a). Crohn's disease (answer b), carcinoid syndrome (answer c), and celiac disease (answer e) do not typically present with macroglossia and hepatomegaly with normal liver function values. If advanced metastatic colon cancer (answer d) with multiple liver lesions was present, one would expect the serum alkaline phosphatase level to be increased.

12. Answer c

The clinical presentation of recurrent oral ulcerations, arthritis, erythema nodosum, and genital ulceration is most consistent with Behçet's syndrome, which in persons from Asia, in contrast to those from the United States, is more likely to include gastrointestinal manifestations, typically Crohn-like enterocolitis. Ocular involvement also often occurs (answer c). An acute gastroenteritis (*Salmonella*, *Yersinia*, answers a and b) should not include changes of chronic colitis on biopsy. Reiter's syndrome in persons who are positive for HLA-B27 can present with arthritis, uveitis, oral ulcers, and distal penile ulceration (circinate balanitis) but not with chronic ileocolitis. Answer d is a good answer but not the best. Sarcoidosis (answer e), which could include arthritis and erythema nodosum, is unlikely to include ileocolic disease or recurrent oral ulceration.

13. Answer e

The clinical history of acute, episodic pain out of proportion to tenderness on physical examination is most consistent with ischemia or neuropathic pain. The patient has never had operation and is not vomiting; hence, early small-bowel obstruction (answer a) is unlikely. Celiac axis-artery compression syndrome (answer b) should include pain, often epigastric, occurring after meals and a bruit on physical examination. Minor findings on Doppler ultrasonography of the celiac artery may be found in otherwise normal persons. Cholecystitis (answer c) and sphincter of Oddi dysfunction (answer d) would more likely produce upper abdominal discomfort and have additional findings and characteristics. Porphyria with abdominal crisis precipitated by alcohol and menstruation (answer e) is the best answer. Mental disturbances and hyponatremia (syndrome of inappropriate antidiuretic hormone) also can occur with abdominal crises.

14. Answer b

A small juvenile polyp (answer a) could present with bleeding, but not pain, and the histologic results, unlike that in the figure, would depict dilated glands with intestinal-type lining cells. The history, age of the patient, and pathologic results are not consistent with colonic adenocarcinoma (answer d), and the pathologic findings are not consistent with metastatic ovarian carcinoma (answer e). Carcinoid tumors (answer c), like all of the choices of answers, can bleed, but usually they are in the rectum, have a distinctive yellow hue, and do not cause pain. Moreover, the pathologic findings are inconsistent with a carcinoid tumor. Endometriosis (answer b) is the best and only correct answer, because the pathologic findings are dilated glands, cuboidal epithelial lining cells, and stroma distinctly different from colonic tissue. Infertility, dyspareunia, and rectosigmoid involvement with pain, diarrhea, and bleeding all can occur with endometriosis. Symptoms often are not cyclic with menstruation.

15. Answer e

The best answer is thyroid storm with sepsis. The long history of progressive weakness, weight loss, and diarrhea is consistent with hyperthyroidism, as is the hair loss. With advanced, untreated, severe hyperthyroidism, jaundice, liver function test abnormalities, and ascites may be found. The increased jugular venous pressure and dyspnea suggest cardiac dysfunction, which may be the cause of ascites in patients with hyperthyroidism; accordingly, the serum-to-ascites albumen gradient is increased, and the total protein value is high. The normal values for platelets, alanine aminotransferase, and aspartate aminotransferase make cirrhosis less likely (answer a). A perforated cecal adenocarcinoma (answer b) could result in infected ascitic fluid and sepsis, but the long (2-week) history and the increased jugular venous pressure make this less likely. Human immunodeficiency virus type 1 and adrenal insufficiency with sepsis also are possible, but they are less likely to explain all of these findings.

16. Answer b

The endoscopic description is typical of Kaposi's sarcoma. Superficial endoscopic mucosal biopsies for Kaposi's sarcoma often are negative, in contrast to lymphoma, cytomegalovirus gastritis, and *Mycobacterium avium-intracellulare*, all of which would be unlikely to have the appearance of purplish nodules with negative biopsy results. A gastrointestinal stromal tumor is unlikely to manifest as three nodules, but it could bleed and biopsy results could be negative because of its submucosal location. The patient is at increased risk for all but gastrointestinal stromal tumor due to his human immunodeficiency virus infection, immunosuppression (previous infections, noncompliance with therapy), and multiple sex partners (human herpesvirus type 8).

17. Answer b

Persons with human immunodeficiency virus are at increased risk for infection with enteroadherent *Escherichia coli*, which is not diagnosed with standard stool cultures for bacteria (unlike enterohemorrhagic *E. coli*), does not cause occult or obvious bleeding (enterohemorrhagic *E. coli* and enteroinvasive *E. coli* often do), does not result in fecal leukocytes (enterohemorrhagic *E. coli* and enteroinvasive *E. coli* can), and often improves with ciprofloxacin. Enteropathogenic *E. coli* most often occurs in newborns and children.

18. Answer c

The best answer is distal esophagitis, Los Angeles grade B. This patient probably has gastroesophageal reflux with nocturnal asthma. Despite her given history of heartburn, she could have esophageal inflammation causing her intermittent dysphagia to solids. Although she had thrush, this most likely was due to her recent use of a corticosteroid inhaler. *Candida* esophagitis would be unlikely given her successful treatment for human immunodeficiency virus and recent fluconazole treatment of thrush. Likewise, cytomegalovirus esophagitis is unlikely in a nonimmunosuppressed patient, and, more often when it does occur, it presents with odynophagia. Pill esophagitis is always possible, but usually it is more acute, often with pain. Esophageal adenocarcinoma is much less likely in an African-American woman than a white male.

19. Answer b

The clinical scenario is most consistent with pancreatitis, and trimethoprim-sulfamethoxazole is a common cause of acute pancreatitis. Choledocholithiasis with pancreatitis in a young man would be less likely. There is no history of odynophagia, which would be likely with an idiopathic esophageal ulcer, and the patient is unlikely to be severely immunosuppressed, which would usually be the case in persons who have human immunodeficiency virus with retroperitoneal B-cell lymphoma or acquired immunodeficiency syndrome cholangiopathy.

20. Answer c

This patient with HIV is at increased risk for enteric infections because of his age (decreased gastric acid production), the HIV (he may not be taking all his medications because of the cost), and perhaps his trip to California. The vegetarian sandwich may have included sprouts, a risk for *Salmonella* infection, which is more common in elderly and immunosuppressed patients and presents 8 to 48 hours after ingestion with cramps, watery diarrhea, and, in HIV-infected persons, bacteremia (fever and chills). *Giardia* would not cause fever and chills. The antiretroviral medications would be unlikely to produce such an acute illness. Enterohemorrhagic *E. coli* would be less common after a vegetarian sandwich, and *Staphylococcus aureus* from mayonnaise would present with acute (within hours) nausea and vomiting.

SECTION V

Colon

CHAPTER 20

Inflammatory Bowel Disease: Clinical Aspects

William J. Tremaine, M.D.

DEFINITIONS

Ulcerative colitis is an idiopathic chronic inflammatory disorder of the colonic mucosa with the potential for extraintestinal inflammation. The disease extends proximally from the anal verge in an uninterrupted pattern to involve all or part of the colon.

Crohn's disease is an idiopathic chronic inflammatory disorder of the full thickness of the intestine, most commonly in the ileum and the colon, with the potential to involve the gastrointestinal tract at any level from the mouth to the anus and perianal region. There is also the potential for extraintestinal inflammation. Typically, there is patchy disease in the gastrointestinal tract, with intervening areas of normal mucosa.

EPIDEMIOLOGY

Men and women are generally at a similar risk for inflammatory bowel disease (IBD). Onset of IBD is highest among adolescents; the peak incidence is between ages 15 and 25 years. IBD is more common among Jews than non-Jews. The incidence and prevalence of ulcerative colitis are similar in a given location, but the numbers vary depending on the patient population of the reporting center. The prevalence of the disease is much higher than the incidence for several reasons: the onset of disease is often in young adults and children, the disease is chronic and lifelong, and the mortality rate associated with the disease is low. In Europe and North America, the incidence of ulcerative colitis and Crohn's disease roughly doubled during the 1960s and 1970s, and the numbers have been relatively stable since then. With this doubling of the incidence, the prevalence also increased, and it will be several more decades before the prevalence levels.

The incidence of ulcerative colitis is 7.3 per 100,000 in Olmsted County, Minnesota, and 14.0 per 100,000 in Winnipeg, Manitoba. The prevalence in Olmsted County, Minnesota, is 181 per 100,000. The proportion of patients with ulcerative proctitis varies in different series from 17% to 49% of the totals.

The incidence of Crohn's disease also varies among different reporting centers. It is 5.8 per 100,000 in Olmsted County and 15.0 per 100,000 in Winnipeg, and the prevalence in Olmsted County is 133 per 100,000.

Mortality rates with IBD are slightly higher than those in the general population. In a study from Stockholm, the standardized mortality ratio was 1.37 for ulcerative colitis and 1.51 for Crohn's disease.

GENETICS

From 10% to 15% of patients with ulcerative colitis have a relative with IBD, mainly ulcerative colitis and less commonly Crohn's disease. About 15% of patients with Crohn's disease have a relative with IBD, mainly Crohn's disease and less commonly ulcerative colitis. Several genetic linkages have been identified, and specific genetic defects have been determined in IBD. The first to be characterized was the *CARD15/NOD2* gene, present in the homozygous form in up to 17% of patients with Crohn's disease and in less than 15% of controls. This genetic defect causes fibrostenotic disease involving the distal ileum. The *MDR1* (multidrug resistance) gene is located on chromosome 7 and is associated with Crohn's disease. Other genetic linkages have been identified, but so far the phenotypes have not been characterized. Three genetic syndromes are associated with IBD: Turner's syndrome, Hermansky-Pudlak syndrome (oculocutaneous albinism, a platelet aggregation defect, and a ceroid-like pigment deposition), and glycogen storage disease type 1B.

DIET

There are no specific diet restrictions for patients with IBD. Although lactose intolerance is more common with Crohn's disease than in the general population, lactose and other milk components do not seem to influence the inflammatory disease. Elemental diets and parenteral hyperalimentation are useful for correction of malnutrition and for growth failure in children with IBD. Corticosteroids are superior to enteral nutrition for the treatment of Crohn's disease. Parenteral nutrition has not been found to be superior to enteral nutrition for Crohn's disease. The role of enteral and parenteral nutrition as primary therapy for Crohn's disease is controversial and is primarily used as an alternative to corticosteroids. There is no convincing evidence that elemental or parenteral nutrition is therapeutic for ulcerative colitis.

PREGNANCY

Fertility is normal in inactive ulcerative colitis and Crohn's disease. Fertility is decreased in some women with active IBD, but most patients are able to conceive. Sulfasalazine causes reversible infertility in men as a result of abnormalities of spermatogenesis and decreased sperm motility. There is controversy about the risk of birth defects in the offspring of a parent with IBD: although most studies do not show an increased risk in association with the disease or the treatments, one study found more birth defects among the offspring of fathers with Crohn's disease who took 6-mercaptopurine. The course of pregnancy is usually normal, although there is an increased chance of a preterm delivery and decreased birth weight. For women with IBD in remission before pregnancy, two-thirds remain in remission through the pregnancy and postpartum. Flares occur most commonly during the first trimester and postpartum. Previous colectomy with an end-ileostomy or with a continent ileal pouch does not preclude pregnancy, and in some women vaginal delivery is still an option.

ENVIRONMENTAL INFLUENCES

Ulcerative colitis is primarily a disease of nonsmokers. Only 13% of patients with ulcerative colitis are current smokers and the rest are nonsmokers or former smokers. Pouchitis after proctocolectomy with an ileal J pouch-to-anal anastomosis for ulcerative colitis is less common among smokers. In contrast, patients with Crohn's disease are more commonly smokers

than the general population, and smoking increases the risk of symptomatic recurrences.

IBD is more common in colder climates than in warmer climates, and it is more common in developed countries than developing countries.

DIAGNOSIS

The diagnosis of IBD is confirmed by a combination of endoscopic, radiographic, and pathologic studies, and the specific diagnostic tests are based on the presenting symptoms and physical examination findings.

CLINICAL PRESENTATIONS

Ulcerative Colitis

The onset may be gradual or sudden, with an increase in bowel movements and bloody diarrhea, fecal urgency, cramping abdominal pain, and fever. The course is variable, with periods of exacerbation, improvement, and remission that may occur with or without specific medical therapy. About half of patients have disease involving the left side of the colon to some extent, including proctitis, proctosigmoiditis, and disease from the splenic flexure distally. Constipation with rectal bleeding is a presenting symptom in about 25% of patients with disease limited to the rectum. Diarrhea may vary from 1 to 20 or more loose or liquid stools a day, usually worse in the morning and immediately after meals, and patients with moderate or severe symptoms often have nocturnal stools. Abdominal pain is usually cramping, worse after meals or bowel movements. Anorexia, weight loss, and nausea in the absence of bowel obstruction are common with severe and extensive disease but uncommon with mild to moderate disease or disease limited to the left colon. In children, urgency, incontinence, and upper gastrointestinal symptoms are more frequent and growth failure is common. Extraintestinal symptoms occur in up to 36% of patients.

Crohn's Disease

Symptoms depend on the anatomical location of the disease. With ileocecal disease, abdominal pain, diarrhea, and fever are typical. With colonic disease, bloody bowel movements with diarrhea, weight loss, and low-grade fever are common. Patients with gastroduodenal Crohn's disease often have burning epigastric pain and early satiety, and these symptoms usually overshadow the symptoms from coexisting ileal or colonic disease. The symptoms of oral or esophageal Crohn's disease include dysphagia, odynophagia, and chest pain, even without eating. The findings of perianal Crohn's disease include perirectal abscess, painful and edematous external hemorrhoids, and anal and perianal fistulas. Enterovesical fistulas can cause pneumaturia and recurrent urinary tract infections. Rectovaginal fistulas occur in up to 10% of women with rectal Crohn's disease and may cause gas or stool to be passed from the vagina. In children, the onset of Crohn's disease often is insidious; weight loss occurs in up to 87% before the diagnosis, and 30% of children have growth failure before the onset of intestinal symptoms.

Physical Examination

Results of the examination often are normal with mildly active ulcerative colitis, or there may be abdominal tenderness, particularly with palpation over the sigmoid colon. Patients with more severe disease may have pallor, dehydration, tachycardia, fever, diminished bowel sounds, and diffuse abdominal tenderness with rebound. Tenderness with rebound is ominous and suggests toxic dilatation or perforation. In Crohn's disease, results of the physical examination may be normal or findings may include one or more of the following: fever, weight loss, muscle wasting, abdominal tenderness (particularly in the lower abdomen), and a palpable mass, usually in the ileocecal region of the right lower abdomen. On rectal examination there may be large, edematous, violaceous external hemorrhoidal tags, fistulas, anal canal fissures, and anal stenosis. Ulcers in Crohn's disease may occur on the lips, gingiva, or buccal mucosa. The physical examination findings due to the extraintestinal manifestations of IBD are discussed in Chapter 22, Inflammatory Bowel Disease: Extraintestinal Manifestations and Cancer.

Laboratory Findings

In mild disease, laboratory study results may be normal. Iron deficiency anemia due to gastrointestinal blood loss may occur in ulcerative colitis and Crohn's disease, and anemia of chronic disease, presumably due to cytokine effects on the bone marrow, may occur with either disorder. Malabsorption of vitamin B_{12} or folate is an additional cause for anemia in patients with Crohn's disease. Hypoalbuminemia, hypokalemia, and metabolic acidosis can occur with severe disease because of potassium and bicarbonate wasting with diarrhea. An increased leukocyte count may be a consequence of active IBD or be due to a complicating abscess.

Acute-phase reactants, including the erythrocyte sedimentation rate, C-reactive protein, and orosomucoid, usually correlate with disease activity but may be normal with mildly active disease. The perinuclear antineutrophil cytoplasmic antibody is positive in about two-thirds of patients with ulcerative colitis and about one-third of patients with Crohn's disease. The anti-*Saccharomyces cerevisiae* antibody is positive in about two-thirds of patients with Crohn's disease and about one-third of patients with ulcerative colitis. These tests may be used together to help distinguish ulcerative colitis from Crohn's disease. However, the positive predictive value of the two tests together is 63.6% for ulcerative colitis and 80% for Crohn's disease; thus, distinguishing the two diseases with these serologic tests is less than ideal (Table 1). With new-onset IBD or at relapse, infection should be ruled out with stool studies, including cultures for bacterial pathogens, examinations for ova and parasites, and *Clostridium difficile* toxin. Patients with systemic symptoms such as fever, malaise, and myalgias should have cytomegalovirus infection excluded by mucosal biopsy.

Endoscopy

Flexible proctosigmoidoscopy or colonoscopy can identify characteristic mucosal changes of ulcerative colitis, including loss of the normal vascular markings, mucosal granularity, friability, mucous exudate, and focal ulceration (Fig. 1). With colonoscopy, the extent of disease can be determined and the terminal ileum can be examined for evidence of backwash ileitis in ulcerative colitis or ileal involvement in Crohn's disease. Patients with left-sided ulcerative colitis may have inflammatory changes around the appendix, called a cecal patch, as a manifestation of the disease, and this finding should not be confused with segmental colitis due to Crohn's disease. Only a limited examination of the rectosigmoid colon should be performed in patients with severely active colitis because of the risk of perforation or hemorrhage with an extensive examination. In Crohn's disease, characteristic lesions at colonoscopy are deep linear ulcers (rake ulcers) with surrounding erythema and granularity and skip areas of normal-appearing mucosa between areas of involvement (Fig. 2). Upper gastrointestinal endoscopy can confirm the presence and distribution of disease in the upper gut and define the mucosal severity. Wireless capsule endoscopy may be useful in some patients with Crohn's disease, but its precise role in the work-up of IBD is yet to be defined.

In Crohn's disease, the endoscopic findings do not correlate closely with clinical disease activity. In patients with extensive involvement with ulcerative colitis (extending proximal to the

Table 1. Positive Predictive Value of Serologic Markers in Patients With Indeterminate Colitis

Disease	Marker	Positive predictive value, %
Ulcerative colitis	pANCA+ ASCA–	63.6
Crohn's disease	pANCA– ASCA+	80

ASCA, anti-*Saccharomyces cerevisiae* antibody; pANCA, perinuclear antineutrophil cytoplasmic antibody.

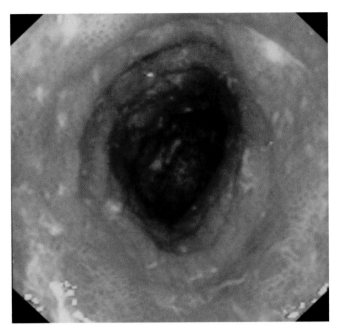

Fig. 1. Diffuse changes of colitis with mucosal granularity and erythema, with mucous exudate. This is typical of moderately active ulcerative colitis.

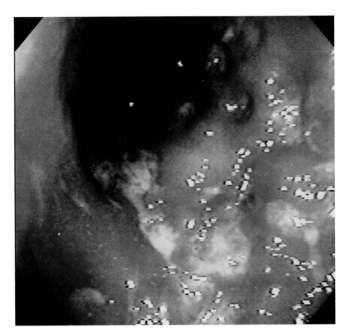

Fig. 2. Linear ulcers and surrounding mucosal erythema, edema, and granularity. This is typical of Crohn's colitis.

splenic flexure), the risk of malignancy is increased above that in the general population after 8 to 10 years of disease. For that reason, periodic colonoscopy with biopsies for surveillance for dysplasia is indicated after 8 to 10 years of disease. The risk of malignancy among patients with less extensive ulcerative colitis (with involvement of the colon distal to the splenic flexure) also is increased, but the magnitude of the risk is not defined. There does not appear to be an increased risk of rectal cancer for ulcerative proctitis without colitis above the rectum. Patients with left-sided ulcerative colitis of 8 to 10 years in duration, or longer, should also undergo periodic surveillance biopsies. The optimal interval between surveillance examinations is undefined, and the examinations are most commonly performed at 1- to 2-year intervals.

Radiologic Features

Plain abdominal films with supine and upright views should be obtained in severely active colitis to examine for complications, including dilatation of the right colon to a diameter more than 5 cm, perforation with free air, and marked mucosal edema with a thumbprint appearance of the mucosa. In Crohn's disease, barium studies, including an air-contrast barium enema and a single-contrast small-bowel follow-through examination (Fig. 3), can identify the location and extent of disease and complications such as fistulas or strictures. In some patients, a small-bowel air-contrast study (enteroclysis) may provide additional information for evaluating jejunal and ileal disease. An upper gastrointestinal barium study may be useful in Crohn's disease with strictures involving the stomach or the duodenum.

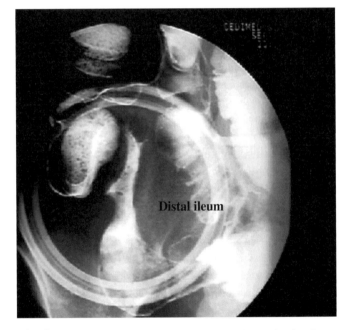

Fig. 3. Spot film of a small-bowel barium radiograph, showing changes consistent with Crohn's ileitis.

Abdominal or pelvic abscesses or masses can be visualized with ultrasonography, either abdominal or transrectal, and computed tomography or magnetic resonance imaging.

Histology

Mucosal biopsies of involved areas of the gastrointestinal tract are useful for excluding self-limited colitis and other infections and noninfectious colitis due to ischemia, collagenous and lymphocytic colitis, drug effect, radiation injury, and solitary rectal ulcer syndrome. Noncaseating granulomas are a feature of Crohn's disease and can be helpful for distinguishing it from ulcerative colitis, but even when multiple sections are taken, granulomas are identified in only 30% of resected Crohn's disease specimens. The presence of focal, patchy inflammation with normal intervening mucosa is characteristic of Crohn's disease but not invariably identifiable.

Differential Diagnosis

Ulcerative colitis and Crohn's disease must be distinguished from infectious causes of colitis and also the noninfectious causes of inflammation in the colon and small intestine (Table 2). Microscopic colitis is a descriptive term for a syndrome of chronic watery diarrhea with characteristic histologic abnormalities but without specific endoscopic or radiographic features. Specific forms of microscopic colitis include lymphocytic colitis, in which there are intraepithelial lymphocytes and chronic inflammatory cells in the lamina propria, and collagenous colitis, which includes the features of lymphocytic colitis plus the presence of a subepithelial collagen band. Diverticular disease-associated chronic colitis is a segmental colitis in which there are chronic inflammatory changes to the mucosa limited to areas of the sigmoid colon where diverticula are present.

Nonsteroidal anti-inflammatory drugs can cause ulcerations throughout the gastrointestinal tract, including the colon and rectum, which can be confused with Crohn's disease. Ischemia more commonly causes segmental colitis that may be confused with Crohn's disease, but occasionally it can cause a diffuse colitis that can appear as ulcerative colitis. Injury to the rectum from radiation for prostate cancer or gynecologic malignancy may appear as ulcerative proctitis or Crohn's disease with fistulas and strictures. Injury to the small intestine and more proximal colon from radiation may cause chronic diarrhea, strictures, malabsorption, and other features that may mimic extensive Crohn's disease. Solitary rectal ulcer syndrome may be confused with Crohn's disease involving the rectum but can be differentiated on the basis of histologic features showing marked subepithelial fibrosis without inflammation. Diverticulitis may mimic Crohn's disease with fistulas, localized abscesses, and segmental colitis. In addition, patients with diverticulitis may have extraintestinal symptoms, just as patients with IBD.

Table 2. Differential Diagnosis of Inflammatory Bowel Disease

Acute self-limited colitis
    Bacteria
        Toxigenic *Escherichia coli*
        Salmonella
        Shigella
        Campylobacter
        Yersinia
        Mycobacterium
        Neisseria gonorrhoeae
        Clostridium difficile
Parasites
    Amebiasis
    Chlamydia
Viruses
    Cytomegalovirus
    Herpes simplex
Collagenous/lymphocytic colitis
Diverticular disease-associated colitis
Medication-induced
    Nonsteroidal anti-inflammatory drugs
    Gold
Ischemic colitis
Radiation enterocolitis
Diverticulitis
Appendicitis
Neutropenic enterocolitis
Solitary rectal ulcer syndrome
Malignancy
    Carcinoma
    Lymphoma
    Leukemia

RECOMMENDED READING

Duerr RH. Update on the genetics of inflammatory bowel disease. J Clin Gastroenterol. 2003;37:358-67.

D'Haens G, Geboes K, Peeters M, Baert F, Ectors N, Rutgeerts P. Patchy cecal inflammation associated with distal ulcerative colitis: a prospective endoscopic study. Am J Gastroenterol. 1997;92:1275-9.

Joossens S, Reinisch W, Vermeire S, Sendid B, Poulain D, Peeters M, et al. The value of serologic markers in indeterminate colitis: a prospective follow-up study. Gastroenterology. 2002;122:1242-7.

Kornbluth A, Legnani P, Lewis BS. Video capsule endoscopy in inflammatory bowel disease: past, present, and future. Inflamm Bowel Dis. 2004;10:278-85.

Loftus EV Jr. Clinical epidemiology of inflammatory bowel disease: incidence, prevalence, and environmental influences. Gastroenterology. 2004;126:1504-17.

Podolsky DK. Inflammatory bowel disease. N Engl J Med. 2002;347:417-29.

CHAPTER 21

Inflammatory Bowel Disease: Therapy

William J. Sandborn, M.D.

Many different medical and surgical therapies are available for inflammatory bowel disease. Medical therapies include anti-inflammatory drugs such as sulfasalazine, olsalazine, balsalazide, and mesalamine; antibiotics; corticosteroids, including budesonide; immunosuppressive medications such as azathioprine, 6-mercaptopurine, methotrexate, cyclosporine, and tacrolimus; and biotechnology medications such as infliximab. Surgical therapies include colectomy with ileostomy, ileoanal pouch, or Kock pouch for ulcerative colitis and surgical resection, stricturoplasty, and placement of setons for Crohn's disease.

Many of the treatments for ulcerative colitis and Crohn's disease are designed to deliver medications topically to the inflamed bowel, with the goal of achieving local efficacy with minimal systemic absorption, thus minimizing toxicity. A thorough understanding of the anatomical classification of both ulcerative colitis and Crohn's disease is required in order to choose the optimal drug delivery system for a patient.

Ulcerative colitis can be divided into ulcerative proctitis (rectal involvement only, with a maximal extent of 10 cm from the anal verge), ulcerative proctosigmoiditis (inflammation is limited to the rectum and sigmoid colon), left-sided ulcerative colitis (inflammation does not extend proximal to the splenic flexure), and extensive colitis or pancolitis (inflammation extends proximal to the splenic flexure or involves the entire colon). Crohn's disease can be divided into Crohn's ileitis (only the small bowel is involved), Crohn's colitis (only the colon is involved), and Crohn's ileocolitis (both the small bowel and colon are involved).

ANTI-INFLAMMATORY MEDICATIONS (5-AMINOSALICYLATES)

Sulfasalazine, oral mesalamine (Pentasa, Asacol), rectal mesalamine (Rowasa), olsalazine, and balsalazide are all drugs that deliver 5-aminosalicylate (mesalamine) to the colon (Table 1). Sulfasalazine, the first drug developed in this class, was designed to combine the anti-inflammatory properties of 5-aminosalicylate with the antibacterial properties of sulfapyridine for the treatment of rheumatoid arthritis. Subsequently, it was discovered that sulfasalazine was effective for ulcerative colitis and served as a prodrug for the active ingredient 5-aminosalicylate. 5-Aminosalicylate is linked to sulfapyridine by an azo bond that is cleaved by bacteria in the colon. Olsalazine and balsalazide are also prodrugs for 5-aminosalicylate. Olsalazine consists of a dimer of two 5-aminosalicylate molecules linked by an azo bond. Balsalazide consists of 5-aminosalicylate linked to an inert carrier by an azo bond. Parent 5-aminosalicylate (mesalamine) can be delivered orally in a capsule covered with the pH-dependent polymer Eudragit-S, which dissolves at pH 7 in the terminal ileum and cecum (Asacol), or as ethylcellulose-coated granules that give a timed release throughout the gastrointestinal tract, beginning in the duodenum, jejunum, and ileum and ending in the colon and rectum (Pentasa). Mesalamine can also be administered as an enema (Rowasa) or a suppository (Canasa).

In placebo-controlled trials, sulfasalazine at doses of 2 to 6 g daily was effective in both inducing remission in mildly to moderately active ulcerative colitis and maintaining remission. In comparative trials, sulfasalazine was less effective than oral corticosteroids for active ulcerative colitis. In contrast,

Table 1. 5-Aminosalicylate Preparations

| Generic name | Proprietary name | Formulation | Site of delivery | Daily dose, g | | Indication |
				Active	Maintenance	
Mesalamine	Rowasa	Enema suspension	Distal to splenic flexure	4	1-4	Active distal UC Remission maintenance distal UC
	Rowasa	Suppository	Rectum	1-1.5	0.5-1	Active proctitis Remission maintenance distal UC
	Asacol	Eudragit-S–coated tablets (release at pH ≥7.0)	Terminal ileum, colon	1.6-4.8	0.8-4.8	Active UC Remission maintenance UC
	Pentasa	Ethylcellulose-coated micro-granules (time- and pH-dependent release)	Duodenum, jejenum, ileum, colon	2-4	1.5-4	Active UC Remission maintenance UC
Olsalazine	Dipentum	5-ASA dimer linked by azo bond	Colon	2-3	1	Remission maintenance UC
Sulfasalazine	Azulfadine	5-ASA linked to sulfapyridine by azo bond	Colon	2-4	2-4	Active UC Remission maintenance UC
Balsalazide	Colazal	5-ASA linked to inert carrier by azo bond	Colon	2-6.75	2-6.75	Active UC Remission maintenance UC

ASA, aminosalicylate; UC, ulcerative colitis.

placebo-controlled trials of sulfasalazine at doses of 3 to 5 g daily for mildly to moderately active Crohn's disease found only modest efficacy for inducing remission (this effect was limited to patients with Crohn's colitis or ileocolitis). In comparative trials, sulfasalazine was less effective than oral corticosteroids for active Crohn's disease. Sulfasalazine at doses of 2.5 to 3 g daily was not more effective than placebo for maintaining remission in Crohn's disease. Drug-associated toxicity occurs in up to 30% of patients treated with sulfasalazine. Commonly observed adverse events include headache, epigastric pain, nausea and vomiting, and rash. Less common but severe adverse events include hepatitis, fever, autoimmune hemolysis, aplastic anemia, leukopenia, agranulocytosis, folate deficiency, pancreatitis, drug-induced lupus, pneumonitis, and Stevens-Johnson syndrome. Reversible male infertility also may occur. Sulfasalazine may be taken during pregnancy and breastfeeding.

Similar to those for sulfasalazine, placebo-controlled trials of mesalamine enemas, 1 to 4 g daily, and mesalamine suppositories, 0.5 to 1.5 g daily, have shown efficacy for both inducing remission in mildly to moderately active left-sided ulcerative colitis and ulcerative proctitis and maintaining remission. Oral mesalamine delivered to the terminal ileum and cecum (Asacol) at doses of 1.6 to 4.8 g daily or throughout the gastrointestinal tract (Pentasa) at doses of 2 to 4 g daily in patients with mildly to moderately active ulcerative colitis is effective for inducing remission, and Asacol, 0.8 to 1.6 g daily, and Pentasa, 4 g daily, are effective for maintaining remission.

The data for use of oral mesalamine in the treatment of Crohn's disease are less clear. Placebo-controlled trials have found that low-dose mesalamine (1-2 g daily) is not effective for inducing remission in mildly to moderately active Crohn's disease. Data from placebo-controlled trials for high-dose mesalamine (3.2-4 g daily) for inducing remission in active Crohn's disease are conflicting (if there is a benefit, it is relatively small). A comparative trial showed that oral mesalamine is less effective than controlled ileal release budesonide, 9 mg daily, for active Crohn's disease. Data from placebo-controlled trials of oral mesalamine, 1 to 4 g daily, for maintenance of medically induced remission or postoperative remission of Crohn's disease are conflicting (however, a meta-analysis has suggested a small benefit for postoperative maintenance of remission). Oral mesalamine, 4 g daily, is not steroid-sparing.

Placebo-controlled trials have shown that olsalazine at doses of 0.75 to 3 g daily is effective for inducing remission in patients with mildly to moderately active ulcerative colitis. Placebo-controlled trials also have found that olsalazine, 1 g daily, is effective for maintaining remission in ulcerative colitis. In comparative trials, balsalazide at a dose of 6.75 g (contains 2.4 g 5-aminosalicylate) daily had an efficacy similar to that of oral mesalamine at a dose of 2.4 g daily for inducing remission in mildly to moderately active ulcerative colitis. In dose-response trials, balsalazide at doses of 4 to 6 g daily was more effective than balsalazide at doses of 2 to 3 g daily for maintaining remission in ulcerative colitis (this evidence of dose response shows a maintenance benefit for balsalazide even though a placebo-controlled trial has not been performed).

Olsalazine, balsalazide, and mesalamine generally are better tolerated than sulfasalazine. Commonly occurring adverse events include headache and gastrointestinal symptoms attributable to underlying inflammatory bowel disease. Rash, alopecia, and a hypersensitivity reaction resulting in a syndrome of worsening diarrhea and abdominal pain sometimes occur. Rarely, serious adverse events, including interstitial nephritis, pericarditis, pneumonitis, hepatitis, and pancreatitis, are observed. Ileal secretory diarrhea can occur with olsalazine, but this problem usually can be avoided by administering olsalazine with food and titrating the dose upward. Olsalazine, balsalazide, and mesalamine may be taken during pregnancy and breastfeeding.

ANTIBIOTICS

Controlled trials of various antibiotics, including vancomycin, metronidazole, ciprofloxacin, and tobramycin, have not shown efficacy for ulcerative colitis. Thus, antibiotics as a primary treatment for ulcerative colitis are not appropriate. The data for use of antibiotics in Crohn's disease are less clear-cut. Three small underpowered comparative studies suggested equivalence of either metronidazole or ciprofloxacin to sulfasalazine, methylprednisolone, and oral mesalamine (Pentasa). However, a placebo-controlled trial of metronidazole, 10 mg/kg daily or 20 mg/kg daily, did not find efficacy in active Crohn's disease. Similarly, a comparative trial of budesonide (9 mg daily) or combination therapy with budesonide (9 mg), metronidazole (1.5 g), and ciprofloxacin (1.0 g daily) did not find an adjunctive role for antibiotics in patients undergoing budesonide therapy for active Crohn's disease. A single controlled trial showed that metronidazole, 1,500 mg daily for 3 months after ileal resection, could delay the occurrence of severe endoscopic lesions for up to 1 year in patients undergoing operation for Crohn's disease. On the basis of the results of these studies, the role of antibiotic therapy for Crohn's disease is controversial. Many clinicians undertake a trial of antibiotic therapy before prescribing corticosteroids for active Crohn's disease.

Uncontrolled studies have reported that metronidazole, 750 to 1,500 mg daily, and ciprofloxacin, 1,000 mg daily, may be effective for fistulizing Crohn's disease, particularly in patients with perianal fistulas. No controlled trials have been performed, but antibiotic therapy is widely used for this indication and is considered to be the first-line therapy.

In small placebo-controlled and comparative trials, metronidazole (750-1,500 mg daily) and ciprofloxacin (1,000 mg daily) were effective for inducing remission in patients with active acute pouchitis after colectomy and ileoanal anastomosis for ulcerative colitis. Uncontrolled clinical observations have suggested that metronidazole and ciprofloxacin also may be effective for maintenance of remission in patients with chronic pouchitis.

Adverse events associated with metronidazole include paresthesias, peripheral neuropathy, yeast vaginitis, anorexia, nausea, a metallic taste, and possible intolerance to alcohol. Adverse events observed with ciprofloxacin include photosensitivity, nausea, rash, increased liver enzyme values, and Achilles tendon rupture (rare). Ciprofloxacin should not be taken during pregnancy or breastfeeding, and metronidazole should be avoided during the first trimester of pregnancy.

CORTICOSTEROIDS

A small number of pharmacologic studies have been conducted with corticosteroids in inflammatory bowel disease, and they can be used to guide dosing and route of administration. A dose-response study in patients with active ulcerative colitis found that prednisone at doses of 40 or 60 mg daily is more effective than prednisone at 20 mg daily. There were more side effects in the 60-mg daily dose group. These results have been extrapolated to patients with Crohn's disease. Most clinicians initiate oral corticosteroid therapy with prednisone at a dose of 40 mg daily and then taper the dose over 2 to 4 months. Pharmacokinetic studies in patients with active ulcerative colitis have shown a decreased bioavailability of prednisolone compared with that in controls. Thus, patients with severely active ulcerative colitis or Crohn's disease who do not have a response to oral corticosteroid therapy are often hospitalized and given corticosteroids intravenously to ensure adequate bioavailability of the corticosteroid dose.

In placebo-controlled trials, orally administered cortisone, 100 mg daily, or prednisone, 40 to 60 mg daily, was effective for inducing remission in mildly to severely active ulcerative colitis. In contrast, placebo-controlled trials have found that low-dose oral corticosteroids (cortisone at 25 mg twice daily, prednisone at 15 mg daily, or prednisone at 40 mg every other day) are not effective for maintaining remission in ulcerative colitis.

No controlled trials of intravenous corticosteroid therapy for severely active ulcerative colitis have been conducted. Uncontrolled studies have suggested that intravenous prednisolone, 60 mg daily, or hydrocortisone, 300 to 400 mg daily, is effective for severely active ulcerative colitis. Most clinicians intravenously administer methylprednisolone, 40 to 60 mg daily, as a single bolus dose, in divided doses (2-4 times daily), or as a continuous infusion.

Placebo-controlled trials have found that hydrocortisone administered rectally as an enema at a dose of 100 mg daily or prednisolone at a dose of 5 mg daily is effective for inducing remission in mildly to moderately active left-sided ulcerative colitis or ulcerative proctitis. Placebo-controlled trials also have shown that hydrocortisone enemas at a dose of 100 mg 2 nights per week are not effective for maintaining remission in left-sided ulcerative colitis or ulcerative proctitis.

Placebo-controlled trials have found that oral prednisone administered at a dose of 60 mg daily and 6-methylprednisolone at 48 mg daily are effective for inducing remission in mildly to moderately active Crohn's disease. In contrast, placebo-controlled trials have reported that low-dose corticosteroids (oral prednisone, 20 mg daily, or 6-methylprednisolone, 8 mg daily) are not effective for maintaining remission in Crohn's disease.

Both short-term and long-term adverse events occur frequently in patients treated with corticosteroids. Short-term adverse events include moon face, acne, ecchymoses, hypertension, hirsutism, petechial bleeding, striae, and psychosis. Long-term adverse events include diabetes mellitus, increased risk of infection, osteonecrosis, osteoporosis, myopathy, cataracts, and glaucoma. Corticosteroids may be taken during pregnancy and breastfeeding.

Budesonide is a newer corticosteroid that has 90% first-pass metabolism in the liver. It can be administered orally as a controlled ileal release formulation (release is pH-dependent) or rectally as an enema. These "topical" formulations result in decreased corticosteroid side effects compared with conventional corticosteroids. In a placebo-controlled trial, controlled ileal release budesonide at doses of 9 to 15 mg daily was effective for inducing remission in mildly to moderately active ileal or right colonic Crohn's disease. Comparative studies have found that oral controlled ileal release budesonide at 9 mg daily is more effective than mesalamine at 4 g daily and equivalent to oral corticosteroids for inducing remission in active Crohn's disease. In contrast, oral controlled ileal release budesonide at 3 to 6 mg daily is not effective for maintaining remission in Crohn's disease.

AZATHIOPRINE AND 6-MERCAPTOPURINE

Azathioprine is a prodrug that is rapidly converted to 6-mercaptopurine after administration. 6-Mercaptopurine is then either inactivated to 6-thiouric acid by xanthine oxidase or to 6-methylmercaptopurine by thiopurine methyltransferase, or it is activated through several enzyme steps to the 6-thioguanine nucleotides, which are thought to be the active metabolites. The enzyme activity of thiopurine methyltransferase is genetically determined: 1 in 300 patients has no enzyme activity, 10% have intermediate enzyme activity, and 90% have normal enzyme activity.

Placebo-controlled trials have shown that azathioprine at doses of 1.5 to 2.5 mg/kg daily is effective for steroid-sparing in patients with steroid-dependent ulcerative colitis. Similarly, a placebo-controlled trial found that azathioprine at 100 mg daily is effective for maintaining remission in ulcerative colitis.

Placebo-controlled trials also have shown that azathioprine at doses of 2 to 3 mg/kg daily and 6-mercaptopurine at a dose of 1.5 mg/kg daily are effective for inducing remission and closing fistulas in patients with active Crohn's disease. Similarly, placebo-controlled trials have found that azathioprine at 2 to 3 mg/kg daily and 6-mercaptopurine at 1.5 mg/kg daily are effective for maintenance of remission and steroid-sparing in Crohn's disease.

Adverse events that have been associated with azathioprine and 6-mercaptopurine include nausea, allergic reactions, pancreatitis, bone marrow suppression, drug hepatitis, and infectious complications. A causal link between azathioprine or 6-mercaptopurine, inflammatory bowel disease, and lymphoma has not been clearly established; however, lymphoma may be a rare complication of these therapies. Azathioprine and 6-mercaptopurine can be administered during pregnancy in selected cases, but routine use during pregnancy is controversial.

METHOTREXATE

As shown in a placebo-controlled trial, methotrexate administered orally at a dose of 12.5 mg weekly is not effective for active ulcerative colitis or for maintaining remission.

Placebo-controlled trials have shown that low-dose oral methotrexate (12.5 mg weekly) is not effective for inducing or maintaining remission in Crohn's disease. In contrast, placebo-controlled trials found that higher-dose methotrexate (25 mg weekly given intramuscularly and possibly 15 mg weekly given orally) is effective for inducing remission in patients with steroid-dependent and steroid-refractory active Crohn's disease. A placebo-controlled trial also showed that methotrexate at doses of 15 to 25 mg weekly given intramuscularly is effective for maintenance of remission and steroid-sparing in Crohn's disease.

The adverse events that may occur with methotrexate therapy include rash, nausea, mucositis, diarrhea, bone marrow suppression, hypersensitivity pneumonitis, increased liver enzyme levels, and liver fibrosis or cirrhosis. Methotrexate is contraindicated for pregnant women.

CYCLOSPORINE AND TACROLIMUS

A placebo-controlled trial of intravenous cyclosporine administered as a continuous infusion at a high dose of 4 mg/kg daily (equivalent to 12-16 mg/kg daily of oral cyclosporine) found it had efficacy for inducing remission in patients with severely active, steroid-refractory ulcerative colitis. A comparative trial reported that monotherapy with moderate-dose intravenous cyclosporine (2 mg/kg as a continuous daily infusion) had efficacy similar to that of high-dose intravenous cyclosporine (4 mg/kg as a continuous daily infusion) for inducing remission in patients with severely active ulcerative colitis. There are no controlled trials of oral cyclosporine for the treatment of active ulcerative colitis or for maintaining remission in ulcerative colitis.

Placebo-controlled trials of cyclosporine administered orally at a low dose of 5 mg/kg daily did not show efficacy for inducing remission in active Crohn's disease or for maintaining remission in Crohn's disease. There are no controlled trials of high-dose intravenously administered cyclosporine for severely active or fistulizing Crohn's disease.

In a placebo-controlled trial, oral tacrolimus, 0.2 mg/kg daily, had efficacy for treatment of fistulizing Crohn's disease.

The toxic effects that may occur with cyclosporine therapy include headache, tremor, paresthesias, seizures, hypertrichosis, gingival hyperplasia, renal insufficiency, hypertension, infections, hepatotoxicity, nausea and vomiting, and anaphylaxis. Those that may occur with tacrolimus therapy include headache, tremor, paresthesias, renal insufficiency, hypertension, infections, and diabetes. Although not absolutely contraindicated, cyclosporine and tacrolimus therapy generally should be avoided for pregnant women.

INFLIXIMAB

Infliximab is a chimeric monoclonal antibody directed toward tumor necrosis factor-α. In controlled trials, infliximab at 5 mg/kg administered 1 to 3 times over 6 weeks as an intravenous infusion was effective for inducing remission and closing fistulas in active Crohn's disease. For patients who have a response to induction therapy with infliximab, re-treatment with infliximab at doses of 5 mg/kg or 10 mg/kg administered intravenously every 8 weeks is effective for maintenance of remission in Crohn's disease and is steroid-sparing. Treatment of ulcerative colitis with infliximab is investigational.

The adverse events that may occur with infliximab therapy include formation of human antichimeric antibodies, infusion reactions, delayed hypersensitivity reactions, autoantibody formation, drug-induced lupus, infection (particularly tuberculosis and fungal infections such as histoplasmosis), and possibly non-Hodgkin's lymphoma. Human antichimeric antibodies frequently lead to higher rates of infusion reactions and loss of efficacy. The frequency of formation of human antichimeric antibodies in patients undergoing infliximab therapy is decreased when patients receive concomitant immunosuppressive therapy with azathioprine, 6-mercaptopurine, or methotrexate; pretreatment with 200 mg intravenously administered hydrocortisone; or 3 induction doses of infliximab followed by systematic maintenance infusions every 8 weeks. Although data are limited, infliximab can be used in pregnant women in selected circumstances.

SURGERY FOR ULCERATIVE COLITIS

The original operation for ulcerative colitis consisted of total proctocolectomy with Brooke ileostomy (Fig. 1). In the 1970s,

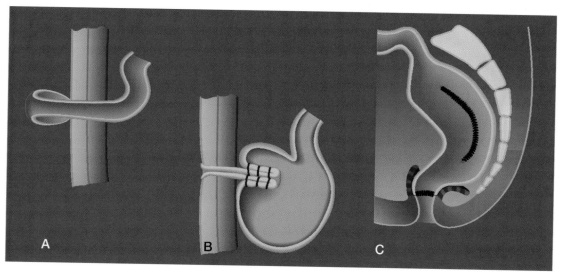

Fig. 1. Surgical options for ulcerative colitis. *A*, Conventional ileostomy (Brooke). *B*, Continent ileostomy (Kock pouch). *C*, Ileoanal anastomosis with reservoir.

the continent ileostomy, or Kock pouch, served as an alternative to ileostomy (Fig. 1). Reoperation frequently was required with the Kock pouch. In the 1980s, the ileoanal pouch largely replaced the Kock pouch for patients with ulcerative colitis who required operation (Fig. 1). Colectomy is indicated for patients with ulcerative colitis who have definite low-grade or high-grade dysplasia, who have colorectal cancer, who are steroid-dependent, or who are refractory to medical therapy (including severely active steroid-refractory ulcerative colitis and toxic megacolon). Pouchitis is inflammation of the ileoanal pouch leading to recurrent symptoms of diarrhea, urgency, and fecal incontinence. The cumulative frequency of acute pouchitis after colectomy with ileoanal pouch approaches 50% by 5 years. The frequency of chronic pouchitis is 5% to 10% by 5 years.

SURGERY FOR CROHN'S DISEASE

The probability of surgical resection in patients with Crohn's disease increases with time. By 15 years after diagnosis, 70% of patients have had at least one operation, and half of these had two or more operations. In patients with extensive stricturing or multiple previous operations (or both), bowel-sparing techniques such as stricturoplasty may be used (Fig. 2). In patients with perianal fistulas, incision and drainage of abscesses, fistulotomy, and placement of setons (drains) may be used in an attempt to avoid proctectomy.

TREATMENT STRATEGIES FOR ULCERATIVE COLITIS

Induction of Remission

Sulfasalazine, oral mesalamine, olsalazine, and balsalazide are effective for inducing remission in patients who have active extensive or pancolonic ulcerative colitis. Active ulcerative proctitis, ulcerative proctosigmoiditis, or left-sided ulcerative colitis may be treated with rectal mesalamine enemas or suppositories, corticosteroid enemas, the oral therapies outlined above for extensive and pancolonic ulcerative colitis, or a combination of oral and rectal therapy. For disease that is moderate to severe and when sulfasalazine, oral or rectal mesalamine, olsalazine, or balsalazide therapy has failed, the next step is second-line therapy with prednisone. Patients with moderately active disease can receive oral prednisone as an outpatient. Patients who require corticosteroid therapy often become steroid-dependent. Patients with persistent symptoms may require oral corticosteroids, azathioprine, or 6-mercaptopurine or colectomy with ileostomy or ileoanal pouch. However, in patients with significantly active ulcerative colitis, azathioprine and 6-mercaptopurine are of limited usefulness as induction agents because of their slow onset of action. Patients who are more severely ill should be hospitalized for intravenous corticosteroid therapy; if the disease does not respond, colectomy should be performed (intravenous cyclosporine may be considered as an alternative to colectomy). Methotrexate is not effective for ulcerative colitis, and infliximab is investigational for ulcerative colitis.

Maintenance of Remission

Sulfasalazine, oral mesalamine, olsalazine, and balsalazide are effective for maintaining remission in patients with extensive or pancolonic ulcerative colitis. Patients with ulcerative proctitis, ulcerative proctosigmoiditis, or left-sided ulcerative colitis can receive maintenance treatment with rectal mesalamine enemas or suppositories or with the oral therapies outlined above for extensive and pancolonic disease. Low-dose prednisone is not effective for maintenance of remission; patients treated with corticosteroids for active ulcerative colitis often become steroid-dependent. Azathioprine and 6-mercaptopurine are effective for maintenance of remission, particularly steroid-induced remission, and for steroid-sparing. Methotrexate is not effective for ulcerative colitis, and infliximab is investigational for ulcerative colitis.

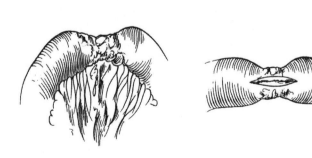

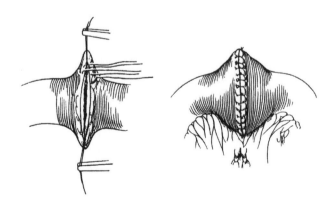

Fig. 2. Stricturoplasty for Crohn's disease.

TREATMENT STRATEGIES FOR CROHN'S DISEASE

Induction of Remission

Sulfasalazine is modestly effective for inducing remission in patients with active Crohn's disease, with the benefit confined largely to patients with Crohn's colitis and ileocolitis. Mesalamine and metronidazole are not consistently effective for inducing remission. Nevertheless, many clinicians continue to use these agents for induction of remission in patients with mildly to moderately active Crohn's disease. Budesonide is more effective than mesalamine and similarly effective to but safer than prednisone. Thus, budesonide is the first-line treatment of choice for inducing remission in patients with mildly to moderately active Crohn's disease involving the terminal ileum or right colon, whereas sulfasalazine is the optimal first-line therapy in patients with Crohn's colitis. Figure 3 shows a traditional treatment algorithm for the first-line therapy of Crohn's disease, and Figure 4 shows a newer evidence-based treatment algorithm for first-line therapy of Crohn's disease.

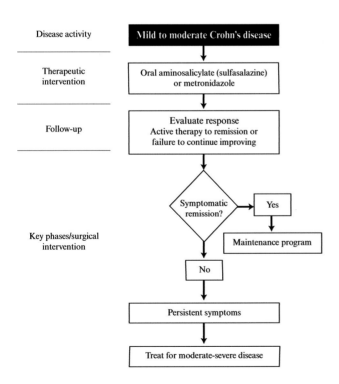

Fig. 3. Suggested treatment algorithm for mildly to moderately active Crohn's disease: traditional approach to induction. (Modified from Sandborn WJ. Medical therapy for Crohn's disease. In: Sartor RB, Sandborn WJ, editors. Kirsner's inflammatory bowel diseases. 6th ed. Edinburgh: Saunders; 2004. p. 530-54. Used with permission.)

For patients who have disease that is moderate to severe, and for patients in whom budesonide or sulfasalazine therapy has failed, the next step is second-line therapy with prednisone. Patients with moderately active disease can receive oral prednisone as an outpatient, whereas patients who are more severely ill should be hospitalized for intravenous corticosteroid therapy. Patients who require corticosteroid therapy often become steroid-dependent. In patients with significantly active Crohn's disease, azathioprine, 6-mercaptopurine, and methotrexate are of limited usefulness as induction agents because of their slow onset of action. Infliximab is effective for the treatment of active Crohn's disease in patients who are refractory to other therapies, usually corticosteroids or immunosuppressive medications. Concomitant immunosuppressive therapy with azathioprine, 6-mercaptopurine, or methotrexate is required to suppress the formation of human antichimeric antibodies against infliximab.

Maintenance of Medically Induced Remission

Sulfasalazine is not effective for maintenance of medically induced remission, and mesalamine is not consistently effective. Metronidazole has not been evaluated for this indication. Low-dose prednisone is not effective for maintenance of remission; patients treated with corticosteroids for active Crohn's disease often become steroid-dependent. Budesonide, 6 mg, prolongs the time to relapse, but a maintenance effect using conventional criteria has not been found. Azathioprine, 6-mercaptopurine, and methotrexate are all effective for maintenance of remission, particularly steroid-induced remission. Infliximab is effective for maintenance of remission in patients who are refractory to other therapies. Concomitant immunosuppression reduces the frequency of human antichimeric antibody formation. Figure 5 shows a treatment algorithm for maintenance therapy in patients with Crohn's disease who are budesonide- or prednisone-dependent or have refractory disease.

Postoperative Maintenance of Remission

Sulfasalazine is not effective for postoperative maintenance of remission. Mesalamine is not consistently effective and is of minimal benefit. Metronidazole, 20 mg/kg for 3 months, reduces recurrence of severe endoscopic lesions at 3 months but does not alter clinical recurrence at 1 year; side effects are common. Low-dose prednisone is not effective for postoperative maintenance therapy, nor is budesonide, 6 mg. Azathioprine and 6-mercaptopurine may be effective, but clinical data are limited. In the absence of definitive data, these agents are currently the treatment of choice in patients who are deemed to be at high risk for recurrence. Methotrexate and infliximab have not been evaluated for postoperative maintenance of remission. Figure 6 shows a treatment algorithm for postoperative maintenance therapy in patients with Crohn's disease.

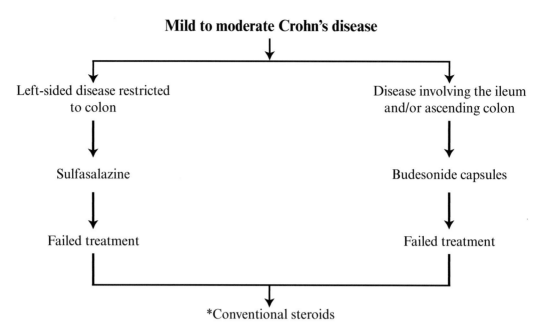

Mild to moderate Crohn's disease

Left-sided disease restricted to colon → Sulfasalazine → Failed treatment

Disease involving the ileum and/or ascending colon → Budesonide capsules → Failed treatment

*Conventional steroids

Fig. 4. Suggested treatment algorithm for mildly to moderately active Crohn's disease: new evidence-based approach to induction. *If the patient is not improving, disease should be reclassified as moderate to severe and treatment with infliximab, immunomodulators, or surgery considered. (From Sandborn WJ, Feagan BG. Review article: mild to moderate Crohn's disease: defining the basis for a new treatment algorithm. Aliment Pharmacol Ther. 2003;18:263-77. Used with permission.)

Closure of Fistulas and Maintenance of Fistula Closure

Antibiotics may be effective for fistula closure, but a placebo-controlled trial has never been performed. Similarly, azathioprine and 6-mercaptopurine may be effective for this treatment indication, but no controlled trials have been conducted in which fistula closure is the primary end point. Uncontrolled studies have suggested that cyclosporine may be effective; controlled trials have not been performed. A placebo-controlled trial of tacrolimus did show effectiveness for fistula closure in patients with refractory fistulizing Crohn's disease. Infliximab is effective for both inducing fistula closure and maintaining fistula closure. Currently, infliximab is the best evidence-based therapy for fistulas. Concomitant immunosuppression is required. Figure 7 shows a treatment algorithm for treatment of perianal Crohn's disease.

CONCLUSIONS

Therapies for different indications in patients with ulcerative colitis and Crohn's disease are summarized in Tables 2 and 3.

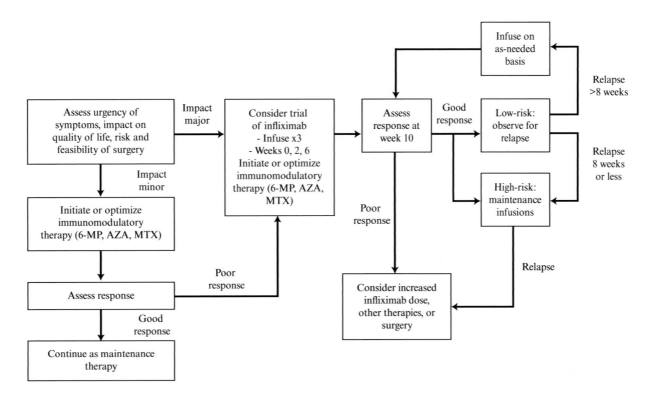

Fig. 5. Suggested treatment algorithm for managing refractory Crohn's disease. AZA, azathioprine; 6-MP, 6-mercaptopurine; MTX, methotrexate. (Modified from Sands BE. Therapy of inflammatory bowel disease. Gastroenterology. 2000;118:S68-S82. Used with permission.)

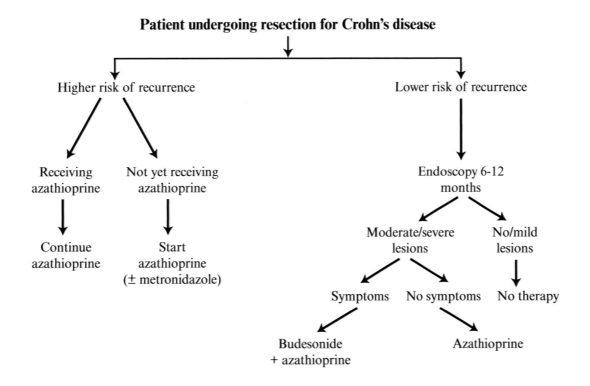

Fig. 6. Suggested treatment algorithm for patients who have had operation for Crohn's disease: new evidence-based approach. (From Sandborn WJ. Medical therapy for Crohn's disease. In: Sartor RB, Sandborn WJ, editors. Kirsner's inflammatory bowel diseases. 6th ed. Edinburgh: Saunders; 2004. p. 530-54. Used with permission.)

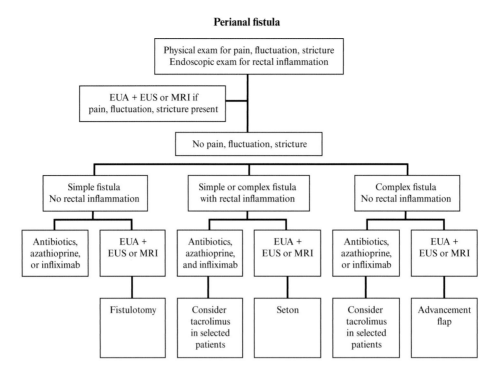

Fig. 7. Treatment algorithm for managing patients with perianal Crohn's disease. EUA, examination under anesthesia; EUS, anorectal endoscopic ultrasonography; MRI, pelvic magnetic resonance imaging. A simple fistula is low, has a single external opening, and does not have associated perianal abscess, rectovaginal fistula, anorectal stricture, or macroscopically evident rectal inflammation. A complex fistula is high or has multiple external openings, perianal abscess, rectovaginal fistula, anorectal stricture, or macroscopic evidence of rectal inflammation. (From Sandborn WJ, Fazio VW, Feagan BG, Hanauer SB, American Gastroenterological Association Clinical Practice Committee. AGA technical review on perianal Crohn's disease. Gastroenterology. 2003;125:1508-30. Used with permission.)

Table 2. Ulcerative Colitis: Treatment, According to Indication

| | Indication | | | | | |
| Drug | Mildly to moderately active | | | | Remission maintenance | |
	Distal	Extensive	Refractory	Severely active	Distal	Extensive
Sulfasalazine	Yes	Yes	Yes*	No†	Yes	Yes
Rectal mesalamine	Yes	No	Yes*	No†	Yes	No
Oral mesalamine	Yes	Yes	Yes*	No†	Yes	Yes
Olsalazine	Yes	Yes	Yes*	No†	Yes	Yes
Balsalazide	Yes	Yes	Yes*	No†	Yes	Yes
Rectal corticosteroids	Yes	No	Yes*	Yes‡	No	No
Oral corticosteroids	Yes	Yes	Yes*	No	No	No
Intravenous corticosteroids	No	No	Yes§	Yes	No	No
Azathioprine/6-mercaptopurine	No	No	Yes	No	Yes	Yes
Cyclosporine	No	No	No	Yes	No	No
Colectomy	No	No	Yes	Yes	No	No

*Typically continued as a carryover of treatment for mildly to moderately active disease when additional agents are added.
†Typically discontinued because of possibility of intolerance to sulfasalazine, mesalamine, or balsalazide.
‡Adjunctive therapy to intravenous corticosteroids.
§Some patients in whom therapy with oral corticosteroids has failed will respond to hospitalization with intravenous administration of corticosteroids.

Table 3. Crohn's Disease: Treatment, According to Indication

Drug	Mildly to moderately active	Refractory	Fistulizing	Severely active	Remission maintenance
Sulfasalazine	Yes	?Yes*	No	No†	?Yes‡
Oral mesalamine	?Yes‡	?Yes*	No	No†	?Yes‡
Antibiotics	?Yes‡	?Yes*	?Yes‡	No	?Yes‡
Budesonide	Yes	?Yes*	No	No	No
Oral corticosteroids	Yes	Yes*	No	No	No
Intravenous corticosteroids	No	Yes§	No	Yes	No
Azathioprine/6-mercaptopurine	No	Yes	Yes	No	Yes
Methotrexate	No	Yes	No	No	Yes
Cyclosporine	No	No	?Yes//	?Yes//	No
Tacrolimus	No	No	Yes	No	No
Infliximab	No	Yes	Yes	?Yes	?Yes
Surgical resection	No	Yes	Yes	Yes	No

Controlled trials do not show an adjunctive benefit for sulfasalazine, mesalamine, or antibiotics in combination with corticosteroids or budesonide. Typically continued as a carryover of treatment for mildly to moderately active disease when additional agents are added.
†*Typically discontinued because of the possibility of intolerance to sulfasalazine or mesalamine.*
‡*Controlled trials do not uniformly show benefit, but treatment commonly is used in clinical practice.*
§*Some patients in whom therapy with oral corticosteroids has failed will respond to hospitalization with intravenous administration of corticosteroids.*
//*No controlled trials conducted; uncontrolled studies suggest benefit.*

RECOMMENDED READING

Camma C, Giunta M, Rosselli M, Cottone M. Mesalamine in the maintenance treatment of Crohn's disease: a meta-analysis adjusted for confounding variables. Gastroenterology. 1997;113:1465-73.

Egan LJ, Sandborn WJ. Methotrexate for inflammatory bowel disease: pharmacology and preliminary results. Mayo Clin Proc. 1996;71:69-80.

Hanauer SB, Sandborn W. Management of Crohn's disease in adults. Am J Gastroenterol. 2001;96:635-43.

Kornbluth A, Sachar DB. Ulcerative colitis practice guidelines in adults: American College of Gastroenterology, Practice Parameters Committee. Am J Gastroenterol. 1997;92:204-11.

Mahadevan U, Sandborn WJ. Diagnosis and management of pouchitis. Gastroenterology. 2003;124:1636-50.

Pearson DC, May GR, Fick GH, Sutherland LR. Azathioprine and 6-mercaptopurine in Crohn disease: a meta-analysis. Ann Intern Med. 1995;123:132-42.

Sandborn WJ. A critical review of cyclosporine therapy in inflammatory bowel disease. Inflamm Bowel Dis. 1995;1:48-63.

Sandborn WJ, Fazio VW, Feagan BG, Hanauer SB, American Gastroenterological Association Clinical Practice Committee. AGA technical review on perianal Crohn's disease. Gastroenterology. 2003;125:1508-30.

Sandborn WJ, Feagan BG. Review article: mild to moderate Crohn's disease: defining the basis for a new treatment algorithm. Aliment Pharmacol Ther. 2003;18:263-77.

Sandborn WJ, Hanauer SB. Antitumor necrosis factor therapy for inflammatory bowel disease: a review of agents, pharmacology, clinical results, and safety. Inflamm Bowel Dis. 1999;5:119-33.

Sutherland LR, May GR, Shaffer EA. Sulfasalazine revisited: a meta-analysis of 5-aminosalicylic acid in the treatment of ulcerative colitis. Ann Intern Med. 1993;118:540-9.

CHAPTER 22

Inflammatory Bowel Disease: Extraintestinal Manifestations and Cancer

Edward V. Loftus, Jr., M.D.

Although ulcerative colitis and Crohn's disease are idiopathic inflammatory bowel diseases (IBDs) that by definition affect the gastrointestinal tract, they are associated with a wide variety of systemic complications. Such extraintestinal manifestations are classically defined as immune-mediated phenomena that affect the joints, eye, skin, or hepatobiliary tract, but they can be more broadly defined to include complications in other organ systems and complications that arise as a direct pathophysiologic consequence of extensive bowel inflammation or resection. This chapter reviews the most common extraintestinal manifestations, their relationship to activity of the underlying bowel disease, and their treatment.

One of the complications of IBD most feared by patients and physicians alike is the development of colorectal cancer. IBD is less commonly associated with other malignancies, such as cholangiocarcinoma. Fortunately, the risk of colorectal cancer can be partially mitigated by the use of colonoscopic surveillance. This chapter reviews risk factors for cancer and an algorithm for surveillance colonoscopy.

ARTHRITIS

The overall prevalence of IBD-related rheumatologic manifestations is thought to be approximately 30%. Several types of arthritis have been identified, each with its own clinical presentation, natural history, and treatment (Table 1).

Arthritis affecting the axial skeleton can be classified into the more common, frequently asymptomatic sacroiliitis and the less common, more progressive, ankylosing spondylitis. Subtle inflammatory changes of the sacroiliac joints may be detected with magnetic resonance imaging in up to 45% of

Table 1. Bone and Joint Manifestations of Inflammatory Bowel Disease

Spondyloarthropathy
  Axial skeleton
    Sacroiliitis
    Ankylosing spondylitis
  Peripheral
    Type 1 (oligoarticular)
    Type 2 (polyarticular) (rare)
Metabolic bone diseases
  Osteoporosis or osteopenia
  Osteomalacia (rare)
  Osteonecrosis (rare)

patients with IBD, but the vast majority of patients are asymptomatic. Typical changes on plain radiographs of the sacroiliac joints include narrowing of the joints and surrounding sclerosis. Symptomatic sacroiliitis presents as low back pain and stiffness, typically worse in the morning and with rest. A subset progresses to ankylosing spondylitis, which involves the vertebral facet joints and associated ligaments, resulting in progressive stiffness and lordosis of the spine. The prevalence of ankylosing spondylitis in IBD ranges between 1% and 6% across studies, with a higher prevalence in Crohn's disease than in ulcerative colitis. The relationship among spondyloarthropathy, intestinal inflammation, and classic inflammatory bowel disease is complex. Many patients with ankylosing spondylitis who have no gastrointestinal symptoms have evidence of subtle ileal inflammation, and symptomatic Crohn's disease eventually develops in 5% to 10% of these patients. Radiographic changes of ankylosing spondylitis include squaring of the vertebral bodies in the early stages followed by the classic "bamboo spine" appearance of syndesmophytes between the vertebral bodies. The HLA-B27 antigen is associated with ankylosing spondylitis occurring in the setting of IBD in 50% to 75% of patients. HLA-B27 positivity in patients with sacroiliitis implies a higher risk of progression to ankylosing spondylitis.

The clinical course of the axial arthritides associated with IBD appears to be unrelated to the activity of the underlying bowel disease. The course of ankylosing spondylitis is typically progressive even if the associated IBD is quiescent. The treatment of ankylosing spondylitis has been revolutionized with the availability of tumor necrosis factor antagonists. First-line therapy consists of physical therapy directed at maintaining spinal mobility, analgesics such as acetaminophen (with or without mild opioid agents such as propoxyphene or hydrocodone), and anti-inflammatory agents if needed. Conventional nonsteroidal anti-inflammatory drugs can be problematic because they may trigger an exacerbation of IBD. In more resistant cases, etanercept and infliximab are indicated.

The peripheral arthritis associated with IBD consists of two subtypes that are associated with different HLA antigens. Type 1, the more common type, is an asymmetric oligoarticular arthritis primarily affecting large joints such as the knees, ankles, wrists, and elbows. The clinical presentation consists of joint pain and swelling with limited range of motion. Plain radiographs typically do not show destructive changes, although they may occur rarely. Type 1 arthritis is usually self-limited and its activity mirrors the activity of the underlying IBD. Rarely, this form of peripheral arthritis becomes more chronic. Type 2 arthritis is a more chronic symmetric polyarthritis, similar to rheumatoid arthritis; however, rheumatoid factor is typically absent. The activity of this arthritis is independent of the associated IBD. Initial treatment of peripheral arthritis consists of physical therapy and analgesics. Nonsteroidal anti-inflammatory drugs may exacerbate the underlying IBD. Sulfasalazine should be considered the aminosalicylate of choice. Corticosteroids, administered either by oral ingestion or by intra-articular injection, may be required. For refractory cases of type 2 arthritis, methotrexate with or without infliximab may be required.

OCULAR MANIFESTATIONS

Inflammatory ocular complications occur in 1% to 13% of patients with IBD (Table 2). The most common forms are anterior uveitis (also known as iritis) and scleritis, although an inflammatory retinopathy or keratitis (corneal inflammation) may occur less frequently. Anterior uveitis occurs in up to

6% of patients with IBD and presents with ocular pain, redness, photophobia, or blurred vision. The presentation may be either acute or chronic. The acute form is associated with HLA-B27 in 50% of patients, and the chronic form is not associated with any particular HLA antigen. If the diagnosis is suspected, it should be confirmed with a slit-lamp examination by an ophthalmologist. (Indeed, any ocular symptoms in a patient with IBD should prompt a referral to an ophthalmologist.) The activity of the HLA-B27–associated form does not necessarily correlate with the activity of the IBD, whereas the activity of the chronic form unrelated to HLA antigens typically mirrors the activity of the bowel disease. One recent retrospective study suggested that sulfasalazine treatment resulted in fewer exacerbations of uveitis in the year after initiation of therapy compared with the previous year (from 3.4 to 0.9 flares per year). If left untreated, uveitis can result in irreversible complications such as adhesions, cataracts, and glaucoma. Initial treatment consists of topical corticosteroids and cycloplegic agents. For more refractory cases, oral corticosteroids may be required. Recent studies have shown the steroid-sparing qualities of methotrexate in this setting, and open-label studies of tumor necrosis factor inhibitors for treatment of uveitis have been promising.

Episcleritis and scleritis result in symptoms of eye irritation (e.g., burning, itching) and conjunctival erythema. The activity of these conditions typically correlates with the activity of the IBD. Initial treatment consists of topical corticosteroids, but oral corticosteroids may be required for refractory scleritis. Again, because an untrained physician cannot differentiate vision-threatening conditions such as scleritis from nonthreatening conditions such as episcleritis, ocular symptoms in a patient with IBD should lead to referral to an ophthalmologist.

Some ocular complications may be treatment-related (Table 2). The most common example is cataract formation after prolonged therapy with corticosteroids. The cumulative incidence of cataract formation may be as high as 85% after 4 years of corticosteroid use. Less commonly, the prolonged use of

Table 2.   Ocular Manifestations of Inflammatory Bowel Disease

Inflammatory
Anterior uveitis (iritis)
Scleritis
Episcleritis
Retinitis (rare)
Treatment-related (corticosteroids)
Cataracts
Glaucoma

corticosteroids may prompt the development of glaucoma. Patients with IBD who have required prolonged courses of corticosteroids (i.e., several years) should undergo periodic eye examinations even if they are asymptomatic.

DERMATOLOGIC MANIFESTATIONS

The two most common dermatologic extraintestinal manifestations are pyoderma gangrenosum and erythema nodosum, although numerous other disorders of the skin have been described in association with IBD (Table 3). Pyoderma gangrenosum is an idiopathic ulcerative skin disease that occurs in up to 12% of patients with IBD. It presents initially as a pustular lesion, which evolves to an ulcer with undermining borders. The lesion often exhibits "pathergy," or a tendency to worsen with trauma. The most common location is the lower extremity, but it can occur anywhere, including peristomal areas in patients with ostomies. Although skin biopsy may be helpful in excluding other conditions, there are no pathognomonic histologic features, and the diagnosis is a clinical one. Bacterial and fungal superinfection should be excluded. The course of pyoderma gangrenosum is independent of the associated IBD. First-line treatment consists of oral corticosteroids. There should be a low threshold for institution of immunosuppressive therapies so that the dose of corticosteroids can be tapered rapidly. The most commonly used immunosuppressive agents are cyclosporine and tacrolimus, although azathioprine and mycophenolate mofetil occasionally have been used for more chronic lesions. Case reports and case series have reported the efficacy of infliximab in both adult and pediatric patients with refractory pyoderma gangrenosum.

Erythema nodosum occurs more commonly in Crohn's disease (up to 15%) but may occur rarely in ulcerative colitis (up to 5%). For reasons that are unclear, this complication is most likely to develop in young women. It presents as painful, tender, erythematous subcutaneous nodules, most typically in the pretibial areas. The activity of erythema nodosum tends to correlate with that of the underlying IBD, and the lesions typically resolve with aggressive treatment of the bowel disease.

Cutaneous Crohn's disease refers to granulomatous lesions of the skin, most commonly in the perianal region. When such changes occur distant to the perineum, they are sometimes called "metastatic" Crohn's disease. These lesions present as erythematous plaques or nodules. The disease activity may not correlate with that of the underlying IBD, and treatment may be difficult. Corticosteroids and immunosuppressive therapy frequently are required.

HEPATOBILIARY MANIFESTATIONS

The most important hepatobiliary condition associated with IBD is primary sclerosing cholangitis (Table 4). This idiopathic chronic cholestatic liver disease is characterized by inflammation and fibrosis of the biliary tree. Approximately 75% to 80% of all patients with primary sclerosing cholangitis have associated IBD, and the vast majority of these have ulcerative colitis. Conversely, 2% to 7% of patients with ulcerative colitis and an even smaller percentage of patients with Crohn's disease have associated primary sclerosing cholangitis. Patients present with pruritus and jaundice in advanced stages of the condition, but with increased diagnostic awareness the most frequent presentation is in an asymptomatic patient with IBD who has abnormal results on hepatic biochemistry tests. The presence of numerous strictures and dilatations of the extrahepatic or intrahepatic biliary tree on endoscopic retrograde cholangiopancreatography most commonly confirms the diagnosis. Liver biopsy may be necessary for diagnosis in small duct primary sclerosing cholangitis (formerly known as pericholangitis). The IBD associated with primary sclerosing cholangitis is commonly mild in activity and almost always pancolonic in extent. Rectal sparing and "backwash ileitis" appear to be more common in primary sclerosing cholangitis-related IBD than in typical

Table 3. Dermatologic Manifestations of Inflammatory Bowel Disease

Common
   Pyoderma gangrenosum
   Erythema nodosum
   Cutaneous ("metastatic") Crohn's disease
Less common
   Bowel-associated dermatosis-arthritis syndrome (bowel
    bypass syndrome)
   Sweet's syndrome (acute neutrophilic dermatosis)
   Epidermolysis bullosa acquisita
   Pyostomatitis vegetans

Table 4. Hepatobiliary Manifestations of Inflammatory Bowel Disease

Biliary
   Primary sclerosing cholangitis (large duct)
   Small duct primary sclerosing cholangitis
    (pericholangitis)
   Cholelithiasis or choledocholithiasis
   Cholangiocarcinoma (rare)
   Primary biliary cirrhosis (rare)
Hepatic
   Fatty liver or steatohepatitis
   Autoimmune hepatitis

ulcerative colitis, suggesting that primary sclerosing cholangitis-associated IBD may be a unique phenotype. The course of primary sclerosing cholangitis is completely independent of the underlying IBD, and even total proctocolectomy is thought to have no effect on its natural history. The disease course is typically progressive, and there are no proven medical therapies, although high-dose ursodeoxycholic acid appears promising. Orthotopic liver transplantation may be required. Complications include acute cholangitis, formation of dominant biliary strictures, choledocholithiasis, and cholangiocarcinoma (see Chapter 35, Cholestatic Liver Disease).

Autoimmune hepatitis is rarely associated with IBD; when such an association exists, it is usually with ulcerative colitis. Some patients may have features of both autoimmune hepatitis and primary sclerosing cholangitis (the so-called overlap syndrome) (see Chapter 36, Autoimmune Hepatitis).

Cholelithiasis is a common consequence of Crohn's disease. Either inflammation or surgical resection of the distal ileum results in impaired enterohepatic recycling of bile salts and a resultant upset in the balance of bile salts, cholesterol, and phospholipids, leading to an increased tendency to form cholesterol crystals and stones. Pigment stones also have been implicated in patients with steatorrhea, most likely due to an impaired enterohepatic circulation of bilirubin.

OSTEOPENIA AND OSTEOPOROSIS

An evolving literature strongly suggests that osteopenia and osteoporosis are highly prevalent in IBD (up to 50%-70%, depending on the patients studied and definitions used) (Table 1). Several factors may play a role, including corticosteroid use, malabsorption of calcium and vitamin D, malnutrition, low body mass index, cigarette smoking, and increased concentrations of cytokines, which contribute to bone resorption. However, conventional risk factors for osteoporosis such as female sex, menopause, and increasing age are equally important in patients with IBD. Although corticosteroid use is thought by some investigators to be the most important risk factor for osteoporosis in IBD, vertebral compression fractures occasionally have been diagnosed in patients with IBD who have never received corticosteroids. Bone loss associated with corticosteroid use is rapid, and the bulk of the loss occurs within the first several months of therapy. Surprisingly, population-based studies of patients with IBD have shown only a modestly increased risk of actual bone fracture relative to the general population. Diagnosis is made with bone mineral densitometry (dual photon absorptiometry). A T score of –2.5 (more than 2 SD below mean bone mass for a young adult) signifies osteoporosis, and a T score between –1 and –2.5 signifies osteopenia. There is as yet no consensus as to which patients with IBD should be screened with densitometry. Treatment consists of calcium

and vitamin D supplementation (1,200 mg calcium and 800 IU vitamin D), sex hormone replacement if deficient, and a bisphosphonate (alendronate or risedronate). For patients who are intolerant of oral bisphosphonates, therapeutic options include intravenous pamidronate, intravenous zoledronic acid, intranasal calcitonin, or parenteral teraparatide.

MISCELLANEOUS COMPLICATIONS

Renal complications are most common in Crohn's disease (Table 5). Nephrolithiasis may occur in up to 10% of patients with Crohn's disease, mostly a result of calcium oxalate stone

Table 5.   Miscellaneous Extraintestinal Manifestations and Complications of Inflammatory Bowel Disease

Renal
    Nephrolithiasis (oxalate, urate)
    Glomerulonephritis (rare)
    Right ureteral obstruction
    Urinary system fistulas (e.g., enterovesical, colovesical, rectourethral)
Hematologic
    Anemia
        Iron deficiency
        Vitamin B_{12} deficiency
        Folic acid deficiency
        Anemia of chronic disease
        Autoimmune hemolytic anemia
    Neoplastic
        Myelodysplastic syndrome (rare)
        Promyelocytic leukemia (rare)
Cardiopulmonary
    Pericarditis (extraintestinal manifestation or drug-induced)
    Myocarditis
    Conduction abnormalities
    Pneumonitis
    Eosinophilic pneumonia
    Bronchiolitis obliterans with organizing pneumonia
Pancreatic
    Acute pancreatitis
        Drug-induced (purine analogs, 5-aminosalicylates)
        Duodenal Crohn's disease
        Granulomatous involvement of pancreas (rare)
    Chronic pancreatitis
        Autoimmune pancreatitis
Thrombophilia
    Multifactorial

formation. Intestinal inflammation or resection results in excessive oxalate absorption. In the setting of fat malabsorption, the intestinal luminal calcium, which normally binds to oxalate, instead binds to fatty acids, leaving oxalate free to be absorbed from the colonic lumen. Patients with ulcerative colitis, especially those who have undergone colectomy, have a slightly increased tendency to form uric acid stones. Other renal complications include glomerulonephritis, right ureteral obstruction due to ileal inflammation, and enterovesical fistula formation.

Hematologic complications such as anemia, thrombocytosis, and leukocytosis are common. Anemia may be multifactorial (e.g., iron or vitamin B_{12} deficiency, anemia of chronic disease), and rarely it is a sign of an associated hematologic disorder such as autoimmune hemolytic anemia, myelodysplastic syndrome, or promyelocytic leukemia.

Various cardiopulmonary complications have been described, including pericarditis, myocarditis, conduction abnormalities, eosinophilic pneumonia, and interstitial pneumonitis. Pericarditis and pneumonitis may arise both as a true extraintestinal manifestation and as an allergic complication of therapy with sulfasalazine or other 5-aminosalicylates.

Pancreatitis most commonly occurs in IBD as a complication of medical therapy. Azathioprine and 6-mercaptopurine are most likely to result in pancreatitis (3%-5%). Acute pancreatitis also has developed rarely after therapy with sulfasalazine or other 5-aminosalicylates. In patients with duodenal Crohn's disease, pancreatitis may develop as a result of a stricture or fistula formation. However, up to 50% of patients with IBD have no obvious cause of pancreatitis, and a subset of these may have a true extraintestinal manifestation. In some patients with Crohn's disease, granulomatous inflammation of the pancreas seems to develop. Furthermore, antipancreatic antibodies have been described in up to 30% of patients with Crohn's disease.

Thromboembolism is more common in patients with IBD, probably due to various factors. Activation of the inflammatory cascade in IBD appears to result in secondary activation of important mediators of thrombosis, such as platelets, fibrinogen, and fibrinopeptide A. A single genetic mutation does not appear to be responsible, but cases of factor V Leiden mutation, protein C deficiency, and protein S deficiency have been described. The risk of thromboembolism was initially tied to the activity of IBD, but there are numerous reports of thromboembolic activity in the absence of active IBD.

COLORECTAL CANCER

Patients with ulcerative colitis, and likely Crohn's colitis, are at increased risk of colorectal cancer, and this remains an important cause of mortality in IBD. In most population-based studies of ulcerative colitis, the relative risk of colorectal cancer is 2 to 8 times higher than that of the general population. Overall,

the absolute risk, or cumulative incidence, of colorectal cancer is 8% to 18% after 20 to 30 years of disease. However, when the risk is stratified by extent of disease, it is clear that more extensive disease confers a higher risk of colorectal cancer (Table 6). The cumulative incidence of colorectal cancer among patients with extensive ulcerative colitis (i.e., extent of disease proximal to splenic flexure) ranges from 6% to 50% after 30 years of disease. Another major risk factor appears to be duration of ulcerative colitis. The cumulative risk of colorectal cancer does not seem to be higher than that in the general population until 8 to 10 years after diagnosis, and the increase in risk is 0.5% to 1% each year thereafter. Whether age at onset of colitis is a risk factor independent of disease duration remains unclear.

Another important risk factor for colorectal cancer in IBD appears to be the presence of primary sclerosing cholangitis. Whether primary sclerosing cholangitis is a truly independent risk factor for colorectal cancer, or whether it functions as a marker for long-standing but asymptomatic pancolitis, remains unclear. Finally, a family history of colorectal cancer in a patient with IBD appears to be a risk factor for cancer independent of the aforementioned factors.

In many studies, prolonged use of 5-aminosalicylates or sulfasalazine appears to reduce the risk of colorectal cancer substantially. Conversely, in the period when non-sulfonamide 5-aminosalicylate agents were not commercially available, the presence of sulfonamide allergy appeared to be a risk factor for colorectal cancer. However, the data are conflicting on this point in that some studies have not found a risk reduction in patients receiving 5-aminosalicylates. Several studies also have suggested that the use of ursodeoxycholic acid is associated with a lower risk of colorectal neoplasia among patients with primary sclerosing cholangitis who have IBD.

Dysplasia frequently precedes or is associated with IBD-related colorectal cancer. Dysplastic change may be flat or polypoid on endoscopy. Surveillance colonoscopy with biopsy

Table 6. Risk Factors for Colorectal Cancer in Inflammatory Bowel Disease

Extent of colitis
Duration of disease
Family history of colorectal cancer
Primary sclerosing cholangitis
Medical noncompliance or lack of follow-up
No or minimal use of sulfasalazine or 5-aminosalicylates
Sulfonamide allergy

at regular intervals is offered to many patients with long-standing and extensive ulcerative colitis in an attempt to manage the increased risk of colorectal cancer. Although surveillance colonoscopy has never been proved to reduce colorectal cancer-related mortality in patients with IBD, several retrospective studies have suggested this to be the case. Surveillance is thought to detect early, curable cancers and to identify patients at increased risk for development of cancer. The use of staining dyes in combination with high-magnification lenses (also known as "chromoendoscopy") may substantially increase the ability of the endoscopist to detect dysplastic lesions, and this technique is being actively studied.

We recommend institution of regular surveillance colonoscopy with biopsies after 8 to 10 years of extensive colitis in both ulcerative colitis and Crohn's disease. This procedure should be performed at least every other year, and some experts advocate yearly procedures. Patients with left-sided disease should begin periodic surveillance after 15 to 20 years of disease. Patients with only proctitis do not have an increased risk of colorectal cancer and do not require surveillance colonoscopy. Patients with primary sclerosing cholangitis should begin surveillance colonoscopy immediately. Random biopsy specimens should be obtained in a consistent fashion ("the more biopsies, the better"). Some experts advocate four-quadrant biopsies every 10 to 15 cm, which results in approximately 40 biopsy specimens. At Mayo Clinic, we obtain at least 32 (4 each from cecum, ascending, proximal transverse, distal transverse, proximal descending, distal descending, sigmoid, and rectum). These are placed in four bottles (eight per bottle). In addition to the 32 random samples, specimens are obtained from suspicious lesions or nodules and placed in separate bottles.

Most investigators agree that patients with flat, high-grade dysplasia are at particularly high risk of either synchronous cancer or metachronous cancer in the near future. Immediate colectomy is recommended. However, there is ongoing controversy about whether patients with flat, low-grade dysplasia should be offered immediate colectomy or more intensive surveillance colonoscopy. At Mayo Clinic we recommend immediate colectomy, because most retrospective studies have suggested that the 5-year risk for progression to high-grade dysplasia, polypoid dysplasia, or cancer after a diagnosis of low-grade dysplasia may be as high as 50%. The management of polypoid dysplasia (formerly known as dysplasia-associated lesion or mass) also is evolving. Previous dogma suggested that all such lesions were an indication for immediate colectomy. However, recent studies suggest that if these lesions are not associated with flat dysplasia in the surrounding mucosa, they can be removed safely with colonoscopic polypectomy and close follow-up.

OTHER CANCERS

Patients with ulcerative colitis are at increased risk of cholangiocarcinoma, likely because of the increased risk of primary sclerosing cholangitis in the population with ulcerative colitis. (Primary sclerosing cholangitis is a risk factor for cholangiocarcinoma.) Patients who have Crohn's disease with small bowel involvement seem to be at increased risk for small bowel adenocarcinoma relative to the general population. However, the absolute risk is low, and surveillance for this lesion is not recommended. Whether IBD is a risk factor for lymphoma remains controversial. In general, population-based studies have not shown an increased relative risk, although this has been suggested by several referral-center–based studies. The question has become more complicated with the more widespread use of immunosuppressive agents such as azathioprine, 6-mercaptopurine, methotrexate, and infliximab. It is well recognized that immunosuppressed states, such as the posttransplantation state and the acquired immunodeficiency syndrome, are associated with an increased risk of lymphoproliferative disorders. Although most studies of patients with IBD who have received immunosuppressive agents have not shown an increased risk of lymphoma, a recent preliminary meta-analysis of lymphoma risk among patients with IBD taking 6-mercaptopurine or azathioprine suggested a threefold increase in lymphoma risk. Again, it is important to emphasize that the absolute risk of lymphoma remains small, and in most situations the benefits of the drug outweigh this potential risk.

RECOMMENDED READING

Bernstein CN, Blanchard JF, Rawsthorne P, Yu N. The prevalence of extraintestinal diseases in inflammatory bowel disease: a population-based study. Am J Gastroenterol. 2001;96:1116-22.

Dayharsh GA, Loftus EV Jr, Sandborn WJ, Tremaine WJ, Zinsmeister AR, Witzig TE, et al. Epstein-Barr virus-positive lymphoma in patients with inflammatory bowel disease treated with azathioprine or 6-mercaptopurine. Gastroenterology. 2002;122:72-7.

De Vos M. Crohn's disease and spondyloarthropathy. Inflamm Bowel Dis Monitor. 2003;5:11-7.

Hoffmann RM, Kruis W. Rare extraintestinal manifestations of inflammatory bowel disease. Inflamm Bowel Dis. 2004;10:140-7.

Jayaram H, Satsangi J, Chapman RW. Increased colorectal neoplasia in chronic ulcerative colitis complicated by primary sclerosing cholangitis: fact or fiction? Gut. 2001;48:430-4.

Judge TA, Su CG, Lichtenstein GR. Pyoderma gangrenosum. Clin Perspect Gastroenterol. 2001;4:325-9.

Loftus EV Jr. Does monitoring prevent cancer in inflammatory bowel disease? J Clin Gastroenterol. 2003;36 Suppl:S79-83.

Loftus EV Jr. Management of extraintestinal manifestations and other complications of inflammatory bowel disease. Curr Gastroenterol Rep. 2004;6:506-13.

Loftus EV Jr, Harewood GC, Loftus CG, Tremaine WJ, Harmsen WS, Zinsmeister AR, et al. PSC-IBD: a unique form of inflammatory bowel disease associated with primary sclerosing cholangitis. Gut. 2005;54:91-6.

Loftus EV Jr, Rubin DT. Managing the complications of chronic inflammatory bowel disease: osteoporosis and colorectal cancer. Semin Inflamm Bowel Dis. 2003;2:1-7.

Loftus EV Jr, Sandborn WJ. Lymphoma risk in inflammatory bowel disease: influences of referral bias and therapy. Gastroenterology. 2001;121:1239-42.

Mintz R, Feller ER, Bahr RL, Shah SA. Ocular manifestations of inflammatory bowel disease. Inflamm Bowel Dis. 2004;10:135-9.

Quera R, Shanahan F. Thromboembolism: an important manifestation of inflammatory bowel disease. Am J Gastroenterol. 2004;99:1971-3.

Smale S, Natt RS, Orchard TR, Russell AS, Bjarnason I. Inflammatory bowel disease and spondyloarthropathy. Arthritis Rheum. 2001;44:2728-36.

Solem CA, Harmsen WS, Zinsmeister AR, Loftus EV Jr. Small intestinal adenocarcinoma in Crohn's disease: a case-control study. Inflamm Bowel Dis. 2004;10:32-5.

Solem CA, Loftus EV, Tremaine WJ, Sandborn WJ. Venous thromboembolism in inflammatory bowel disease. Am J Gastroenterol. 2004;99:97-101.

Talwalkar JA, Lindor KD. Primary sclerosing cholangitis. Inflamm Bowel Dis. 2005;11:62-72.

CHAPTER 23

Microscopic Colitis and *Clostridium difficile*-Associated Disease

Darrell S. Pardi, M.D.

MICROSCOPIC COLITIS

The term "microscopic colitis" was used originally in 1980 to describe a condition of chronic watery diarrhea and normal findings on barium enema and colonoscopy but colon biopsy specimens with microscopic inflammation. Collagenous colitis is a closely related condition, with similar clinical and histologic features, but in addition the subepithelial collagen band is thickened. It is unclear whether these conditions represent separate disease entities or are part of the spectrum of a single disease process. Therefore, "microscopic colitis" currently is used as an umbrella term, covering two major subsets: collagenous colitis, with a thickened subepithelial collagen band, and lymphocytic colitis, without collagen thickening.

Case Presentation

A 61-year-old woman has a 6-month history of eight watery bowel movements per day, including several nocturnal stools, often with crampy abdominal and rectal pain. She has lost 10 lb. She occasionally passes mucus per rectum but does not have melena, hematochezia, greasy or oily stools, incontinence, or fever. She has not done any traveling, drunk well water, eaten contaminated food, or recently taken antibiotics or new medications. She has no past medical history, and the physical examination findings are normal.

The results of laboratory investigations were normal except for the presence of fecal leukocytes; stool studies did not show pathologic bacteria, parasites, or *Clostridium difficile* toxin. The results of colonoscopy were unremarkable, but biopsy specimens showed an increase in intraepithelial lymphocytes, with a mixed inflammatory cell infiltrate in the lamina propria, consistent with lymphocytic colitis.

Epidemiology

Microscopic colitis represents about 10% of cases of chronic watery diarrhea. According to European reports, collagenous colitis has an annual incidence of 0.6 to 5.2/100,000 population and a prevalence of 10 to 15.7/100,000, whereas lymphocytic colitis has an incidence of 3.4 to 4.0/100,000 and a prevalence of 14.4/100,000. In a recent study from North America, from 1994-2001, both lymphocytic colitis and collagenous colitis were more common than previously reported, with incidences of 9.8 and 5.1/100,000 and prevalences of 64 and 36/100,000, respectively. That study also reported that the incidence of microscopic colitis is increasing substantially over time, from 0.8/100,000 in 1985-1989 to 19.1/100,000 in 1998-2001. The reasons for the increase are not known.

There is a female predominance, as high as 9:1, that appears to be more striking for collagenous colitis than for lymphocytic colitis. Microscopic colitis typically presents in the sixth to eighth decade, although a wide age range has been reported.

Clinical Features

Microscopic colitis is characterized by chronic or intermittent watery diarrhea, and up to 50% of patients have abdominal pain or mild weight loss. Self-limited single attacks and spontaneous resolution have been reported. Of patients without full remission, many have intermittent symptoms and do not require continuous therapy. Fecal leukocytes may be present, and mild steatorrhea has been reported. Dehydration is unusual, and marked fever, nausea, vomiting, or hematochezia should raise the possibility of an alternative diagnosis. Arthralgias and various autoimmune conditions can occur in microscopic colitis, as can an increased erythrocyte sedimentation rate and a positive antinuclear antibody or other autoimmune markers.

Of particular interest is the apparent association between microscopic colitis and celiac sprue. In patients with celiac sprue, up to one-third have colon biopsy results consistent with microscopic colitis. However, the prevalence of small-bowel spruelike changes in patients with microscopic colitis ranges from 2% to 9% in the largest series. Thus, microscopic colitis and celiac disease often coexist. This association should be considered in patients with sprue who do not respond to a gluten-free diet or for those with microscopic colitis who do not respond to the usual therapies.

Endoscopic and radiologic evaluations of the colon are normal or show mild nonspecific changes such as erythema or edema. Histologic findings include a mixed inflammatory cell infiltrate in the lamina propria, with an increased number of intraepithelial lymphocytes (Fig. 1 and 2). These inflammatory changes are often accompanied by focal or diffuse surface epithelial damage. In collagenous colitis, the subepithelial collagen band is abnormally thickened (Fig. 3). Microscopic colitis can be distinguished from inflammatory bowel disease by the absence of distortion of crypt architecture.

The reliability of left-sided colon biopsy (i.e., flexible sigmoidoscopy) for making the diagnosis of microscopic colitis is somewhat controversial. Some studies have reported that collagen thickening and intraepithelial lymphocytosis become less evident from the cecum to the rectum and that rectosigmoid biopsy can miss the diagnosis in up to 40% of cases. Others report that sigmoid biopsy is very reliable, missing the diagnosis in only 0% to 5%. Despite these mixed results, it is generally accepted that biopsy from the descending colon should be reasonably sensitive and that flexible sigmoidoscopy is sufficient to make the diagnosis of microscopic colitis in most cases. If left-sided colon biopsy is nondiagnostic and clinical suspicion remains high, a colonoscopy with proximal biopsy can be considered.

Pathophysiology

Data on the mechanisms involved in microscopic colitis come from studies on a small number of patients, and no consistent mechanism has been established. Postulated mechanisms include bile acid malabsorption, altered fluid and electrolyte absorption or secretion, unidentified infection, immunologic reaction to a luminal antigen (food, microorganism, other), medication side effect (including nonsteroidal anti-inflammatory drugs), autoimmunity, and alteration in collagen synthesis or degradation. The clinicopathologic term "microscopic colitis" likely encompasses several different etiologic or pathophysiologic mechanisms with similar histologic phenotypes.

Treatment

Use of nonsteroidal anti-inflammatory drugs and agents that might exacerbate diarrhea (e.g., excessive caffeine or alcohol) should be discontinued. Nonspecific antidiarrheal therapy such as loperamide or diphenoxylate-atropine should be prescribed. If treatment with these agents is unsuccessful, bismuth subsalicylate can be considered at a dose of two tablets (262 mg each) three or four times daily.

If diarrhea does not respond to bismuth, the next therapeutic intervention considered is often mesalamine or sulfasalazine. However, several large retrospective series have reported benefit in fewer than half of the patients treated with these drugs. Cholestyramine may be more effective, although many patients do not tolerate it because of its texture.

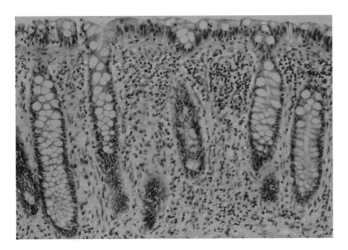

Fig. 1. Lymphocytic colitis. Note mixed inflammatory infiltrate in lamina propria, with an increased number of intraepithelial lymphocytes. The crypt architecture is normal, unlike that in ulcerative colitis or Crohn's colitis. (From Pardi DS, Smyrk TC, Tremaine WJ, Sandborn WJ. Microscopic colitis: a review. Am J Gastroenterol. 2002;97:794-802. Used with permission.)

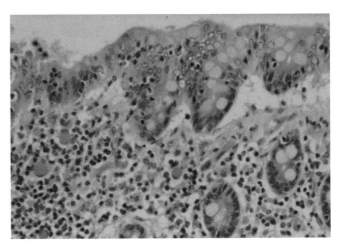

Fig. 2. Lymphocytic colitis. This higher power view emphasizes intraepithelial lymphocytes.

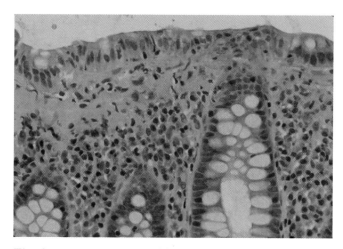

Fig. 3. Collagenous colitis. In addition to inflammatory infiltrate, note thickened subepithelial collagen band. (From Pardi DS, Smyrk TC, Tremaine WJ, Sandborn WJ. Microscopic colitis: a review. Am J Gastroenterol. 2002;97:794-802. Used with permission.)

Disease refractory to these medications may respond to corticosteroids, which are among the best therapies in the largest uncontrolled series. Budesonide is a synthetic corticosteroid with low systemic bioavailability and less risk of corticosteroid side effects which has been effective in controlled studies of collagenous colitis. However, relapse after discontinuation of therapy is common, and many patients become corticosteroid-dependent. Furthermore, corticosteroid therapy should not be given long term because of the risk of side effects. Thus, before corticosteroid therapy is initiated, the diagnosis should be reevaluated and alternative diagnoses, such as coexistent celiac sprue or hyperthyroidism, should be excluded, if not done already.

The goal of corticosteroid therapy is to induce remission, and then therapy is tapered after 4 to 6 weeks in an attempt to maintain remission with another of the medications mentioned above. For corticosteroid-refractory or corticosteroid-dependent cases, immune modifiers such as azathioprine or 6-mercaptopurine can be used, although side effects are frequent and may be treatment-limiting in some patients. Clinicians are gaining experience with chronic low-dose (3-6 mg/day) budesonide therapy for patients with corticosteroid-dependent microscopic colitis. However, the safety and effectiveness of this strategy remain to be proved in clinical trials.

Other management options include antibiotics, calcium channel blockers, octreotide, other immune modifiers, or, rarely, surgery (ileostomy with or without colectomy). The medications typically used to treat microscopic colitis are listed in Table 1.

Clinical Course

Most patients with microscopic colitis have chronic watery diarrhea, although the course can be waxing and waning. Spontaneous resolution has been reported. There does not appear to be a risk for progression to more overt forms of inflammatory bowel disease or colon cancer. Most patients have a response to the treatment algorithm suggested above, but it is not clear how long therapy should be continued. For example, patients given treatment with bismuth subsalicylate for 8 weeks have entered remissions lasting longer than 2 years. Thus, when an agent is found to control the diarrhea, treatment should be continued for 8 to 12 weeks, after which an attempt to taper therapy can be considered. For patients who have recurrent symptoms, chronic maintenance therapy can be used.

- Collagenous colitis and lymphocytic colitis are two subtypes of microscopic colitis.
- Diarrhea is the typical symptom, sometimes with abdominal pain or mild weight loss.
- Microscopic colitis is associated with various autoimmune diseases, including celiac sprue.
- Microscopic colitis may be associated with use of nonsteroidal anti-inflammatory drugs.
- Histologic features include mixed lamina propria inflammation, intraepithelial lymphocytosis, and, in collagenous colitis, a thickened subepithelial collagen band.
- Treatment with nonspecific antidiarrheal medications is often successful.
- Remission (drug-induced or spontaneous) is not uncommon, and prolonged therapy may not be necessary.

Table 1. Medications Used to Treat Microscopic Colitis

Medication	Dose
Loperamide	2-16 mg daily
Diphenoxylate-atropine	1-8 tablets daily
Cholestyramine	4 g 1-4 times daily
Bismuth subsalicylate	2 tablets 3-4 times daily
Budesonide	9 mg daily
Prednisone	30-60 mg daily
Sulfasalazine	2-4 g daily
Mesalamine (Asacol)	2.4-4.8 g daily
Mesalamine (Pentasa)	2-4 g daily
Azathioprine	2 mg/kg daily
Mercaptopurine	1-1.5 mg/kg daily

Modified from Pardi DS, Smyrk TC, Tremaine WJ, Sandborn WJ.
Microscopic colitis: a review. Am J Gastroenterol.
2002;97:794-802. Used with permission.

CLOSTRIDIUM DIFFICILE-ASSOCIATED DISEASE

Background

The first case of pseudomembranous colitis was reported in 1893 as "diphtheritic colitis," and the *Clostridium difficile* organism was described in 1935. It was not until the 1970s that *C. difficile* was implicated as a causative factor in pseudomembranous colitis. Although *C. difficile*-associated disease was described before antibiotics were used, most current cases are associated with antibiotic use. Other conditions that can predispose to *C. difficile*-associated disease include bowel ischemia, surgery, malnutrition, chemotherapy, and critical illness. The spectrum of disease associated with *C. difficile* includes an asymptomatic carrier state, diarrhea without colitis, and variable degrees of colitis with or without pseudomembranes.

Epidemiology

During the past 25 years, there has been an increase in the occurrence rate and a more modest clinical spectrum of *C. difficile*-associated disease, trends thought to be due to increased antibiotic use, more aggressive testing, and early intervention. Recent data reflect the health care burden of *C. difficile* infection: an additional hospital cost of more than $3,000 per patient and an extra length of stay of 3.6 days, leading to an estimated cost in the United States in excess of $1 billion per year.

C. difficile is detected in very few (1%-3%) healthy adults. It is more common in hospitalized adults and in patients receiving antibiotic therapy. Up to 50% of infants and children carry the bacterium, but pseudomembranous colitis is rare in this age group. The incidence of antibiotic-associated diarrhea varies from 5% to 39% depending on the antibiotic used, and most cases are due to the antibiotic and not to infection with *C. difficile*, particularly in outpatients. Pseudomembranous colitis occurs in only 10% of cases of antibiotic-associated diarrhea. In contrast to antibiotic-associated diarrhea, most cases of pseudomembranous colitis are due to *C. difficile*.

Populations at high risk for *C. difficile*-associated disease include the elderly, patients with uremia, burns, abdominal surgery, or cancer, and patients in an intensive care unit. It is not known whether these groups are more exposed to nosocomial infections or are more susceptible to *C. difficile*-associated disease because of their specific illnesses.

- Most cases of *C. difficile*-associated disease occur after antibiotic use, although other risk factors exist.
- *C. difficile*-associated disease ranges from asymptomatic carriage to diarrhea without colitis to colitis with or without pseudomembranes.
- *C. difficile* can be found in healthy infants but is uncommon in healthy adults.

- Most antibiotic-associated diarrhea is due to the antibiotic and not to *C. difficile*.
- Most pseudomembranous colitis is due to *C. difficile* infection.

Case Presentation

A 75-year-old man presented with a 2-day history of crampy lower abdominal pain, nonbloody diarrhea, tenesmus, and fever. He recently completed a course of antibiotic therapy for pneumonia. On physical examination, he appeared ill, with a temperature of 101°F, normal blood pressure, and a pulse rate of 98 beats/min. The abdomen was mildly distended and tender without guarding or rebound. Laboratory studies showed leukocytosis of 13.4 cells × 10⁹/L, with 15% band forms. Stool analysis showed many leukocytes, and *C. difficile* toxin was detected. Abdominal radiography showed mild ileus but no dilatation of the colon. Treatment with metronidazole, 500 mg three times daily by mouth, promptly improved his symptoms.

Clinical Presentation

The time between starting antibiotic therapy and the appearance of clinical symptoms varies from 1 day to 6 weeks, most commonly 3 to 9 days. However, symptoms may occur after a single dose of antibiotics (including topical antibiotics) or they may not begin until several weeks after antibiotic therapy has been discontinued.

Presentation may range from only loose stools to toxic megacolon (nausea, vomiting, high-grade fever, ileus) and colonic perforation. Typically, the disease presents with watery or mucoid diarrhea along with abdominal pain and low-grade fever. Stools may contain small amounts of blood. Extraintestinal manifestations, such as arthritis, are rare. Diarrhea may cause dehydration and electrolyte depletion. Overall mortality is low (2%-3%), although it is higher among elderly or debilitated patients (10%-20%) and with fulminant colitis or toxic megacolon (30%-80%). In some patients (5%-19%), disease is localized to the proximal colon and may present with an acute abdomen, localized rebound tenderness, no diarrhea, and normal findings on sigmoidoscopy.

Despite successful treatment, 10% to 25% of patients have disease relapse, regardless of the therapeutic agent used. These patients usually respond well to re-treatment with metronidazole or vancomycin, but the risk of additional recurrences is high.

- *C. difficile*-associated disease usually occurs within 1 to 2 weeks after antibiotic therapy is started.
- In about 10% of patients, the disease is localized above the splenic flexure and can present atypically.
- From 10% to 25% of patients have recurrent disease.

Differential Diagnosis

Staphylococcal enterocolitis and typhlitis can occur in patients receiving chemotherapy and can have a presentation similar to that of *C. difficile*-associated disease. Crohn's disease and ulcerative colitis exacerbations can simulate *C. difficile*-associated disease, and, importantly, *C. difficile* infection can cause a symptom flare in patients with inflammatory bowel disease. Other disorders in the differential diagnosis include chemical colitis (chemotherapy, gold), ischemic colitis, and other infections (*Campylobacter*, *Salmonella*, *Shigella*, *Escherichia coli*, *Entamoeba*, *Listeria*, cytomegalovirus).

Pathophysiology

The development of *C. difficile*-associated disease requires an alteration in the normal gut flora or mucosal immunity, the acquisition and germination of spores, overgrowth of *C. difficile*, and the production of toxin. Toxin A binds to mucosal receptors and causes cytotoxicity by disrupting cytoplasmic microfilaments and inducing apoptosis. Toxin B can then enter the damaged mucosa and cause further cytotoxicity, resulting in hemorrhage, inflammation, and cellular necrosis. The toxins also interfere with protein synthesis, stimulate granulocyte chemotaxis, increase capillary permeability, and promote peristalsis. In severe cases, inflammation and necrosis may involve deeper layers of the colon and result in toxic dilatation or perforation.

Diagnostic Testing

Diagnosis is based on a combination of clinical findings, laboratory test results, and sometimes endoscopy. Leukocytosis and hypoalbuminemia are not uncommon. Fecal leukocytes can be seen, but their absence does not exclude colitis. Stool culture for *C. difficile* is relatively demanding and has low predictive value.

Cytotoxicity assays are considered positive when cultured cells show cytopathic changes when exposed to stool filtrates. The result is then confirmed by neutralizing these effects with specific antitoxins. This is considered the standard diagnostic method because of its high sensitivity and specificity. However, cytotoxicity assays are expensive and time-consuming.

Enzyme-linked immunosorbent assay (ELISA) for the detection of toxin A or B is less expensive and faster than tissue culture and, thus, is preferred at many centers. Sensitivity is lower (75%-85%) than for cytotoxic assays, but performing the test on two or three separate stools should increase sensitivity to 90% to 95%. In addition, proper storage and handling may prevent toxin degradation and improve sensitivity. A newer ELISA to detect the presence of either toxin (TOX A/B test) has excellent specificity and improved sensitivity compared with testing for either toxin alone, because some strains of *C. difficile* may produce only one toxin or the other.

Although endoscopic findings may be normal in patients with mild *C. difficile*-associated disease, most patients have abnormal mucosa. Flexible sigmoidoscopy is diagnostic in most cases, but colonoscopy may be required in about 10% of cases when disease is localized above the splenic flexure. Endoscopy may be the fastest means of suggesting the diagnosis, but in patients with severe disease, it is hazardous and should be avoided. Colitis may range from minimal erythema or edema to ulceration, often with nodular exudates that may coalesce to form yellow "pseudomembranes" consisting of mucus and fibrin filled with dead leukocytes and mucosal cells (Fig. 4).

- *C. difficile*-associated disease is toxin-mediated.
- Stool cytotoxicity assay is the standard diagnostic test, but it is expensive and time-consuming.
- ELISA for toxin A or B is used in most laboratories because it is faster and less expensive than tissue culture. Its relatively poor sensitivity can be improved by testing two or three stool samples.
- In many patients, endoscopy is not necessary for diagnosis.

Treatment of Primary Infection

For mild disease, supportive therapy alone (without antibiotic treatment) may be sufficient, including rehydration and discontinuation of use of the offending antibiotic. Antidiarrheal agents and narcotics should be avoided because they may prolong exposure to toxins and result in more severe colitis. Specific antibiotic therapy should be given if supportive therapy fails, if treatment with the offending antibiotic cannot be discontinued, or if symptoms are severe. For severe disease, hospitalization for antibiotic therapy and intravenous hydration may be necessary. When *C. difficile*-associated disease is

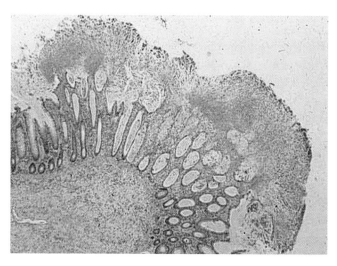

Fig. 4. Typical histologic appearance of pseudomembranous colitis.

suspected in elderly and severely ill patients, empiric antibiotic therapy should be started before test results are known.

Metronidazole is inexpensive and effective and has response and relapse rates comparable to those of vancomycin. The usual oral dose is 250 to 750 mg three or four times daily for 7 to 10 days. Because of concerns about cost and resistance with vancomycin, metronidazole is the preferred first-line therapy. However, metronidazole has more side effects and is not recommended for children or pregnant women. If the patient's condition does not improve promptly (2 or 3 days), the situation should be reassessed and, if the diagnosis is secure, vancomycin should be substituted for metronidazole.

Vancomycin is a reliable but more expensive treatment, with response rates of 90% to 100%, and is the preferred treatment for severely ill patients. Because oral vancomycin is poorly absorbed, high stool concentration can be achieved without systemic side effects. The usual dose is 125 mg every 6 hours for 7 to 14 days. A higher dose, 250 to 500 mg four times daily, can be given to severely ill patients.

Parenteral therapy is less effective than oral therapy, but when necessary (e.g., paralytic ileus), intravenous metronidazole, 500 to 750 mg three or four times daily, is recommended, perhaps supplemented by vancomycin, 500 mg four times daily, through a nasogastric tube or by enema.

Anion exchange resins work by binding toxin. Cholestyramine, 4 g four times daily, can help decrease symptoms in mild disease, but when it has been given alone, results have been disappointing, with variable but generally low cure rates. Obstipation is the most common side effect. Because cholestyramine binds vancomycin, they should not be given simultaneously.

Treatment of Recurrent Infection

Recurrent disease usually responds well to re-treatment with metronidazole or vancomycin at standard doses. For multiple or refractory recurrences, several therapeutic options are available. One is a prolonged course of vancomycin therapy, followed by gradual tapering, for example, 125 mg four times daily for 4 to 6 weeks, 125 mg twice daily for 1 week, 125 mg daily for 1 week, and 125 mg every other day for 1 week, followed by 125 mg every 72 hours for 2 weeks. A similar prolonged, tapering course of metronidazole can be considered, although side effects may increase with longer treatment.

Another option is to give antibiotic and anion exchange resin for 5- to 7-day periods, alternating with periods when antibiotic treatment is withheld. Treatment with a combination of vancomycin and rifampin has also been successful. Other regimens aim to suppress *C. difficile* with the use of oral *Lactobacillus* GG or nonpathogenic yeast (*Saccharomyces boulardii*) or with enemas containing feces from healthy subjects. However, none of these agents have been proved superior.

Surgical Treatment

Surgical treatment usually is not necessary for *C. difficile*-associated disease. Diverting ileostomy or colectomy is performed for severe refractory disease or for complications such as perforation or megacolon. Because the risk of complications increases markedly after several days of ineffective therapy, some advocate surgery for severe disease that does not respond after 2 to 7 days of treatment.

Prevention

C. difficile spores can survive for up to 5 months in the environment, and a primary mode of infection is the hands of hospital personnel or contaminated objects. Therefore, prevention has a crucial role in disease management and can be facilitated by the prudent use of antibiotics, routine hand-washing, disinfection of potentially contaminated objects, and isolation of infected patients, including the use of gloves for patient contact.

Treatment of asymptomatic carriers is not recommended because it may prolong the carrier state, which usually resolves spontaneously. Restricting the use of broad-spectrum antibiotics has decreased the rate of *C. difficile*-associated disease at some institutions.

- Metronidazole and vancomycin are equally effective, particularly for mild-to-moderate disease.
- If oral therapy is not possible, intravenous metronidazole may be useful. Intravenous vancomycin is not useful.
- Cholestyramine works by binding toxins, but it can bind vancomycin.
- Multiple recurrences of disease may require prolonged tapering or pulses of antibiotics, with or without additional therapy.

Summary

C. difficile is a spore-forming toxigenic bacterium that causes diarrhea and colitis, typically after the use of antibiotics. The clinical presentation ranges from self-limited diarrhea to fulminant colitis and toxic megacolon. Although in most cases the disease is mild and responds quickly to treatment, *C. difficile* colitis may be severe, especially if diagnosis and treatment are delayed. Recurrence can be a serious problem. Prevention is best accomplished by limiting the use of broad-spectrum antibiotics and by following good hygienic techniques and universal precautions to limit the transmission of the bacteria. A high index of suspicion results in early diagnosis and treatment and potentially decreases the incidence of complications.

RECOMMENDED READING

Microscopic Colitis

Bohr J, Tysk C, Eriksson S, Abrahamsson H, Jarnerot G. Collagenous colitis: a retrospective study of clinical presentation and treatment in 163 patients. Gut. 1996;39:846-51.

Pardi DS, Ramnath VR, Loftus EV Jr, Tremaine WJ, Sandborn WJ. Lymphocytic colitis: clinical features, treatment, and outcomes. Am J Gastroenterol. 2002;97:2829-33.

Pardi DS, Smyrk TC, Tremaine WJ, Sandborn WJ. Microscopic colitis: a review. Am J Gastroenterol. 2002;97:794-802.

Clostridium difficile-Associated Disease

McFarland LV. Epidemiology, risk factors and treatments for antibiotic-associated diarrhea. Dig Dis. 1998;16:292-307.

Pothoulakis C. Pathogenesis of *Clostridium difficile*-associated diarrhoea. Eur J Gastroenterol Hepatol. 1996;8:1041-7.

Yassin SF, Young-Fadok TM, Zein NN, Pardi DS. *Clostridium difficile*-associated diarrhea and colitis. Mayo Clin Proc. 2001;76:725-30.

CHAPTER 24

Colorectal Neoplasms

Lisa A. Boardman, M.D.
Paul J. Limburg, M.D.

Colorectal cancer (CRC) is primarily a disease of urban, industrialized societies. In the United States, the lifetime risk for development of CRC is approximately 6%. Recent data have suggested that the incidence rates for CRC may be gradually decreasing in some subgroups of the population. However, the mechanisms underlying these favorable trends are poorly understood. Several national organizations have adopted CRC screening and surveillance guidelines. Through widespread application of and appropriate compliance with these recommendations, CRC prevention may become increasingly achievable.

CLINICAL FEATURES

Definition
Most cases (98%) of CRC are adenocarcinomas. Less common cancer subtypes include lymphoma, carcinoid, and leiomyosarcoma. Metastatic lesions to the colorectum include lymphoma, leiomyosarcoma, malignant melanoma, and adenocarcinomas of the breast, ovary, prostate, lung, and stomach. Because of the relative rarity of these other malignancies, "CRC" is used throughout the rest of this chapter to refer to primary adenocarcinoma.

Presentation
Clinical manifestations of CRC often are related to tumor size and location. Common signs and symptoms of proximal neoplasms (cecum to splenic flexure) include ill-defined abdominal pain, weight loss, and occult bleeding. Distal neoplasms (descending colon to rectum) may present with altered bowel habits, decreased stool caliber, or hematochezia

(or a combination of these). Colonoscopy is the test of choice for diagnosis because tissue specimens can be obtained at the time of the examination. Surgical intervention, either for cure or palliation, is the standard initial therapeutic approach in the absence of prohibitive coexisting conditions. Regional lymph node metastases are detected in 40% to 70% of patients at the time of surgical resection. Distant metastases are found in 25% to 30% of patients and typically occur in the liver, peritoneal cavity, and lung. Less common sites of CRC metastases are the adrenal glands, ovaries, and bone. Central nervous system metastases are rare. Rectal cancers have higher local recurrence rates and may recur first in the lungs, whereas colon cancers tend to recur in the liver.

Adenoma-Carcinoma Sequence
Most CRCs are thought to develop through an ordered series of events: normal colonic mucosa→mucosa at risk→adenoma→ adenocarcinoma. Indirect evidence to support this adenoma-carcinoma sequence includes the following: 1) prevalence rates cosegregate within populations, 2) distribution patterns within the colorectum are similar, 3) benign adenomatous tissue is often juxtaposed with invasive cancer in early-stage malignancies, and 4) CRC incidence rates are reduced by endoscopic polypectomy. An increasing number of genetic events have been correlated with different phases of colorectal carcinogenesis (Fig. 1). The *APC* gene is considered the "gatekeeper" and is mutated in approximately 85% of CRCs. DNA mismatch repair genes, including *hMSH2*, *hMLH1*, *hPMS1*, *hPMS2*, and *hMSH6*, maintain nucleic acid sequence integrity during replication and have been termed "caretaker" genes. Mutations in these genes are found in 10% to 15% of sporadic CRCs and are

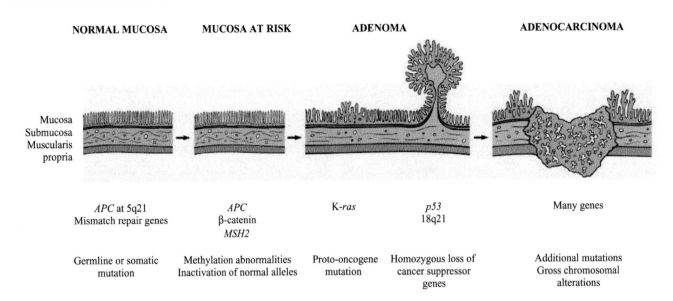

NORMAL MUCOSA   MUCOSA AT RISK   ADENOMA   ADENOCARCINOMA

Mucosa
Submucosa
Muscularis
propria

APC at 5q21 Mismatch repair genes	APC β-catenin MSH2	K-ras	p53 18q21	Many genes
Germline or somatic mutation	Methylation abnormalities Inactivation of normal alleles	Proto-oncogene mutation	Homozygous loss of cancer suppressor genes	Additional mutations Gross chromosomal alterations

Fig. 1. Adenoma-carcinoma sequence. (Modified from Crawford JM. The gastrointestinal tract. In: Cotran RS, Kumar V, Collins T, editors. Robbins pathologic basis of disease. 6th ed. Philadelphia: WB Saunders; 1999. p. 775-843. Used with permission.)

associated with microsatellite instability. K-*ras* is the most frequently activated oncogene in colorectal neoplasms and is mutated in approximately 50% of large (≥1 cm) adenomas and adenocarcinomas. The *p53* gene appears to be mutated later in carcinogenesis because chromosomal loss is relatively more common in malignant (70%-80%) than benign neoplasms.

Polyp Subtypes

As described above, adenomatous polyps are considered to have malignant potential, whereas hyperplastic, inflammatory, and hamartomatous (juvenile) polyps generally are not. Adenomas can be further classified as tubular (70%-85%), villous (<5%), or tubulovillous (10%-25%) on the basis of their glandular histologic features and classified as low-grade or high-grade on the basis of their degree of dysplasia. Features associated with an increased risk of CRC are categorized as "advanced" adenomas and include 1) size (≥1 cm), 2) villous histologic features, and 3) high-grade dysplasia. Multiple (three or more) synchronous adenomas are also associated with an increased risk of CRC.

Staging and Prognosis

The TNM classification is the basis of the preferred CRC staging system (Table 1). The extent of disease is determined primarily with computed tomography and surgical exploration. For rectal cancer, endoscopic ultrasonography also can be used preoperatively to assess the depth of tumor invasion and regional lymph node status. Stage is the most important predictor of survival. Within-stage comparisons show a lower 5-year

survival for patients with rectal cancer than for those with colon cancer. Regardless of stage, histologically well-differentiated CRCs (grades 1 and 2) may portend a better prognosis than poorly differentiated ones (grades 3 and 4).

EPIDEMIOLOGY

General Distribution

CRC ranks fourth worldwide in cancer incidence (excluding nonmelanoma skin cancer) and cancer mortality. Peak incidence rates are reported in the Czech Republic, Australia, and New Zealand. Incidence rates are exceptionally low in central African countries. In the United States, CRC ranks fourth in cancer incidence and second in mortality. Age-adjusted incidence and mortality rates for women are 36.8/100,000 and 14.3/100,000, respectively, and for men, the rates are higher at 51.8/100,000 and 20.9/100,000. From 1992 to 1998, the incidence rates decreased by an estimated 0.6% per year, and annual mortality rates decreased by 1.8%.

Race and Ethnicity

Of the five racial-ethnic population subgroups recognized by the Surveillance Epidemiology and End Results (SEER) program, African Americans have the highest incidence and mortality rates for CRC, and the 5-year survival rate is less than that of whites. Although this is explained partly by differences in stage of disease at the time CRC is diagnosed, the survival gap persists when within-stage comparisons are made.

Table 1. Colorectal Cancer Staging

Stage	TNM classification*	5-year survival, %
0	Tis N0 M0	100
I	T1 N0 M0	95
	T2 N0 M0	90
II	T3 N0 M0	80
	T4 N0 M0	75
III	Any T N1 M0	72
	Any T N2 M0	60
	Any T N3 M0	40
IV	Any T Any N M1	5

*Tis, carcinoma in situ, intraepithelial or invasion of the lamina propria; T1, invasion of submucosa; T2, invasion of muscularis propria; T3, invasion through muscularis propria into subserosa or nonperitonealized pericolic/perirectal tissue; T4, perforation of visceral peritoneum or direct invasion into adjacent organs or tissue.

N0, no regional lymph node metastases; N1, metastases in 1-3 pericolic/perirectal lymph nodes; N2, metastases in ≥4 lymph nodes; N3, metastases in lymph nodes along a named vascular trunk or tumor invasion of adjacent organs.

M0, distant metastases absent; M1, distant metastases present.

Modified from Goldberg RM. Gastrointestinal tract cancers. In: Casciato DA, Lowitz BB, editors. Manual of clinical oncology. 4th ed. Philadelphia: Lippincott Williams & Wilkins; 2000. p. 172-217. Used with permission.

Anatomical Subsite

Anatomical subsites of the colorectum differ in their embryologic origin, physiologic function, and vascular supply. Differences in the morphology, histology, and genetics of CRC have been observed across regions within the large bowel. Subsite-specific incidence rates also differ, and the proportion of cases of CRC located in the proximal colon appears to be increasing relative to that in the distal colon and rectum.

HOST AND ENVIRONMENTAL FACTORS

Age

As with most malignancies, the incidence rates of CRC increase with advancing age. Fewer than 5% of cases occur among persons younger than 45 years. SEER data suggest that age-specific CRC incidence rates begin to increase more rapidly during the fifth decade. The prevalence of adenomatous polyps also increases with age, with estimates of 30% at 50 years, 40% to 50% at 60 years, and 50% to 65% at 70 years. Also, several important clinical features of adenomas may be age-related. In the National Polyp Study, the risk of having a polyp with high-grade dysplasia was 80% higher among subjects 60 years or older than among younger subjects.

Personal History of Colorectal Neoplasia

Individuals with a personal history of colorectal adenomas or adenocarcinomas are at increased risk (threefold to sixfold) for metachronous neoplasms. Adenoma characteristics associated with future tumor development include large size (> 1 cm), villous histology, and increased multiplicity. Neither hyperplastic polyps nor small, solitary tubular adenomas are strong risk factors for metachronous neoplasms. Patients who have had surgical resection for CRC are prone to the development of recurrent primary cancers, second primary cancers, and adenomatous polyps. The median time to detection of metachronous adenomas ranges from 19 to 32 months after surgical resection in this group, whereas most (85%) recurrent adenocarcinomas are diagnosed within 3 years.

Family History of Colorectal Neoplasia

Familial clustering is observed in approximately 15% of all cases of CRC, including patients with heritable cancer syndromes (see below). Large epidemiologic investigations have reported remarkably consistent risk estimates of a 1.5- to 2-fold increase in the risk of CRC among persons with a family history of colorectal neoplasia. Although less thoroughly investigated, colorectal cancer in a second- or third-degree relative also appears to be associated with a modestly increased risk.

Inflammatory Bowel Disease

Chronic ulcerative colitis is associated with a substantially increased risk of CRC over time. Cumulative incidence rates range from 1.8% after 20 years to 43% after 35 years of disease. Pancolitis appears to confer a greater risk than proctitis or distal colitis; however, disease activity does not appear to be a major risk factor. Primary sclerosing cholangitis in conjunction with chronic ulcerative colitis may confer additional risk, but this association is controversial. Fewer data exist about the association between Crohn's disease and CRC, but the risk appears to be comparable to that of chronic ulcerative colitis among patients with inflammatory bowel disease of similar duration. Current data do not support an increased risk for CRC among patients with lymphocytic or collagenous colitis. Recent studies suggest that inflammatory bowel disease-related tumors may develop through a different molecular pathway than sporadic neoplasia, with aneuploidy occurring early in the carcinogenic process.

Dietary Components

Dietary fats induce the excretion of primary bile acids, which may be converted to secondary bile acids by colonic bacteria. Select subtypes of dietary fat also may affect epithelial mitogenesis, serum concentrations of insulin, prostaglandin E_2 levels, and host immunocompetence—all of which may promote CRC. However, the available data about an association with CRC risk are inconclusive.

Red meat, particularly when consumed with a heavily browned surface, may be an independent risk factor for both benign and malignant colorectal neoplasia.

Vegetables and fruits contain a wide array of potentially anticarcinogenic substances that may function through one or several independent or codependent mechanisms. Generally, vegetable consumption has been one of the most consistent predictors of reduced CRC risk, but fruit consumption appears to be less strongly associated with reductions in large-bowel tumorigenesis.

Fiber enhances stool bulk, decreases the concentration of procarcinogenic secondary bile acids, and increases the concentration of anticarcinogenic short-chain fatty acids. Although multiple case-control studies initially suggested a protective effect by increased dietary fiber, subsequent intervention trials have not observed appreciable reductions in CRC risk.

Calcium binds to intraluminal toxins and also influences mucosal proliferation within the colorectum. In a recent large clinical trial, calcium supplementation was associated with a statistically significant 19% decrease in adenoma recurrence among postpolypectomy patients after 4 years.

Antioxidants (including retinoids, carotenoids, ascorbic acid, α-tocopherol, and selenium) have been hypothesized to prevent carcinogen formation by neutralizing free radical compounds. So far, observational and experimental data have been unimpressive, with the exception that selenium decreased CRC risk by 58% when measured as a secondary end point in a skin cancer prevention study.

Folate and methionine supply methyl groups necessary for critical cellular functions such as nucleotide synthesis and gene regulation. Particularly in the context of excess alcohol consumption, dietary deficiencies of these compounds may be a risk factor for CRC.

Lifestyle

Alcohol induces cellular proliferation, blocks methyl group donation, and inhibits DNA repair. Many observational studies have suggested a twofold to threefold increase in CRC risk with excess alcohol consumption, although a meta-analysis of 27 case-control and cohort studies found only a 10% increase in risk among daily alcohol users.

Tobacco smoke contains several putative carcinogens, including polycyclic aromatic hydrocarbons, nitrosamines, and aromatic amines. On the basis of data from three large cohort studies, smoking appears to be a CRC risk factor after a prolonged latency of 20 or more years.

Physical activity has been consistently associated with a 40% to 50% decrease in CRC risk, particularly in the distal colon, through the stimulation of intestinal transit, decreased prostaglandin E_2 levels, or other as yet undefined mechanisms.

Other

Type 2 diabetes mellitus has been associated with CRC in some, but not all, epidemiologic investigations. In the largest study to date, a statistically significant 30% increase in CRC risk among 7,229 male patients with diabetes and a smaller, non-statistically significant 16% increase among 8,258 female patients with diabetes was observed.

Persons with acromegaly may be predisposed metabolically or anatomically to higher risks of CRC. Because of the relative rarity of this condition, most observational studies have lacked adequate statistical power, but the preponderance of evidence supports a positive risk association.

Cholecystectomy results in an altered fecal bile acid composition. Two meta-analyses have reported moderately increased risks of 11% to 34% for CRC (mainly in the proximal colon) after gallbladder surgery.

HERITABLE SYNDROMES

Cases of hereditary colorectal cancer account for approximately 15% of all large-bowel malignancies. Several well-defined syndromes have been recognized, as discussed below. It is important to remember that patients with germline abnormalities are also at increased risk for target organ cancers outside the colorectum. Guidelines for genetic testing in the context of possible hereditary CRC were approved by the Clinical Practice and Practice Management and Economics committees of the American Gastroenterological Association in 2001.

Familial Adenomatous Polyposis

Germline mutations in the *APC* gene form the basic molecular foundation for familial adenomatous polyposis (FAP) (autosomal dominant). As many as one in five cases may represent new-onset spontaneous mutations. The estimated prevalence is 1/5,000 to 7,500 persons. Additional genetic and environmental factors, as yet unidentified, seem likely to influence the clinical manifestations of FAP because phenotypic features vary widely despite similar inherited *APC* mutations. The hallmark lesion of FAP is diffuse colorectal polyposis, with typically hundreds to thousands of adenomas developing sometime during adolescence. Other findings include duodenal adenomas, gastric (fundic) gland hyperplasia, mandibular osteomas, and supernumerary teeth. In the absence of prophylactic colectomy, CRC is inevitably diagnosed in FAP patients at a mean age approximating 40 years. Even after colectomy, increased cancer risks remain, particularly in the periampullary region of the duodenum and in the retained rectal remnant (if partial colectomy was performed).

Gardner's syndrome is a variant of FAP in which individuals with *APC* mutations have the same phenotypic features as classic FAP, but in addition osteomas of the skull and long bones, congenital hypertrophy of the retinal pigmented epithelium, desmoid tumors, epidermoid cysts, fibromas, and lipomas can develop.

Familial Adenomatous Polyposis Variants

Attenuated FAP is associated with relatively fewer adenomas (< 100 adenomas) and later onset of CRC (approximate age, 55 years) than in classic FAP. Roughly 40% of these cases can be found to be associated with germline *APC* mutations. Because both the adenomas and the cancers appear to arise in the proximal colon, at-risk family members should have screening with a full colonoscopy, rather than flexible sigmoidoscopy as recommended for screening in classic FAP kindreds.

Turcot's syndrome refers to a familial predisposition for both colonic polyposis and central nervous system tumors and likely represents a constellation of molecular features that can be variants of either FAP or hereditary nonpolyposis colorectal cancer (HNPCC). Individuals with early-onset colonic polyposis associated with *APC* mutations tend to have medulloblastomas (FAP variant), whereas those with DNA mismatch repair gene mutations are prone to development of glioblastoma multiforme (HNPCC variant). Interestingly, glioblastoma multiforme arising in the setting of Turcot's syndrome tends to occur at an earlier age and has a better prognosis than the sporadic form of this tumor.

Hereditary Nonpolyposis Colorectal Cancer

HNPCC (autosomal dominant) is characterized by early-onset CRC (usually located in the proximal colon) and increased risks for extracolonic (uterus, ovaries, stomach, urinary tract, small bowel, and bile duct) malignancies. Although HNPCC is traditionally recognized with the use of clinical criteria (Table 2), it has been associated recently with mutations in at least five DNA mismatch repair genes. Presumably because the

mechanistic abnormality relates more to processes underlying tumor progression rather than to initiation, patients with HNPCC do not manifest the large number of colorectal adenomas typical of FAP. Nonetheless, adenomas are believed to precede carcinomas in most instances, and colorectal cancer develops in 75% to 80% of persons with HNPCC at a median age of 46 years. Jarvinen et al. reported that regularly performed colonoscopy with polypectomy can decrease the risk of large-bowel adenocarcinoma in HNPCC by approximately 60%. Other experts have argued that prophylactic colectomy may be the preferred preventive approach, but this strategy is controversial.

Hereditary Nonpolyposis Colorectal Cancer Variants

Patients with Muir-Torre syndrome have sebaceous neoplasms, urogenital malignancies, and gastrointestinal tract adenocarcinomas in association with defective DNA mismatch repair. The ratio of affected men to women is 2:1.

Hamartomatous Polyposis Syndromes

Peutz-Jeghers syndrome is an autosomal dominant condition characterized by multiple hamartomatous polyps scattered throughout the gastrointestinal tract. Up to 60% of cases of the syndrome are related to germline mutations in the *LKB1* (*STK11*) gene. Melanin deposits usually can be seen around the lips, buccal mucosa, face, genitalia, hands, and feet, although occasionally the skin and intestinal lesions are inherited separately. Foci of adenomatous epithelium can develop within Peutz-Jeghers polyps and may be directly associated with increased CRC risk. Extracolonic malignancies include other gastrointestinal cancers (duodenum, jejunum, ileum, pancreas, biliary tree, gallbladder), ovarian sex cord tumors, Sertoli cell testicular tumors, and breast cancer.

Tuberous sclerosis (autosomal dominant) is associated with hamartomas, mental retardation, epilepsy, and adenoma sebaceum. Adenomatous polyps may occur, particularly in the distal colon.

Juvenile polyposis syndrome is an autosomal dominant condition in which juvenile mucous retention polyps (misnamed hamartomata) can arise in the colon, stomach, or elsewhere in the gastrointestinal tract. Both *PTEN* and *SMAD4* mutations have been implicated as genetic causes for the syndrome. Symptoms of bleeding or obstruction may arise during childhood and may warrant surgery of affected intestinal segments for treatment of anemia or obstruction or for cancer prevention. The risk for CRC is increased when synchronous adenomas or mixed juvenile-adenomatous polyps are present. If prophylactic or therapeutic colonic resection is performed, ileorectostomy or total proctocolectomy should be considered because of an increased risk for recurrent juvenile polyps within the retained

Table 2. Clinical Criteria for Diagnosing Hereditary Nonpolyposis Colorectal Cancer (HNPCC)

Amsterdam criteria I	Amsterdam criteria II
≥3 relatives with colorectal cancer	≥3 relatives with HNPCC-related cancers*
≥1 case is a first-degree relative of 2 other cases	≥1 case is a first-degree relative of 2 other cases
≥2 successive generations affected	≥2 successive generations affected
≥1 case diagnosed before age 50 years	≥1 case diagnosed before age 50 years

Including cancer of the colorectum, endometrium, small bowel, ureter, or renal pelvis.

colorectal segment. Of note, fewer than five juvenile polyps (including solitary polyps) in an individual with no family history of juvenile polyposis syndrome does not indicate a heritable syndrome and, on the basis of current knowledge, does not warrant further diagnostic testing or aggressive cancer surveillance.

Cowden disease is an autosomal dominant condition in which persons with *PTEN* mutations may have trichilemmomas, other skin lesions, and alimentary tract polyps that are histologically similar to the polyps of juvenile polyposis syndrome. Patients with Cowden disease are at increased risk for breast cancer (often bilateral) and papillary thyroid cancer. CRC risk is not well-defined in this syndrome, but colonoscopy should be included in the original diagnostic evaluation.

Cronkhite-Canada syndrome refers to a noninherited condition manifested by signs and symptoms of malnutrition or malabsorption. Gastrointestinal hamartomas may be present and can exhibit foci of adenomatous epithelium. Characteristic clinical features include alopecia and hyperkeratosis of the fingernails and toenails. In the United States and Europe, Cronkhite-Canada syndrome typically develops in men, whereas in Asian countries, women appear to be affected more often.

PREVENTION

Screening

Established screening tools include the fecal occult blood test, flexible sigmoidoscopy, barium enema, and colonoscopy. Computed tomography colonography and DNA-based stool testing are novel early detection methods with considerable promise. The algorithm for CRC screening endorsed by most national gastrointestinal and oncology organizations is provided in Figure 2. As noted, screening should begin at age 50 years for asymptomatic adults with no CRC risk factors. For high-risk patients, the following recommendations have been adopted:

- FAP—flexible sigmoidoscopy annually at the onset of puberty for gene carriers and indeterminate cases
- HNPCC—colonoscopy biennially at age 20 years and annually after age 40 years
- Peutz-Jeghers syndrome—colonoscopy beginning in the second decade of life, with surveillance intervals determined by examination findings
- Family history of colorectal neoplasia (excluding FAP, HNPCC, or other identifiable syndromes)—colonoscopy or alternate testing at age 40 years (or 5 years before the youngest case diagnosis, whichever is earlier)
- Inflammatory bowel disease—annual colonoscopy with surveillance biopsies, beginning 8 years after the onset of pancolitis or 15 years after the onset of distal colitis

Surveillance

After a complete clearing colonoscopy has been performed, repeat examinations can be delayed for 5 years for low-risk persons (those with one or two tubular adenomas < 1 cm at baseline and no family history of CRC). Surveillance colonoscopy is indicated at 3 years for patients with advanced or multiple adenomas at baseline or a family history of CRC. After a negative surveillance examination has been documented, subsequent surveillance colonoscopies may be deferred for 5 years.

Patients with previously resected large (> 2 cm), sessile adenomas should have endoscopy again in 3 to 6 months. Residual adenomatous tissue after 2 or 3 therapeutic colonoscopies should prompt a surgical consultation. Malignant polyps, defined as neoplasms with dysplastic cells invading through the muscularis mucosa, can be treated endoscopically if 1) the lesion has been excised completely and fully examined by a pathologist, 2) the depth of invasion, grade of differentiation, and completeness of excision can be determined accurately, 3) poor differentiation, vascular invasion, and lymphatic involvement are not present, and 4) the margin of excision is free of cancer cells. Follow-up colonoscopy should be performed at 3 months for sessile malignant polyps with favorable prognostic criteria.

Among patients with a history of curatively resected CRC, clearing colonoscopy should be performed within 1 year of the initial operation. The first surveillance colonoscopy is then recommended at 3 years; if negative, surveillance colonoscopy should be repeated in 5 years.

Chemoprevention

"Chemoprevention" is the use of chemical compounds to prevent, inhibit, or reverse carcinogenesis before the invasion of dysplastic epithelial cells across the basement membrane. In its broadest sense, chemoprevention includes both nutritional and pharmaceutical interventions. Several promising nutritional interventions are discussed above. With regard to pharmaceutical agents, nonsteroidal anti-inflammatory drugs are structurally diverse, yet appear to share abilities to decrease proliferation, slow cell cycle progression, and stimulate apoptosis. Extensive epidemiologic data uphold a negative risk (40%-60%) association between regular use of nonsteroidal anti-inflammatory drugs and colorectal tumors. The chemopreventive effects of these drugs are thought to be derived through cyclooxygenase-2 inhibition, and agents that selectively block this enzyme isoform (celecoxib, rofecoxib) are being investigated as CRC prevention agents. Of note, cardiovascular toxicities associated with these agents may limit their chemopreventive applications outside of high-risk clinical settings (such as FAP).

Estrogen compounds cause a decrease in bile acid synthesis, leading to lower concentrations of secondary (potentially toxic)

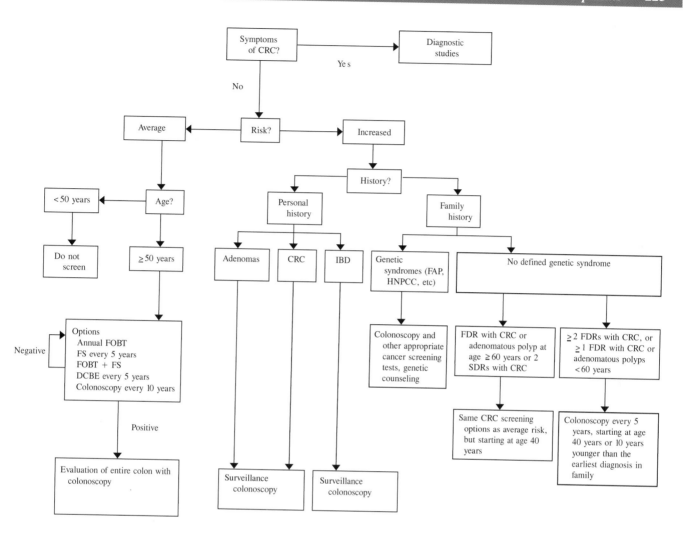

Fig. 2. Screening and surveillance guidelines for colorectal cancer (CRC). DCBE, double-contrast barium enema; FAP, familial adenomatous polyposis; FDR, first-degree relative; FOBT, fecal occult blood test; FS, flexible sigmoidoscopy; HNPCC, hereditary nonpolyposis colorectal cancer; IBD, inflammatory bowel disease; SDR, second-degree relative. (Modified from Winawer SJ, Fletcher RH, Miller L, Godlee F, Stolar MH, Mulrow CD, et al. Colorectal cancer screening: clinical guidelines and rationale. Gastroenterology. 1997;112:594-642. Used with permission.)

bile acids within the colorectal lumen. The estrogen receptor may also be involved in the regulation of growth of large-bowel mucosa. At least 28 observational studies have examined the relationship between hormone replacement therapy and the risk of colorectal neoplasia. In most, a negative risk association was reported when "ever-users" were compared with "never-users." According to a recent meta-analysis of these studies, estrogen compounds appear to be associated with approximately a 20% decrease in CRC risk.

Ursodeoxycholic acid, a hydrophilic epimer of cheno-deoxycholate, is noncytotoxic, stimulates expression of major histocompatibility complex antigens on premalignant tissues, and may beneficially modulate epithelial cell growth and differentiation through a protein kinase C-mediated pathway. When used to treat liver disease, it is extremely well tolerated and appears to be virtually free of serious side effects. Ursodeoxycholic acid has shown strong chemopreventive potential in animal models, and clinical trial data are pending.

TREATMENT

Surgery

Currently, surgical excision is the only potentially curative treatment of CRC. Surgical resection can be performed with an open incision or laparoscopically if technically feasible. For cancers above the rectum, at least a 5-cm margin of grossly uninvolved tissue should be obtained and regional lymph nodes should be sampled aggressively. Most colonic lesions can be resected with a primary anastomosis. Adenocarcinomas in the middle and upper rectum are usually removed by anterior resection. Cancers in the lower rectum (0-5 cm above the anal verge) may require preoperative chemoradiation therapy or abdominoperineal resection with a permanent colostomy (or both). The need for preoperative chemoradiation therapy is determined by computed tomography or endoscopic ultrasound staging to assess the depth of tumor invasion and presence or absence of involved lymph nodes. For tumors that are staged as $\geq$T3 or $\geq$N1, preoperative chemoradiation is generally recommended to minimize potential complications associated with irradiating the surgical anastomosis. Radiation treatment has not been proved to be useful for locally recurrent colon cancer, but it does have potential application for locally recurrent (i.e., within the pelvis) rectal cancer. In cases of isolated or few hepatic or lung metastases, surgical resection of distant disease can be considered with curative intent. Other treatment options include chemoembolization, radiofrequency ablation, or multi-agent chemotherapy, although these interventions should be considered palliative rather than curative.

Adjuvant Therapy

Although dosages differ slightly from center to center, adjuvant chemotherapy for stage III colon cancer typically includes 5-fluorouracil (5-FU) and leucovorin. Additional drugs, such as oxaliplatin, may provide further benefit. Some patients with stage II colon cancer have a prognosis similar to that of patients with stage III colon cancer. Research studies are ongoing to identify which subset of patients with stage II might benefit from adjuvant chemotherapy. When indicated, adjuvant chemotherapy is usually initiated 3 to 5 weeks postoperatively and administered over a total of 6 months. Stomatitis, diarrhea, and neutropenia are common adverse effects. Dermatologic complications (hand-foot syndrome) can occur with continuous intravenous infusion of 5-FU. Also, patients with dihydropyrimidine dehydrogenase (the rate-limiting enzyme in 5-FU metabolism) deficiency can experience severe or even fatal adverse effects at standard chemotherapy doses. At most U.S. institutions, adjuvant therapy for stage II and stage III rectal cancer includes a combination of 5-FU and radiotherapy. Newer biological therapies, such as bevacizumab and cetuximab, are typically reserved for patients with stage IV CRC or recurrent disease.

RECOMMENDED READING

Bond JH, Practice Parameters Committee of the American College of Gastroenterology. Polyp guideline: diagnosis, treatment, and surveillance for patients with colorectal polyps. Am J Gastroenterol. 2000;95:3053-63.

Compton C, Fenoglio-Preiser CM, Pettigrew N, Fielding LP. American Joint Committee on Cancer Prognostic Factors Consensus Conference: Colorectal Working Group. Cancer. 2000;88:1739-57.

Crawford JM. The gastrointestinal tract. In: Cotran RS, Kumar V, Collins T, editors. Robbins pathologic basis of disease. 6th ed. Philadelphia: WB Saunders Company; 1999. p. 775-843.

Giardiello FM, Brensinger JD, Petersen GM. AGA technical review on hereditary colorectal cancer and genetic testing. Gastroenterology. 2001;121:198-213.

Goldberg RM. Gastrointestinal tract cancers. In: Casciato DA, Lowitz BB, editors. Manual of clinical oncology. 4th ed. Philadelphia: Lippincott Williams & Wilkins; 2000. p. 172-217.

Greenlee RT, Hill-Harmon MB, Murray T, Thun M. Cancer statistics, 2001. CA Cancer J Clin. 2001;51:15-36.

Janne PA, Mayer RJ. Chemoprevention of colorectal cancer. N Engl J Med. 2000;342:1960-8.

Jarvinen HJ, Aarnio M, Mustonen H, Aktan-Collan K, Aaltonen LA, Peltomaki P, et al. Controlled 15-year trial on screening for colorectal cancer in families with hereditary nonpolyposis colorectal cancer. Gastroenterology. 2000;118:829-34.

Macdonald JS, Astrow AB. Adjuvant therapy of colon cancer. Semin Oncol. 2001;28:30-40.

Parkin DM, Pisani P, Ferlay J. Global cancer statistics. CA Cancer J Clin. 1999;49:33-64.

Potter JD. Colorectal cancer: molecules and populations. J Natl Cancer Inst. 1999;91:916-32.

Vasen HF, Watson P, Mecklin JP, Lynch HT. New clinical criteria for hereditary nonpolyposis colorectal cancer (HNPCC, Lynch syndrome) proposed by the International Collaborative Group on HNPCC. Gastroenterology. 1999;116:1453-6.

Winawer SJ, Fletcher RH, Miller L, Godlee F, Stolar MH, Mulrow CD, et al. Colorectal cancer screening: clinical guidelines and rationale. Gastroenterology. 1997;112:594-642.

Winawer SJ, Zauber AG, Gerdes H, O'Brien MJ, Gottlieb LS, Sternberg SS, National Polyp Study Workgroup. Risk of colorectal cancer in the families of patients with adenomatous polyps. N Engl J Med. 1996;334:82-7.

CHAPTER 25

Irritable Bowel Syndrome

G. Richard Locke III, M.D.

Irritable bowel syndrome (IBS) is a common condition that contributes substantially to health care costs. Because the cause of IBS is not known and no curative therapy is available, IBS historically has been managed symptomatically. Recent discoveries in the physiology of the enteric nervous system have led to the development of new agents that are targeted at potential pathophysiologic mechanisms of IBS. In addition, the role of psychologic issues has been well recognized, and therapy directed at behavioral intervention has been used more extensively than in the past. The overall goal is to improve the patient's symptoms and overall quality of life and, ideally, to prevent the suffering that patients experience.

DEFINITION

The symptom criteria for IBS are provided in Table 1. The Rome criteria were developed in conjunction with the World Congress of Gastroenterology held in Rome, Italy, in 1988 and were revised (Rome II) in 1999, and further revision (Rome III) is in progress. The Rome II criteria are similar to the criteria established by Manning et al. in 1978. However, a goal of the Rome criteria was to incorporate constipation-type symptoms into the IBS definition.

As with any set of criteria, there is a trade-off between sensitivity and specificity depending on the threshold used. In clinical practice, this can be helpful. The more criteria a specific patient meets, the more likely the patient is to have IBS. Nonetheless, the diagnosis of IBS can be made only if there are not any structural or metabolic abnormalities that explain the symptoms.

Table 1. Symptom Criteria for Irritable Bowel Syndrome

Rome II criteria	Manning criteria
In the past 12 months, at least 12 weeks of abdominal pain or discomfort that has 2 of the following 3 features: Relieved with defecation Associated with a change in frequency of stool Associated with a change in form (appearance) of stool	Pain eased after bowel movement Looser stools at onset of pain More frequent bowel movements at onset of pain Abdominal distention Mucus per rectum Feeling of incomplete emptying

EPIDEMIOLOGY

IBS is thought to be a common condition. Many population-based surveys have assessed the individual symptoms of IBS. The prevalence rates for symptom reporting have varied between 8 and 22 per 100 adults. It is simplest to think of the prevalence of IBS as 10% (1 in 10).

Although many studies have assessed the prevalence of IBS, data on incidence are more difficult to obtain. Because not everyone with IBS seeks medical care, data on incidence need to come from a population-based study. The exact numbers have varied among surveys, but about 10% of the general population report the onset of IBS symptoms over a 1-year period. However, it is not known whether these people had IBS in the past. Thus, this is an onset rate rather than a true incidence rate. Approximately a third of persons with IBS report that symptoms resolve over time. A recent estimate of the incidence of clinically diagnosed IBS is 196 per 100,000 person-years. This clinical incidence figure is lower than the 10% onset figure, which likely reflects both the fluctuating pattern of symptoms and the limited seeking of health care by persons with IBS. Still, this is much higher than the incidence of colon cancer (50 per 100,000 person-years) and inflammatory bowel disease (10 per 100,000 person-years).

RISK FACTORS

Multiple risk factors have been proposed for IBS. In clinic-based studies, there is a strong association with sex. However, the female-to-male ratio in the community is approximately 2:1. Thus, sex may have a role not only in the onset of IBS but also in health care-seeking behavior. The prevalence of IBS decreases slightly with age. However, the new onset of symptoms may occur in the elderly. Prevalence estimates now are available from around the world. No consistent racial or ethnic differences have been identified.

Multiple studies have assessed the role of personality characteristics, psychiatric illness, and physical and sexual abuse in the development of IBS. These problems are common in patients with IBS evaluated in academic centers. However, persons in the community who have IBS are much less distressed.

Many patients with IBS report that a family member also has the condition. Familial aggregation of IBS exists, and twin studies have suggested a genetic component. However, other studies have shown that seeking health care for gastrointestinal problems is increased among children of parents with gastrointestinal symptoms. Additional study is needed to separate nature from nurture in the development of IBS.

IBS symptoms can occur after acute inflammatory conditions such as *Salmonella* infection. The propensity for development of postinfectious IBS is associated with sex, duration of illness, and the psychologic state of the person at the time of infection. Inflammatory markers have been identified in the colons of people with postinfectious IBS. This concept of postinfectious IBS is being actively investigated.

Food allergies or sensitivities also may play a role in the development of IBS. Patients with IBS symptoms report more sensitivity to food than people without symptoms. However, the data on exclusion diets have not convincingly shown food to be a cause of the symptoms. Most recently, a trial of dietary modification based on immunoglobulin G antibodies to food antigens did show an effect.

PATHOGENESIS

The etiology of IBS is not completely understood. However, IBS has been associated consistently with visceral hypersensitivity. Balloon distention studies have shown that patients with IBS feel discomfort at a lower volume than do subjects without IBS. Patients with IBS and subjects without IBS do equally well on tests of somatic pain such as cold water immersion, a suggestion that IBS is a disorder specific to the gut. Balloon distention studies also have suggested that patients with IBS have hypersensitivity throughout the gastrointestinal tract. The frequent overlap between IBS and fibromyalgia and urinary symptoms suggests that the problem may be an even more diffuse visceral hypersensitivity.

More recently, imaging studies of the central nervous system during balloon distention have shown that a different part of the brain is activated during balloon distention in patients with IBS than in healthy controls. Considerable advances have been made in understanding this brain-gut axis. The concept of a "big brain" in the cranial vault and a "little brain" in the abdomen has gained widespread acceptance. With this understanding, research has been undertaken to evaluate compounds that have central nervous system activity to determine whether they have a role in the management of IBS. Currently, serotonin is being investigated most intensively. The pathophysiologic state of carcinoid diarrhea shows that serotonin has a role in gastrointestinal physiology. Other studies have shown that serotonin has a role in visceral hypersensitivity, which increasingly is viewed as the primary pathophysiologic mechanism of IBS. Several serotonin receptor agonists and antagonists have been identified, although the number of receptor subtypes identified changes rapidly. Most investigations have focused on type 1, type 3, and type 4 serotonin receptors. The roles of opioid receptors, cholecystokinin receptors, dopamine receptors, cannabinoid receptors, and α-adrenergic agonists are being actively investigated.

DIAGNOSIS

A diagnosis of IBS is made on the basis of symptom criteria (Table 1) in the absence of structural or metabolic abnormalities that can explain the symptoms. Many disorders can cause abdominal pain. However, the combination of abdominal pain and abnormal defecation has a more limited differential diagnosis. Colon cancer, inflammatory bowel disease, thyroid disorders, celiac disease, and giardiasis are all relatively common conditions that can have similar symptoms. Carcinoid syndrome, microscopic colitis, bacterial overgrowth, and eosinophilic gastroenteritis also can have similar symptoms, but they are less common. The problem is that IBS is so common that it is difficult to justify performing extensive diagnostic tests on a large proportion of the population. All tests will have a very low yield.

Young patients with classic IBS symptoms do not necessarily need any tests when they present to their primary care provider. The American Gastroenterological Association recommends simple blood tests, stool tests for ova and parasites, and an anatomical evaluation of the colon. Flexible sigmoidoscopy is sufficient for patients younger than 50 years, but those older than 50 need a full colonic evaluation to exclude colorectal cancer.

Recent studies have heightened the awareness about celiac sprue. Although much needs to be learned about how common the diagnosis of sprue is among patients presenting with IBS symptoms, clinicians should consider some form of testing for sprue in these patients.

Another area of discussion is related to bacterial overgrowth. In one center, this was found in a high proportion of patients with IBS. It remains to be seen whether this finding is replicated elsewhere.

PROGNOSIS

The natural history of IBS is becoming better understood. In approximately 30% of patients, IBS symptoms resolve over the course of a year. This contributes to the placebo response rate, which has made evaluation of investigative agents difficult. Although IBS symptoms may resolve, symptoms of another functional gastrointestinal disorder develop in some patients. Thus, the degree to which the gastrointestinal symptoms resolve completely is not clear.

MANAGEMENT

Although IBS often is managed with a high-fiber diet and antispasmodic agents, an approach that considers the patient's predominant symptom is recommended (Fig. 1). Does the patient complain primarily of constipation, diarrhea, or abdominal pain? Constipation can be treated with laxatives and a high-fiber diet, and diarrhea may be treated with loperamide, especially when taken before meals. A high-fiber diet may be helpful for patients who alternate between constipation and diarrhea, but the role of a high-fiber diet in diarrhea-predominant IBS is uncertain. Antispasmodic agents are appropriate for patients who have primarily abdominal pain. These agents have been prescribed because of the belief that the pathophysiologic mechanism of IBS is spasms and irregular contractility. The

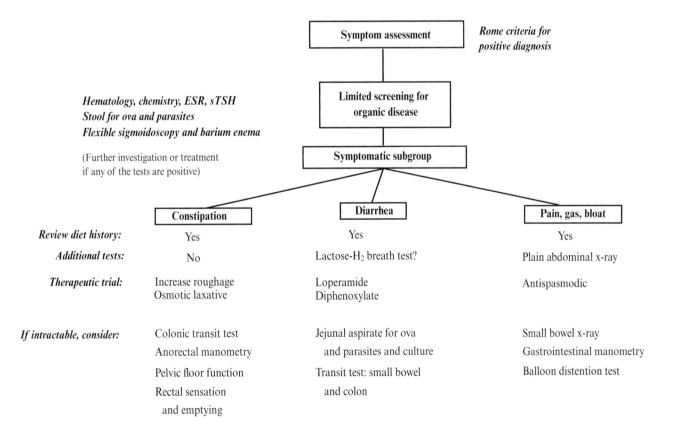

Fig. 1. Management of irritable bowel syndrome. ESR, erythrocyte sedimentation rate; sTSH, sensitive thyroid-stimulating hormone. (Modified from Drossman DA, Whitehead WE, Camilleri M. Irritable bowel syndrome: a technical review for practice guideline development. Gastroenterology. 1997;112:2120-37. Used with permission.)

clinical trial data on the effectiveness of antispasmodic agents are mixed. However, with the absence of alternative medications, antispasmodic agents have been used widely. In each case, a dietary history is important to ensure that the patient is not consuming products that may inadvertently cause diarrhea, constipation, or abdominal gas. Further evaluation should be withheld until the initial treatment program is undertaken (3-6 weeks).

The hope is that the patient will be reassured about the diagnosis and will have a response to the initial therapy. However, some patients continue to have pronounced symptoms and seek care. What are the options for these patients? Tegaserod, a type 4 serotonin receptor agonist, is available for IBS with constipation. Tegaserod accelerates colonic transit. A modest benefit over placebo was shown in clinical trials. Otherwise, further testing and treatment are based on the predominant symptom. Patients with refractory constipation need to be evaluated for problems of colonic transit and pelvic floor dysfunction (see Chapter 26, Constipation and Disorders of Pelvic Floor Function). Patients with pelvic floor dysfunction may benefit from biofeedback. Those with colonic transit disorders require escalating doses of laxatives.

Patients with documented delay in colonic transit may be considered for colonic resection. However, if the patient has symptoms of IBS, surgery for colonic inertia needs to be considered most carefully because the abdominal pain may persist postoperatively.

For patients with diarrhea, stool chemistry tests for surreptitious laxative abuse, duodenal aspirate for bacterial overgrowth, colonic biopsies for microscopic colitis, determination of urinary 5-hydroxyindoleacetic acid for carcinoid syndrome, and a small-bowel colonic transit study may all be considered. The yield of these tests is low, but they are useful for evaluating patients who have chronic diarrhea. High-dose loperamide (up to 16 mg daily), cholestyramine, clonidine, verapamil, or even octreotide may be considered. Alosetron, a type 3 serotonin receptor antagonist, was shown to help nonconstipated women who had IBS. The main side effect was constipation. Because of reports of ischemic colitis and severe constipation requiring surgery among patients with IBS taking alosetron, the agent was temporarily withdrawn from the market. Alosetron is available but requires special prescribing. Other type 3 receptor antagonists may be available in the near future.

Many physicians consider pain-predominant IBS the most challenging to manage. A plain radiograph of the abdomen obtained during a time of severe pain may help to exclude obstruction. In academic centers, pseudo-obstruction or other motility disorders may be evaluated, but pain is not common in these conditions. Often, the next step is a course of treatment with a low dose of a tricyclic antidepressant. The goal is not to alleviate depression but rather to reduce visceral sensation.

The association between psychologic distress and IBS is well established. When formal psychiatric disorders are present, appropriate therapy directed toward treating the underlying disorder is mandatory. Even when there is no diagnosis of a psychiatric disorder, the approach of using psychologic intervention is helpful in the management of IBS. When traditional symptomatic measures have not been adequate, treatment with low doses of tricyclic antidepressants or selective serotonin reuptake inhibitors has provided improvement for many patients. The pathophysiologic mechanism of tricyclic antidepressants is not clear. The dosages used are much less than those used to treat depression. In a recent randomized clinical trial, tricyclic antidepressants were helpful in people who did not experience side effects (per protocol analysis). In the intention-to-treat analysis, cognitive behavioral therapy was shown to be effective. Patients with IBS refractory to other treatment may benefit from formal pain management approaches.

HEALTH CARE UTILIZATION

Annually, IBS accounts for 3.5 million physician visits, 2.2 million prescriptions, and 35,000 hospitalizations. Primary care physicians provide most care for patients with IBS, although a survey of gastroenterologists indicated that 28% of their patient population had IBS. The exact expenditures accountable to IBS are difficult to determine. In one study, subjects with IBS in the community were found to incur an extra $300 annually in health care expenditures. Extrapolated to the U.S. population, this is equal to $8 billion. IBS also is associated with absenteeism. This and other indirect costs to patients and their families make the total cost of IBS considerable.

SUMMARY

During the past few years, important changes have occurred in the management of IBS. The traditional approach of reassurance and a high-fiber diet is no longer adequate for everyone. Symptomatic care likely will remain the appropriate treatment for patients with mild symptoms. However, for patients with pronounced gastrointestinal symptoms, more aggressive approaches will be necessary. In time, the role of newer medications will be established. Similarly, the adjunctive use of behavioral intervention will gain wider use.

RECOMMENDED READING

Brandt LJ, Bjorkman D, Fennerty MB, Locke GR, Olden K, Peterson W, et al. Systematic review on the management of irritable bowel syndrome in North America. Am J Gastroenterol. 2002;97 Suppl 11:S7-26.

Camilleri M, Thompson WG, Fleshman JW, Pemberton JH. Clinical management of intractable constipation. Ann Intern Med. 1994;121:520-8.

Cash BD, Chey WD. Irritable bowel syndrome: an evidence-based approach to diagnosis. Aliment Pharmacol Ther. 2004;19:1235-45.

Clouse RE. Antidepressants for functional gastrointestinal syndromes. Dig Dis Sci. 1994;39:2352-63.

Cremonini F, Delgado-Aros S, Camilleri M. Efficacy of alosetron in irritable bowel syndrome: a meta-analysis of randomized controlled trials. Neurogastroenterol Motil. 2003;15:79-86.

Drossman DA, Camilleri M, Mayer EA, Whitehead WE. AGA technical review on irritable bowel syndrome. Gastroenterol. 2002;123:2108-31.

Drossman DA, Corazziari E, Talley NJ, Thompson WG, Whitehead W, editors. Rome II: the functional gastrointestinal disorders: diagnosis, pathophysiology, and treatment; a multinational consensus. 2nd ed. McLean (VA): Degnon and Associates; 2000.

Drossman DA, Toner BB, Whitehead WE, Diamant NE, Dalton CB, Duncan S, et al. Cognitive-behavioral therapy versus education and desipramine versus placebo for moderate to severe functional bowel disorders. Gastroenterology. 2003;125:19-31.

Evans BW, Clark WK, Moore DJ, Whorwell PJ. Tegaserod for the treatment of irritable bowel syndrome. Cochrane Database Syst Rev. 2004;CD003960.

Inadomi JM, Fennerty MB, Bjorkman D. Systematic review: the economic impact of irritable bowel syndrome. Aliment Pharmacol Ther. 2003;18:671-82.

Kim DY, Camilleri M. Serotonin: a mediator of the brain-gut connection. Am J Gastroenterol. 2000;95:2698-709.

Locke GR III. The epidemiology of functional gastrointestinal disorders in North America. Gastroenterol Clin North Am. 1996;25:1-19.

Manning AP, Thompson WG, Heaton KW, Morris AF. Towards positive diagnosis of the irritable bowel. Br Med J. 1978;2:653-4.

Whitehead WE. Behavioral medicine approaches to gastrointestinal disorders. J Consult Clin Psychol. 1992;60:605-12.

CHAPTER 26

Constipation and Disorders of Pelvic Floor Function

Adil E. Bharucha, M.D.

CONSTIPATION

Colonic Motor Physiology and Pathophysiology: Salient Aspects

Function

Colonic functions include water and electrolyte absorption, storage of intraluminal contents until elimination is socially convenient, and nutrient salvage from bacterial metabolism of carbohydrates that are not absorbed in the small intestine. The colon absorbs all but 100 mL of fluid and 1 mEq of sodium and chloride from approximately 1,500 mL of chyme received over 24 hours. Absorptive capacity can increase to 5 to 6 L and 800 to 1,000 mEq of sodium and chloride daily. In healthy subjects, the average mouth-to-cecum transit time is approximately 6 hours, and the average regional transit time through the right, left, and sigmoid colon is about 12 hours each, yielding an average total colonic transit time of 36 hours. (The physiology of defecation is discussed in the section on "Disorders of Pelvic Floor Function.")

Regional Differences in Colonic Motor Function

The right colon is a reservoir that mixes and stores contents and absorbs fluid and electrolytes. The left colon is primarily a conduit, whereas the rectum and anal canal are responsible for continence and defecation. The ileocolic sphincter regulates the intermittent transfer of ileal contents into the colon, a process that normalizes in response to augmented storage capacity in the residual transverse and descending colon within 6 months after right hemicolectomy.

Motor Patterns

Colonic motor activity is extremely irregular, ranging from quiescence (particularly at night) to isolated contractions, bursts of contractions, or propagated contractions. In contrast to the small intestine, rhythmic migrating motor complexes do not occur. Contractions are tonic or sustained, lasting several minutes to hours, and shorter or phasic. Propagated phasic contractions propel colonic contents over longer distances than nonpropagated phasic contractions. High-amplitude propagated contractions are greater than 75 mm Hg in amplitude, occur about 6 times daily (frequently after awakening and after meals), are responsible for mass movement of colonic contents, and frequently precede defecation. Stimulant laxatives such as bisacodyl (Dulcolax) and glycerol induce high-amplitude propagated contractions.

Colonic Contractile Response to a Meal

Neurohormonal mechanisms are responsible for increased colonic motor activity beginning within a few minutes after ingestion of a meal of 500 kcal or more. The term "gastrocolic reflex" is a misnomer because this response, induced by gastric distention and chemical stimulation by nutrients, is observed even after gastrectomy. This response may explain postprandial urgency and abdominal discomfort in patients with irritable bowel syndrome.

Colonic Relaxation

Colonic relaxation resulting from sympathetic stimulation or opiates may cause acute colonic pseudo-obstruction, or Ogilvie's syndrome. Stimulation of α_2-adrenergic receptors decreases the release of acetylcholine from excitatory cholinergic terminals in the myenteric plexus, thereby inhibiting gastrointestinal motility. Conversely, reduced tonic sympathetic inhibition impairs the net absorption of water and electrolytes and accelerates transit in patients who have diabetic neuropathy with diarrhea. Clonidine restores the sympathetic brake, reducing diarrhea.

Colocolonic Inhibitory Reflexes

Peristalsis is a local reflex mediated by intrinsic nerve pathways and characterized by contraction proximal to and relaxation distal to the distended segment. In addition, rectal or colonic distention can inhibit motor activity in the stomach, small intestine, or colon. These inhibitory reflexes are mediated by extrinsic reflex pathways with synapses in the prevertebral ganglia, independent of the central nervous system. They may account for delayed left colonic or small intestinal (or both) transit in patients with obstructive defecation.

Serotonin and the Gut

About 95% of the body's serotonin (5-hydroxytryptamine [5-HT]), a monoamine neurotransmitter, is in the gut: 90% in enterochromaffin cells and 10% in enteric neurons. The effects of serotonin are mediated by receptors located on gut neurons, smooth muscle, and enterochromaffin cells. There are seven families of 5-HT receptors; 5-HT_3 and 5-HT_4 receptors and, to a lesser degree, 5-HT_{1p}, 5-HT_{1a}, and 5-HT_2 receptors are important targets of pharmacologic modulation in the gut. Serotoninergic 5-HT_4 receptor agonists include cisapride, prucalopride, and tegaserod (Zelnorm). Alosetron and cilansetron are more potent 5-HT_3 receptor antagonists than ondansetron.

The effects of 5-HT are as follows:

Motor—Stimulation of serotoninergic 5-HT_4 receptors may facilitate both components of the peristaltic reflex, that is, proximal excitation coordinated with distal inhibition. Thus, stimulation of 5-HT_4 receptors located on cholinergic enteric neurons induces acetylcholine release and enhances contractility, whereas 5-HT_4 receptor-mediated stimulation of inhibitory neurons releases inhibitory neurotransmitters, for example, nitric oxide or vasoactive intestinal polypeptide, which relax smooth muscle.

Sensory—5-HT_3 and 5-HT_4 receptors are also located on *intrinsic* primary afferent neurons, which initiate peristaltic and secretory reflexes. 5-HT_3 receptors also are located on *extrinsic* sensory afferents and vagal afferents, partly explaining why 5-HT_3 antagonists reduce nausea.

Other—Central 5-HT has a role in the regulation of appetite, sexual function, and mood.

Assessment of Colonic Transit

The radiopaque marker technique using commercially available markers (Sitz capsule) is simple and inexpensive, and the results correlate well with those of scintigraphic methods. There are several variations in the methodologic details; however, a practical approach is to administer a capsule containing 24 markers at the same time on 3 consecutive days. Plain abdominal radiographs are taken on the fourth and seventh days. The number of markers remaining in the abdomen at a preset date after ingestion reflects colonic transit. With this technique, the average normal colonic transit time is 36 hours and the maximum is 72 hours.

With scintigraphy, the isotope (generally ^{99m}Tc or ^{111}In) is delivered into the colon by orocecal intubation or within a delayed-release capsule. The delayed-release capsule contains radiolabeled activated charcoal covered with a pH-sensitive polymer (methacrylate) designed to dissolve in the alkaline pH of the distal ileum. This releases the radioisotope within the ascending colon. Gamma camera scans taken 4, 24, and, if necessary, 48 hours after ingestion of the isotope show the colonic distribution of isotope. Regions of interest are drawn around the ascending, transverse, descending, and sigmoid colon and the rectum; counts in these areas are weighted by factors 1-4, respectively, and stool counts are weighted by a factor of 5. Thus, colonic transit may be summarized as an overall geometric center (Fig. 1). The 4-hour scan identifies rapid colonic transit, and the 24-hour and 48-hour scans show slow colonic transit.

- Colonic transit assessments made with radiopaque markers correlate with those made with scintigraphy.
- Scintigraphy permits simultaneous assessment of gastric, small intestinal, and colonic transit.

Constipation

Definition

A committee of experts developed symptom-based criteria for diagnosing functional gastrointestinal disorders. These criteria are used infrequently in clinical practice, but they are essential for entering patients into research studies. "Chronic constipation" is defined by two or more of the following symptoms for at least 12 weeks, not necessarily consecutive, in the preceding 12 months: fewer than 3 defecations per week, straining with more than one-fourth of defecations, lumpy or hard stools with more than one-fourth of defecations, sensation of incomplete evacuations with more than one-fourth of defecations, sensation of anorectal obstruction or blockage with more than one-fourth of defecations, and manual maneuvers to facilitate more than one-fourth of defecations (e.g., digital evacuation, support of the pelvic floor). Constipation-predominant irritable bowel syndrome is defined by abdominal discomfort and at least two of the following three symptoms for at least 12 weeks, not necessarily consecutive, in the preceding 12 months: abdominal

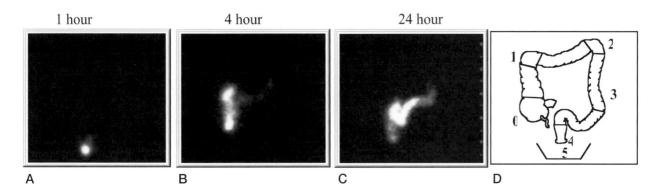

Fig. 1. Scintigraphic assessment of colonic transit. Note isotope progression through, *A*, cecum (1 hour), *B*, ascending colon (4 hours), and, *C*, transverse colon (24 hours). *D*, Numbers represent average isotope distribution corresponding to a geometric center of 1-5. In this patient, the geometric center at 24 hours was 1.7 (normal, 1.7-4.0). (From Bharucha AE, Klingele CJ. Autonomic and somatic systems to the anorectum and pelvic floor. In: Dyck PJ, Thomas PK, editors. Peripheral neuropathy. Vol 1. 4th ed. Philadelphia: Elsevier; 2005. p. 279-98. Used with permission.)

discomfort associated with change in stool form, abdominal discomfort associated with change in stool frequency, and abdominal discomfort relieved by defecation.

Clinical Assessment

Clinical assessment should focus on identifying secondary causes of 1) constipation (Tables 1 and 2), 2) inadequate dietary calorie and fiber intake, 3) a history of physical, emotional, or sexual abuse, and 4) obstructive defecation. Evaluating bowel habits from stool diaries should be considered; these are more accurate than self-reported bowel habits. Symptoms that suggest obstructive defecation include a history of prolonged straining, a tendency to facilitate defecation by assuming different positions, difficulty in evacuating soft stool, and induction of evacuation by rectal or vaginal pressure. The examination may demonstrate anismus, inadequate perineal descent, or, conversely, ballooning of the perineum with excessive descent.

Practical Classification of Constipation

The classification of functional constipation shown in Table 3 facilitates a rational algorithmic therapeutic approach to this symptom. Most patients with normal-transit constipation respond to dietary fiber supplementation. Therefore, assessment of colonic transit and pelvic floor function should be restricted to patients who do not have a response to dietary fiber supplementation. A subset of patients with normal-transit constipation have abdominal discomfort or bloating (or both) suggestive of irritable bowel syndrome.

Pelvic floor function should be assessed in refractory constipation because symptoms alone cannot distinguish among constipation resulting from pelvic floor dysfunction, normal transit, and slow transit. Most patients with obstructive defecation

also have delayed colonic transit. Consequently, delayed colonic transit does not imply slow-transit constipation.

"Colonic inertia" refers to severe colonic motor dysfunction that is identified by reduced colonic contractile responses to a meal and stimulants such as bisacodyl or neostigmine, as assessed by intraluminal measurements of pressure activity or tone.

Management of Constipation

Principles

Reassurance and education about normal bowel habits, the need for adequate caloric intake and dietary fiber supplementation, and the absence of a "serious disorder" are vital. Deficient caloric intake can cause or exacerbate constipation, whereas refeeding may restore colonic transit.

Medical Therapy

Dietary fiber supplementation either in foods or as a fiber supplement increases stool weight and accelerates colonic transit.

Table 1. Common Secondary Causes of Constipation

Structural—colonic or anorectal (e.g., colon cancer or stricture, large rectocele)
Endocrine—diabetes mellitus, hypothyroidism
Metabolic—hypokalemia, hypercalcemia, hypocalcemia, uremia
Infiltrative—scleroderma, amyloidosis
Neurologic—Parkinson's disease, spinal cord disease, autonomic neuropathy, multiple sclerosis
Psychological—anorexia nervosa

Table 2.   Common Medications That Cause Constipation

Analgesics—opiates, nonsteroidal anti-inflammatory drugs
Antihypertensives—calcium channel blockers, α_2-agonists, diuretics ($\downarrow$ potassium)
Antacids containing aluminum, calcium
Anticholinergics, antidepressants, antihistaminics, antiparkinsonian agents
Long-term laxative use
Others—iron, cholestyramine

Table 3.   Classification of Functional Constipation

Transit	Normal	Delayed	Normal/delayed
Pelvic floor function	Normal	Normal	Abnormal
Category	Normal-transit	Slow-transit	Obstructive defecation
Management	Fiber supplementation	Fiber supplementation Laxatives Surgery	Biofeedback therapy

Fiber intake should be increased gradually to 12 to 15 g daily: psyllium (Konsyl, Metamucil), daily with fluid, or methylcellulose (Citrucel), 1 tsp up to 3 times daily; Konsyl, 2 tsp twice daily; calcium polycarbophil (FiberCon), 2 to 4 tablets daily; bran, 1 cup daily. Fiber supplements should be part of any regimen, but they are more effective in normal-transit or "fiber-deficiency" constipation than in slow-transit constipation or pelvic floor dysfunction. Fiber supplementation should start at a small dose administered twice daily (AM and PM) with fluids or meals, increasing the dose gradually after 7 to 10 days. Patients should be reassured that although fiber supplements may increase gaseousness, this often subsides with time. A response to fiber supplements is evident over several weeks, not over days, as with a laxative. Bloating may be reduced by gradually titrating the dose of dietary fiber to the recommended dose or by switching to a synthetic fiber preparation such as methylcellulose. Bran impairs absorption of iron and calcium. Fiber supplements are contraindicated for patients with intestinal obstruction, fecal impaction, or severe vomiting.

• Dietary fiber content should be increased gradually to 12 to 15 g daily for constipated patients.
• In normal-transit constipation, ≥85% to 90% of patients have a symptomatic response to dietary fiber supplementation.

Hyperosmolar agents, sorbitol or lactulose, 15 to 30 mL once or twice daily, are nonabsorbable disaccharides metabolized by colonic bacteria into acetic and other short-chain fatty acids. Lactulose and sorbitol accelerate proximal colonic transit in healthy subjects. Lactulose and sorbitol may cause transient abdominal cramps and flatulence. They are equally effective for treating constipation in the elderly. However, lactulose ($1.20-$2.40 per dose) is extremely sweet and more expensive than sorbitol ($0.15-$0.30 per dose). Polyethylene glycol (Miralax), 17 g daily ($1.90), is a potent agent generally reserved for patients who do not respond to other agents.

Saline laxative, milk of magnesia (15-30 mL once or twice daily), draws fluid osmotically into the lumen, stimulates the release of cholecystokinin, and accelerates colonic transit. It may cause hypermagnesemia, particularly in patients with renal insufficiency.

• Patients with slow-transit constipation can take saline laxatives or hyperosmolar agents daily and stimulant laxatives on an as-needed basis.
• Sorbitol is as effective but less expensive and less sweet than lactulose.

Stimulant laxatives affect mucosal transport and motility and include surface-active agents (docusate sodium [Colace] 100 mg orally twice daily), diphenylmethane derivatives, ricinoleic acid, anthraquinones, glycerin (suppository), and bisacodyl (Dulcolax) (10-mg tablet or suppository). Stool softeners such as docusate sodium are of limited efficacy. Glycerin and bisacodyl, taken up to once every other day, work by inducing colonic high-amplitude propagated contractions. Bisacodyl tablets take effect in 6 to 8 hours, and suppositories should be administered 30 minutes after eating to maximize synergism with the gastrocolic reflex. Of the diphenylmethane derivatives, phenolphthalein was withdrawn from the U.S. market after animal studies suggested that it may be carcinogenic; there is no epidemiologic evidence to support this claim. The anthraquinone compounds may cause allergic reactions, electrolyte depletion, melanosis coli, and cathartic colon. "Melanosis coli" refers to brownish black colorectal pigmentation of unknown composition associated with apoptosis of colonic epithelial cells. "Cathartic colon" refers to altered colonic structure observed on barium enema studies and associated with long-term use of stimulant laxatives. The altered structure includes colonic dilatation, loss of haustral folds, strictures, colonic redundancy, and wide gaping of the ileocecal valve. Early reports implicating laxative-induced destruction of myenteric plexus neurons in cathartic colon have been disputed. Although anthraquinones may induce colorectal tumors in animal models, several cohorts and a recent case-control study failed to find an association between anthraquinones and colon cancer.

- Bisacodyl and glycerin facilitate defecation by inducing colonic high-amplitude propagated contractions.
- Melanosis coli indicates recent laxative use. The evidence linking anthraquinones to colon cancer and destruction of the myenteric plexus is inconclusive.

Tegaserod (Zelnorm) is a partial 5-HT$_4$ receptor agonist that accelerates small bowel transit and tends to accelerate colonic transit in patients with constipation-predominant irritable bowel syndrome. On the basis of four phase III trials, the U.S. Food and Drug Administration approved tegaserod for short-term therapy of constipation-predominant irritable bowel syndrome in women. In the trials, the response rates for tegaserod and placebo were approximately 46% and 34%, respectively; the response measure was a weekly self-administered questionnaire for overall symptoms of irritable bowel syndrome. Stool frequency increased within the first week with tegaserod treatment and then returned toward the pretrial range. More recently, the U.S. Food and Drug Administration approved tegaserod for treatment of chronic constipation for patients younger than 65 years. The primary end point was an increase in one complete (i.e., feeling of complete evacuation), spontaneous (i.e., not preceded by laxative use within 24 hours) bowel movement per week during the first 4 weeks compared with baseline. Taken together, the response rates at 4 and 12 weeks were 25% and 28% for placebo, 39% and 38% for tegaserod 2 mg twice daily, and 43% and 45% for tegaserod 6 mg twice daily. Differences between tegaserod 6 mg twice daily and placebo were significant at 4 and 12 weeks; for tegaserod 2 mg twice daily, differences were significant at 4 weeks only. Subgroup analyses did not show significant therapeutic benefit for patients older than 65 years. The main side effect is diarrhea (6.6% for tegaserod 6 mg twice daily compared with 3% for placebo). No causal relationship between tegaserod and major complications (e.g., abdominal surgery, ischemic colitis) has been established.

Enemas, including mineral oil retention enema (100–250 mL daily per rectum), phosphate enema (Fleet) (1 unit per rectum), tap water enema (500 mL per rectum), and soapsuds enema (1,500 mL per rectum), are especially useful in patients with fecal impaction in the rectosigmoid colon, as may occur in obstructive defecation. All the preparations are contraindicated for patients with rectal inflammation, and phosphate enemas are contraindicated for patients with hyperphosphatemia or hypernatremia. Mineral oil taken orally is associated with lipid pneumonia, malabsorption of fat-soluble vitamins, dehydration, and fecal incontinence.

- Enemas may be used judiciously on an as-needed basis for constipation.

Other pharmacologic approaches that have been used to manage constipation include colchicine and misoprostol (Cytotec). Colchicine (0.6 mg orally 3 times daily) and misoprostol (1,200 µg daily) cause diarrhea. Colchicine should be used cautiously, if at all, for treating constipation because long-term use may be associated with neuromyopathy. Other side effects include hypersensitivity reactions, bone marrow suppression, and renal damage. The use of misoprostol to treat constipation should be avoided because it is expensive, may cause miscarriage in pregnant women, and may exacerbate abdominal bloating. Moreover, its beneficial effects appear to decrease with time.

- Colchicine and misoprostol are unproven, potentially deleterious agents for treating slow-transit constipation.

Surgical Therapy
Subtotal colectomy with ileorectal anastomosis is effective and occasionally indicated for patients with medically refractory severe slow-transit constipation, provided that pelvic floor dysfunction has been excluded or treated. In patients with megarectum, the rectum is also resected. Postoperative ileus and delayed mechanical small-bowel obstruction each occur in approximately 10% of patients. Diarrhea is common shortly after the operation but tends to resolve with time. The importance of identifying and treating pelvic floor dysfunction with biofeedback therapy preoperatively in patients with slow-transit constipation cannot be overemphasized.

- Subtotal colectomy is necessary and beneficial for patients with slow-transit constipation who do not have a response to medical management.

Diverticular Disease
In Western society, acquired diverticulosis affects approximately 5% to 10% of the population older than 45 years and almost 80% of those older than 85. Because uninflamed diverticula are asymptomatic, symptoms such as abdominal discomfort and altered bowel habits in patients with diverticulosis should be ascribed to coincident irritable bowel syndrome rather than to "painful diverticulosis." Approximately 20% of patients with diverticula have an episode of symptomatic diverticulitis. After vascular lesions, diverticular hemorrhage is the second commonest cause of colonic bleeding.

- Colonic diverticula occur commonly but do not cause symptoms unless infected or bleeding.

Pathology

In the West, diverticulosis affects predominantly the sigmoid colon, but it may involve the entire colon. Diverticula are formed by the protrusion of mucosa through weak areas where the vasa recta penetrate the bowel wall. Consequently, diverticula are arranged in rows between the mesenteric and lateral taeniae coli. Light microscopy often shows the thickening of colonic smooth muscle in diverticulosis. If undigested food blocks the neck of a diverticulum, the diverticulum may distend and perforate. Generally, the perforation is walled off by the adjacent mesocolon or appendices epiploicae. Colovesical and, less frequently, colovaginal and colocutaneous fistulae may occur. In contrast to colitis, the colonic mucosa is grossly and microscopically normal in acute diverticulitis, despite considerable inflammation of the pericolonic tissue.

- Diverticula form predominantly in the sigmoid colon by the protrusion of mucosa through weak spots in the bowel wall.
- Diverticulitis is not accompanied by mucosal inflammation.

Pathophysiology

It is believed that high intraluminal pressures prompt mucosal protrusion through weak areas in the bowel wall to cause diverticula. There is an association between diverticulosis and a Western diet high in refined carbohydrates and low in dietary fiber. Whether this represents a cause and effect is unproven. The potentially deleterious effects of an inadequate content of dietary fiber, including delayed gastrointestinal transit and higher intraluminal colonic pressure, are reversible by dietary fiber supplementation.

Diverticulitis

Classification

Stage I diverticulitis is characterized by small confined pericolonic abscesses. Stage II disease includes larger confined pericolonic collections. Stage III is generalized suppurative peritonitis ("perforated diverticulitis"); however, because the diverticular neck usually is obstructed by a fecalith, peritoneal contamination by feces may not occur. In contrast, tearing of an uninflamed diverticulum causes fecal peritonitis, or stage IV disease.

- Virtually all patients with diverticulitis have a microperforation.
- Stage I, small confined abscess; stage II, large confined abscess; stage III, suppurative but not fecal peritonitis; stage IV, fecal peritonitis.

Clinical Features

Symptoms of diverticulitis include lower abdominal pain and altered bowel habits, typically diarrhea. Although the stool may contain trace blood, profuse lower gastrointestinal tract bleeding is uncommon in acute diverticulitis. Dysuria, urinary frequency, and urgency reflect bladder irritation, whereas pneumaturia, fecaluria, or recurrent urinary tract infection suggests a colovesical fistula. Physical findings include fever, left lower quadrant tenderness, or a lower abdominal or rectal mass (or a combination of these).

Complications

Rupture of a peridiverticular abscess or uninflamed diverticulum causes peritonitis. This occurs more commonly in elderly and immunosuppressed persons and carries a high mortality rate. Repeated episodes of acute diverticulitis may lead to colonic obstruction. Small-bowel obstruction occurs more frequently, especially in the presence of a large peridiverticular abscess. Jaundice or liver abscesses should raise concern about pylephlebitis. A massively dilated (> 10 cm) cecum, signs of cecal necrosis (air in the bowel wall) on abdominal radiography, or marked tenderness of the right lower quadrant associated with a moderately dilated cecum mandates immediate surgery.

- Elderly and immunosuppressed persons are at a higher risk for complications from diverticulitis. Also, their initial symptoms and signs may be less pronounced, and they are less likely to have a response to medical therapy. Furthermore, free perforation is more frequent, and postoperative morbidity and mortality are greater.

Diagnostic Studies

A contrast enema will show diverticula but not diverticular inflammation. Moreover, contrast studies may dislodge an obstructing fecalith and cause perforation. If the clinical features are highly suggestive of acute diverticulitis, imaging studies are unnecessary. If the diagnosis cannot be made on the basis of clinical features alone or if an intra-abdominal abscess is suspected, computed tomography (CT) is the imaging method preferred. Also, CT-guided percutaneous drainage of an abscess can control systemic sepsis, permitting a single-stage surgical procedure at a later stage, if necessary. CT results are false-negative in up to 20% of patients with acute diverticulitis. Although ultrasonography also may show diverticular inflammation, it is more operator-dependent than CT. Furthermore, abdominal tenderness may preclude application of sufficient external pressure to visualize the intra-abdominal contents. Flexible sigmoidoscopy is necessary only if carcinoma or colitis is a diagnostic possibility, but it is contraindicated during possible acute diverticulitis.

- Contrast radiographs demonstrate diverticula but not inflammation.
- Indications for CT: uncertain clinical diagnosis and diagnosis and drainage of a suspected intra-abdominal abscess.

- Flexible sigmoidoscopy is necessary only to exclude carcinoma or colitis, after acute diverticulitis has resolved.

Differential Diagnosis

The presence of a stricture or signs of extraluminal compression occasionally make it difficult to differentiate diverticulitis from carcinoma; however, the clinical distinction between diverticulitis and nonperforating carcinoma is not usually subtle. Right-sided diverticulitis, which occurs rarely in the West, may simulate acute appendicitis.

Treatment of Acute Diverticulitis

The therapeutic approach is influenced by the severity of the clinical features, the ability to tolerate oral hydration, and a previous history of complicated diverticulosis.

For a mild first attack in patients who tolerate oral hydration: outpatient therapy with a liquid diet and a 10-day course of oral broad-spectrum antimicrobial therapy, including coverage against anaerobic microorganisms (ciprofloxacin and metronidazole). After the acute attack has resolved, a high dietary fiber content and colonoscopy are advisable to exclude a diagnosis of cancer. Approximately 5% of patients have a second attack within 2 years after medical treatment for the first attack; others have noted higher rates of recurrence.

For severe pain, inability to tolerate oral hydration, persistent symptoms despite adequate outpatient therapy: hospitalization, nothing by mouth, and broad-spectrum intravenous antibiotics. Preferred antibiotics include ampicillin, gentamicin, and metronidazole or monotherapy with newer broad-spectrum antibiotics (piperacillin or tazobactam). For pain relief, meperidine is preferred to morphine sulfate, which causes colonic spasm. Imaging studies should be considered if there is no improvement after 2 or 3 days of antibiotic therapy.

Peridiverticular abscesses larger than 5 cm in diameter are managed with radiologically assisted percutaneous drainage.

For surgical intervention, *emergency surgery* is reserved for generalized peritonitis, uncontrolled sepsis, visceral perforation, and acute clinical deterioration. *Urgent surgery* is necessary for immunocompromised hosts or when the diagnosis of carcinoma cannot be excluded definitively. Indications for *elective surgery* include fistula formation or recurrent diverticulitis.

If surgical therapy can be deferred until the acute inflammation heals, then a single-stage primary resection and reanastomosis procedure, potentially with a laparoscopic approach, can be accomplished with minimal morbidity and less than 1% mortality. For emergency indications, the first stage of a two-stage procedure involves resection of the diseased segment and creation of an end colostomy with oversewing of the distal colonic or rectal stump (Hartmann procedure). Colonic continuity is reestablished in the second operation. Only 30% to 75% of patients who undergo the first-stage resection eventually have colostomy closure.

Diverticular Hemorrhage

Nearly 50% of patients who are hospitalized for acute lower gastrointestinal tract bleeding are bleeding from uninflamed colonic diverticula, generally in the right colon. Diverticular hemorrhage is usually of minor importance clinically, but massive bleeding may occur in 5% of patients with diverticulosis. Patients with severe lower gastrointestinal tract hemorrhage, especially those taking nonsteroidal anti-inflammatory drugs, should first have emergency upper endoscopy to exclude the possibility of a bleeding duodenal ulcer after fluid resuscitation. Urgent colonoscopy after thorough bowel lavage is indicated to identify stigmata of a recent hemorrhage, that is, active bleeding (e.g., arterial spurting), nonbleeding visible vessels appearing as discrete pigmented or nonpigmented protuberances, and focally adherent clots. These stigmata occur in up to 20% of patients who have acute diverticular hemorrhage and are associated with a higher risk of recurrent bleeding. In this group of patients, endoscopic therapy decreases the risk of recurrent bleeding during the same admission. The risk of recurrent hemorrhage is not known, but it is estimated to be 20% to 30% after one episode and to increase to more than 50% after a second diverticular hemorrhage. Emergency angiography and nuclear scanning techniques with ^{99m}Tc sulfur colloid and ^{99m}Tc-tagged blood cells are alternatives to colonoscopy in patients with brisk (0.5-1 mL blood/min) and low (0.1 mL/min) bleeding rates, respectively. Angiography also permits intra-arterial infusion of vasopressin or selective embolization. Urgent surgical treatment, generally subtotal colectomy, is indicated for patients with continued severe bleeding and negative findings on angiography. Elective colonic resection should be considered after two or more bleeding episodes that require transfusion if the source of bleeding has been identified clearly and the operative risk is acceptable.

- A majority of bleeding diverticula are located in the right colon and are not inflamed; diverticular bleeding is usually minor.
- In patients with rectal bleeding and hemodynamic instability, upper gastrointestinal endoscopy should be performed first.
- Colonoscopy should be performed after thorough colonic lavage with the intention of identifying and treating diverticula with stigmata of bleeding.
- The risk of recurrent bleeding is approximately 20% to 30% after the first and more than 50% after the second clinically important episode of bleeding. Colonic resection, generally subtotal colectomy, should be considered after two or more episodes of diverticular bleeding.

DISORDERS OF PELVIC FLOOR FUNCTION

Disorders of pelvic floor function include obstructive defecation and fecal incontinence. Fecal incontinence, or involuntary leakage of stool from the anus, is a common symptom, particularly in the elderly. In community-based surveys, the prevalence of fecal incontinence among women 50 years or older approaches 15%. The prevalence among nursing home residents is as high as 40%. The prevalence of obstructive defecation in the community is unknown. At Mayo Clinic, 50% of patients with chronic constipation had a component of pelvic floor dysfunction or obstructive defecation.

Physiology of Defecation

Rectal distention evokes the desire to defecate and induces relaxation of the internal anal sphincter by an involuntary reflex (Fig. 2). Defecation is completed by adoption of a suitable posture, contraction of the diaphragm and abdominal muscles to increase intra-abdominal pressure, and relaxation of the puborectalis and external anal sphincter, both striated muscles. Relaxation of the puborectalis muscle allows widening and lowering of the anorectal angle, with perineal descent (Fig. 3). The coordination between abdominal contraction and pelvic floor relaxation is crucial to the process. Although defecation may be preceded by colonic high-amplitude propagated contractions, the contribution of rectal contraction to defecation is unclear.

Obstructive Defecation

Patients with obstructive defecation strain excessively in futile attempts to overcome the functional obstruction resulting from inadequate relaxation of the external anal sphincter or puborectalis sling (or both). The distinction between these two components (puborectalis and external anal sphincter) is often blurred by the use of the term "anismus" to describe pelvic floor dyssynergia. Other, generally older patients with obstructive defecation cannot generate rectal forces adequate to expel stool. Symptoms considered suggestive of obstructive defecation include frequent straining, a sensation of incomplete evacuation, dyschezia, and digital evacuation of feces. These symptoms are not sufficiently specific for distinguishing among obstructive defecation, normal transit, and slow transit constipation.

Tests

Various tests are available to confirm the clinical suspicion of obstructive defecation.

High resting anal sphincter pressure: The 3- to 5-cm-long anal canal generates a resting pressure predominantly attributable to the internal anal sphincter. Normal values for anal sphincter pressures measured with manometric sensors are technique-dependent and influenced by age, sex, and perhaps parity.

Failure of anal sphincter relaxation during simulated defecation: Normal relaxation of the anal sphincter during defecation argues strongly against obstructive defecation (Fig. 4). However, the results of this test are false-positive in up to 20% of healthy controls, limiting its diagnostic usefulness in constipated patients.

Balloon expulsion test: This is a highly sensitive and specific functional assessment of pelvic expulsion. Patients with obstructive defecation require abnormal (excessive) traction to expel a rectal balloon (Fig. 5).

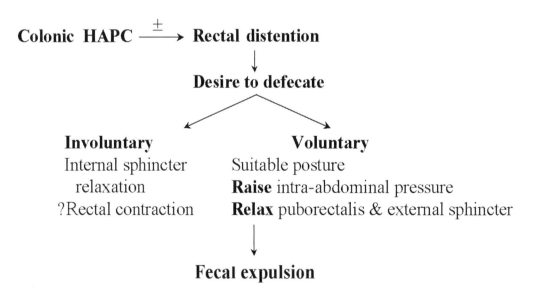

Fig. 2. Physiology of defecation. HAPC, high-amplitude propagated contraction. (From Bharucha AE, Camilleri M. Physiology of the colon. In: Zuidema GD, Yeo CJ, editors. Shackelford's surgery of the alimentary tract. Vol IV. 5th ed. Philadelphia: WB Saunders Company; 2002. p. 29-39. Used with permission.)

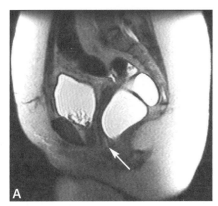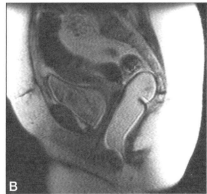

Fig. 3. Magnetic resonance fluoroscopic images of the pelvis at rest (*A*) and during simulated defecation (*B*). Defecation is accompanied by opening of the anorectal junction (*arrow*), pelvic descent, and widening of the anorectal angle from 101° at rest to 124° during defecation. The rectum was filled with ultrasound gel.

Defecography: This visualizes the anorectum at rest, during squeeze, and during simulated defecation. Abnormal findings in obstructive defecation include inadequate (< 1 cm) perineal descent, widening of the anorectal angle, opening of the anal canal, pelvic descent, and barium expulsion. Rectoceles are particularly common in multiparous subjects but obstruct defecation only in a small proportion. Clinically important rectoceles are generally large and fail to empty completely during defecation. Moreover, women with clinically important rectoceles often apply posterior vaginal pressure to facilitate defecation. Barium defecography involves exposure to radiation, and the pubis and sacrum—landmarks for measuring pelvic descent—often are not visible on radiographs. Moreover, the interobserver variability for anorectal angle measurements is poor, limiting the diagnostic usefulness of this test.

Colonic transit: Up to 70% of patients with pelvic floor dysfunction have delayed colonic transit. Thus, the finding of slow colonic transit does not exclude the diagnosis of obstructive defecation.

Treatment

Pelvic floor retraining using biofeedback therapy improves symptoms in 70% of patients with obstructive defecation. Symptomatic improvement may be associated with objective evidence of improved pelvic floor function, that is, external anal sphincter pressures, anorectal angle changes, and rectal evacuation during defecation. Pelvic floor retraining facilitates pelvic floor relaxation and improves the coordination between abdominal wall and diaphragmatic contraction and pelvic relaxation during defecation. The specific protocols for biofeedback training vary among centers.

Fecal Incontinence

Fecal continence is maintained by anatomical factors and complex sensory and motor interactions among the sphincters, the anorectum, central and peripheral awareness, mental awareness,

Fig. 4. Anal sphincter relaxation during bearing down. Bar at top denotes period (30 s) of bearing down.

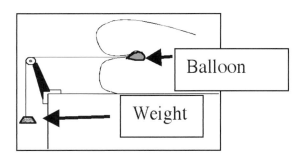

Fig. 5. Balloon expulsion test. (From Bharucha AE, Klingele CJ. Autonomic and somatic systems to the anorectum and pelvic floor. In: Dyck PJ, Thomas PK, editors. Peripheral neuropathy. Vol 1. 4th ed. Philadelphia: Elsevier; 2005. p. 279-98. Used with permission.)

and the physical ability to get to a toilet. Patients with chronic fecal incontinence lead a restricted lifestyle (constantly in fear of having an embarrassing episode) and often miss work. The symptom frequently coexists with urinary incontinence and contributes to institutionalization.

Etiology

Important factors that contribute to fecal incontinence include the following:

Sphincter damage: This includes obstetric and postsurgical (e.g., posthemorrhoidectomy) damage. Known obstetric risk factors for sphincter damage include forceps delivery, median episiotomy, and high birth weight.

Neurologic causes: These include multiple sclerosis, Parkinson's disease, Alzheimer's disease, stroke, diabetic neuropathy, and cauda equina or conus medullaris lesions. Cauda equina lesions that cause fecal incontinence usually are accompanied by other neurologic symptoms and signs.

Pudendal neuropathy: This may be attributable to obstetric trauma. Also, constipated patients may strain excessively during defecation and cause stretch injury to the pudendal nerve, soft tissue laxity, and excessive perineal descent. Ultimately, sphincter weakness develops, predisposing to fecal incontinence.

Other local causes: Examples are perianal sepsis, radiation proctitis, and systemic sclerosis. In radiation proctitis, the entry of stool into a noncompliant (stiff) rectum may overwhelm continence mechanisms and cause incontinence. Scleroderma is associated with fibrosis of the internal anal sphincter and weak resting pressures.

Assessment

Patients with diarrhea must be asked specifically about fecal incontinence because they may not volunteer the symptom. Physician interview assesses the severity, risk factors (obstetric history, perineal surgery), and circumstances of incontinence and the effect of incontinence on lifestyle. Patients with "urge incontinence" generally are incontinent only to liquid stools, have a brief warning time, and are unable to reach the toilet in time. In contrast, patients with "passive incontinence" are only aware of stool leakage after the episode. Patients with urge incontinence have decreased squeeze pressures or squeeze duration (or both), whereas those with passive incontinence have lower resting pressures of the anal sphincters. Nocturnal incontinence occurs in patients with diabetes mellitus or scleroderma and is suggestive of internal sphincter weakness.

A complete physical examination should include perianal assessment to identify common causes of perianal soiling, such as hemorrhoidal prolapse, perianal fistula, rectal mucosal prolapse, fecal impaction, anal stricture, and rectal mass. The perianal area must be inspected closely, both with the patient in the left lateral position and seated on the toilet. The digital examination should include assessment of the external anal sphincter response to voluntary squeezing and perineal descent when the patient tries to expel the examiner's finger. Flexible sigmoidoscopy, with or without anoscopy, is the final component in this phase of evaluation.

Tests

A combination of tests is necessary to evaluate the various components of anorectal anatomy and function. For each patient, the intensity of investigation depends on the patient's age, severity of incontinence, and clinical assessment of risk factors and anal sphincter pressures (Fig. 6).

Anorectal manometry: This test assesses the average and maximal anal canal pressures at rest and during squeeze. Maximal squeeze pressure had the greatest sensitivity and specificity in discriminating incontinent patients from controls and continent patients; a pressure less than 60 mm Hg had a sensitivity of 60% and a specificity of 78% in women. Thus, other factors such as disturbed rectal compliance or rectoanal sensation (or both) may further compromise and compound sphincter weakness in fecal incontinence.

Anal ultrasonography: This reliably identifies anatomical defects or thinning of the internal sphincter, which occur frequently in fecal incontinence. Reports have suggested that ultrasonography identifies external sphincter defects that are often clinically unrecognized or amenable to surgical repair (or both). However, the interpretation of external sphincter images is more subjective, operator-dependent, and confounded by normal anatomical variations of the external sphincter.

Evacuation proctography: This involves imaging the rectum with contrast material and observing the process, rate, and completeness of evacuation with fluoroscopy. The term "evacuation proctography" is preferred to "barium defecography" because the test simulates, but is not identical to, normal defecation. Evacuation proctography has been criticized on several grounds: 1) interobserver agreement for anorectal angle measurements during squeeze and defecation is poor, 2) some findings, especially rectocele, excessive pelvic floor descent, and internal intussusception, occur in asymptomatic persons, and 3) rectal evacuation often does not correlate with symptoms. Therefore, evacuation proctography is useful for corroborating the results of other anorectal diagnostic tests and for confirming the clinical diagnosis. It also is useful for showing rectoceles larger than 2 cm or those that empty incompletely.

Sphincter denervation measurements: The pudendal nerve may be injured (with or without damaging the sphincter) during vaginal delivery or by repetitive straining in patients with chronic constipation. Pudendal nerve terminal motor latency (PNTML) can be measured by placing the examining finger, covered by a glove containing stimulating and recording electrodes, as close

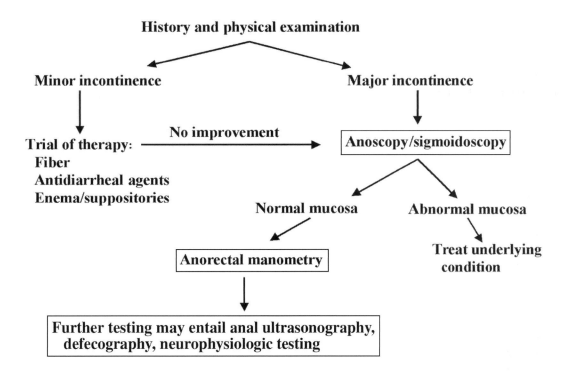

History and physical examination

Minor incontinence   **Major incontinence**

Trial of therapy: — **No improvement** → **Anoscopy/sigmoidoscopy**
Fiber
Antidiarrheal agents
Enema/suppositories

Normal mucosa   **Abnormal mucosa**

Treat underlying condition

Anorectal manometry

Further testing may entail anal ultrasonography, defecography, neurophysiologic testing

Fig. 6. Algorithmic approach to fecal incontinence.

as possible to the pudendal nerve as it courses around the pelvic brim. PNTML measures the function of the fastest conducting fibers. Initial studies showed prolonged PNTML in fecal incontinence. However, PNTML measurements are operator-dependent and lack adequate sensitivity and specificity for identifying pudendal nerve damage. Patients with prolonged PNTML may have normal anal canal squeeze pressures. In contrast to earlier studies, recent data have suggested that prolonged PNTML does not predict success after surgical repair of sphincter defects. Needle electromyographic examination of the external sphincter provides a sensitive measure of denervation and usually can identify myopathic, neurogenic, or mixed injury.

Rectal sensation: Sensation is assessed by asking subjects to rate the threshold or intensity of perception during rectal balloon distention. The three commonly assessed sensations are the first detectable sensation, the desire to defecate (or urgency), and maximal tolerable discomfort. The balloon can be distended physically with a handheld syringe or a barostat, a continuous-infusion pump. Normal values for these thresholds vary among laboratories, and they are influenced by balloon size, shape, and composition and by the type (phasic or continuous) and speed of inflation. This variability can be reduced by using a high-compliance balloon and the barostat. Pronounced loss of the ability to perceive rectal distention reduces the cue for contracting the external anal sphincter. Moreover, improved ability to detect rectal sensation may be the most important component of biofeedback training for fecal incontinence.

Pelvic magnetic resonance imaging: Magnetic resonance imaging is a relatively new method for imaging anal sphincter anatomy and pelvic floor motion during defecation and squeeze without radiation exposure. The anal sphincters also can be visualized, preferably with an endoanal magnetic resonance imaging coil. Magnetic resonance imaging is superior to ultrasonography for visualizing external sphincter morphologic features, particularly atrophy. In contrast to evacuation proctography, dynamic magnetic resonance imaging does not entail radiation exposure and it directly visualizes the pelvic floor, including the anterior (bladder) and middle (uterus) compartments.

Treatment

Medical treatment is directed at making stools more solid. This may be the most important approach for patients with functional diarrhea. Other potential approaches include the diagnosis and treatment of associated malabsorption, the correction of dietary indiscretions, and treatment of bacterial overgrowth in intestinal pseudo-obstruction. Antidiarrheal agents must be prescribed in adequate doses to solidify stools in functional diarrhea. Loperamide hydrochloride (4 mg), diphenoxylate hydrochloride with atropine sulfate (5 mg), or codeine sulfate (30-60 mg) may need to be taken regularly, preferably 30 minutes before meals, perhaps up to several times daily. For patients with fecal impaction and overflow incontinence, scheduled rectal emptying with suppositories or enemas is often useful.

Biofeedback therapy is effective for some patients with fecal incontinence, particularly those with partially preserved rectal sensation. In uncontrolled studies, success rates up to 70% have been reported. The technique can improve rectal sensation (thereby alerting patients to the need for evacuation and improving coordination between rectal sensation and external sphincter contraction) and can augment external anal sphincter contraction; success is more likely attributable to improvement in rectal sensation rather than augmented contraction. Poor prognostic factors include total absence of rectal sensation, dementia, sphincter denervation, and megarectum. Success is highly dependent on the motivation of the patient and the therapist. Although resting and squeeze pressures increased to a variable degree after biofeedback therapy, the magnitude of improvement was relatively small and not correlated with symptom improvement; perhaps these modest effects are attributable to inadequate biofeedback therapy, lack of reinforcement, and assessment of objective factors at an early stage after biofeedback therapy. In contrast, sensory assessments (i.e., preserved baseline sensation and improved sensory discrimination after biofeedback therapy) are more likely to be associated with improved continence after biofeedback therapy.

A recent study randomized 171 incontinent patients to four groups: standard medical and nursing care (i.e., advice only), advice and verbal instruction on sphincter exercises, hospital-based computer-assisted sphincter pressure biofeedback, or hospital biofeedback and use of a home electromyographic biofeedback device. Overall, 75% reported improved symptoms and 5% were cured, improvement was sustained at 1 year after therapy, and symptoms and resting and squeeze pressures improved to a similar degree in all four groups. These results underscore the importance that patients attach to understanding the condition, practical advice regarding coping strategies (e.g., diet and skin care), and nurse-patient interaction.

For surgical therapy, in contrast to encouraging early reports, long-term results after anterior overlapping repair of sphincter defects are disappointing. More complicated procedures, such as the anal neosphincter or dynamic graciloplasty, may be effective in selected patients but are complicated by considerable morbidity, particularly wound infections.

Colon

Questions and Answers

Multiple Choice (choose the one best answer)

1. A 26-year-old woman presents with a 4-month history of diarrhea that began 1 week after returning from a camping trip. She initially had crampy abdominal pain with bloating and six nonbloody bowel movements per day. After several weeks the stools became more bulky and malodorous and appeared somewhat greasy. Three weeks ago, her primary care physician performed a stool analysis for fecal leukocytes, bacterial culture, and ova and parasites. These tests were all negative. She has lost 5 lb and is without fever or nausea or vomiting. Which of the following is *least* appropriate in the management of this patient?
   a. Repeat stool analysis for ova and parasites
   b. Upper endoscopy with small-bowel biopsy and aspirate
   c. An empiric trial of metronidazole, 250 mg three times a day for 7 days
   d. Fecal analysis for *Giardia* antigen
   e. Loperamide, 2 mg after each bowel movement

2. A 1-year-old boy is brought to his pediatrician having had watery diarrhea for 10 days. He has no fever or evidence for blood in his stools. Which of the following viruses is most likely to explain his diarrhea?
   a. Rotavirus
   b. Enteric adenovirus
   c. Astrovirus
   d. Norwalk virus
   e. Hepatitis A virus

3. A 47-year-old man has had crampy lower abdominal pain, low-grade fever, and bloody stools that contain pus and mucus for 3 days. He has had no recent travel, antibiotics, or exposure to sick people or animals. He cannot recall any potential contaminated food exposures, although he did eat a hamburger at a fast-food restaurant last week. Which of following organisms is *least* likely to cause this presentation?
   a. *Shigella*
   b. *Escherichia coli* O157:H7
   c. *Salmonella*
   d. *Vibrio cholerae*
   e. *Campylobacter*

4. A 6-year-old girl is brought for evaluation of diarrhea. Her symptoms began 2 days after a family picnic. She initially had watery diarrhea with abdominal pain and nausea and vomiting. Three days later, the volume of diarrhea decreased and the stools became bloody with mucus. Besides *Escherichia coli* O157:H7, which other organism causes a typical progression from watery diarrhea to dysentery?
   a. *Salmonella*
   b. *Shigella*
   c. Enterotoxigenic *E. coli*
   d. *Vibrio cholerae*
   e. *Cryptosporidium*

5. Which of the following is true regarding extraintestinal manifestations of infectious diarrhea?

a. Hemolytic uremic syndrome, an uncommon complication of bacterial infections such as *Escherichia coli* O157:H7, primarily occurs in young adults

b. Postinfectious reactive arthritis primarily occurs in patients who are positive for HLA DQ2

c. Patients with liver cirrhosis are at increased risk for sepsis and death from *Vibrio vulnificus* infection and therefore should avoid eating raw seafood

d. Although typhoid fever is characterized by recurrent bacteremia, distant infection is uncommon

e. Pregnant women are at increased risk for disseminated *Bacillus cereus* infection with associated significant mortality

6. Fecal incontinence developed in a 45-year-old woman after she sustained a fourth-degree perineal tear during a vaginal delivery 20 years ago. Her symptoms improved after an external anal sphincter defect was surgically repaired 15 years ago, but they have since recurred and worsened during the past 3 years. Her undergarments are stained with a small amount of stool on several days every week. Her bowel movements are regular, but she occasionally has increased rectal urgency and her stools are often semiformed. Digital rectal examination disclosed reduced anal resting tone and no external sphincter contraction or puborectalis contraction to voluntary command. Endoanal ultrasonography showed an anterior tear involving 50% of the circumference of the internal and external anal sphincters. What is the most appropriate next step?

a. Taking of a careful dietary history for consumption of caffeinated products and sugars (e.g., fructose, sorbitol) and consider an empiric trial of eliminating these products from her diet

b. Assessment of pudendal nerve terminal motor latency to evaluate for pudendal neuropathy

c. Surgical repair of anal sphincter defects

d. Colostomy

e. Implantation of an artificial anal sphincter

7. A 55-year-old woman has had symptoms of constipation for the past 3 years. Despite straining excessively, applying manual abdominal pressure, and bending over, 15 minutes or longer is required to evacuate stool from the rectum. She uses enemas and occasionally complains of abdominal bloating. She has used various laxatives and adequate dietary fiber supplements during this time; these seem to work initially, but the effects wear off with time. Currently she uses tegaserod (6 mg twice daily) and milk of magnesia (twice weekly), expelling small, semiformed-to-liquid stools the day after. Her appetite and weight are stable, and there is no history of gastrointestinal bleeding. On physical

examination, she appears well. Results of abdominal examination are unremarkable. Digital rectal examination shows normal anal resting tone, hesitant squeeze to voluntary command, and reduced perineal descent during simulated defecation. Complete blood count and routine chemistry panel (including serum calcium and thyroid-stimulating hormone) are normal. A colonoscopy was normal 1.5 years ago. What is the most appropriate next step to evaluate this patient's symptoms?

a. Repeat colonoscopy

b. Assess colonic transit with radiopaque markers or scintigraphy and anorectal functions by manometry

c. Refer to a surgeon for subtotal colectomy

d. Increase the dietary fiber content

e. Double the dose of tegaserod to 12 mg twice daily

8. A 51-year-old disabled registered nurse has had long-standing alternating constipation and diarrhea. The diarrhea is postprandial, is preceded by relatively modest abdominal cramps that are completely relieved by defecation, and is not associated with gastrointestinal bleeding or mucus. When she has diarrhea, she has a minute or less to get to the toilet. When she does leave home, she has typical urge incontinence approximately once a week. She always wears a pad. To a lesser degree, she also has passive incontinence, primarily attributable to an inability to discriminate between the sensation of gas from stool in the rectum. These episodes occur approximately 5 times a week and are associated with leakage of a small amount of stool, perhaps slightly larger than a quarter. She eats less on days she has diarrhea and misses a bowel movement for the next 1 to 3 days. After this 1- to 3-day period, lower abdominal bloating and minimal rectal urgency develop, and she goes to the toilet, strains for 5 to 10 minutes to pass a "small plug," and passes soft stool thereafter. She occasionally uses a finger to retrieve stool from her rectum and applies manual abdominal pressure to facilitate that process, but generally she feels satisfied thereafter. The past medical history is particularly significant for disability related to a myocardial infarction in 2001. She has relatively mild stress urinary incontinence and considerable urinary urgency and urge urinary incontinence. On physical examination she appears well but depressed. The abdominal examination is unremarkable. Rectal examination shows a patulous anal sphincter at rest, poorly sustained weak puborectalis lift to voluntary command, and reduced perineal descent during simulated evacuation. Which of the following statements is correct with regard to pelvic floor retraining by biofeedback therapy for fecal incontinence?

a. Biofeedback therapy is based on the principle of operant conditioning (i.e., patients are taught how to control the activity of their own muscles by providing them feedback from the muscles)

b. Pelvic floor retraining only works by improving anal sphincter tone at rest and during squeeze

c. Controlled studies have shown that pelvic floor retraining is superior to other conservative measures (i.e., education, dietary modification) in fecal incontinence

d. Pelvic floor retraining can improve the latency between perception of rectal sensation and contraction of the external anal sphincter

e. Options a, b and c are correct

9. You are asked to see a 49-year-old man who has experienced left-sided upper abdominal and lower chest discomfort during the past 4 to 5 years. The discomfort initially was intermittent, but currently it occurs daily, generally beginning shortly after awakening and worsening during the course of the day. He is relatively uncomfortable by the time he gets home and has to lie on his abdomen or in the genu valgus position to evacuate the gas, maneuvers that are accompanied by considerable relief. However, there are no features of an acute abdomen during this period. Although his appetite is excellent, he tends to eat less than he did previously. His bowel habits are unchanged, and defecation is painless. He has never noticed blood in his stool. He is otherwise well. There is no history of fevers, pruritus, jaundice, or other medical conditions. On physical examination, he appears well. The abdomen is soft and nontender, and bowel sounds are normal. A barium enema shows marked dilatation of the distal transverse and proximal descending colon, and the proximal descending colon is up to 12 cm in maximal diameter. There is a smooth transition to normal-caliber colon in the mid descending colon without evidence for an obstructing lesion. Results of colonoscopy are normal. Anal manometry shows a normal recto-anal inhibitory reflex. On the basis of these features, what is the most appropriate next step?

a. Recommend a laxative agent

b. Prescribe acetaminophen with codeine for pain

c. Repeat colonoscopy

d. Place a colonic decompression tube colonoscopically

e. Consider subtotal colectomy for chronic megacolon

10. With regard to surgery for fecal incontinence, which of the following statements is correct?

a. Fecal continence improves in approximately 70% of patients in the short term (i.e., up to about 2 years) after surgical repair of anal sphincter defects, but improvement is not sustained over time

b. Fecal continence improves in approximately 70% of patients in the short term (up to about 2 years) after surgical repair of anal sphincter defects, and this improvement is sustained over time

c. Artificial anal sphincter is associated with a low risk (<10%) of significant complications

d. Dynamic graciloplasty is used widely for treating fecal incontinence in the United States

e. Patients with fecal incontinence should not be offered a colostomy

11. A 20-year-old man had development of bloody diarrhea 4 weeks ago. He had eaten dinner at a friend's home the day before, and one other person who was at the dinner also had diarrhea develop. A stool culture was positive for *Campylobacter jejuni*. He was treated with ciprofloxacin for 7 days and the rectal bleeding improved. He continues to have loose stools with some rectal bleeding 2 weeks after completing the course of antibiotics. Stool culture was repeated, the results of which are pending. Colonoscopy shows mild erythema and granularity throughout the entire colon. A sample of random colonoscopic biopsies is shown in the Figure. Which of the following is true?

a. The biopsy findings are probably due to infectious colitis

b. The colonoscopic finding could be due to *Giardia lamblia*

c. The biopsy findings are consistent with idiopathic inflammatory bowel disease

d. The colon biopsy is diagnostic of Crohn's disease

e. There is no need to repeat a stool culture for bacterial pathogens

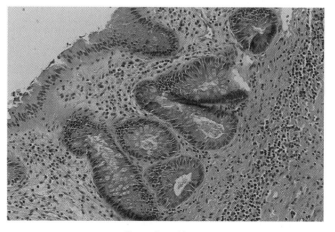

Question 11

12. A 28-year-old woman has a 3-year history of Crohn's disease involving the ileum and the colon. Her disease is in symptomatic remission with 6-mercaptopurine, 50 mg daily. She is contemplating pregnancy and she asks you for information about pregnancy and Crohn's disease. Which of the following is *not* true?
    a. If her disease flares during pregnancy, methotrexate could be used as an alternative to 6-mercaptopurine
    b. She likely will be able to get pregnant if her disease is active
    c. 6-Mercaptopurine therapy may be continued through pregnancy, if clinically indicated
    d. Her child will have an increased risk for development of either Crohn's disease or ulcerative colitis
    e. Worsening of her symptoms is most likely to occur during the first trimester or postpartum

13. A 45-year-old man has had ulcerative coliltis for 20 years. He currently is asymptomatic, receiving mesalamine 2.0 g daily. He underwent colonoscopy with biopsy throughout the colon for surveillance for dysplasia, and the abnormality shown in the Figure was identified in biopsy from the ascending colon. Which one of the following statements is true?
    a. He should be advised to undergo colectomy
    b. He does not need to have surveillance colonoscopies in the future
    c. It is unlikely that he has ulcerative colitis
    d. He should have repeat colonoscopy with biopsies of the same area in 4 weeks
    e. The mesalamine dose should be increased to 4.8 g/d

14. In a 30-year-old man, chronic colitis was diagnosed 2 years ago on the basis of findings of a flexible sigmoidoscopy with biopsy. He has had mild intermittent symptoms for 3 years, including 0 to 3 loose stools a day without blood, despite treatment with sulfasalazine 1 g twice daily. He has smoked 1 pack of cigarettes daily for 12 years. He has arthritis involving only his left knee and takes rofecoxib, 25 mg daily. Laboratory studies included a negative result for perinuclear antineutrophil cytoplasmic antibodies (pANCA) and an anti-saccharomyces cytoplasmic antibody (ASCA). Which of the following statements is true?
    a. The negative pANCA and ASCA results exclude a diagnosis of Crohn's disease
    b. It is unlikely that the patient has ulcerative colitis
    c. Use of a cyclooxygenase-2 (COX-2) inhibitor such as rofecoxib does not pose a risk of worsening the colitis
    d. The patient should undergo yearly colonoscopy with biopsies for surveillance for dysplasia
    e. Because the arthritis is unilateral, it is likely due to

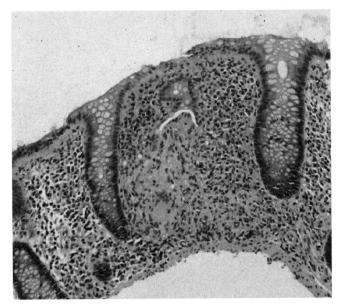

Question 13

degenerative joint disease and not colitic arthritis, which is usually symmetric

15. A 27-year-old woman has had Crohn's disease for 6 years and has undergone four previous resections, with a total of 150 cm of ileum removed and near-total resection of the colon. She has an ileosigmoid anastomosis. She has severe diarrhea that is not controlled with loperamide and opium tincture. She is losing weight. Which of the following statements about her is *not* true?
    a. Her diet should be fat-restricted
    b. She should be evaluated for recurrence of Crohn's disease
    c. She should receive parenteral vitamin B_{12} injections even if her serum vitamin B_{12} level is normal
    d. Her diarrhea will likely improve with cholestyramine
    e. Intestinal bacterial overgrowth could be worsening her diarrhea

16. A 50-year-old man with extensive small intestinal Crohn's disease is referred to you with complaints of diarrhea and abdominal cramping. He has a history of terminal ileal and cecal resection, with 55 cm of small bowel resected previously. A barium small-bowel radiograph shows 50 cm of ileal and jejunal inflammation and long areas of narrowing but no pre-stenotic dilatation. The patient has received prednisone for the past 2 years. He responds to prednisone at doses of 20 to 60 mg per day but has relapse when the prednisone dose is tapered to 10 mg per day or less. Which of the following medications is not appropriate for corticosteroid-sparing in this patient?

a. Oral mesalamine and metronidazole or ciprofloxacin
b. Azathioprine
c. Methotrexate
d. Infliximab
e. 6-Mercaptopurine

17. A 23-year-old woman with a 2.5-month history of diarrhea and rectal bleeding comes to your clinic for evaluation. Flexible sigmoidoscopy shows friability and loss of vascular pattern from the anal verge up to 22 cm with a sharp demarcation to normal-appearing mucosa. The colonic mucosa from 22 cm through 70 cm is endoscopically normal. Biopsy specimens show active chronic colitis in the distal colon and normal colonic mucosa in the more proximal uninvolved colon. Which of the following treatments is *not* appropriate as induction therapy in this patient?
    a. Rectal mesalamine 4,000 mg per day
    b. Rectal corticosteroids (cortisone 100 mg per day)
    c. Balsalazide 6.75 g per day
    d. Oral prednisone 40 mg per day tapered over 2.5 months
    e. Azathioprine 2-3 mg/kg per day

18. A 32-year-old man with a history of Crohn's ileocolitis and perianal fistulas presents for evaluation. He complains of perianal pain. He is not having cramping or diarrhea. Perianal examination shows a draining fistula to the right of the anus and a tender fluctuant mass on rectal examination on the left. All of the following treatment recommendations regarding treatment of Crohn's disease in this patient are correct *except*:
    a. Colorectal surgical consultation for examination under anesthesia with incision and drainage of a suspected perianal abscess
    b. Treatment with an antibiotic such as metronidazole or ciprofloxacin
    c. Initiation of therapy with azathioprine or 6-mercaptopurine
    d. Initiation of therapy with infliximab after surgical drainage of perianal abscess
    e. Treatment with oral prednisone 40 mg per day tapered over 2.5 months

19. Which of the following statements is true regarding 5-aminosalicylate drugs used for the treatment of inflammatory bowel disease?
    a. Mesalamine is commonly associated with headache, dyspepsia, and rash
    b. Balsalazide consists of a dimer of two 5-aminosalicylate molecules linked by an azo bond
    c. The oral mesalamine formulation, Pentasa, is comprised of ethylcellulose-coated granules that give a timed release

throughout the gastrointestinal tract beginning in the duodenum and ending in the colon and rectum
    d. The oral mesalamine formulation, Asacol, begins release in the mid small bowel (distal jejunum and proximal ileum)
    e. Sulfasalazine, osalazine, and balsalazide are all activated at pH 7 in the terminal ileum

20. A 42-year-old woman with a 6-year history of left-sided ulcerative colitis presents to your clinic with a 3-week history of bloody diarrhea with up to 15 stools per day and incontinence. She has lost 25 lb. She is pale, and her pulse is 110 beats/min supine. You decide to hospitalize her for treatment of severe colitis. Her only medication is oral mesalamine 4.0 g per day, which she has taken since diagnosis for induction and then maintenance of remission. Which of the following treatment options is *not* appropriate for this patient?
    a. Initiate therapy with intravenous methylprednisolone 40 mg daily
    b. Initiate therapy with rectal corticosteroids with cortisone 100 mg daily as adjunctive therapy
    c. Continue oral mesalamine as adjunctive therapy
    d. Obtain colorectal surgical consultation for possible colectomy
    e. Initiate therapy with intravenous cyclosporine if there is no response to intravenous corticosteroids in 5 to 7 days

21. A 45-year-old man with a 4-year history of ulcerative colitis has a 6-week history of a painful sore on the left leg. The patient recalls having bumped his shin, and this incident was followed by the development of a small "boil," which then developed into an open sore. The ulcer has been slowly enlarging. He takes mesalamine 2.4 g daily as maintenance therapy for his minimally active ulcerative colitis. Physical examination shows a 6-cm lesion in the left pretibial area, with violaceous, undermining borders. Specimens for bacterial, fungal, and mycobacterial cultures were obtained 3 weeks ago by the primary care physician, and these have not yielded any pathogens thus far. Biopsy of the lesion showed a neutrophilic infiltrate. Therapy with oral prednisone 60 mg daily was begun 2 weeks ago, but this has had no effect on the lesion; in fact, it has enlarged. Which of the following treatments is appropriate as the next step?
    a. Metronidazole 500 mg orally three times daily
    b. Increase mesalamine dosage to 1.6 g orally three times daily
    c. Azathioprine 2 mg/kg body weight daily
    d. Tacrolimus 0.15 to 0.20 mg/kg body weight daily
    e. Wound debridement

22. A 38-year-old woman with ulcerative colitis seeks evaluation for 2 days of pain in the left knee. She recently experienced more diarrhea, rectal bleeding, and tenesmus. In the previous week, flexible sigmoidoscopy showed erythema, friability, and edema of the mucosa as far as the extent of the examination (descending colon). The mesalamine dose was increased to 4.8 g daily, but the symptoms persist. The left knee joint is tender and has limited range of motion, and there are signs of an effusion on physical examination. The joint was aspirated. Gram stain was negative, and crystal analysis showed no crystals. Which therapy is most appropriate?

    a. Infliximab 5 mg/kg body weight by intravenous infusion over 2 hours
    b. Indomethacin 50 mg orally three times daily
    c. Prednisone 60 mg orally daily for 2 weeks followed by a taper
    d. Sulfasalazine 1 g orally three times daily
    e. Glucosamine-chondroitin supplementation

23. A 34-year-old man is noted to have abnormal hepatic biochemistry values at the time of his first blood donation. Viral hepatitis serologic results are negative. The alkaline phosphatase level is 3 times the upper limit of normal, and the alanine aminotransferase and aspartate aminotransferase values are 2 times the upper limit of normal. Ultrasonography of the liver and gallbladder is normal. The hepatic biochemical abnormalities persist during the next 9 months. Endoscopic retrograde cholangiopancreatography shows multiple diffuse strictures of the extrahepatic and intrahepatic ducts. The patient is questioned again about his bowel habit. He has noted a stable bowel pattern of two semiformed bowel movements daily for many years. He occasionally notes wipe bleeding, however. Sigmoidoscopy is recommended and shows subtle changes as far as the procedure extended (sigmoid), characterized by loss of vascular pattern and granularity. Small hemorrhoids are noted. Biopsies show mildly active chronic colitis. Which of the following would you recommend?

    a. Computed tomography (CT) colonography to evaluate the proximal colon
    b. Colonoscopy with surveillance biopsies now, followed by repeat colonoscopy every 1 to 2 years
    c. Surveillance colonoscopy in 8 years, followed by an examination every 1 to 2 years
    d. Folic acid supplementation
    e. Fecal DNA sampling

24. A 41-year-old woman with a 25-year history of ulcerative colitis is seen for a "checkup." During the first 5 years of her condition, she required several courses of prednisone and also sulfasalazine, but she has been in clinical remission without medications for the past 20 years. She is having a checkup mostly at her spouse's urging. She has two bowel movements daily. Physical examination is unremarkable. At colonoscopy, mildly active pancolitis is noted. Random surveillance biopsy specimens are obtained. In the ascending colon, three small sessile polyps are noted, and these are all removed with electrocautery. Histologic analysis of these polyps shows fragments of colonic mucosa with low-grade dysplasia and fragments without dysplasia. The random biopsy specimens show low-grade dysplasia in the ascending colon and no dysplasia elsewhere. What is your recommendation to the patient?

    a. Proctocolectomy with ileal pouch-anal anastomosis
    b. Repeat surveillance colonoscopy with biopsies in 3 months
    c. Mesalamine 1.6 g orally three times daily and folic acid 1 mg orally daily
    d. Repeat colonoscopy now with argon plasma coagulation treatment of the ascending colon
    e. Right hemicolectomy with ileotransverse colonic anastomosis

25. Which of the following statements is true with regard to dual-energy x-ray absorptiometry (DEXA) screening for osteoporosis in patients with inflammatory bowel disease?

    a. Patients who do not have bone or joint pain do not require DEXA
    b. All patients with Crohn's disease and ulcerative colitis should undergo DEXA testing at diagnosis
    c. Patients who are not currently treated with corticosteroids do not require DEXA testing
    d. Patients with inflammatory bowel disease (IBD) who are older than 60 years or who are postmenopausal women should undergo DEXA testing
    e. Patients with IBD who are older than 50 years should undergo DEXA testing

26. You have recommended initiation of azathioprine therapy for a 24-year-old woman with Crohn's ileocolitis in whom prednisone could not be tapered for the past 2 years. She has read the product labeling and is very concerned about the risk of neoplasia, specifically lymphoma. Which of the following statements is true with regard to lymphoma risk in Crohn's disease?

    a. Most population-based studies suggest that there is an increased "baseline" risk of lymphoma in Crohn's disease
    b. The risk of lymphoma associated with azathioprine or 6-mercaptopurine is increased 4 times relative to the risk in the general population

c. The absolute risk of lymphoma in a patient receiving azathioprine or 6-mercaptopurine is between 1% and 5% per year

d. Lymphomas containing Epstein-Barr virus are less common among users of azathioprine or 6-mercaptopurine

e. The risk of lymphoma associated with azathioprine or 6-mercaptoprine is increased 14 times relative to the risk in the general population

27. A 35-year-old man with Crohn's colitis who is currently in clinical remission while receiving delayed-release mesalamine complains of low-back pain and morning stiffness. Exertion improves the pain and stiffness, and rest worsens the symptoms. He has no symptoms of peripheral arthritis. Plain radiographs of the pelvis and lumbar spine show sacroiliitis and early ankylosing changes of the spine. Because a flare of Crohn's disease developed when the patient was treated with a conventional nonsteroidal anti-inflammatory drug (NSAID) in the past, you start therapy with a cyclooxygenase (COX-2) inhibitor. Although this helps the back pain and stiffness to a degree, diarrhea and abdominal cramping develop after 2 weeks. These persist after use of the anti-inflammatory medication is discontinued, and a flexible sigmoidoscopy shows numerous aphthous and superficial ulcerations in the rectosigmoid. He has an allergy to sulfonamides. Which medical therapy would be most appropriate at this point?

a. Combination therapy with a combination of diclofenac and misoprostol

b. Methotrexate 7.5 mg by mouth weekly

c. Etanercept 25 mg subcutaneously twice weekly

d. Infliximab 5 mg/kg intravenously at 0, 2, and 6 weeks and every 8 weeks thereafter

e. Glucosamine and chondroitin supplements by mouth daily

28. Which of the following statements regarding collagenous colitis is *false*?

a. It can cause strictures or fistulas

b. It is most common in the sixth to eighth decades of life

c. It is less common in men than in women

d. It can resolve spontaneously

e. It may be associated with use of a nonsteroidal anti-inflammatory drug

29. Which of the following statements about microscopic colitis is true?

a. Collagenous colitis can be distinguished from lymphocytic colitis because collagenous colitis has a thickened subepithelial collagen band, whereas lymphocytic colitis has increased intraepithelial lymphocytes

b. Abdominal pain or weight loss would be unusual for microscopic colitis

c. Microscopic colitis is associated with an increased risk of colon cancer, although less than that with ulcerative colitis

d. Most patients with microscopic colitis respond to nonspecific antidiarrheal medications (e.g., loperamide, bismuth)

e. Thickening of the subepithelial collagen band is specific for collagenous colitis and should not be found in other conditions or in subjects without diarrhea

30. Which of the following statements is true?

a. Collagenous colitis is associated with an increased risk of colon cancer, but only in patients who have had disease for more than 15 years

b. Patients with microscopic colitis often have alternating diarrhea and constipation

c. Fecal leukocytes should strongly suggest an alternative diagnosis

d. Collagenous colitis is due to dysregulation of the gene for fibroblast growth factor

e. In patients with microscopic colitis who do not respond to antidiarrheal agents and mesalamine, celiac sprue should be considered

31. Which of the following statements regarding *Clostridium difficile*-associated disease is true?

a. Most cases of antibiotic-associated diarrhea are not due to *C. difficile*

b. Normal results of flexible sigmoidoscopy exclude pseudomembranous colitis

c. Healthy infants rarely are asymptomatic carriers of *C. difficile*

d. Healthy adults often are asymptomatic carriers of *C. difficile*

e. Stool enzyme-linked immunosorbent assay (ELISA) sensitivity for *C. difficile* toxin approaches 95%

32. Which of the following is *not* necessary for *Clostridium difficile*-associated disease?

a. A source of the organism

b. Exposure to antibiotics

c. Alteration of the normal flora

d. Activation of spores

e. Toxin production

33. Which of the following statements regarding treatment of *Clostridium difficile*-associated disease is *false*?

a. Mild disease may require no specific treatment other than stopping use of the offending antibiotic

b. Antibiotic treatment of mild disease does not decrease the risk of recurrence

c. Cholestyramine works by binding toxin

d. Metronidazole is equivalent to vancomycin for mild-to-moderate disease

e. For patients unable to take medications orally, intravenous metronidazole or vancomycin is an effective alternative

34. Abdominal pain and diarrhea develop in a 42-year-old woman during a course of antibiotics for a urinary tract infection. *Clostridium difficile* toxin is found in her stools with enzyme-linked immunosorbent assay. The symptoms resolve during a 10-day course of metronidazole 500 mg three times daily. One week after completing the metronidazole therapy, she has a recurrence of diarrhea and mild abdominal pain without fever or hematochezia. Which is the most appropriate step in her management?

a. Metronidazole 500 mg three times daily for 10 days

b. Vancomycin 125 mg four times daily for 10 days

c. Colonoscopy, followed by antibiotics if pseudomembranes are seen

d. Metronidazole 1,000 mg four times daily for 10 days

e. Metronidazole 500 mg three times daily for 30 days

35. A 36-year-old man schedules an appointment with you to discuss a 6-month history of intermittent hematochezia. He has also noticed a "bump" on his left eyelid which seems to be getting larger. Lower gastrointestinal symptoms are described as bright red blood on the toilet tissue and in the toilet water after bowel movements. No melena has been observed. Other pertinent history includes a recent 10-lb weight loss that he attributes to being on a low-carbohydrate diet. The patient's mother underwent hysterectomy for endometrial cancer at age 42 years. His maternal grandmother died of colorectal cancer at age 38 years, and colorectal polyps were diagnosed in his maternal uncle at age 28 years (and kidney cancer at age 34 years). Other family history information is currently unavailable. Which test(s) is most appropriate?

a. Fecal occult blood test (to confirm gastrointestinal bleeding)

b. Flexible sigmoidoscopy

c. Colonoscopy

d. Abdominopelvic computed tomography

e. All of the above are appropriate

36. A 42-year-old man presents to your office to discuss long-standing constipation (one bowel movement every third day) that has been present throughout his adult life. On review of his family history, the patient mentions that colorectal adenomas were diagnosed in his father at age 57 years. A paternal cousin died of colorectal cancer at age 54 years. No other relatives are known to have had colorectal polyps, colorectal cancer, or other forms of malignant disease. On the basis of currently endorsed screening guidelines for colorectal cancer, what testing should be performed?

a. Fecal occult blood test

b. Flexible sigmoidoscopy

c. Fecal occult blood test and flexible sigmoidoscopy

d. Double-contrast barium enema

e. Colonoscopy

37. A 73-year-old woman with no family history of colorectal neoplasia returns to your office to discuss the results of her recent screening colonoscopy. Findings included a 12-mm tubular adenoma with low-grade dysplasia in the ascending colon, a 6-mm tubular adenoma with low-grade dysplasia at the hepatic flexure, a 3-mm hyperplastic polyp in the sigmoid colon, and pancolonic diverticuli. The preparation was excellent, and more than 90% of the mucosal surface was well seen. When should you perform her next surveillance colonoscopy?

a. 3 months

b. 1 year

c. 3 years

d. 5 years

e. Because all polyps were removed, the patient does not need another colonoscopy

38. A 34-year-old woman with familial adenomatous polyposis (FAP) comes to see you for her annual evaluation. She is currently asymptomatic from a gastrointestinal standpoint. Past surgical history is remarkable for total protocolectomy with ileoanal pouch anastomosis, performed 18 years ago. You recommend extended esophagogastroduodenoscopy (including examination of the periampullary region with a side-viewing instrument), and seven duodenal adenomas are identified. They range in size from 5 mm to 4 cm. On histologic review, several of the adenomas have villous morphology (low-grade or mild dysplasia). What is the severity of the duodenal polyp burden according to the Spigelman classification system?

a. Stage 0

b. Stage I

c. Stage II

d. Stage III

e. Stage IV

39. Which of the following does *not* represent "poor" prognostic features of a malignant polyp?

a. Poor differentiation
b. Vascular involvement
c. Cancer cells present at the margin of excision
d. Lymphatic involvement
e. Cancer cells within the stalk of a pedunculated polyp

40. Which of the following symptoms is *not* included in the diagnostic criteria of irritable bowel syndrome?
    a. Pain relieved by defecation
    b. More frequent stools with onset of pain
    c. Looser stool with onset of pain
    d. Alternating periods of diarrhea and constipation
    e. Less frequent stools with onset of pain

41. A 55-year-old woman is referred for evaluation of abdominal pain and diarrhea. She has had symptoms for 10 years, but they are worse now. She has never seen a physician for this problem or had any evaluation previously. The pain occurs after meals and leads to a loose bowel movement that promptly relieves the pain. There is no bleeding, and she has not lost weight. Examination shows active bowel sounds and slight tenderness in the left lower quadrant. What testing is warranted?
    a. Abdominal computed tomography
    b. Pelvic ultrasonography
    c. Colonoscopy
    d. Urine 5-hydroxyindoleacetic acid test
    e. Esophagogastroduodenoscopy with duodenal biopsy and aspirate

42. A 25-year-old woman is referred to you for abdominal pain and diarrhea. She has had symptoms for 5 years. Her symptoms are classic for irritable bowel syndrome and her examination results are unremarkable. She wants to know what this diagnosis means. You tell her which of the following?
    a. Her risk of colon cancer is increased

b. It will progress to the point of colon surgery
c. It will lead to weight loss and gut failure
d. It may never go away
e. It will increase her risk of complicated pregnancies

43. A 55-year-old woman with a long history of constipation-predominant irritable bowel syndrome comes for care because her symptoms have changed. She feels bloated, has abdominal distention and anorexia, and has lost weight. On examination her abdomen is distended without organomegaly. What is the best approach?
    a. Explore the stressors in her life and consider a psychiatric referral
    b. Review the fiber in her diet and consider increasing the strength of her laxatives
    c. Initiate investigation
    d. Discuss air swallowing and methods for reducing intestinal gas
    e. Begin antispasmodic treatment

44. A 35-year-old man has had chronic pain in his abdomen for 2 years, anorexia, and alternating bowel habit. He is tired and is not sleeping, and his joints hurt all over. His weight is stable. Examination is remarkable only for a flat affect. His hemoglobin and albumin values are normal. What should you do?
    a. Tell him that he does not have a gastrointestinal problem and refer him back to his primary care provider
    b. Start therapy with a tricyclic antidepressant 25 mg at bedtime
    c. Perform esophagogastric duodenoscopy, colonoscopy, and abdominal computed tomography, and obtain a rheumatology consultation
    d. Refer to a surgeon for laparoscopy
    e. Educate him about irritable bowel syndrome, schedule a consultation with a psychologist, and set up a return appointment

ANSWERS

1. Answer e

This patient's history is highly suggestive of giardiasis. The initial stool analysis for ova and parasites was performed in a chronic phase of illness, at which time this test is relatively insensitive. Repeating the analysis for ova and parasites increases the sensitivity of this test. In the chronic phase, small-bowel biopsy or fecal analysis for *Giardia* antigen may be more sensitive. Alternatively, an empiric trial of metronidazole for 7 days also is appropriate. Given the suggestion of steatorrhea, empiric loperamide is not appropriate.

2. Answer b

Rotavirus, Norwalk virus, and astrovirus all typically cause diarrhea that resolves within 5 days. Enteric adenovirus typically lasts 7 to 14 days. Prolonged diarrhea would be unusual with hepatitis A.

3. Answer d

V. cholerae causes diarrhea by enterotoxin-mediated stimulation of secretion. Thus, the stools are nonbloody. The other organisms can cause bloody stools with pus and mucus (i.e., dysentery).

4. Answer b

E. coli O157:H7 and *Shigella* may produce a biphasic diarrheal illness that begins as watery diarrhea and progresses to dysentery. In shigellosis, the initial diarrhea is due to an enterotoxin, whereas the bloody diarrhea reflects mucosal invasion. The other organisms do not typically cause a biphasic disease. *Salmonella* typically causes either gastroenteritis (nonbloody) or colitis (can be bloody) but usually not both. *Vibrio* and *Cryptosporidium* usually cause nonbloody diarrhea.

5. Answer c

Patients with chronic illness, including liver cirrhosis, are at increased risk for sepsis and death from *V. vulnificus*. Therefore, they should be discouraged from eating raw seafood, particularly oysters. Hemolytic uremic syndrome occurs in 5% of *E. coli* O157:H7 infections and can result in significant morbidity and mortality, particularly in the very young and very old. Young, otherwise healthy adults seem to be at less risk. Postinfectious arthritis typically occurs in patients who are positive for HLA-B27. Typhoid fever commonly is associated with disseminated metastatic infections. Pregnant women are at risk for disseminated infection with *Listeria monocytogenes*, which can result in significant mortality. There is no evidence that pregnant women are at risk for disseminated *B. cereus* infection.

6. Answer a

In this patient, fecal incontinence is probably attributable to semiformed stools and pelvic floor weakness. Measures to regulate stool consistency and frequency often improve continence. Contrary to early studies, more recent studies suggest that pudendal nerve latencies are not reliable for diagnosing a pudendal neuropathy. Continence improves in about 80% of patients shortly after surgical repair of anal sphincter defects, but it deteriorates over time; less than 50% of patients benefit from the operation in the long term. The artificial anal sphincter is associated with considerable morbidity, particularly wound infections, often requiring device explantation. A colostomy is a last resort for patients with severe fecal incontinence.

7. Answer b

After exclusion of a secondary cause for constipation, colonic transit and anorectal functions should be assessed in patients with constipation that has not responded to dietary fiber supplements and laxatives. Patients with slow-transit constipation unresponsive to laxatives and without pelvic floor dysfunction may require a subtotal colectomy.

8. Answer c

Uncontrolled studies suggest that pelvic floor retraining restores coordinated contraction of the external anal sphincter when rectal distention is perceived. In contrast, pelvic floor retraining has relatively modest, if any, effects on anal resting and squeeze pressures. A recent study randomized 171 incontinent patients to four groups: standard medical and nursing care (i.e., advice only), advice and verbal instruction on sphincter exercises, hospital-based computer-assisted sphincter pressure biofeedback, or hospital biofeedback and use of a home electromyographic biofeedback device. Overall, 75% reported improved symptoms and 5% were cured, improvement was sustained at 1 year after therapy, and symptoms and resting and squeeze pressures improved to a similar degree in all four groups. These results underscore the importance that patients attach to understanding the condition and the importance of practical advice regarding coping strategies (e.g., diet and skin care) and patient interactions with health care providers. Further controlled studies are necessary to define the effect of pelvic floor retraining in patients who do not respond to advice only and of anorectal sensory retraining in incontinent patients.

9. Answer e

The clinical features and barium enema indicate that this patient has chronic megacolon; an intact recto-anal inhibitory reflex excluded Hirschprung's disease. Recent studies suggest a marked depletion in nerve fibers and interstitial cells of Cajal, the pacemaker cells of the gut, in chronic megacolon. In this condition, laxatives are unlikely to improve colonic distention; opiates may increase colonic distention. Colonic decompression is used to relieve distention in acute colonic pseudo-obstruction (i.e., Ogilvie's syndrome), not chronic megacolon.

10. Answer a

Continence improves in up to 85% of patients with sphincter defects after an overlapping anterior sphincteroplasty. However, less than 50% of patients remain continent up to 5 years after the operation. Dynamic graciloplasty and artificial anal sphincter devices are available in a handful of centers worldwide, are effective in selected patients, and are associated with considerable morbidity (e.g., device problems, wound infection) in one-third of patients, and reoperation often is required. The hardware for dynamic graciloplasty is not approved for use in the United States. A colostomy is useful for patients with severe fecal incontinence unresponsive to other measures.

11. Answer c

The colonoscopic biopsy shows a branching crypt, consistent with chronic colitis due to inflammatory bowel disease. This patient likely had underlying inflammatory bowel disease with a superimposed acute infectious colitis. Acute bacterial colitis due to *C. jejuni* or other bacterial pathogen does not cause branching crypts in the lamina propria, thus answer a is incorrect. *G. lamblia* does not cause colonic injury, thus answer b is incorrect. Although the biopsy is compatible with a diagnosis of Crohn's colitis, the biopsy is not diagnostic and is also consistent with ulcerative colitis, thus answer d is incorrect. *C. jejuni* infection possibly was not eradicated with the course of ciprofloxacin, so it is appropriate to repeat the stool culture. However, even if *Campylobacter* infection is still present, the patient probably has underlying ulcerative colitis as the cause of his current symptoms.

12. Answer a

Methotrexate is teratogenic and should not be used in pregnancy. Answer b is correct; although fertility may be slightly decreased in Crohn's disease, the majority of patients are able to conceive. Answer c is correct; 6-mercaptopurine and azathioprine can be used throughout pregnancy if clinically indicated. Answer d is correct; first-degree relatives of patients with Crohn's disease have a 10% to 15% risk for development of Crohn's disease or ulcerative colitis. Answer e is correct; about a third of patients have worsening of symptoms during pregnancy, most commonly during the first trimester or postpartum.

13. Answer c

The abnormality shown on the photomicrograph is a non-caseating granuloma, found on mucosal biopsies in about half of patients with Crohn's disease and rarely (and as isolated lesions) in patients with ulcerative colitis. Answer a is incorrect; there is no dysplasia on the biopsy specimen and colectomy is not indicated. He should have regular colonoscopic surveillance, but there is no need for prophylactic colectomy at this time. Answer b is incorrect; he has had colitis for 20 years and is at an increased risk for development of colon cancer, with either a diagnosis of ulcerative colitis or Crohn's disease of the colon. Answer d is incorrect; there is no need to repeat the colonoscopy with biopsy in 4 weeks because the presence or absence of the granuloma will not change the management in this asymptomatic patient. Answer e is incorrect; there is no need to increase the dose of mesalamine in this asymptomatic patient.

14. Answer b

The patient is a long-time and current cigarette smoker; because only 13% of patients with ulcerative colitis are current smokers, it is unlikely he has ulcerative colitis. Cigarette smoking is associated with Crohn's disease, thus it is more likely that this patient with long-standing colitis has Crohn's disease. Answer a is incorrect; although most patients with ulcerative colitis are positive for pANCA and most patients with Crohn's disease are positive for ASCA, a small proportion of patients with either condition do not have these antibodies present. Answer c is incorrect; although the COX-2 inhibitor drugs, such as rofecoxib, have less risk of gastrointestinal side effects than other nonsteroidal anti-inflammatory drugs, there is still some risk that the COX-2 inhibitors can worsen colitis symptoms. Answer d is incorrect; the risks of dysplasia and cancer of the colon increase after 8 to 10 years of disease in patients with idiopathic inflammatory bowel disease. There is no need for this man, who has had symptoms of disease for only 3 years, to undergo colonoscopy for surveillance for dysplasia. Answer e is incorrect; colitic arthritis usually involves the large joints, such as the knees, ankles, or elbows, and often is asymmetric, as in this patient.

15. Answer d

Cholestyramine is unlikely to help the diarrhea because the patient probably has fat malabsorption and not bile acid diarrhea, in view of the long length of the bowel resected with relative depletion of the total bile acid pool. Patients with less than 100 cm of distal ileum resected are at risk for bile acid diarrhea. Answer a is correct; she has had more than 100 cm of the distal ileum resected and should be receiving a diet restricted in long-chain fatty acids. Diet supplements with oral medium-chain triglycerides are appropriate. Answer b is correct; the diarrhea could be due to recurrent Crohn's disease in the small intestine or rectosigmoid, and she should be evaluated for a recurrence. Answer c is correct; the extensive resection of the terminal ileum eventually will cause vitamin B_{12} deficiency unless she receives parenteral B_{12} supplements. Answer e is correct; she has had the ileocecal valve and proximal colon resected and could have intestinal bacterial overgrowth due to retrograde propagation of bacteria from the colon.

16. Answer a

Oral mesalamine is not corticosteroid-sparing for patients with corticosteroid-dependent Crohn's disease. Antibiotics have not been carefully studied for this indication, but, in general, they have not been consistently effective in patients with mildly to moderately active Crohn's disease. Azathioprine, 6-mercaptopurine, methotrexate, and infliximab have all been shown to be corticosteroid-sparing in randomized controlled trials and would be appropriate treatment agents for this patient.

17. Answer e

Rectal corticosteroids and rectal mesalamine are effective for inducing remission in patients with mildly to moderately active ulcerative proctosigmoiditis. In patients who respond, rectal mesalamine can be continued for maintenance, whereas rectal corticosteroids are not effective for maintenance. Balsalazide, olsalazine, and oral mesalamine are also effective for inducing remission in patients with ulcerative proctosigmoiditis, as are oral corticosteroids. Azathioprine and 6-mercaptopurine have a slow onset of efficacy over 4 to 12 weeks and are more useful as maintenance drugs and for corticosteroid-sparing in patients in whom induction or maintenance therapy with one of the 5-aminosalicylate class of drugs fails.

18. Answer e

Patients with suspected perianal abscess should undergo colorectal surgical evaluation with examination under anesthesia and incision and drainage of any perianal abscess that is identified. Although antibiotics have not been studied in controlled trials for perianal fistulas, they are considered to be effective and to be the first-line medical therapy. Uncontrolled studies, and a meta-analysis of secondary end points from controlled trials, have suggested that the immunosuppressive medications azathioprine and 6-mercaptopurine are of benefit in patients with perianal Crohn's disease. Infliximab is effective for perianal Crohn's disease, but many clinicians reserve it for patients in whom other therapies have failed and for those with a severe presentation. If an abscess is present, it should be drained before beginning treatment with infliximab. Corticosteroids are not effective therapy for perianal Crohn's disease.

19. Answer c

Mesalamine is well tolerated in most patients. The sulfapyridine component of sulfasalazine is commonly associated with headache, dyspepsia, and rash. Osalazine is a dimer of two 5-aminosalicylate molecules linked by an azo bond. Balsalazide is a single 5-aminosalicylate molecule linked to an inert carrier by an azo bond. The oral mesalamine formulation, Pentasa, is an ethylcellulose-coated formulation that gives a timed release throughout the gastrointestinal tract beginning in the duodenum and ending in the colon and rectum. The oral mesalamine formulation, Asacol, is designed to release in the terminal ileum and cecum at pH 7, not in the mid small bowel. Controlled ileal-release budesonide is designed to release in the mid small bowel. Sulfasalazine, olsalazine, and balsalazide all have azo bonds, which are cleaved by colonic bacteria, releasing active 5-aminosalicylate. Thus, these drugs are activated and release 5-aminosalicylate in the colon, not in the terminal ileum and not at pH 7, and they are not dependent on achieving a pH of 7.

20. Answer c

Patients with severely active ulcerative colitis should be hospitalized, given treatment with intravenous corticosteroids, and evaluated by a colorectal surgeon in case their condition urgently worsens or they fail to respond to medical therapy. Many experts advocate the use of rectal corticosteroids as adjunctive therapy. There is no evidence that continuing oral mesalamine therapy is beneficial in the short term in patients with severely active ulcerative colitis, and most experts advocate discontinuing therapy with sulfasalazine and other drugs in the mesalamine class because of the possibility of a drug-associated allergic reaction presenting as worsening colitis. Cyclosporine is effective as monotherapy in patients with severe ulcerative colitis. However, because of the toxicity profile of cyclosporine, it should be reserved for patients in whom therapy with intravenous corticosteroids for 5 to 7 days has failed and who do not want to pursue colectomy immediately.

21. Answer d

The patient has pyoderma gangrenosum that has been refractory to 2 weeks of therapy with high-dose oral corticosteroids. Answers a and b are incorrect; metronidazole and mesalamine will have no effect whatsoever on this lesion. Answer c is incorrect; azathioprine eventually may be effective but will take at least 1 to 2 months to take effect. Answer e is incorrect; surgical debridement of the lesion will worsen pyoderma gangrenosum, because the lesion typically exhibits pathergy, or a tendency to worsen with trauma. Either tacrolimus or cyclosporine would be appropriate for this refractory lesion. Both are rapidly acting; tacrolimus, which has more predictable oral bioavailability, does not require initial intravenous infusion. (Incidentally, early uncontrolled series suggest that infliximab may be efficacious in the healing of pyoderma gangrenosum.)

22. Answer c

The patient appears to have a type 1 peripheral arthritis. This form of large-joint pauciarticular arthritis typically mirrors the activity of the bowel disease, and in most cases its course is self-limited. Treatment of the ulcerative colitis should result in resolution. Septic arthritis, gout, and pseudogout, which are in the differential diagnosis, have been excluded by the joint fluid analysis. Answer a is incorrect; infliximab is not indicated for the peripheral arthritis of inflammatory bowel disease, although it does seem to be efficacious for ankylosing spondylitis. (Currently, there is no compelling evidence that infliximab is effective for ulcerative colitis, although clinical trials are under way.) Answer b is incorrect; the concern with indomethacin would be its deleterious effects on this patient's active colitis. Prednisone would not only treat the colitis exacerbation but also likely would result in resolution of the knee synovitis. Answer d is incorrect; sulfasalazine may be helpful for the arthritis but likely would be ineffective for the colitis flare, because the patient's condition has already failed to respond to high-dose mesalamine. Answer e is also incorrect; there is no evidence that supplementation with glucosamine and chondroitin would be beneficial for arthritis related to inflammatory bowel disease.

23. Answer b

This patient with newly diagnosed primary sclerosing cholangitis (PSC) turns out to have relatively asymptomatic ulcerative colitis. A significant portion of patients with PSC who do not have bowel symptoms will prove to have mild pancolitis on endoscopy. Because patients with PSC and associated inflammatory bowel disease (IBD) are more likely to have development of dysplasia and colorectal cancer, they should begin colonoscopic surveillance immediately. Answer a is incorrect; CT colonography does not allow histologic sampling of the mucosa for neoplastic change. Answer c is incorrect; because PSC-associated colitis is often mild and asymptomatic, the onset of IBD is unknown, and a delay of 8 years before surveillance is started could prove fatal. Answer d is incorrect; although folic acid supplementation may ultimately be proved to reduce the risk of dysplasia and cancer in IBD, it does not address the more pressing concern of the immediate risk. Likewise, answer e is incorrect; fecal DNA sampling may prove to be useful for detecting dysplastic or cancerous changes in IBD, but at this time there is no evidence.

24. Answer a

This patient has polypoid dysplasia *and* flat low-grade dysplasia. The flat dysplasia was found in an area adjacent to the polyp. This condition raises the possibility of a true dysplasia-associated lesion or mass not amenable to endoscopic therapy rather than a mere adenoma that can be treated with

polypectomy. Moreover, this patient's dysplasia is multifocal, a trait that most experts agree justifies colectomy. Thus, there are two indications for surgery. Answer b is incorrect; surveillance colonoscopy in 3 months leaves the patient at risk for progressive neoplasia. Answer c is incorrect; mesalamine and folic acid may be chemopreventive, but there is no evidence they cause regression of existing dysplasia. Answer d is incorrect; there is no role for argon plasma coagulation of this lesion. Answer e is incorrect; right hemicolectomy would address the existing dysplasia, but this surgical option leaves the patient at risk for metachronous neoplasia in the colonic remnant.

25. Answer d

It has been increasingly recognized that osteoporosis and osteopenia are more prevalent among patients with IBD than in the general population. Although the prevalence of these conditions of decreased bone density is as high as 70% in referral-based studies, studies in unselected populations suggest that osteoporosis occurs in up to 15% of patients with Crohn's disease, and osteopenia occurs in up to 45% (these figures generally are lower for ulcerative colitis). This higher prevalence means that the risk of osteoporotic fracture of between 15% and 45% is higher than that in the general population. Both the American Gastroenterological Association and the American College of Gastroenterology recently published guidelines for the evaluation and management of osteoporosis in IBD. DEXA scanning of the lumbar spine, hip, or wrist is considered the standard diagnostic tool. The guidelines suggest that patients with IBD should be tested if they have at least one of the following risk factors: age older than 60 (not 50) years, low body mass index (<20), hypogonadism (postmenopausal in women or low testosterone in men), corticosteroid treatment for at least 3 months, recurrent courses of corticosteroids, family history of osteoporosis, history of heavy smoking, or personal history of osteoporotic fracture. Answer a is incorrect because osteoporosis is asymptomatic before development of fracture. Although some patients with IBD do indeed have low bone density at diagnosis (suggesting that inflammation itself may contribute to the condition), this decreased density does not occur frequently enough to warrant blanket testing of everyone at diagnosis. Thus, answer b is incorrect. Patients not currently receiving corticosteroids may nevertheless provide a history of corticosteroid therapy for a cumulative duration of more than 3 months; therefore, answer c is incorrect.

26. Answer b

Most population-based studies of lymphoma risk in inflammatory bowel disease (IBD) have not shown an increased risk, although several referral-based studies have suggested it. A recent meta-analysis of all studies of lymphoma risk among patients with IBD receiving azathioprine or 6-mercaptopurine estimated a fourfold increase in *relative* risk. Nevertheless, the *absolute* risk of lymphoma remains low in these patients (estimated incidence of much less than 1% per year—actually, 1 case per 350 to 4,500 person-years). In most clinical situations, the benefits of azathioprine or 6-mercaptopurine are thought to outweigh this risk. One study from Mayo Clinic showed that Epstein-Barr virus was noted in 5 of 6 patients with lymphoma receiving the drugs and in 2 of 12 patients with lymphoma who were not. The presence of Epstein-Barr virus in lymphoma often implies that the lymphoma arose in the setting of immunosuppression, similar to that of posttransplantation and human immunodeficiency virus infection.

27. Answer d

First-line therapy of ankylosing spondylitis usually consists of NSAIDs and physical therapy. This man already had had adverse events with two different NSAIDs, including a COX-2 inhibitor. Although methotrexate has been used in ankylosing spondylitis, it usually is reserved for patients who have a concomitant peripheral arthritis, in which the peripheral symptoms predominate. A consensus conference sponsored by the Canadian Rheumatology Association analyzed evidence from clinical trials and concluded that either infliximab or etanercept is indicated for moderately to severely active ankylosing spondylitis when therapy with at least two different NSAIDs has been unsuccessful. In this patient the Crohn's colitis is currently active; therefore, infliximab, which is efficacious in Crohn's disease, is indicated, whereas etanercept, which is not efficacious in Crohn's disease, is not.

28. Answer a

Collagenous colitis, unlike Crohn's disease, does not cause strictures, fistulas, or abscesses. The remaining choices are correct.

29. Answer d

Answer a is incorrect because collagenous colitis also has increased intraepithelial lymphocytes, in addition to a thickened collagen band. The symptoms listed in answer b can occur in up to 50% of patients. The risk of colon cancer has not been well studied, but it does not seem to be significantly increased. Finally, a thickened collagen band has been reported in other settings, including patients without diarrhea.

30. Answer e

Coexistent celiac sprue can be the cause of failure to respond to the usual therapies. Answers a and d have no data to support them, and c is incorrect because up to 50% of patients with microscopic colitis have fecal leukocytes. Constipation is not a recognized symptom of microscopic colitis.

31. Answer a

Most antibiotic-associated diarrhea is due to the antibiotic itself and not to *C. difficile* infection. The remaining choices are false: flexible sigmoidoscopy may miss the unusual case of pseudomembranous colitis localized above the splenic flexure, infants, but not adults, are often carriers of *C. difficile* without symptoms, and stool ELISA sensitivity is relatively low, reaching 95% only if three or four samples are analyzed.

32. Answer b

C. difficile-associated disease (CDAD) often follows antibiotic use, although other factors, such as chemotherapy or critical illness, can cause disease. The other factors are thought to be critical for the development of CDAD.

33. Answer e

Intravenous vancomycin is not effective in *C. difficile*-associated disease.

34. Answer a

This patient responded well to the initial course of metronidazole and would therefore be expected to respond well again. Antibiotic resistance is uncommon in *C. difficile*, so it is not necessary to switch to vancomycin if the recurrence is mild, as in this case. Colonoscopy and high-dose or prolonged metronidazole are not indicated in this patient.

35. Answer c

The patient's family history fulfills Amsterdam II criteria for hereditary nonpolyposis colorectal cancer (HNPCC) syndrome. The "bump" on the eyelid may well be a sebaceous carcinoma of the upper eyelid, which is consistent with the Muir-Torre variant of HNPCC syndrome. The Muir-Torre variant is more common in men than in women, and colorectal cancers tend to be located in the proximal rather than the distal colorectum. Therefore, full structural evaluation with colonoscopy should be performed. Additional information regarding when and how to screen patients at risk for heritable colorectal cancer syndromes can be found in the review article by Winawer et al. (Gastroenterology. 2003;124:544-60).

36. Answer e

Because the available family history includes a first-degree relative with an adenomatous polyp diagnosed before age 60 years, colonoscopy every 5 years is recommended, beginning at age 40 (or 10 years younger than the earliest diagnosis in the family, whichever comes first). The additional family history of a third-degree relative with colorectal cancer does not influence current guidelines. Additional information regarding screening tests and screening or surveillance intervals among patients with a family history of adenomatous polyps can be found in the review article by Winawer et al. (Gastroenterology. 2003;124:544-60).

37. Answer c

Because the adenoma in the ascending colon was larger than 1 cm in diameter, the patient should be considered at high risk for development of metachronous (recurrent) neoplasia. Colonoscopy is the preferred surveillance test in this clinical setting and should be performed in 3 years. Additional information on postpolypectomy surveillance strategies can be found in the American College of Gastroenterology Practice Guidelines published by Bond (Am J Gastroenterol. 2000;95:3053-63).

38. Answer e

The Spigelman classification system for duodenal adenomas is based on number, size, histology, and degree of dysplasia. Patients with stage IV disease are at the highest risk for development of duodenal adenocarcinoma and should be monitored with more comprehensive endoscopic surveillance or treated with prophylactic pancreaticoduodenectomy. Further details regarding the Spigelman classification system and duodenal cancer in patients with FAP can be found in the articles by Spigelman et al. (Lancet. 1989;2:783-5) and Groves et al. (Gut. 2002;50:636-41).

39. Answer e

By definition, malignant polyps contain cancer cells that have invaded into the submucosa. Stalk invasion of a pedunculated polyp does not qualify as an unfavorable prognostic criterion as long as the cancer cells do not extend to the margin of stalk resection. Findings of poor differentiation, vascular or lymphatic involvement, or cancer cells present at the margin of excision should prompt consideration of surgical resection. Additional details regarding management of malignant polyps can be found in the American College of Gastroenterology Practice Guidelines published by Bond (Am J Gastroenterol. 2000;95:3053-63).

40. Answer d

Although for some clinicians an alternating bowel pattern is sine qua non for irritable bowel syndrome, this symptom has not been supported in factor analyses and is not a part of the diagnostic criteria for irritable bowel syndrome.

41. Answer c

This woman has typical symptoms of irritable bowel syndrome and likely has an exaggerated gastrocolic reflex. The yield of any diagnostic test is low, and extensive diagnostic testing is discouraged. However, evaluation of the colon has been considered cost-effective for screening for colorectal cancer in asymptomatic patients and thus should be cost-effective in people presenting with symptoms. Certainly, bacterial overgrowth and carcinoid tumor are possibilities but are unlikely, and thus testing for these conditions should be reserved for people who do not respond. Celiac disease is recognized as presenting with symptoms similar to those of irritable bowel syndrome. Blood tests can serve as an initial screening rather than going directly to small-bowel biopsy.

42. Answer d

Although irritable bowel syndrome has a significant impact on a person's quality of life, it does not increase the risk of cancer or lead to complications that require surgery or nutritional support or have an impact on pregnancies. The natural history is to fluctuate over time with changes in symptoms and can include times of quiescence. It may never go away.

43. Answer c

Although irritable bowel syndrome is a chronic relapsing condition, one needs to be wary when an affected patient older than 50 years has a change in symptoms. The risk of malignancy in irritable bowel syndrome is not increased, yet affected patients are not protected against malignancy such as ovarian cancer. Thus, a change in symptoms, especially with alarm symptoms such as weight loss, should be evaluated before they are assumed to be a continuation of irritable bowel syndrome.

44. Answer e

Patients with irritable bowel syndrome frequently have concurrent mood disorders. These need to be acknowledged and managed appropriately. Studies in these patients have shown that the quality of the physician-patient relationship improves outcome. Aggressive investigation in this situation is low-yield and may well raise patient expectations regarding an alternative diagnosis.

SECTION VI

Liver I

CHAPTER 27

Approach to the Patient With Abnormal Liver Tests and Fulminant Liver Failure

John J. Poterucha, M.D.

The management of patients who have abnormal liver tests or fulminant liver failure depends on many clinical factors, including the chief complaints of the patient, patient age, risk factors for liver disease, personal or family history of liver disease, medications, and physical examination findings. Because of all these factors, standard algorithms for the management of liver test abnormalities are often inefficient. Nevertheless, with some basic information, gastroenterologists should be able to evaluate liver test abnormalities in an efficient, cost-effective manner and appropriately manage patients who have acute liver failure. To achieve this goal, this chapter includes the following:

1. General discussion of commonly used liver tests
2. Differential diagnosis and discussion of diseases characterized by an increase in hepatocellular enzyme levels
3. Differential diagnosis and discussion of diseases characterized by an increase in cholestatic enzyme levels
4. Evaluation of a patient who has jaundice
5. Diagnostic algorithms for patients with abnormal liver tests
6. Management of patients who have fulminant liver failure

COMMONLY USED LIVER TESTS

Aminotransferases (Alanine and Aspartate Aminotransferases)

The aminotransferases (also referred to as "transaminases") are located in hepatocytes and, thus, are markers of liver cell injury (hepatocellular disease). Injury of the hepatocyte membrane allows these enzymes to "leak" out of hepatocytes, and within a few hours after liver injury, the serum levels of these enzymes increase. Aminotransferases consist of alanine aminotransferase (ALT) and aspartate aminotransferase (AST). ALT is relatively specific for liver injury, whereas AST is found not only in hepatocytes but also in skeletal and cardiac muscle and in other organs. Marked muscle injury can produce striking increases in AST levels and, in some cases, in ALT levels.

Alkaline Phosphatase

Alkaline phosphatase is an enzyme located on the hepatocyte membrane bordering bile canaliculi (the smallest branches of the bile ducts). Because alkaline phosphatase is found also in bone and placenta, an increase in its level without other indication of liver disease should prompt further testing to discover if the increase is from liver or other tissues; determining the concentration of alkaline phosphatase isoenzymes is one way. Another is determining the level of γ-glutamyltransferase, an enzyme of intrahepatic biliary canaliculi. Other than to confirm the liver origin of an increased level of alkaline phosphatase, γ-glutamyltransferase has little role in the evaluation of diseases of the liver because its synthesis can be induced by many medications, thus decreasing its specificity for clinically important liver disease.

Bilirubin

Bilirubin is the water-insoluble product of heme metabolism that is taken up by the hepatocyte and conjugated with glucuronic acid to form monoglucuronides and diglucuronides. Conjugation makes bilirubin water-soluble, allowing it to be excreted in bile. The serum concentration of bilirubin is measured in direct (conjugated) and indirect (unconjugated) fractions. Diseases characterized by overproduction of bilirubin, such as hemolysis or resorption of a hematoma, are characterized by hyperbilirubinemia that is 20% or less conjugated bilirubin. Hepatocyte dysfunction or impaired bile flow produces hyperbilirubinemia that is usually 50% or more conjugated bilirubin. Because conjugated bilirubin is water-soluble and may be excreted in urine, patients with conjugated hyperbilirubinemia may note dark urine. In these patients, the stools are lighter in color because of the absence of bilirubin pigments.

Prothrombin Time and Albumin

Prothrombin time and serum albumin are true markers of liver synthetic function. Abnormalities of prothrombin time and albumin imply severe liver disease and should prompt immediate evaluation. Prothrombin time is a measure of the activity of factors II, V, VII, and X, all of which are synthesized in the liver. These factors also are dependent on vitamin K for synthesis. Vitamin K deficiency may be produced by antibiotics, prolonged fasting, small-bowel mucosal disorders such as celiac disease, or severe cholestasis with an inability to absorb fat-soluble vitamins. Hepatocellular dysfunction is characterized by an inability to synthesize clotting factors despite adequate stores of vitamin K. A simple way to differentiate vitamin K deficiency from hepatocellular dysfunction in a patient with a prolonged prothrombin time is to administer vitamin K. Administration of vitamin K improves prothrombin time within 2 days in a vitamin K-deficient patient but has no effect if the prolonged prothrombin time is due to liver disease with poor synthetic function.

Because albumin has a half-life of 21 days, decreases due to liver dysfunction do not occur acutely; however, the serum level of albumin can decrease relatively quickly in a patient who has a severe systemic illness such as bacteremia. This rapid decrease is likely caused by the release of cytokines, with accelerated metabolism of albumin. Other causes of hypoalbuminemia include urinary or gastrointestinal tract losses, and these should be considered in a hypoalbuminemic patient without overt liver disease.

HEPATOCELLULAR DISORDERS

Diseases that primarily affect hepatocytes are termed "hepatocellular disorders" and are characterized predominantly by increased levels of aminotransferases. The disorders are best categorized as "acute" (generally less than 3 months) or "chronic." Acute hepatitis may be accompanied by malaise, anorexia, abdominal pain, and jaundice. Common causes of acute hepatitis are listed in Table 1.

The pattern of increase in aminotransferase levels may be helpful in making a diagnosis. Acute hepatitis caused by viruses or drugs generally produces a marked increase in the levels of aminotransferases, often more than 1,000 U/L. Generally,

ALT increases more than AST. Aminotransferase levels above 3,000 U/L are usually due to acetaminophen hepatotoxicity, ischemic hepatitis ("shock liver"), or hepatitis caused by unusual viruses, such as herpesvirus. Ischemic hepatitis occurs in patients after an episode of hypotension. Aminotransferase levels improve within a few days. Another cause of a transient increase in aminotransferase levels is transient obstruction of the bile duct, usually from a stone. These increases can be as high as 1,000 U/L, but the levels decrease dramatically within 24 to 48 hours. In patients with pancreatitis, a transient increase in AST or ALT suggests gallstone pancreatitis. Alcoholic hepatitis is characterized by more modest increases in aminotransferase levels, nearly always less than 400 U/L, with an AST:ALT ratio greater than 2:1. Patients with alcoholic hepatitis frequently have a markedly increased level of bilirubin out of proportion to the increase in aminotransferase levels.

Diseases producing sustained (>3 months) increases in aminotransferase levels are included in the category of "chronic hepatitis." The increase in aminotransferase levels generally is more modest (2-5 times) than that in acute hepatitis. Although patients may be asymptomatic, they occasionally complain of fatigue and right upper quadrant pain. The differential diagnosis for chronic hepatitis is relatively lengthy, but the most important and common disorders are listed in Table 2.

Risk factors for hepatitis C include a history of blood transfusions or intravenous drug use. Patients with hepatitis B may give a history of illegal drug use or frequent sexual contacts or they may be from an endemic area such as Asia or Africa. Patients with nonalcoholic fatty liver disease are usually

Table 1. Common Causes of Acute Hepatitis

Disease	Clinical clue	Diagnostic test
Hepatitis A	Exposure history	IgM anti-HAV
Hepatitis B	Risk factors	HBsAg, IgM anti-HBc
Drug-induced	Compatible medication	Improvement after withdrawal of agent
Alcoholic hepatitis	History of alcohol excess, AST:ALT >2, AST <400 U/L	Liver biopsy, improvement with abstinence
Ischemic hepatitis	History of severe hypotension	Rapid improvement of aminotransferase levels

ALT, alanine aminotransferase; AST, aspartate aminotransferase; HAV, hepatitis A virus; HBc, hepatitis B core; HBsAg, hepatitis B surface antigen.

Table 2. Common Causes of Chronic Hepatitis

Disease	Clinical clue	Diagnostic test
Hepatitis C	Risk factors	Anti-HCV, HCV RNA
Hepatitis B	Risk factors	HBsAg
Nonalcoholic fatty liver disease	Obesity, diabetes mellitus, hyperlipidemia	Ultrasonography, liver biopsy
Hemochromatosis	Arthritis, diabetes mellitus, family history	Iron studies, gene test, biopsy
Alcoholic liver disease	History, AST:ALT >2	Liver biopsy, improvement with abstinence
Autoimmune hepatitis	ALT 200-1,500 U/L, usually female, other autoimmune disease	Antinuclear or anti-smooth muscle antibody, biopsy

ALT, alanine aminotransferase; AST, aspartate aminotransferase; HBsAg, hepatitis B surface antigen; HCV, hepatitis C virus.

obese or have diabetes mellitus or hyperlipidemia. A complete history is needed to help diagnose drug-induced or alcohol-induced liver disease. Genetic hemochromatosis is a common disorder that affects about 1/300 people of Northern European ancestry. Many patients with genetic hemochromatosis have normal liver enzyme levels. The disease is transmitted in an autosomal recessive manner, so patients may have a family history of liver disease or hepatocellular carcinoma. Genetic hemochromatosis also causes diabetes mellitus, hypogonadism, and joint complaints. Autoimmune hepatitis may present as acute or chronic hepatitis. Patients usually have higher levels of aminotransferases than do patients with other disorders that cause chronic hepatitis. Autoantibodies, hypergammaglobulinemia, and other autoimmune disorders are helpful clues to the diagnosis of autoimmune hepatitis.

CHOLESTATIC DISORDERS

Diseases that affect predominantly the biliary system are termed "cholestatic diseases." These can affect the microscopic ducts (e.g., primary biliary cirrhosis), large bile ducts (e.g., pancreatic cancer causing common bile duct obstruction), or both (e.g., primary sclerosing cholangitis). In these disorders, the predominant abnormality generally is in alkaline phosphatase. Although diseases that produce increased bilirubin levels are often called "cholestatic," it is important to remember that

severe hepatocellular injury, as in acute hepatitis, also produces hyperbilirubinemia because of hepatocellular dysfunction. Common causes of cholestasis are listed in Table 3.

Primary biliary cirrhosis generally occurs in middle-aged women who may complain of fatigue or pruritus. Primary sclerosing cholangitis has a strong association with ulcerative colitis. Patients with primary sclerosing cholangitis often are asymptomatic but may have jaundice, fatigue, or pruritus. Large bile duct obstruction often is due to stones or benign or malignant strictures. Remember that acute large bile duct obstruction from a stone may produce marked increases in aminotransferase levels. Intrahepatic mass lesions should be considered if a patient has cholestatic liver test abnormalities and a history of malignancy. Infiltrative disorders such as amyloidosis, sarcoidosis, or lymphoma should also be considered. A clue to a possible infiltrative disorder is a markedly increased alkaline phosphatase level with a normal bilirubin concentration. Any systemic inflammatory process such as infection or immune disorder may produce nonspecific liver test abnormalities. The abnormalities usually are a mixed cholestatic (alkaline phosphatase) and hepatocellular (ALT or AST) pattern.

JAUNDICE

Jaundice is visibly evident hyperbilirubinemia and occurs when the bilirubin concentration is more than 2.5 mg/dL. It is

Table 3. Common Causes of Cholestasis

Disease	Clinical clue	Diagnostic test
Primary biliary cirrhosis	Middle-aged woman	Antimitochondrial antibody
Primary sclerosing cholangitis	Association with ulcerative colitis	ERCP, MRCP
Large bile duct obstruction	Jaundice and pain are common	Ultrasonography, ERCP, MRCP
Drug-induced	Compatible medication/timing	Improvement after withdrawal of agent
Infiltrative disorder	History of malignancy, amyloidosis, sarcoidosis	Ultrasonography, computed tomography
Inflammation-associated	Symptoms of underlying inflammatory disorder	Blood cultures, appropriate antibody tests

ERCP, endoscopic retrograde cholangiopancreatography; MRCP, magnetic resonance cholangiopancreatography.

important to determine whether the increase is predominantly conjugated or unconjugated bilirubin. A common disorder that produces unconjugated hyperbilirubinemia (but not usually jaundice) is Gilbert syndrome. Total bilirubin is generally less than 3.0 mg/dL, whereas direct bilirubin is 0.3 mg/dL or less. The level of bilirubin generally is higher when a patient is fasting or is ill. A presumptive diagnosis of Gilbert syndrome can be made in an otherwise well patient who has unconjugated hyperbilirubinemia, normal liver enzyme values, and a normal concentration of hemoglobin (to exclude hemolysis).

Direct hyperbilirubinemia is more common than indirect hyperbilirubinemia in patients with jaundice. Patients can be categorized as those with a nonobstructive condition and those with an obstructive condition. Abdominal pain, fever, or a palpable gallbladder (or a combination of these) is suggestive of obstruction. Risk factors for viral hepatitis, a bilirubin concentration more than 15 mg/dL, and persistently high aminotransferase levels suggest that the jaundice is due to hepatocellular dysfunction. In patients with acute hepatocellular dysfunction, improvement in bilirubin concenration often lags the improvement in aminotransferase level. A sensitive, specific, and noninvasive test to exclude an obstructive cause of jaundice is liver ultrasonography. In diseases characterized by large bile duct obstruction, the intrahepatic bile ducts generally are dilated, especially if the bilirubin concentration is more than 10 mg/dL and the patient has had jaundice for longer than 2 weeks. Acute large bile duct obstruction, usually from a stone, may not cause dilatation of the bile ducts, and if the clinical suspicion is strong for bile duct obstruction despite normal-sized bile ducts on ultrasonography, the extrahepatic duct should be imaged with endoscopic retrograde cholangiopancreatography (ERCP), magnetic resonance cholangiopancreatography (MRCP), or endoscopic ultrasonography.

GENERAL APPROACH TO ABNORMAL LIVER TESTS

When a patient has abnormal liver tests at presentation, it is helpful to classify the patient's condition as one of the clinical syndromes listed in Table 4. The overlap among these categories is considerable. Patients with acute hepatitis or cirrhosis often have jaundice. The approach to patients with acute hepatitis, chronic hepatitis, cholestasis, and jaundice is outlined above. Patients with a "first-time" increase in liver enzyme levels are generally asymptomatic, and liver test abnormalities are found incidentally. As long as 1) no risk factors for liver disease are identified, 2) liver enzyme levels are less than three times normal, 3) liver function is preserved, and 4) the patient feels well, observation is reasonable, with the test repeated in a few months. If the repeat test results are still abnormal, the patient's condition fits the category of chronic hepatitis or cholestasis

and appropriate evaluation should be initiated. A similar approach can be taken for patients with incidentally discovered abnormal liver tests who are taking medications that only rarely cause liver disease.

Patients also may present with cirrhosis or portal hypertension. Most patients with portal hypertension have cirrhosis, although occasionally patients present with noncirrhotic portal hypertension that is idiopathic or due to portal vein thrombosis. The evaluation of a patient with cirrhosis is similar to that of a patient with chronic hepatitis and cholestasis (as shown above). Alpha$_1$-antitrypsin deficiency, genetic hemochromatosis, and alcoholic liver disease frequently present with cirrhosis, with or without portal hypertension, as the first manifestation of liver disease. If a patient has clinical features that strongly suggest cirrhosis, confirmatory liver biopsy is not necessary.

ALGORITHMS FOR PATIENTS WITH ABNORMAL LIVER TESTS

At best, algorithms for abnormal liver tests are guidelines, and at worst, they are misleading. Always remember that in evaluating (or not evaluating) abnormal liver tests, the patient's clinical presentation should be considered. Generally, a patient with liver test abnormalities that are less than twice normal may be followed as long as the patient is asymptomatic and the albumin level, prothrombin time, or bilirubin concentration is normal. Persistent abnormalities should also be evaluated. Algorithms for evaluating increased ALT, alkaline phosphatase, and conjugated bilirubin levels are shown in Figures 1 to 3.

MANAGEMENT OF FULMINANT LIVER FAILURE

"Fulminant liver failure" has been defined traditionally as the presence of acute liver failure, including the development of hepatic encephalopathy, within 8 weeks after the onset of jaundice in a patient without a previous history of liver disease. Because not all patients with severe acute liver disease meet this strict definition, some authors have proposed the term "acute liver failure," which encompasses other clinical scenarios, including fulminant liver failure. There are about 2,000

Table 4.   Abnormal Liver Tests: Clinical Syndromes

"First-time" increase in liver enzymes
Acute hepatitis
Chronic hepatitis
Cholestasis without hepatitis or jaundice
Jaundice
Cirrhosis or portal hypertension

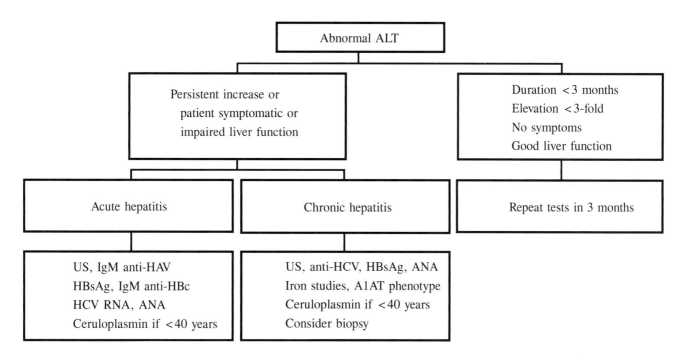

Fig. 1. Evaluation of abnormal alanine aminotransferase (ALT). A1AT, alpha₁-antitrypsin; ANA, antinuclear antibody; HAV, hepatitis A virus; HBc, hepatitis B core; HBsAg, hepatitis B surface antigen; HCV, hepatitis C virus; US, ultrasonography.

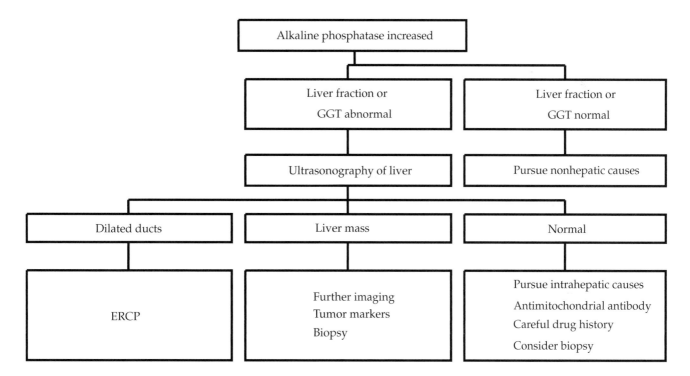

Fig. 2. Evaluation of increased alkaline phosphatase levels. ERCP, endoscopic retrograde cholangiopancreatography; GGT, γ-glutamyltransferase.

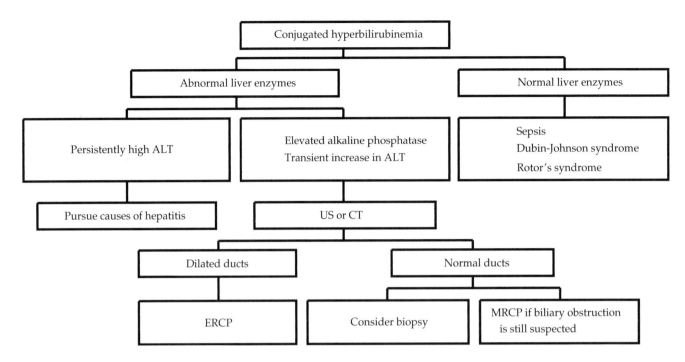

Fig. 3. Evaluation of conjugated hyperbilirubinemia. ALT, alanine aminotransferase; CT, computed tomography; ERCP, endoscopic retrograde cholangiopancreatography; MRCP, magnetic resonance cholangiopancreatography; US, ultrasonography.

cases of fulminant liver failure in the United States annually. The overall mortality of fulminant liver failure without liver transplantation is high. Because many of the patients are young and previously healthy, the outcomes of this relatively unusual condition are particularly tragic. Specific management, including liver transplantation, is available, and knowledge of management strategies is important.

Determining the cause of fulminant liver failure is important for two reasons: one, specific therapy may be available, as for acetaminophen hepatotoxicity or herpes hepatitis, and, two, the prognosis differs depending on the cause. For instance, the spontaneous recovery rate for fulminant liver failure due to acetaminophen or hepatitis A is more than 50%; consequently, a more cautious approach would be advised before proceeding with liver transplantation. In comparison, spontaneous recovery from fulminant liver failure due to Wilson's disease is unusual and early liver transplantation would be recommended. Also, identifying a specific cause may have implications for other patients. The identification of a hepatotoxic agent is helpful in monitoring other patients receiving the same drug treatment. Identification of a viral cause of fulminant liver failure has implications for other patients who have been exposed to the transmissible agent.

The U.S. Acute Liver Failure Study Group has coordinated the effort of several centers that have attempted to better define the causes and outcome of acute liver failure in the United States. The most common identifiable causes are acetaminophen hepatotoxicity, idiosyncratic drug reactions, hepatitis A and B, and ischemia (Fig. 4).

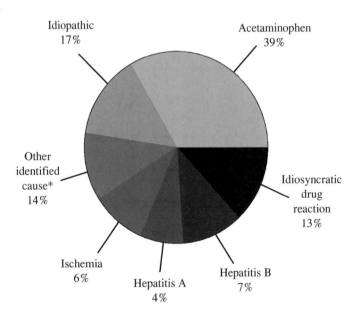

Fig. 4. Cause of fulminant liver failure in the United States, 1998-2001. *Includes autoimmune hepatitis, Wilson's disease, Budd-Chiari syndrome, pregnancy-associated, malignancy, heat stroke, sepsis, and giant cell hepatitis.

The presenting symptoms of fulminant liver failure are usually those of acute hepatitis, including malaise, nausea, and jaundice. Portal systemic encephalopathy is a required feature of the syndrome, and manifestations may range from subtle mental status changes, such as difficulty with concentration, to coma (Table 5). Because encephalopathy in a patient with acute liver disease is an ominous sign, the mental status of patients with acute hepatitis should be assessed frequently. Laboratory features of fulminant liver failure are consistent with severe liver dysfunction. Aminotransferase levels are variably increased, although they usually are quite high. Fulminant Wilson's disease is characterized by only modest increases in aminotransferase levels and a normal or only minimally increased alkaline phosphatase level despite other, more typical laboratory evidence of liver failure. Evidence of hepatocellular dysfunction includes a prolonged prothrombin time and high bilirubin concentration.

The encephalopathy associated with fulminant liver failure is likely different from that of chronic liver disease. The major difference is the propensity of encephalopathy of acute liver disease to progress to cerebral edema. The mechanisms for the development of cerebral edema have not been clarified but may involve disruption of the blood-brain barrier and interference with mechanisms of cellular osmolarity. Clinically, the encephalopathy often is associated with an increase in the serum level of ammonia, although alterations in neurotransmitters likely are involved in causing mental status changes.

Cerebral edema is estimated to cause about 20% of deaths of patients with fulminant liver failure; however, autopsy studies of patients who died of fulminant liver failure have showed that only 50% of them had cerebral edema. Cerebral edema leads to death by causing brain ischemia and cerebral herniation. Because the signs and symptoms of cerebral edema are not specific, intracranial pressure monitoring often is necessary. Computed tomography (CT) of the brain is relatively insensitive for detecting cerebral edema but is useful for excluding other causes of mental status changes, particularly intracerebral bleeding.

Hypoglycemia is a frequent manifestation of fulminant liver failure, and the glucose level should be monitored carefully in all patients. The hypoglycemia is likely due to both inadequate degradation of insulin and diminished production of glucose by the diseased liver.

Infections are another common cause of death of patients with fulminant liver failure. Reasons for the infections are multiple but likely reflect severe illness and the need for numerous interventions and monitoring. The clinical features typical of infection, such as fever and leukocytosis, are not reliable in patients with fulminant liver failure. A high index of suspicion needs to be maintained, and any clinical deterioration should mandate a search for infection.

Table 5. Stages of Hepatic Encephalopathy

Stage	Features
I	Changes in behavior, with minimal change in level of consciousness
II	Gross disorientation, gross slowness of mentation, drowsiness, asterixis, inappropriate behavior, able to maintain sphincter tone
III	Sleeping most of the time, arousable to vocal stimuli, marked confusion, incoherent speech
IV	Comatose, unresponsive to pain, includes decorticate or decerebrate posturing

A hyperdynamic circulation and decrease in systemic vascular resistance frequently accompany fulminant liver failure. Although these features may be well tolerated by patients, occasionally hemodynamic compromise can develop. Monitoring parameters may mimic sepsis. Fluid resuscitation often is necessary, although caution is advised because the administration of excessive fluid may worsen intracranial pressure.

Renal and electrolyte abnormalities occur because of underlying disease such as Wilson's disease, functional renal failure due to sepsis or hepatorenal syndrome, or acute tubular necrosis. Renal dysfunction may be more common when fulminant liver failure is due to acetaminophen hepatotoxicity. Monitoring of electrolytes, including sodium, potassium, bicarbonate, magnesium, and phosphorus, is important. Lactic acidosis also is common in fulminant liver failure, likely because of hypoperfusion and the inability of the diseased liver to clear lactate. The presence of acidosis is a risk factor for poor outcome in fulminant liver failure and has been incorporated into prognostic models.

Several models have attempted to predict outcome of fulminant liver failure. These have been developed to facilitate optimal timing of liver transplantation before the patient becomes so ill that transplantation is contraindicated. The most well known and widely used are the King's College criteria (Table 6). Liver transplantation likely improves mortality, but improved outcomes have been assessed only by comparison with historical controls.

The appearance of encephalopathy precedes cerebral edema; therefore, patients with acute hepatitis and evidence of liver failure need to be monitored carefully for mental status changes. Patients with encephalopathy should receive lactulose, although this agent is not as effective in acute liver failure as in chronic liver disease and may not prevent cerebral edema developing later. Patients with stage II encephalopathy are generally admitted to an intensive care unit for close monitoring of mental status and vital signs. It is especially important that sedatives be avoided at this point to allow close monitoring of mental

Table 6.   King's College Criteria for Liver Transplantation in Fulminant Liver Failure*

1. Fulminant liver failure due to Wilson's disease or Budd-Chiari syndrome
2. Acetaminophen-induced if either of the following are met:
   a. pH < 7.3 24 hours after overdose
   b. Creatinine > 3.4 mg/dL and prothrombin time > 100 s and grade 3-4 encephalopathy
3. Nonacetaminophen if either
   a. INR > 6.5 *or*
   b. Any three of the following: INR > 3.5, more than 7 days from jaundice to encephalopathy, indeterminate or drug-induced cause, age < 10 years, age > 40 years, bilirubin > 17.5 mg/dL

INR, *international normalized ratio.*
*Any one of the three criteria.

status. Also, at most centers, CT of the head is performed to exclude an alternative cause of mental status changes.

Patients who reach stage III encephalopathy are at considerable risk for progression to cerebral edema. Because clinical signs and CT are insensitive for detecting increased intracranial pressure, many centers institute intracranial pressure monitoring when patients reach stage III encephalopathy. Endotracheal intubation and mechanical ventilation usually precede placement of the intracranial pressure monitor. Various such monitors are used, all of which can be complicated by infection and bleeding. The goal of intracranial pressure monitoring is to allow treatment of high pressure and also to identify which patient is too ill for liver transplantation because of a prolonged period of excessively high intracranial pressure. Generally, the goal is to maintain intracranial pressure less than 40 mm Hg and cerebral perfusion pressure (the difference between mean arterial pressure and intracranial pressure) between 60 and 100 mm Hg. Excessively high cerebral perfusion pressures (above 120 mm Hg) can result in worsening cerebral edema.

Maneuvers that cause straining, including tracheal suctioning, should be avoided or limited. Paralyzing agents and sedatives may be necessary although they may limit further assessment of neurologic status. For intracranial pressure more than 20 mm Hg or cerebral perfusion pressure less than 60 mm Hg, elevation of the head to 20 degrees, hyperventilation to a $PaCO_2$ of 25 mm Hg, and mannitol (if renal function is intact) are advised. Barbiturate-induced coma or hypothermia can be used for refractory cases. A prolonged increase in intracranial pressure above mean arterial pressure may signify brain death and generally is a contraindication to liver transplantation. A sudden decrease in intracranial pressure may indicate brain herniation.

The prolonged prothrombin time seen in patients with fulminant liver failure is a simple noninvasive measure to follow, and coagulopathy generally is not corrected unless there is bleeding or a planned intervention such as placement of a monitoring device. If bleeding occurs or an invasive procedure is necessary, fresh frozen plasma generally is administered first. Administration of platelets and fibrinogen may be necessary in certain circumstances. Continuous infusion of 5% or 10% dextrose is used to keep the plasma glucose level between 100 and 200 mg/dL. The plasma glucose level should be monitored at least twice daily. Both bacteremia and fungemia are sufficiently frequent that periodic blood cultures are advised and prophylaxis with antimicrobials may be used, although this practice has not been shown to affect survival.

Liver transplantation has revolutionized the management of fulminant liver failure, which is the indication for 6% of liver transplants in the United States. Even though survival with transplantation for fulminant liver failure is lower than that for transplantation for other indications, outcomes are an improvement over the dismal survival rates for fulminant liver failure when prognostic criteria such as the King's College criteria indicate a poor outcome. Transplantation should be performed when a poor outcome is anticipated, yet before the patient has uncontrolled sepsis or prolonged periods of increased intracranial pressure that prevent recovery even with a functioning transplanted liver.

RECOMMENDED READING

Green RM, Flamm S. AGA technical review on the evaluation of liver chemistry tests. Gastroenterology. 2002;123:1367-84.

Kamath PS. Clinical approach to the patient with abnormal liver test results. Mayo Clin Proc. 1996;71:1089-94.

O'Grady JG, Alexander GJ, Hayllar KM, Williams R. Early indicators of prognosis in fulminant hepatic failure. Gastroenterology. 1989;97:439-45.

Ostapowicz G, Fontana RJ, Schiodt FV, Larson A, Davern TJ, Han SH, et al, U.S. Acute Liver Failure Study Group. Results of a prospective study of acute liver failure at 17 tertiary care centers in the United States. Ann Intern Med. 2002;137:947-54.

Poterucha JJ. Fulminant hepatic failure. In: Johnson LR, editor. Encyclopedia of gastroenterology. Vol 2. Amsterdam: Elsevier Academic Press; 2004. p. 70-4.

Pratt DS, Kaplan MM. Evaluation of abnormal liver-enzyme results in asymptomatic patients. N Engl J Med. 2000;342:1266-71.

Viggiano TR, Sedlack RE, Poterucha JJ. Gastroenterology and hepatology. In: Habermann TM, editor. Mayo Clinic internal medicine board review 2004-2005. Philadelphia: Lippincott Williams & Wilkins; 2004. p. 253-330.

CHAPTER 28

Chronic Viral Hepatitis

John J. Poterucha, M.D.

Viral infections are important causes of liver disease worldwide. The five primary hepatitis viruses that have been identified are A, B, C, D (or delta), and E. Other viruses such as cytomegalovirus or Epstein-Barr virus can also result in hepatitis as part of a systemic infection. In addition, medications, toxins, autoimmune hepatitis, or Wilson's disease may cause acute or chronic hepatitis.

It is useful to divide hepatitis syndromes into "acute" and "chronic" forms. Acute hepatitis can last from weeks up to 6 months and is often accompanied by jaundice. Symptoms of acute hepatitis tend to be similar regardless of the cause and include anorexia, malaise, dark urine, fever, and mild abdominal pain. Patients with chronic hepatitis are often asymptomatic but may complain of fatigue. Occasionally, they have manifestations of cirrhosis (ascites, variceal bleeding, or encephalopathy) as the initial presentation of chronic hepatitis. Each hepatitis virus causes acute hepatitis, but only hepatitis B, C, and D viruses can cause chronic hepatitis.

The purpose of this chapter is to review the primary hepatitis viruses. A more comprehensive discussion of acute hepatitis is found in other chapters. The primary hepatitis viruses are compared in Table 1, and the effects of the three most important viruses in the United States are summarized in Table 2.

HEPATITIS A

Epidemiology

Hepatitis A virus (HAV) causes about 40% of cases of acute viral hepatitis in the United States. The major routes of transmission of HAV are ingestion of contaminated food or water and contact with an infected person. Groups at particularly high risk include people living in or traveling to underdeveloped countries, children in day care centers, homosexual men, and perhaps persons who ingest raw shellfish. Outbreaks of HAV infection in communities are frequently recognized, although an exact

Table 1. Comparison of Four Primary Hepatitis Viruses

Feature	HAV	HBV	HDV	HCV
Incubation, d	15-50	30-160	Unknown	14-160
Jaundice	Common	30% of patients	Common	Uncommon
Course	Acute	Acute or chronic	Acute or chronic	Acute or chronic
Transmission	Fecal-oral	Parenteral	Parenteral	Parenteral
Test for diagnosis	IgM anti-HAV	HBsAg	Anti-HDV	HCV RNA

HAV, hepatitis A virus; HBV, hepatitis B virus; HBsAg, hepatitis B surface antigen; HCV, hepatitis C virus; HDV, hepatitis D virus.

Table 2. Clinical Effect of Hepatitis Viruses in the United States*

	HAV	HBV	HCV
Acute infections, (× 1,000)/y	93,000	78,000	25
Fulminant, deaths/y	50	100	Rare
Chronic infections	0	1-1.25 million	2.8-4 million
Chronic liver disease, deaths/y	0	5,000	8,000-10,000

HAV, hepatitis A virus; HBV, hepatitis B virus; HCV, hepatitis C virus.
*The Centers for Disease Control and Prevention estimates, 2001.

source may not be found. The incubation period for HAV is 2 to 6 weeks.

Clinical Presentation and Natural History

The most important determinant of the severity of acute hepatitis A is the age at which infection occurs. Persons infected when younger than 6 years have nonspecific symptoms that rarely include jaundice. Adolescents or adults who acquire HAV infection usually have jaundice. Hepatitis A is almost always a self-limited infection. There may be a prolonged cholestatic phase characterized by persistence of jaundice for up to 6 months. Rarely, acute hepatitis A presents as fulminant hepatitis that may require liver transplantation. HAV does *not* cause chronic infection and should not be in the differential diagnosis of chronic hepatitis.

Diagnostic Tests

The diagnosis of acute hepatitis A is established by the presence of IgM hepatitis A antibody (anti-HAV), which appears at the onset of the acute phase of the illness and disappears in 3 to 6

months. The IgG anti-HAV also becomes positive during the acute phase, but it persists for decades and is a marker of immunity from further infection. A patient with IgG anti-HAV, but not IgM anti-HAV, has had an infection in the remote past or has been vaccinated.

Treatment and Prevention

The treatment of acute hepatitis A is supportive. Immune serum globulin should be administered to all household and intimate (including day care) contacts within 2 weeks after exposure. Hepatitis A vaccine should be offered to travelers to underdeveloped countries, homosexual men, intravenous drug users, and patients with chronic liver disease. Widespread vaccination of health care workers or food handlers has not been advised.

HEPATITIS B

Epidemiology

Hepatitis B virus (HBV) is a DNA virus that causes about 30% of cases of acute viral hepatitis and 15% of cases of chronic viral hepatitis in the United States. Major risk factors for disease acquisition in the United States are sexual promiscuity and intravenous drug use. HBV infection is also common in Asia and Africa, where it is usually acquired perinatally or in early childhood. Many infected immigrants to the United States from high endemic areas probably acquired HBV by these routes.

Diagnostic Tests

A brief guide to serologic markers for hepatitis B is provided in Table 3. The interpretation of serologic patterns is found in Table 4. The best serologic test for acute hepatitis B is IgM antibody to hepatitis B core (anti-HBc). Occasionally, a patient with acute hepatitis B (usually with a severe presentation such as fulminant hepatitis) lacks hepatitis B surface antigen (HBsAg) and has only IgM anti-HBc as the marker for recent infection.

Increasingly sensitive tests for HBV DNA are now available. Nearly all patients with HBsAg have HBV DNA in serum when

Table 3. Hepatitis B Serologic Markers

Test	Significance
Hepatitis B surface antigen (HBsAg)	Current infection
Antibody to hepatitis B surface (anti-HBs)	Immunity (immunization or resolved infection)
IgM antibody to hepatitis B core (IgM anti-HBc)	Usually recent infection, occasionally "reactivation" of chronic infection
IgG antibody to hepatitis B core (IgG anti-HBc)	Remote infection
Hepatitis B e antigen (HBeAg) and/or HBV DNA > 10^5 viral copies/mL	Active viral replication (high infectivity)

Table 4.   Interpretation of Hepatitis B Serologic Patterns

HBsAg	Anti-HBs	IgM anti-HBc	IgG anti-HBc	HBeAg	Anti-HBe	HBV DNA	Interpretation
+	–	+	–	+	–	+	Usually acute infection, occasionally acute flare of chronic hepatitis B
–	+	–	+	–	±	–	Previous infection with immunity
–	+	–	–	–	–	–	Vaccination with immunity
+	–	–	+	–	+	$< 10^5$	Chronic hepatitis B without replication
+	–	–	+	+	–	$> 10^5$	Chronic hepatitis B with replication
+	–	–	+	–	+	$> 10^5$	HBeAg-negative chronic hepatitis B (often "precore" or "core promoter" variants)

HBc, hepatitis B core; HBe, hepatitis B e; HBeAg, hepatitis B e antigen; HBsAg, hepatitis B surface antigen; HBV, hepatitis B virus.

measured by a highly sensitive test such as the polymerase chain reaction (PCR). Commercially available tests now quantify HBV DNA. HBV DNA levels greater than 10^5 copies/mL are generally considered to indicate active viral replication. Lower levels in a patient with cirrhosis may also be clinically important.

Occasionally, patients have IgG anti-HBc as the only positive hepatitis B serologic marker. There are several possible explanations. The most common reason in a low-risk population is a false-positive test (although the test is often repeatedly positive). Another explanation is a previous, resolved HBV infection in which the antibody to hepatitis B surface (anti-HBs) has decreased below the limit of detection. This can be documented indirectly by demonstrating an anamnestic type of response to hepatitis B vaccine. Finally, patients with hepatitis B may have HBsAg levels that are below the level of detection so that IgG anti-HBc is the only marker of infection.

Although the significance of this low-level infection is unclear, these patients can be identified by the presence of HBV DNA (sensitive assays such as PCR may be necessary) in the serum or liver.

The usefulness of serologic tests obviates the need for liver biopsy in the diagnosis of hepatitis B; however, liver biopsy is useful for grading inflammatory activity and determining the stage of fibrosis. Histologic features of hepatitis B are inflammation that usually is around the portal tract, variable fibrosis that initially is also portocentric, and the presence of ground-glass hepatocytes. Ground-glass hepatocytes are hepatocytes whose cytoplasm has a hazy, eosinophilic appearance. With immunostaining, these cells are positive for HBsAg (Fig. 1). Even though liver biopsy is the "gold standard" for diagnosing cirrhosis, biopsy generally is not necessary in patients who have other features of cirrhosis such as portal hypertension.

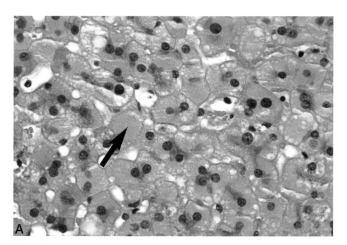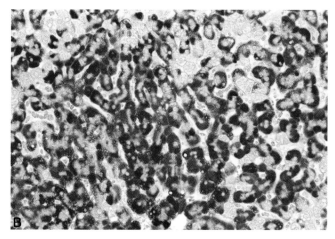

Fig. 1. Liver biopsy specimen from patient with hepatitis B. *A*, Ground-glass hepatocyte (*arrow*). (Hematoxylin-eosin.) *B*, Immunostain for hepatitis B surface antigen showing positive staining of hepatocyte cytoplasm.

Clinical Presentation and Natural History

The incubation period after HBV infection ranges from 30 to 160 days, and the clinical outcome varies. Acute hepatitis B in an adolescent or adult is icteric in about 30% of cases. Complete recovery with subsequent life-long immunity occurs in 95% of infected adults. About 5% of infected adults have persistence of HBsAg for longer than 6 months and are referred to as "chronically infected." Immunosuppressed persons with acute HBV infection are more likely to become chronically infected, presumably because of an insufficient immune response against the virus.

The outcome of chronic infection with HBV is also variable (Fig. 2). Patients with normal liver enzyme levels and normal findings on liver biopsy despite the persistence of HBsAg are referred to as "inactive carriers." Persons with inactive disease have a good prognosis, although they still carry an increased risk of hepatocellular carcinoma. Their overall survival is not very different from that of the noninfected population. Persons with chronic HBV infection, abnormal liver tests, active viral replication, and abnormal liver biopsy findings have "chronic hepatitis B" and are at higher risk for the development of cirrhosis and hepatocellular carcinoma than are inactive carriers. Seroconversion from hepatitis B e antigen (HBeAg)-positive to HBeAg-negative and anti-HBe–positive occurs in about 10% of patients per year. This seroconversion is followed by a decrease in alanine aminotransferase (ALT) and HBV DNA level and an improved prognosis. Patients with chronic hepatitis B may also experience spontaneous flares of disease characterized by markedly abnormal aminotransferase levels, deterioration in liver function, and often seroconversion of HBeAg. The differential diagnosis for acute hepatitis in patients with chronic hepatitis B is listed in Table 5. HBsAg clears spontaneously in about 1% of chronically infected patients annually, although this rate is lower in endemic areas where HBV is acquired at a very young age.

Patients with chronic hepatitis B and cirrhosis are at high risk for the development of hepatocellular carcinoma, and surveillance with ultrasonography and alpha fetoprotein every 6 to

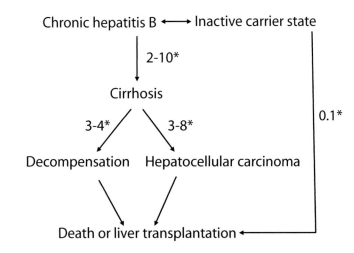

Fig. 2. Natural history of chronic hepatitis B. *Per 100 patient-years.

12 months is advised. Surveillance should also be considered for patients without cirrhosis who meet one of the following criteria: family history of hepatocellular carcinoma, Asian male older than 40 years, Asian female older than 50 years, and black Africans older than 20 years.

Treatment

Generally, hepatitis B is treated if the patient is at risk for progression. This includes patients who have liver enzyme levels more than twice the upper limit of normal, active viral replication (as defined by HBV DNA more than 10^{4-5} copies/mL), and active disease identified in liver biopsy specimens.

Hepatitis B can be treated with interferon or one of the oral agents (lamivudine, adefovir, or entecavir). These agents are compared in Table 6. Pegylated interferon will likely replace standard interferon because of once-weekly dosing and better efficacy. Seroconversion may occur months or even years after completion of treatment. Predictors of greater likelihood of

Table 5. Causes of Acute Hepatitis in Patients With Chronic Hepatitis B

Cause	Clinical clues
Spontaneous "reactivation" of hepatitis B	Seroconversion of HBeAg, reappearance of IgM anti-HBc
Flare due to immune suppression	Chemotherapy, antirejection therapy, corticosteroids
Induced by antiviral therapy	Interferon (common), oral agents (rare)
Superimposed infection with other viruses, especially hepatitis D virus	Exposure to hepatitis D (usually due to illicit drug use), A, or C
Other causes of acute hepatitis	History of alcohol excess, medications, illegal drugs

HBc, hepatitis B core; HBeAg, hepatitis B e antigen.

Table 6. Agents for Treatment of Hepatitis B

Treatment	Pegylated interferon	Lamivudine	Adefovir	Entecavir
Length, mo	12	Often indefinite	Often indefinite	Often indefinite
Side effects	Many	Minimal	Rare renal	Minimal
Cost/mo, $US	1,700	230	630	700
Disease flare	Common	Rare	Rare	Rare
HBeAg seroconversion, % of patients	30	20	15	20
HBsAg seroconversion, % of patients	10	Rare	Rare	Rare
Resistance, %/y	None	15	1-4	Unknown
Durability of response, % of patients	90	50	Unknown	Unknown

HBeAg, hepatitis B e antigen; HBsAg, hepatitis B surface antigen.

response include higher ALT level, lower HBV DNA level, shorter duration of disease, and female sex. Patients treated with interferon may experience a flare of hepatitis (likely due to immune system activation) about 4 to 8 weeks after beginning treatment. Treatment should be continued despite this flare unless there is clinical or biochemical evidence of decompensation. Patients with Child-Pugh class B or C cirrhosis should not be treated with interferon because of the risk of precipitating decompensation with this flare. Side effects of interferon are common and are considered below (HEPATITIS C).

The oral agents have become popular for the treatment of chronic hepatitis B. These drugs are remarkably free of side effects, although adefovir can occasionally cause nephrotoxicity. The oral agents are particularly useful in patients with decompensated cirrhosis because these drugs may improve liver function. The flare of hepatitis that may occur during interferon therapy is unusual with the oral agents. Lamivudine treatment is complicated by resistant mutations at a rate of about 10% to 15% per year. Resistance to adefovir occurs at a rate of about 1% to 4% per year. Resistance to entecavir is uncommon, although data with long-term treatment are needed. Adefovir and entecavir are effective against lamivudine-resistant strains. About 15% to 20% of patients treated with oral agents have seroconversion of HBeAg after 1 to 2 years of therapy, and treatment should be continued for at least 6 months after seroconversion. Patients without seroconversion of HBeAg need to continue treatment indefinitely. Seroconversion of HBsAg with the oral agents occurs only rarely and should not be considered a reasonable treatment goal.

The choice of therapeutic agent for hepatitis B depends on several factors. As noted above, only active hepatitis should be treated. Interferon is reasonable for patients without cirrhosis who have an ALT level less than 200 U/L and who are able to tolerate the numerous side effects of the drug. The oral agents are preferred for patients with cirrhosis, particularly if there is evidence of decompensation. Patients with long-standing hepatitis B, such as adults who acquired the disease in the perinatal period, are not likely to have a response to interferon treatment, and the oral agents are advised. Oral agents are also preferred for patients who are immunosuppressed, for example, after organ transplantation or infection with human immunodeficiency virus (HIV). Finally, oral agents are probably more effective for HBeAg-negative chronic hepatitis B, although courses of interferon longer than the usual 4 to 6 months show promise. Patients with hepatitis B who need a course of chemotherapy have an increased risk of disease flare, and treatment with one of the oral agents is advised.

For patients with end-stage liver disease due to hepatitis B, liver transplantation is advised. Listing for transplantation is recommended when a patient has seven Child-Pugh points or hepatocellular carcinoma complicating cirrhosis. Patients with hepatitis B who have HBeAg or high HBV DNA levels (or both) before liver transplantation are at particularly high risk for recurrence after transplantation. For these patients, oral agents are recommended before transplantation and a combination of hepatitis B immune globulin and an oral agent after transplantation. Even in patients without active viral replication, recurrence rates are sufficiently high that both preoperative and postoperative therapy is still given by most transplant groups.

Prevention

Hepatitis B immune globulin should be given to household and sexual contacts of patients with acute hepatitis B. Infants and previously unvaccinated 10- to 12-year-old children (who are reaching the age when they will be at highest risk for acquiring disease) should receive hepatitis B vaccine. The marker of immunity is anti-HBs. Neonates often acquire hepatitis B peri-natally if the mother is infected. Because infected neonates are at high risk for the development of chronic infection, HBsAg testing should be performed on all pregnant women. If a pregnant woman is HBsAg-positive, the infant should receive both hepatitis B immune globulin and hepatitis B vaccine.

HEPATITIS D

Hepatitis D virus (HDV or the delta agent) is a defective virus that requires the presence of HBsAg to replicate. Consequently, there is no reason to search for HDV unless HBsAg is present. HDV infection can occur simultaneously with HBV (coinfection) or as a superinfection in persons with established hepatitis B. Hepatitis D is diagnosed by antibodies to HDV (anti-HDV) and should be suspected if a patient has acute hepatitis B or an acute exacerbation of chronic hepatitis B. In the United States, intravenous drug users are the group of HBV patients at highest risk for acquiring HDV.

HEPATITIS C

Hepatitis C virus (HCV) is the cause of the most common chronic blood-borne infection in the United States. It has been estimated that 3 to 4 million Americans are infected with the virus; about 70% of them have abnormal ALT levels. Although the number of new cases of HCV infection is decreasing, the number of deaths is increasing because of the propensity of the virus to cause chronic infection. HCV is a factor in 40% of all cases of chronic liver disease and is the leading indication for liver transplantation.

Diagnostic Tests

Antibodies to HCV (anti-HCV) indicate exposure to the virus and are not protective. The presence of anti-HCV can indicate either current infection or a previous infection with subsequent clearance. Even after clearance of the infection, only about 10% of patients lose anti-HCV. The presence of anti-HCV in a patient who has an abnormal ALT level and risk factors for acquiring hepatitis C is strongly suggestive of current HCV infection. The initial test for identifying anti-HCV is enzyme-linked immunoassay. False-positive results for anti-HCV by this test are unusual but can occur in patients with hypergam-maglobulinemia (e.g., patients with autoimmune hepatitis). The specificity (but not sensitivity) of enzyme-linked immunoassay for anti-HCV is improved with the addition of the recombinant immunoblot assay for anti-HCV. A guide to the interpretation of anti-HCV tests is provided in Table 7.

The "gold standard" for the diagnosis of hepatitis C infection is the presence of HCV RNA in serum as determined by PCR. Most reference laboratories are able to reproducibly perform this HCV RNA assay with a sensitivity limit of 50 viral copies/mL. HCV RNA by PCR is now the preferred next test (bypassing anti-HCV by recombinant immunoblot assay) for patients with abnormal liver enzyme levels or for those at high risk for HCV infection who are found to be anti-HCV–positive by enzyme-linked immunoassay. A proposed diagnostic algorithm is shown in Figure 3.

Levels of HCV RNA do not correlate with disease severity or prognosis, and the major use of quantitative assays is to stratify response to therapy. Patients with viral levels more than 2 million copies/mL are less likely to have a response to treatment. Determination of HCV genotype is also helpful in assessing the likelihood of treatment response. Patients with HCV genotype 1 (which comprises about 70% of U.S. patients) are less likely to have a response to therapy. Liver biopsy is not necessary for the diagnosis of hepatitis C, but it is helpful in assessing severity of disease for prognostication and in making decisions about treatment and screening. Typical biopsy findings include a mononuclear (predominantly lymphocytic) portal hepatitis with lymphoid follicles and mild steatosis (Fig. 4).

Clinical Presentation and Natural History

The incubation period of HCV ranges from 2 to 22 weeks (mean, 7.5 weeks). Infection with HCV rarely presents clinically as acute hepatitis, although retrospective studies have suggested that 10% to 20% of patients have an icteric illness with acute infection. Of those who acquire hepatitis C, 60% to 85% develop chronic infection (Fig. 5). Once chronic infection has been established, subsequent spontaneous loss of the virus is rare. Consequently, most patients with hepatitis C present with chronic hepatitis, with a mild-to-moderate increase in ALT levels. For patients with abnormal ALT levels, the degree of increase correlates poorly with histologic severity of disease. Some patients have fatigue or vague right upper quadrant pain (or both). Patients may also come to attention because of complications of

Table 7. Interpretation of Anti-HCV Results

Anti-HCV		Interpretation
By EIA	By RIBA	
+	−	False-positive EIA, patient does not have true antibody
+	+	Patient has antibody*
+	Indeterminate	Uncertain antibody status

EIA, enzyme-linked immunoassay; HCV, hepatitis C virus; RIBA, recombinant immunoblot assay.
*Anti-HCV does not necessarily indicate current HCV infection (see text).

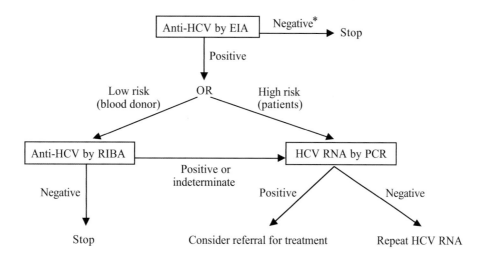

Fig. 3. Algorithm for diagnosing hepatitis C. *Rarely, patients (especially if immunosuppressed) may have hepatitis C without a positive anti-HCV. If clinical suspicion remains high, HCV RNA may be performed. EIA, enzyme-liked immunoassay; HCV, hepatitis C virus; PCR, polymerase chain reaction; RIBA, recombinant immunoblot assay.

end-stage liver disease or, rarely, extrahepatic complications such as cryoglobulinemia or porphyria cutanea tarda (PCT). Patients with hepatitis C-associated cryoglobulinemia should be treated for hepatitis C. PCT presents as a rash on sun-exposed areas, particularly the back of the hands. Many patients also have abnormal iron test results. The response of PCT to anti-hepatitis C therapy is more uncertain than the response of cryoglobulinemia. Phlebotomy improves the rash of PCT and generally is considered first-line therapy.

Up to 30% of patients chronically infected with HCV have a persistently normal level of ALT. These patients generally have less aggressive histologic features and a lower risk of disease progression than do patients with hepatitis C and abnormal ALT levels. The role of liver biopsy and the treatment of hepatitis C patients with normal ALT levels are debated, but most hepatologists manage patients with normal ALT levels similarly to those with abnormal ALT levels.

Nearly all mortality and most morbidity associated with hepatitis C are due to cirrhosis. About 20% to 30% of patients with chronic hepatitis C develop cirrhosis over a 10- to 20-year period (Fig. 5). Multiple factors have been studied to identify the subgroup of patients likely to develop progressive liver disease. Important factors are duration of infection, alcohol intake of more than 50 g/d, steatosis, coinfection with HIV or HBV, and male sex. Patients with cirrhosis due to HCV generally have had the disease longer than 20 years.

Perhaps the most important predictive factor for the development of cirrhosis is the severity of the histologic features of the liver at presentation. Histologic specimens need to be interpreted with knowledge of the duration of infection (if known). Patients who have only mild portal hepatitis without fibrosis

despite 20 years of infection have a significantly lower risk of progression than those who have more active disease with a similar duration of infection. Histologic markers of more active disease include moderate degrees of inflammation and necrosis and the presence of periportal or septal fibrosis. Liver biopsy should be performed in most patients being considered for treatment of hepatitis C to assist in decisions about treatment.

Treatment

The mortality and morbidity of chronic hepatitis C are related largely to cirrhosis. Consequently, treatment should be given to patients who are at highest risk for the development of cirrhosis: an anticipated long duration of hepatitis C, a history of

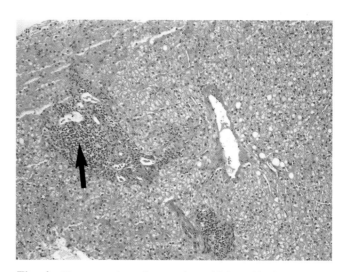

Fig. 4. Biopsy specimen from patient with hepatitis C. Note portal infiltrate, lymphoid follicle (*arrow*), and mild steatosis.

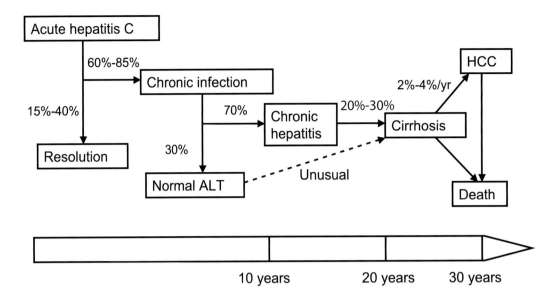

Fig. 5. Natural history of hepatitis C. ALT, alanine aminotransferase; HCC, hepatocellular carcinoma. Percent values refer to patients.

alcohol use, or active disease with at least periportal fibrosis seen in liver biopsy specimens. Patients who have a high probability of having a response to treatment, for example, those with genotype 2 or 3, may be considered candidates for treatment regardless of liver biopsy findings. Thus, biopsy is not always necessary before treatment. It is important to know whether patients have cirrhosis because if they do, they need to be monitored for the development of esophageal varices and hepatocellular carcinoma. For patients with clear evidence of portal hypertension, biopsy to confirm cirrhosis is not necessary. Therapy also should be offered to patients who have extrahepatic manifestations of hepatitis C, such as vasculitis related to cryoglobulinemia. In addition, patients who have an anticipated long lifespan, such as those younger than 40 years, might be offered treatment independently of liver biopsy findings. Treatment may be indicated to reduce potential transmission, for example, a health care worker who performs invasive procedures.

Currently, pegylated interferon in combination with the oral agent ribavirin is the standard of care for patients with hepatitis C who are deemed treatment candidates. This combination therapy, given for 6 to 12 months, results in a sustained clearance of HCV RNA from serum in about 55% of patients. Baseline variables associated with a sustained response to combination therapy include HCV genotype 2 or 3, HCV RNA levels less than 2.0 million copies/mL, no or only portal fibrosis, female sex, and age younger than 40 years. Patients who receive at least 80% of the planned dose of interferon and ribavirin for the duration of therapy are more likely to have a response, especially if HCV genotype 1.

Hepatitis C genotype and viral level should be determined before the initiation of treatment. When treating patients with genotypes 1 or 4, the HCV RNA level should be determined after 12 weeks of therapy (Fig. 6). Patients who do not achieve a 2 $\log_{10}$ decrease in HCV RNA level from the pretreatment value have a very low rate of sustained response and treatment may be discontinued. Those with a 2 $\log_{10}$ decrease (or HCV RNA-negative) at 12 weeks should continue to receive treatment, and HCV RNA determined at 24 weeks. Those who are HCV RNA-positive at 24 weeks will not achieve a sustained response, and treatment can be stopped. Patients who are HCV RNA-negative at 24 weeks should complete a total of 48 weeks of treatment.

Patients with genotype 2 or 3 have a high rate of response, and determining the HCV RNA level at 12 weeks probably is not cost-effective (Fig. 7). If therapy is poorly tolerated and a decision needs to be made about continuing therapy, the 12-week stop rule described for genotype 1 may be applied. Otherwise, treatment should be continued for a total of 24 weeks.

The most troublesome side effects of hepatitis C therapy are hematologic and neuropsychiatric. Anemia is the most common reason for prematurely discontinuing hepatitis C combination therapy. Ribavirin causes a dose-dependent, reversible hemolysis that is evident within 4 weeks after treatment is initiated. Interferon, because of its bone-marrow–suppressive effects, interferes with erythropoiesis that may otherwise compensate for the ribavirin-induced hemolysis. Fatigue, dyspnea, or symptoms of cardiovascular disease may accompany anemia. Because ribavirin-induced hemolysis is dose-dependent, dose reduction usually improves the hemoglobin level but perhaps at the expense of treatment efficacy.

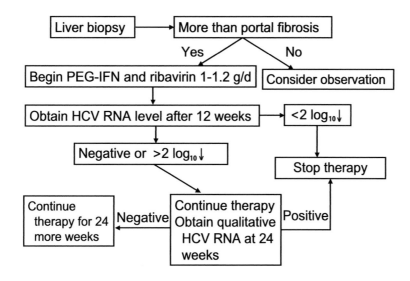

Fig. 6. Management of HCV genotype 1. HCV, hepatitis C virus; PEG-IFN, pegylated interferon.

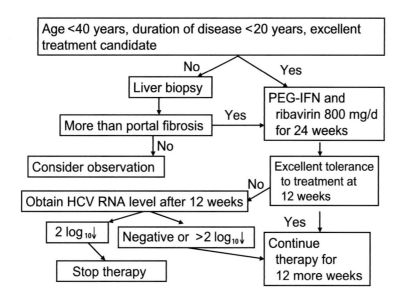

Fig. 7. Management of HCV genotype 2 or 3. HCV, hepatitis C virus; PEG-IFN, pegylated interferon.

Erythropoietin has been used to maintain hemoglobin levels (and therefore ribavirin doses) in patients treated for hepatitis C. Whether erythropoietin-induced improvements in hemoglobin level and ribavirin dosing will lead to improved hepatitis C response rates has not been demonstrated. Patient age, symptoms associated with anemia, risk factors for or presence of cardiovascular disease, and body size should be considered when deciding whether to use erythropoietin.

Neutropenia that occurs during hepatitis C therapy is due to interferon. An absolute neutrophil count less than 500 cells/mL occurs rarely. Serious infections are extremely rare except perhaps in patients with other risk factors for infection, for example, decompensated cirrhosis. Consequently, neutropenia seldom requires intervention in interferon-treated patients.

Most neuropsychiatric side effects of hepatitis C therapy are due to interferon, although anemia and other side effects of ribavirin may potentiate symptoms. The prevalence of neuropsychiatric side effects among patients with hepatitis C is high even before treatment, and baseline mood status may influence the likelihood of dose-limiting neuropsychiatric manifestations of interferon. Pretreatment education for patients and family members about the potential for these side effects is helpful. Reassurance is also important because many patients are able to deal with the neuropsychiatric manifestations by realizing that they are related to treatment and will resolve once treatment has been discontinued. Nevertheless, 30% of patients treated for HCV require the introduction or addition of medications for the treatment of these side effects. Routine "preemptive" therapy is not necessary because 70% to 80% of patients treated for hepatitis C will not require antidepressants during therapy.

Patients with suicidal ideation should discontinue interferon therapy and be referred to psychiatry. For patients with notable depression without suicidal ideation, a selective serotonin reuptake inhibitor such as citalopram can be prescribed. For patients with a prominent anxiety or irritability component of depression, a less activating selective serotonin reuptake inhibitor such as paroxetine, fluvoxamine, or mirtazapine may be helpful. Mirtazapine is also useful for patients who have considerable weight loss with interferon therapy. Fluoxetine, sertraline, venlafaxine, and bupropion are more activating and, thus, may be preferred for patients who have fatigue or cognitive slowing. Patients who have persistent depression despite treatment with antidepressants are referred to psychiatry.

Patients who are not candidates for treatment should be evaluated annually with routine liver tests. For those with early-stage disease, repeat liver biopsy in 3 to 5 years may be indicated to assess for histologic progression. Patients with cirrhosis are at increased risk for hepatocellular carcinoma, particularly if they have a history of alcohol excess. The risk of hepatocellular carcinoma complicating hepatitis C with cirrhosis is 1.4% to 4% per year. Screening with alpha fetoprotein and liver ultrasonography every 6 to 12 months is advised for patients with cirrhosis who are candidates for treatment of hepatocellular carcinoma with liver transplantation, liver resection, or percutaneous ablation.

Patients with HCV and cirrhosis (including those with hepatocellular carcinoma) should be considered for liver transplantation. Currently, patients with 7 Child-Pugh points are eligible for listing and should be referred if there are no contraindications. In patients who received a liver transplant for hepatitis C, posttransplant viremia is nearly universal and histologic changes in the allograft due to recurrent disease are common. Nevertheless, the survival rate is good, and hepatitis C is the leading indication for liver transplantation in the United States.

Prevention

No vaccine is available for hepatitis C. Transmission by needlestick injury is rare, although monitoring after inadvertent exposure is advised. Baseline anti-HCV testing with subsequent HCV RNA 4 weeks after exposure is recommended. Documented acute infections probably should be treated to prevent chronic infection. Perinatal exposure is also uncommon, but it may be more likely if the mother is also infected with HIV. Maternally derived anti-HCV may be found in the neonate for up to 18 months after birth, thus limiting the usefulness of serologic assays for diagnosis; instead, HCV RNA testing should be used.

For patients infected with HCV, donation of blood is prohibited. Precaution needs to be taken when caring for open sores of HCV-infected patients. Sexual transmission is unusual, but condoms are advised for those with multiple sex partners. For patients in a monogamous long-term relationship, the partner should be tested and the couple counseled about the possibility of transmission. The decision about the use of condoms is left to the infected person and partner.

HEPATITIS E

Hepatitis E causes large outbreaks of acute hepatitis in underdeveloped countries. Physicians in the United States are unlikely to have a patient with hepatitis E. Rarely, a patient may become infected during foreign travel. Clinically, hepatitis E virus infection is similar to HAV infection. Resolution of the hepatitis is the rule, and chronic infection does not occur. Women who acquire hepatitis E during pregnancy may present with fulminant liver failure.

RECOMMENDED READING

Alberti A, Fattovich G. Natural history of chronic hepatitis B [abstract]. Curr Hepatitis Rep. 2004;3:54-60.

Liang TJ, Rehermann B, Seeff LB, Hoofnagle JH. Pathogenesis, natural history, treatment, and prevention of hepatitis C. Ann Intern Med. 2000;132:296-305.

Lok AS, Heathcote EJ, Hoofnagle JH. Management of hepatitis B: 2000: summary of a workshop. Gastroenterology. 2001;120:1828-53.

Lok AS, McMahon BJ, Practice Guidelines Committee, American Association for the Study of Liver Diseases. Chronic hepatitis B. Hepatology. 2001;34:1225-41.

Lok AS, McMahon BJ, Practice Guidelines Committee, American Association for the Study of Liver Diseases (AASLD). Chronic hepatitis B: update of recommendations. Hepatology. 2004;39:857-61.

Poterucha JJ. Hepatitis A. In: Johnson LR, editor. Encyclopedia of gastroenterology. Amsterdam: Elsevier Academic Press; 2004. p. 311-5.

Russo MW, Fried MW. Side effects of therapy for chronic hepatitis C. Gastroenterology. 2003;124:1711-9.

Strader DB, Wright T, Thomas DL, Seeff LB, American Association for the Study of Liver Diseases. Diagnosis, management, and treatment of hepatitis C. Hepatology. 2004;39:1147-71. Erratum in: Hepatology. 2004;40:269.

CHAPTER 29

Liver Mass Lesions

Gregory J. Gores, M.D.

A CLINICAL QUESTION-BASED APPROACH TO THE EVALUATION OF LIVER MASS LESIONS

Liver mass lesions are a common diagnostic and management problem in clinical practice. Despite the myriad diagnostic possibilities (Table 1) and plethora of management approaches, the evaluation of these lesions is straightforward. This chapter emphasizes a clinical question-based approach useful in the evaluation of these lesions. The approach follows standard clinical practice routines and is easily adaptable to bedside practices. The overall goal of the clinician is to distinguish rapidly between benign and malignant lesions. In particular, the clinician wants to know if the lesion is a simple liver cyst, a cavernous hemangioma, focal fatty change, or focal nodular hyperplasia. Patients with these diagnostic entities can be given reassurance, and intervention or monitoring is not warranted. Other lesions, including abscesses, hepatic adenomas, cystadenomas, cholangiocarcinomas, hepatocellular carcinomas, and metastases, need either further investigation or other definitive treatment approaches.

Is the Patient Symptomatic?

Neither the presence nor absence of abdominal discomfort ensures that the lesion is either benign or malignant. Indeed, imaging studies that initially identify the mass lesion frequently are performed for evaluation of abdominal discomfort. Aside from pain or abdominal discomfort, certain symptoms help in distinguishing between benign and malignant disease. Symptoms such as night sweats, low-grade fever, involuntary weight loss, anorexia, and diarrhea often signify malignant disease. Night sweats and fevers support the diagnosis of malignancy or liver abscess. In the absence of fever, the diagnosis of liver abscess

Table 1. Liver Mass Lesions

Benign lesions
Angiolipoma
Cavernous hemangioma
Cystadenoma
Echinococcal cyst
Focal fatty change
Focal nodular hyperplasia
Hepatic adenoma
Inflammatory pseudotumor
Liver abscess
Simple liver cyst
Malignant lesions
Cystadenocarcinoma
Fibrolamellar hepatocellular carcinoma
Hepatic epithelioid hemangioendotheliomatosis
Hepatocellular carcinoma
Intrahepatic cholangiocarcinoma
Metastases
Mixed hepatic tumor
Mixed hepatocellular cholangiocarcinoma
Sarcomas

is extremely unlikely. Occasionally, hepatocellular carcinomas present with a syndrome of fever and leukocytosis, simulating an infectious process. Diarrhea is common in hepatocellular carcinoma and with neuroendocrine tumors metastatic to the liver. Anorexia and weight loss are common symptoms of advanced malignancy. Abdominal discomfort is a less useful symptom in making a diagnosis. Many patients have unexplained right upper quadrant abdominal discomfort; thus, this symptom is less specific. Furthermore, large benign tumors occasionally distend the capsule of the liver, causing abdominal discomfort. Patients with hepatic adenomas associated with intra-adenoma or intrahepatic hemorrhage also can present with acute and severe abdominal pain. Occasionally, a hepatocellular carcinoma ruptures through the capsule and causes a pain syndrome indistinguishable from biliary colic; the pain is abrupt in onset, lasts several hours, and then recedes, leaving the patient pain-free. Hemorrhage into the peritoneum from an adenoma or hepatocellular carcinoma causes an acute abdomen, often with hypotension, and is a medical emergency. Most early primary and metastatic tumors to the liver are pain-free and asymptomatic. When patients with malignant liver disease have pain, it is often epigastric and signifies advanced disease with regional lymph node metastases.

Other important aspects of the history are whether the patient has a history of chronic liver disease and whether imaging studies have been performed. A history of inflammatory bowel disease or primary sclerosing cholangitis (or both) favors the diagnosis of cholangiocarcinoma. A history of noncholestatic chronic liver disease (especially viral, alcohol, and hemochromatosis) makes hepatocellular carcinoma a high diagnostic possibility. It is important to obtain previous imaging studies. The presence of a new lesion or an enlarging mass suggests a malignant process.

What Are the Key Features of the Physical Examination When Evaluating Liver Mass Lesions?

When evaluating liver mass lesions, focus the examination on the issue of whether the patient has evidence of chronic liver disease or signs of metastatic disease outside the liver. Evidence of chronic liver disease includes cutaneous stigmata (spider angiomas and palmar erythema), splenomegaly, and bilobar enlargement of the liver. Jaundice, peripheral edema, and ascites are less specific because they may occur also with advanced metastatic disease. The author has not observed peripheral adenopathy in a patient with hepatocellular carcinoma or cholangiocarcinoma, and the presence of peripheral adenopathy is virtually diagnostic of metastatic disease. A bruit over the liver is most consistent with hepatocellular carcinoma and usually indicates advanced disease.

What Is an Appropriate Laboratory Evaluation for a Patient With a Liver Mass?

The laboratory evaluation is outlined in Table 2. Briefly, the evaluation should include a liver panel (i.e., aspartate aminotransferase, alanine aminotransferase, alkaline phosphatase, bilirubin, albumin, and prothrombin time). Marked increases in the levels of aminotransferases suggest either an active

necroinflammatory liver disease or an extensive infiltrative neoplastic disease of the liver (see below). A cholestatic biochemical profile is most consistent with a mass effect or bile duct obstruction (or both). Screening tests for hepatitis C and B should be performed because the presence of viral markers makes the diagnosis of hepatocellular carcinoma likely. Iron studies are useful to screen for hemochromatosis, a risk factor for hepatocellular carcinoma, and to check for gastrointestinal tract blood loss, a finding that raises the possibility of metastatic colorectal carcinoma. Serum tumor markers for hepatocellular carcinoma (i.e., alpha fetoprotein), cholangiocarcinoma (i.e., CA 19-9), and gastrointestinal metastatic adenocarcinoma (i.e., carcinoembryonic antigen) also are useful.

After the history, physical examination, and laboratory evaluation, the physician should be able to answer the following questions:

- Is the patient symptomatic, and do the symptoms help distinguish between benign and malignant disease?
- Does the patient have chronic liver disease, making the diagnosis of hepatocellular carcinoma likely (or cholangiocarcinoma if the patient has primary sclerosing cholangitis)?
- Are viral markers present or are tumor marker levels increased?

What Are the Imaging Characteristics of the Mass Lesion?

The imaging characteristics of liver mass lesions are critical for making diagnostic and management decisions. Because the

Table 2.   Laboratory Evaluation of Liver Mass Lesions

Liver panel
    Aspartate aminotransferase (AST)
    Alanine aminotransferase (ALT)
    Alkaline phosphatase
    Albumin
    Bilirubin
    Prothrombin time
Viral markers
    Hepatitis C virus antibody
    Hepatitis B surface antigen (HBsAg)
    Antibody to hepatitis B core antigen (Anti-HBcAg)
    Antibody to hepatitis B surface antigen (Anti-HBsAg)
Tumor markers
    Alpha fetoprotein
    Carcinoembryonic antigen
    CA 19-9
Iron studies

distinction between benign and malignant lesions frequently can be made radiographically, the common benign and liver mass lesions are reviewed in the following sections, along with clinical management. However, a detailed discussion of the management of hepatocellular carcinoma is beyond the scope of this chapter.

BENIGN LIVER MASS LESIONS

Cavernous Hemangiomas

Cavernous hemangiomas are extremely common, occurring in 7% of adults in autopsy studies. A female predilection (1.5-5:1) has been noted. Although usually single, hemangiomas may be multicentric in up to 30% of patients. They also frequently coexist with focal nodular hyperplasia (see below). Histologically, these tumors consist of an extensive network of vascular spaces lined by endothelial cells and separated by a thin, fibrous stroma. Thrombosis, scarring, and calcifications may be present in large hemangiomas. These processes are responsible for the atypical imaging features of cavernous hemangiomas. Small cavernous hemangiomas are asymptomatic. Giant hemangiomas (> 10 cm) may cause fever, weight loss, anemia, and other associated systemic findings of inflammation. Malignant transformation does not occur. In the usual clinical situation, the goal of the clinician is to not mistake a cavernous hemangioma for a more serious lesion.

Imaging studies of cavernous hemangiomas usually are diagnostic, allowing the clinician to dismiss the lesion as a health concern. Ultrasonography shows a well-circumscribed, homogeneously hyperechoic lesion with smooth margins. Technetium Tc 99m–labeled red blood cell scintigraphy, dynamic bolus computed tomography (CT), and magnetic resonance imaging (MRI) are useful in confirming the diagnosis of cavernous hemangioma. The diagnosis can be made with a high degree of specificity (100%) and sensitivity (80%) using technetium Tc 99m–labeled red blood cell scintigraphy for lesions 3 cm or larger. Cavernous hemangiomas demonstrate decreased perfusion on early images and a high concentration of isotope within the lesion on late images (1 hour). This mismatch between early and late scintigraphic images is highly diagnostic of cavernous hemangiomas. Peripheral nodular enhancement during the arterial phase of contrast-enhanced CT and gadolinium MRI studies is also characteristic of cavernous hemangiomas (Fig. 1). Cavernous hemangiomas also are sharply demarcated, hyperintense lesions on T_2-weighted spin echo MRI scans. Biopsy of these lesions is seldom necessary. However, small lesions may show uniform enhancement, resembling metastases or primary tumors, and large lesions may be so scarred that the enhancement patterns are atypical. If the need to know is absolute, biopsy of the lesion can be

performed. A "skinny" needle biopsy can be performed safely by an experienced radiologist. Because of the scarring, the biopsy specimen may be relatively acellular with occasional vascular elements. This relatively "dry aspirate" is diagnostic and should not prompt another biopsy. Most cavernous hemangiomas do not require intervention and can be observed. Occasionally, symptomatic giant cavernous hemangiomas require surgical enucleation or resection.

Focal Nodular Hyperplasia

Focal nodular hyperplasia (FNH) is thought to occur by reaction of the liver to an intrahepatic arterial malformation. The reaction consists of a proliferation of hepatocytes separated by fibrous septa. The arterial malformation is associated with a vascular stellate scar of connective tissue and bile ductules. The presence of benign hepatic parenchyma with bile ductules in fibrous septa is the diagnostic histologic feature. Although FNH occurs predominantly in women of childbearing age, it is not related to oral contraceptive use. FNH may be multiple (10% of patients), and it may be associated with cavernous hemangiomas (22% of patients). It is associated rarely with fibrolamellar hepatocellular carcinoma and occasionally with arterial venous malformations elsewhere in the body.

Most patients with FNH are asymptomatic. Occasional patients with large lesions may have abdominal discomfort or an abdominal mass. The major decision to be made when evaluating a young woman who has a primary liver mass but

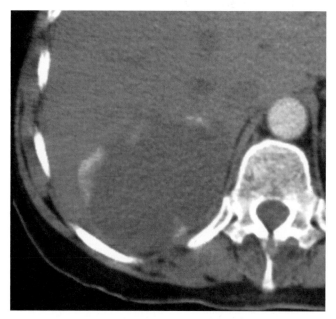

Fig. 1. Computed tomogram of a cavernous hemangioma in the posterior aspect of the right posterior liver lobe. The scan was taken early in the arterial phase of the study (contrast in the aorta). Note the peripheral nodular enhancement of the lesion; this is virtually diagnostic of cavernous hemangioma.

no underlying liver disease is whether the lesion is a cavernous hemangioma, FNH, hepatic adenoma, or fibrolamellar hepatocarcinoma. The distinction between FNH and hepatic adenoma is the most common important clinical diagnostic dilemma (Table 3). FNH does not rupture or have the risk of malignant transformation, but hepatic adenomas do. Thus, FNH lesions can be observed, but hepatic adenomas should be resected. The diagnosis of FNH can be made with radiologic imaging studies in 70% of cases. On ultrasonography, the lesions are ischemic or hypoechoic except for a linear hyperechoic central scar that contains the spider network of the arterial malformation. Color flow Doppler studies may show increased blood flow in the central stellate scar.

The classic features on contrast-enhanced CT include a hyperdense appearance during arterial phase studies and an isodense appearance during venous phase studies (Fig. 2). Indeed, the contrast enhancement with a rapid washout is virtually diagnostic. Furthermore, many FNH lesions have a lobulated contour that is also characteristic. On unenhanced MRI studies, FNH is typically isointense on T1-weighted images and either isointense or slightly hyperintense on T2-weighted studies. The central scar is usually hypointense on T1-weighted images but hyperintense on T2-weighted ones. Gadolinium contrast studies are similar to those described for CT images—rapid and intense contrast enhancement during arterial phase studies and a rapid washout. Technetium Tc 99m sulfur colloid scintigraphy demonstrates hyperintense or isointense uptake in 50% to 60% of cases of FNH because of the presence of Kupffer cells; uptake of colloid seldom occurs in hepatic adenomas, which usually are devoid of Kupffer cells. Also, labeled iminodiacetic acid derivatives used in biliary tract scintigraphy are taken up by the biliary elements of FNH, but the specificity of this observation is not clear. If FNH is diagnosed on the basis of classic radiographic imaging studies and the patient is asymptomatic and has normal serum levels of liver enzymes, no medical or surgical intervention is warranted. Fine-needle

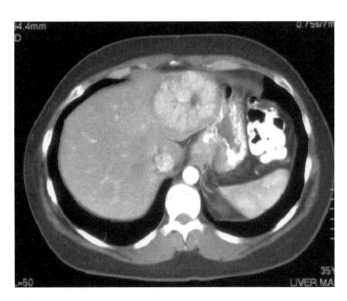

Fig. 2. Focal nodular hyperplasia. Computed tomogram obtained during the arterial phase. A markedly contrast-enhancing lesion is present in the left lobe of the liver. Contrast is not present in the center of the lesion (central scar). Also note that the lesion is relatively round. The imaging characteristics are those of focal nodular hyperplasia.

aspirates from these lesions are seldom helpful because the aspirates usually contain only hepatocytes and the clinician still does not know whether the lesion is an adenoma. Core biopsy specimens containing hepatocytes and biliary elements can be diagnostic in an appropriate clinical context.

Hepatic Adenomas

Hepatic adenomas are benign tumors consisting solely of hepatocytes, without bile ductules, fibrous septa, portal tracts, or central veins. They occur predominantly in young women; a strong association with oral contraceptives has been described. Hepatic adenomas also occur in patients with glycogen storage disease type IA, in patients who take methandrostenolone and methyltestosterone, and as a familial condition associated with diabetes mellitus. Multiple hepatic adenomatosis occurs and is usually an idiopathic disorder.

Most patients with hepatic adenoma are women of childbearing age. The tumors often are identified as incidental liver masses. However, hepatic adenomas have a propensity to rupture, presenting with intrahepatic hemorrhage or hemoperitoneum and shock. Limited intrahepatic hemorrhage causes pain. Aside from a mild increase in the serum level of alkaline phosphatase, the serum level of liver enzymes and the concentration of alpha fetoprotein are normal. The results of radiographic imaging studies are nonspecific, and the lesions cannot be differentiated from hepatocellular carcinoma by ultrasonography, CT, or MRI. Indeed, heterogeneity within a

Table 3. Comparison of Focal Nodular Hyperplasia (FNH) and Hepatic Adenoma (HA)

	FNH	HA
Young women	+	+
Estrogen-stimulated growth	–	+
Rupture	–	+
Malignant transformation	–	+
Central stellate scar on CT or MRI	+	–
Increased or normal uptake on scintigraphy	+	–
Bile ducts in fibrous septa	+	–

CT, computed tomography; MRI, magnetic resonance imaging.

lesion in regard to echogenicity, contrast enhancement, and density is the most characteristic finding. Moreover, small adenomas can demonstrate contrast enhancement because of neovascularity and thus can resemble hypervascular metastases or primary hepatocellular cancer. However, the presence of intratumoral hemorrhage favors the diagnosis of hepatic adenoma. Hepatic adenomas usually are single, but they may be multiple, especially in patients with glycogen storage disease. Hepatic adenomas have been observed to decrease in size after withdrawal of oral contraceptives, but this is infrequent. Moreover, despite withdrawal of oral contraceptives, growth occurs, and adenomas have been observed with foci of malignancy. Therefore, most experienced hepatologists and hepatobiliary surgeons favor resection or ablation of hepatic adenomas because of the risk of rupture and associated malignancy.

Simple Liver Cysts

Solitary and even multiple liver cysts are common, usually asymptomatic, and often coexist with other mass lesions in the liver. The female-to-male ratio is 4:1. The prevalence of simple liver cysts in the general population is approximately 3.6%, and it increases with age. Histopathologically, simple cysts are characterized as thin-walled structures lined by cuboidal bile duct epithelia. They are filled with isotonic fluid. Simple cysts are easy to diagnose radiographically because they are lucent on ultrasonography and have a water density on CT. The lesions are hyperintense on T2-weighted images and, if small, may be difficult to differentiate from a cavernous hemangioma. In the opinion of the author, ultrasonography is best for demonstrating wall thickness and, if present, internal septations in large cysts. Thick-walled cysts with nodularity or irregular septations suggest the diagnosis of cystadenoma or, rarely, cystadenocarcinoma. Simple, thin septations, however, are common in large cysts and should not cause alarm or concern regarding the diagnosis. Occasionally, cysts accumulate proteinaceous material over time, making the distinction between a single cyst and a cystadenoma difficult. Large symptomatic cysts that cause pressure symptoms can be treated with surgical fenestration or percutaneous aspiration, followed by instillation of ethanol to ablate the cyst.

Pseudomass Lesions Due to Fatty Infiltration of the Liver

Fatty infiltration of the liver is common and can give the appearance of mass lesions by two processes. First, fatty infiltration can be focal in the liver, producing the appearance of a mass lesion on imaging studies (Fig. 3). Second, focal sparing of the liver in diffuse fatty liver syndromes can suggest the presence of a mass lesion.

Focal fatty infiltration of the liver is common and occurs with obesity and diabetes mellitus and in patients with heavy alcohol consumption and, most problematic, in patients who are given chemotherapeutic drugs and develop an altered nutritional status. Focal fat in the liver is hypodense on CT, but because the fat is dispersed in normal tissue, the fat density is not as low as that of adipose tissue. On ultrasonography, focal fat appears as a hyperechoic region. MRI is relatively insensitive to fat, unless in- and out-of-phase gradient imaging is used, in which case decreased signal intensity on out-of-phase imaging is diagnostic of focal fat. Occasionally, focal fat may be hyperintense on T_1- and T_2-weighted images, giving the impression of a mass. However, focal fat does not distort the contour of the liver, and if normal vessels, especially veins, can be identified coursing through the region of concern, the diagnosis of focal fat is likely. Focal fat often occurs in areas of a vascular watershed, especially along the falciform ligament. In problematic cases, biopsy is reasonable to exclude metastases on an absolute need-to-know basis.

Skip areas of normal liver on the background of diffuse fatty infiltration also may resemble a mass lesion, especially on ultrasonography because normal liver has a prominent hypoechoic appearance. Regions adjacent to the gallbladder fossa, subcapsular areas of the liver, and the posterior aspect of segment 4 often are spared in diffuse fatty liver syndromes. On CT, fatty liver is recognized by a density less than that of the spleen, and the venous structures are easily seen on venous

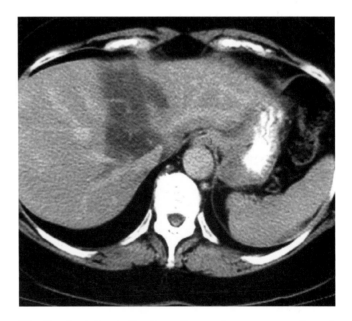

Fig. 3. Focal fatty infiltration. Computed tomogram, performed in late venous phase of the study, demonstrates a low-density lesion between right and left lobes. The lesion does not distort liver architecture. Note normal venous structures coursing through lesion. A low-density lesion that does not distort liver architecture and has normal venous structures is highly suggestive of focal fatty infiltration.

phase studies. The area of normal liver should not have contrast enhancement on arterial phase studies, should have the density of normal liver, and should not distort the liver architecture or vessels. Now that focal fat is recognized as a cause of pseudotumors and the radiographic features generally are appreciated, focal fat usually is recognized by radiologists and does not create a diagnostic problem.

MALIGNANT LIVER LESIONS

Hepatocellular Carcinoma

Hepatocellular carcinoma is one of the most common cancers worldwide. The incidence varies widely, with a relatively low incidence in the United States of 4/100,000 population annually. Hepatocellular carcinoma occurs predominantly in men, with a male-to-female ratio of approximately 3:1. Hepatocellular carcinoma is unique among human cancers because in most instances its cause is well understood. This cancer occurs predominantly in patients who have cirrhosis and viral hepatitis. The most common causes of cirrhosis associated with hepatocellular carcinoma include hepatitis B and hepatitis C. However, hepatocellular carcinoma may occur in cirrhosis of any cause. The risk of hepatocellular carcinoma developing in patients with cirrhosis due to hepatitis C needs to be emphasized because hepatitis C is extremely prevalent (0.5%-1.5% of the population) and has replaced hepatitis B as the leading cause of hepatocellular carcinoma in many areas of the world. Patients with hepatocellular carcinoma may present with 1) decompensation of their cirrhosis, 2) systemic or local symptoms (or both) referable to the cancer, 3) paraneoplastic manifestations, 4) symptoms due to metastases, or 5) a liver mass lesion identified incidentally on a radiographic study.

Liver decompensation is a relatively common presentation of hepatocellular carcinoma and must be considered in anyone who presents with sudden and rapid decompensation of liver disease. As with any neoplastic condition, advanced hepatocellular carcinoma is frequently associated with anorexia, early satiety, malaise, weakness, nausea, vomiting, and weight loss. Local symptoms due to the tumor mass also are common in advanced hepatocellular carcinoma. In particular, a self-limited, single episode of right upper quadrant abdominal pain resembling biliary colic is a common presenting symptom. The pain results either from an abrupt extension of the tumor through the liver capsule or limited hemorrhage and necrosis within the tumor. Various other local complications have been reported in advanced hepatocellular carcinoma, including chronic abdominal pain, abdominal mass, hemoperitoneum from rupture of the tumor, hepatic vein obstruction leading to Budd-Chiari syndrome, inferior vena cava obstruction with peripheral edema, shoulder pain and pleural effusions from

diaphragmatic extension of the tumor, and jaundice or hemobilia due to invasion of the bile ducts by the tumor. Paraneoplastic manifestations are rare and include fever, leukocytosis, hypercalcemia, erythrocytosis, hypoglycemia, hypercholesterolemia, porphyria cutanea tarda, and hypertrophic pulmonary osteoarthropathy. However, it should be emphasized that the finding of asymptomatic hepatocellular carcinoma is becoming increasingly more common as patients have radiographic imaging procedures of the liver to evaluate known liver disease.

The physical findings observed in hepatocellular carcinoma depend on the stage of disease. Firm or tender (or both) hepatomegaly, a palpable liver mass, a liver bruit, a friction rub over the liver, jaundice, ascites, peripheral edema, and splenomegaly may be observed in hepatocellular carcinoma. However, in the United States, physical examination findings frequently are unrevealing in patients with hepatocellular carcinoma, except for the physical findings commonly observed in cirrhosis.

The ultrasonographic appearance of hepatocellular carcinoma varies. Small lesions can be hyperechoic because of fatty infiltration of the tumor. An isoechoic lesion with a hypoechoic halo is another appearance of small tumors. Larger lesions are hypoechoic or mixed, with a mosaic pattern. Vascular infiltration of the portal venous structures is common in hepatocellular carcinoma, and Doppler ultrasonography is useful for identifying this feature. Indeed, metastases do not invade vessels but displace them by a mass effect. Thus, the finding of vascular invasion by a neoplasm in the liver goes a long way toward confirming the diagnosis of hepatocellular cancer. On CT, hepatocellular carcinomas often are hypodense on precontrast images. Small tumors (<5 cm) usually demonstrate contrast enhancement on arterial phase studies because they are hypervascular (Fig. 4). However, larger tumors have a more mosaic pattern because of necrosis in focal areas of the tumor. MRI characteristics parallel those observed on CT. The classic hepatocellular cancer is hypointense on T1-weighted images and hyperintense on T2-weighted ones. The reverse is true for a macroregenerative nodule which, because of the accumulation of iron, may be hyperintense on T1-weighted images and hypointense on T2-weighted ones. However, this finding is not absolute, and no imaging characteristics can universally distinguish between a dysplastic nodule and well-differentiated hepatocellular carcinoma.

Percutaneous fine-needle biopsy of the liver can be used to diagnose hepatocellular carcinoma. However, several caveats must be recognized by the clinician before having this procedure performed. First, hepatocellular carcinomas are highly vascular, increasing the risk of hemorrhage. Second, the pathologist cannot distinguish between low-grade hepatocellular carcinoma and a benign lesion in the material usually obtained with fine-needle biopsy. Third, highly anaplastic hepatocellular

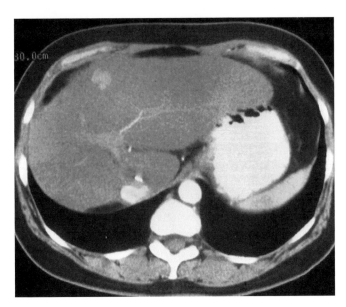

Fig. 4. Hepatocellular carcinoma. Computed tomogram of a patient with cirrhotic stage hepatitis C. The scan, obtained during arterial phase of the study, shows a hypervascular lesion in the anterior aspect of the liver (segment 4). A contrast-enhancing lesion larger than 2 cm in a cirrhotic liver is virtually diagnostic of hepatocellular carcinoma.

carcinomas are frequently interpreted as metastatic cancers by even experienced pathologists. Fourth, the biopsy may promote vascular invasion and peritoneal seeding by the cancer. Fifth, the information obtained by biopsy should alter therapy. If the patient is a candidate for liver transplantation (the best therapy for small unicentric lesions) or for resection, most transplant centers and hepatobiliary surgeons prefer that biopsy of the lesion not be performed. Indeed, the European Association for the Study of Liver Diseases has developed the following noninvasive criteria for the diagnosis of hepatocellular carcinoma: 1) two imaging studies demonstrating a lesion in a cirrhotic liver, with at least one study showing contrast enhancement and 2) a mass in a cirrhotic liver and an alphafetoprotein concentration greater than 100 ng/mL.

Fibrolamellar Hepatocellular Carcinoma

Fibrolamellar hepatocellular carcinoma is an unusual variant of hepatocellular carcinoma with unique histologic features that include deeply eosinophilic malignant cells interspersed between laminated strands of collagen. This cancer accounts for up to 7% of all hepatocellular carcinomas in the Western world. It does not have a sex predilection and occurs predominantly (90% of cases) in persons younger than 40 years. Cirrhosis, viral hepatitis, alcohol use, or a history of contraceptive pill use is unusual in fibrolamellar hepatocellular carcinoma. These tumors are thought to be slow-growing cancers that metastasize late in their development. They have no special ultrasonographic

characteristics. CT demonstrates a hypodense lesion with marked enhancement in the contrast phases of the study. Fibrolamellar cancers may have a central scar caused by hemorrhage, necrosis, and calcification. This feature needs to be considered when determining whether a lesion may be FNH by CT criteria. On MRI, fibrolamellar cancers are hypointense or isointense with normal liver on T1-weighted images. Because of its purely fibrous nature and lack of vascularity, the central scar, if present, is hypointense on both T1- and T2-weighted images.

Because of slow growth, fibrolamellar hepatocellular carcinomas usually are resectable more often (50%-80% of tumors) at presentation than hepatocellular carcinomas are. The 5-year survival rate after liver resection is 56%. If the cancer is not amenable to resection because of anatomic considerations, liver transplantation is indicated. The 2-year survival rate after liver transplantation for fibrolamellar hepatocellular carcinoma is 60%. If the tumor is not amenable to resection or transplantation, the disease apparently has progressed to a more virulent stage and median survival is only 13 months.

Intrahepatic Cholangiocarcinoma

Intrahepatic cholangiocarcinoma is an adenocarcinoma arising from intrahepatic bile ducts. It is the second most common primary malignancy arising within the liver, accounting for approximately 10% to 20% of primary liver malignancies. Because intrahepatic cholangiocarcinoma is an adenocarcinoma, it is frequently misdiagnosed as metastatic adenocarcinoma of an unknown primary source. This misdiagnosis often precludes appropriate attempts to surgically excise the cancer. Patients with primary sclerosing cholangitis are at risk for intrahepatic cholangiocarcinoma, but most patients have no identifiable risk factors. The mean age at presentation is 55 years, and there is no sex predilection. On ultrasonography, the lesions are hypoechoic. The major distinguishing CT feature is peripheral enhancement of a hypodense lesion during the venous phase after the administration of contrast agent. As with most malignancies, intrahepatic cholangiocarcinomas are hypointense on T1-weighted images and hyperintense on T2-weighted ones.

Surgical excision is indicated for patients without extrahepatic disease, vascular invasion, and disease that permits an anatomic resection without compromising liver function. The median survival of patients undergoing curative resection is 3 years, with occasional long-term survivors. The results of orthotopic liver transplantation for intrahepatic cholangiocarcinoma masses are dismal, with virtually 100% of patients having recurrence of disease. Thus, most transplant centers have abandoned orthotopic liver transplantation for this malignancy. No chemotherapy has proved effective in treating this tumor.

Liver Metastases

Liver metastases are common. They are usually multicentric, and the patient often has a history of cancer elsewhere or has additional pulmonary metastases. In this respect, the diagnosis of metastases is not difficult. It is important to realize that some metastases can be hypervascular and can be confused with a primary liver lesion, such as hepatocellular carcinoma, whereas others can be hyperechoic and resemble a cavernous hemangioma (Tables 4 and 5). Vascular forms of liver metastases need to be kept in mind when evaluating liver masses.

Table 4. Hypervascular Liver Metastases

Breast cancer
Choriocarcinoma
Melanoma
Neuroendocrine tumors
Renal cell carcinoma
Thyroid cancer

Table 5. Ultrasonographic Pattern of Liver Metastases

Hypoechoic
  Lung
  Lymphoma
  Pancreas
Hyperechoic
  Choriocarcinoma
  Colon
  Neuroendocrine
  Renal cell carcinoma
  Thyroid
Mixed echogenicity
  Anaplastic cancers
  Breast
  Lung
  Stomach

RECOMMENDED READING

Bennett WF, Bova JG. Review of hepatic imaging and a problem-oriented approach to liver masses. Hepatology. 1990;12:761-75.

Cherqui D, Rahmouni A, Charlotte F, Boulahdour H, Metreau JM, Meignan M, et al. Management of focal nodular hyperplasia and hepatocellular adenoma in young women: a series of 41 patients with clinical, radiological, and pathological correlations. Hepatology. 1995;22:1674-81.

Ichikawa T, Federle MP, Grazioli L, Marsh W. Fibrolamellar hepatocellular carcinoma: pre- and posttherapy evaluation with CT and MR imaging. Radiology. 2000;217:145-51.

Llovet JM, Burroughs A, Bruix J. Hepatocellular carcinoma. Lancet. 2003;362:1907-17.

Mathieu D, Kobeiter H, Maison P, Rahmouni A, Cherqui D, Zafrani ES, et al. Oral contraceptive use and focal nodular hyperplasia of the liver. Gastroenterology. 2000;118:560-4.

Peterson MS, Baron RL. Radiologic diagnosis of hepatocellular carcinoma. Clin Liver Dis. 2001;5:123-44.

Pol B, Disdier P, Le Treut YP, Campan P, Hardwigsen J, Weiller PJ. Inflammatory process complicating giant hemangioma of the liver: report of three cases. Liver Transpl Surg. 1998;4:204-7.

Reddy KR, Schiff ER. Approach to a liver mass. Semin Liver Dis. 1993;13:423-35.

Ros PR, Davis GL. The incidental focal liver lesion: photon, proton, or needle? Hepatology. 1998;27:1183-90.

Rust C, Gores GJ. Locoregional management of hepatocellular carcinoma: surgical and ablation therapies. Clin Liver Dis. 2001;5:161-73.

Schlinkert RT, Nagorney DM, Van Heerden JA, Adson MA. Intrahepatic cholangiocarcinoma: clinical aspects, pathology and treatment. HPB Surg. 1992;5:95-101.

Siegelman ES, Rosen MA. Imaging of hepatic steatosis. Semin Liver Dis. 2001;21:71-80.

Torzilli G, Minagawa M, Takayama T, Inoue K, Hui AM, Kubota K, et al. Accurate preoperative evaluation of liver mass lesions without fine-needle biopsy. Hepatology. 1999;30:889-93.

Trotter JF, Everson GT. Benign focal lesions of the liver. Clin Liver Dis. 2001;5:17-42.

CHAPTER 30

Alcoholic Liver Disease

Vijay H. Shah, M.D.

EPIDEMIOLOGY AND CLINICAL SPECTRUM

Public Health Significance

Alcoholic liver disease is a major cause of morbidity and mortality in the United States. Alcohol is implicated in more than 50% of liver-related deaths in the United States, and complications of alcoholism contribute to one-quarter of a million deaths annually. Also, alcoholic liver disease is a major health care cost expenditure, accounting for nearly $3 billion annually.

Clinical Spectrum

The clinical spectrum of alcoholic liver disease includes fatty liver, alcoholic hepatitis, and alcoholic cirrhosis. Fatty liver develops in response to short periods (days) of alcohol abuse. It is generally asymptomatic and reversible with abstinence. More advanced liver injury usually requires prolonged alcohol abuse over a period of years. Of note, the majority of people who abuse alcohol for extended periods do not develop more advanced lesions of alcoholic liver disease. However, approximately 20% of these patients do develop alcoholic hepatitis or alcoholic cirrhosis (or both).

Risk Factors

Alcohol Ingestion

Although alcoholic fatty liver may develop in response to short periods of alcohol abuse, even only a few days, more advanced and morbid liver injury requires prolonged alcohol abuse. In most cases, the level of ethanol consumption required for the development of advanced forms of alcoholic liver disease is 60 to 80 g of alcohol daily for men, or the equivalent of 6 to 8

drinks per day for several years. In women, half of this amount may cause clinically significant alcoholic liver disease. The quantity of alcohol necessary for liver injury probably does not depend on the type of alcohol consumed. However, there is considerable individual variability in the threshold of alcohol necessary for advanced alcoholic liver disease to develop, and clearly factors other than absolute ethanol consumption are important in determining which persons develop alcoholic liver disease. A recently identified risk factor is obesity. Other risk factors are described below.

Genetic and Hereditary Factors

The interindividual variability in the correlation between alcohol consumption and development of liver disease highlights the role of genetic factors that may predispose a person to alcohol-induced liver toxicity. Specific genetic polymorphisms have been detected in patients who have alcoholic liver disease, most notably mutations in the tumor necrosis factor promoter and in alcohol-metabolizing enzyme systems. In addition to the genetic factors predisposing certain alcoholic persons to liver disease, there also is strong evidence that genetic factors predispose persons to alcoholism.

Sex

Although alcoholic liver disease is observed more commonly in men than women, women are predisposed to the development of this disease and develop more severe disease with less alcohol consumption than men. The reason for this greater risk in women is not clear; however, despite weight adjustment, a similar level of alcohol consumption results in higher blood alcohol levels in women than in men. Theories to explain this include a relative deficiency of gastric alcohol dehydrogenase in women, sex differences in alcohol bioavailability, and female hormone-related effects.

- Alcoholic liver disease encompasses a clinicohistologic spectrum (fatty liver, hepatitis, cirrhosis).
- Although there is considerable variability among persons, the toxic dose of alcohol necessary for advanced liver injury to develop is probably 60 to 80 g daily for several years, with a significantly lower threshold for women.
- Genetic factors contribute to alcoholic liver disease by predisposing a person to alcoholism as well as to alcohol-induced liver injury.
- Although fatty liver occurs nearly uniformly with excess alcohol consumption, more advanced liver injury occurs in only 15% to 20% of persons who continue to abuse alcohol.
- Alcoholic hepatitis may occur in the presence or absence of preexisting liver cirrhosis.

ETHANOL METABOLISM AND PATHOPHYSIOLOGY

More than one enzyme system is capable of metabolizing alcohol in the liver. Enzymes that have received the greatest attention include alcohol dehydrogenase, aldehyde dehydrogenase, and the microsomal ethanol oxidizing system (MEOS) (Fig. 1). The relative importance of each of these pathways is being investigated. When physiologic circumstances are normal and blood levels of alcohol are low, the enzyme of major importance apparently is alcohol dehydrogenase. This enzyme catalyzes the conversion of alcohol to acetaldehyde, and aldehyde dehydrogenase subsequently catalyzes the conversion of acetaldehyde into acetate. Alcohol dehydrogenase catalysis changes the oxidation-reduction state in the cell by increasing the ratio of reduced nicotinamide adenine dinucleotide (NADH) to the oxidized form (NAD), which has important implications for other cellular processes, including the generation of free radicals, inhibition of other enzyme systems, and fat accumulation. Also, an isoform of alcohol dehydrogenase occurs within the gastric mucosa, although the clinical importance of the gastric component of alcohol metabolism is debated.

MEOS is localized in the endoplasmic reticulum instead of the cytosol, where the alcohol dehydrogenase system operates, and appears to be important in alcohol metabolism when blood levels of alcohol are moderate to high. Under normal conditions when these levels are low, the role of MEOS is much smaller than that of the alcohol dehydrogenase system. As explained by its enzyme kinetics, MEOS has a greater role in cases of chronic alcohol use because it is induced by alcohol, thereby allowing progressively increased ethanol metabolism in alcoholics. MEOS also converts alcohol to acetaldehyde, requiring aldehyde dehydrogenase for further metabolism. Importantly, the specific MEOS enzyme CYP2E1 is responsible for the metabolism of various other compounds. The induction of CYP2E1 by alcohol importantly affects blood levels of these compounds and accounts for the increased tolerance of alcoholics to sedatives. Compounds that are rapidly metabolized in alcoholics by this process include isoniazid and acetaminophen. Importantly, nearly one-half of Far East Asians are deficient in aldehyde dehydrogenase activity because of the inheritance of a mutant allele. This can result in excess aldehyde accumulation, accounting for alcohol-induced flushing symptoms in these persons, who may also be more susceptible to alcohol-induced liver injury. Although the peroxisomal catalase enzyme also is capable of ethanol metabolism, its physiologic role in alcohol metabolism appears to be minor.

Experimental evidence suggests that the alcohol metabolite acetaldehyde may be a toxic mediator of alcohol-induced liver injury. The mechanism by which alcohol and acetaldehyde cause liver injury is being investigated. The initiation of fat

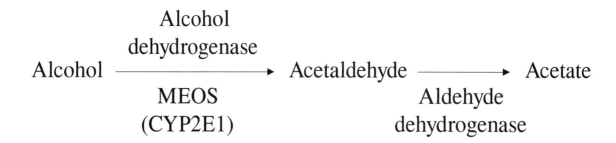

Fig. 1. Alcohol metabolism. Alcohol is metabolized to acetaldehyde by alcohol dehydrogenase and CYP2E1. In most persons, the alcohol dehydrogenase pathway is dominant; however, in alcoholic persons and those with high blood levels of alcohol, CYP2E1 is induced and has a major role in metabolism. Acetaldehyde derived from both these pathways is metabolized by aldehyde dehydrogenase to acetate. MEOS, microsomal ethanol oxidizing system.

accumulation within the liver appears to occur in response to decreased fatty acid oxidation and increased fatty acid accumulation. These events may be linked to changes in the liver oxidation-reduction state induced by ethanol metabolism. Other important physiologic events that mediate liver injury include increased oxidative stress, hepatocyte apoptosis and necrosis, and deposition of collagen, with ensuing fibrosis through activation of liver stellate cells. Various cytokines, transcription factors, and intracellular signaling pathways have been implicated in these events, including tumor necrosis factor, a cytokine whose blood levels appear to correlate with the severity of liver disease in patients with alcoholic hepatitis.

- Alcohol dehydrogenase is the primary alcohol-metabolizing pathway, particularly when blood alcohol levels are low.
- MEOS is important in alcoholics, especially when blood levels of alcohol are high. Induction of this system importantly affects the metabolism of various xenobiotics.
- Diminished aldehyde dehydrogenase activity accounts for the flushing syndrome detected in a large proportion of Asians who consume alcohol.

FATTY LIVER

Case Presentation

A 22-year-old male college student has a series of laboratory tests performed during a routine checkup at the student health clinic. He is asymptomatic, and the physical examination findings are normal. He takes no medications and has no family history of liver disease. He is not sexually active and says he does not use intravenous or intranasal drugs, has not traveled recently, and has not had blood transfusions. Laboratory findings include the following: aspartate aminotransferase (AST), 65 U/L; alanine aminotransferase (ALT), 43 U/L (AST is mildly elevated); γ-glutamyltransferase (GGT), 336 U/L; mean corpuscular volume and total bilirubin and alkaline phosphatase levels are normal. On further questioning, the patient admits to having had 6 to 10 drinks per day over the past week during student orientation.

This patient has the clinical features suggestive of alcoholic fatty liver. The diagnosis and treatment are discussed below.

History and Physical Examination

Fatty liver may develop in response to only a transient alcohol insult, over a period of days. The most salient historical feature is an alcohol binge. The patient may be asymptomatic or may complain of mild nonspecific symptoms, including fatigue, malaise, abdominal discomfort, and anorexia. On physical examination, tender hepatomegaly may be prominent. Stigmata of chronic liver disease are absent, and in many patients, the physical examination findings are normal.

Laboratory and Radiographic Features

Laboratory studies may show mild to moderate increases in the serum levels of aminotransferases, predominantly an increase in AST. Minor increases in alkaline phosphatase or bilirubin (or both) may be observed. Prothrombin time is normal. As in the above case, laboratory abnormalities often are noted incidentally in an asymptomatic person.

Histologic Features

Generally, liver biopsy is not necessary to establish the diagnosis of alcoholic fatty liver because the condition is benign and reversible. However, biopsy may be performed to determine whether the patient has more advanced alcoholic liver disease or another condition. The principal feature of alcoholic fatty liver in biopsy specimens is macrovesicular steatosis within hepatocytes (Fig. 2). There are no inflammatory cells or collagen deposition. Because biopsy specimens from patients with Wilson's disease occasionally have the features of steatosis, Wilson's disease should always be excluded in young persons with abnormal levels of liver enzymes.

Prognosis and Treatment

No specific treatment other than abstinence is required for management of alcoholic fatty liver. If abstinence is achieved, alcoholic fatty liver is entirely reversible. However, 20% to 30% of patients who continue to abuse alcohol chronically develop more advanced forms of alcoholic liver disease, including alcoholic hepatitis and cirrhosis.

- Alcoholic fatty liver may develop in response to short periods of alcohol abuse, although it is more common with chronic alcohol abuse.
- Treatment is focused on abstinence or more judicious consumption of alcohol.

ALCOHOLIC HEPATITIS

Clinical Presentation

A 36-year-old man complains of fatigue, dark urine, and abdominal swelling. He admits to drinking a few beers a day since his teen years, but he has never had a major medical problem. Recently, he has been drinking more heavily while unemployed. He states that he has not had blood transfusions and does not use intravenous drugs. Physical examination findings are remarkable for tachycardia and low-grade fever. Prominent scleral icterus is noted, and the abdominal examination reveals shifting dullness. The liver span is increased on percussion.

This patient has the clinical features typical of alcoholic hepatitis. The diagnosis and treatment are discussed below.

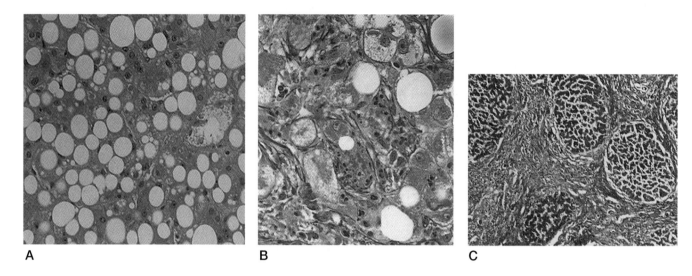

A   B   C

Fig. 2. Histopathologic features of alcoholic liver disease. *A*, Fatty liver. Note macrovesicular steatosis and lack of inflammation and collagen deposition. *B*, Alcoholic hepatitis. Note polymorphonuclear infiltrates, hepatocyte necrosis, steatosis, Mallory bodies, and variable amounts of fibrosis. *C*, Alcoholic cirrhosis. Note characteristic micronodular cirrhosis, although a mixed nodularity pattern is often observed. Frequently, there is prominent secondary hemosiderosis. (From Kanel GC, Korula J. Liver biopsy evaluation: histologic diagnosis and clinical correlations. Philadelphia: WB Saunders Company; 2000. p. 39, 89, 94. Used with permission.)

History and Physical Examination

Although alcoholic fatty liver is predominantly an asymptomatic condition, a constellation of clinical symptoms, often nonspecific, frequently are observed in patients with more advanced lesions, such as alcoholic hepatitis. Persons who drink more than 60 to 80 g of alcohol daily for a period of years are at risk for the development of alcoholic hepatitis; the threshold is lower for women. Also, alcoholic hepatitis may develop in the presence or absence of underlying liver cirrhosis. The clinical presentation of alcoholic hepatitis includes constitutional symptoms such as weakness, anorexia, and weight loss and other nonspecific symptoms such as nausea and vomiting (Fig. 3). Severe alcoholic hepatitis may include more advanced symptoms related to portal hypertension, including gastrointestinal tract bleeding, ascites, and hepatic encephalopathy. It is important to identify risk factors for concomitant or alternative forms of acute and chronic hepatitis, such as viral hepatitis, Wilson's disease, and drug-induced hepatitis.

The diagnosis of alcoholic hepatitis is contingent on determining whether the patient is abusing alcohol. This is not always easy because alcoholic persons and even their family members often minimize or hide their alcohol use. An independent history from multiple family members is often necessary to corroborate the patient's alcohol history, and different caregivers may obtain a different history from the same interviewee because of the type of relation between the patient and caregiver and the approach and persistence of different history takers. Questionnaires have been used to clarify alcohol use and abuse

syndromes; however, because of their length, many of them are limited to research purposes. The most useful screening questionnaire in clinical practice is the CAGE questionnaire, which includes the following inquiries: Has the patient felt the need to **c**ut back on alcohol use? Has the patient become **a**nnoyed with other persons' concerns about his or her alcohol use? Does the patient feel **g**uilty about his or her alcohol use? Does the patient use alcohol in the morning as an **e**ye-opener? Although two positive responses have a high sensitivity and positive predictive value for alcohol dependency, any positive response to these inquiries requires a more detailed investigation and should heighten the suspicion of alcohol abuse.

In patients with alcoholic hepatitis, physical examination findings are most notable for tender hepatomegaly, fever, and tachycardia (Fig. 3). Other findings depend on the severity of liver insult, the presence or absence of concomitant cirrhosis, and the presence or absence of portal hypertension. These findings may include jaundice, splenomegaly, collateral vessels, hypogonadism, palmar erythema, asterixis, and ascites in patients with severe alcoholic hepatitis and portal hypertension. Evidence for concomitant infection is common and may be detected on examination, including signs of spontaneous bacterial peritonitis, pneumonia, or cellulitis.

Laboratory and Radiographic Features

Laboratory abnormalities reflect the extrahepatic adverse effects of alcohol as well as alcohol-induced liver injury (Table 1). Mean corpuscular volume usually is increased, reflecting the adverse effect of alcohol on erythrocytes. The levels of

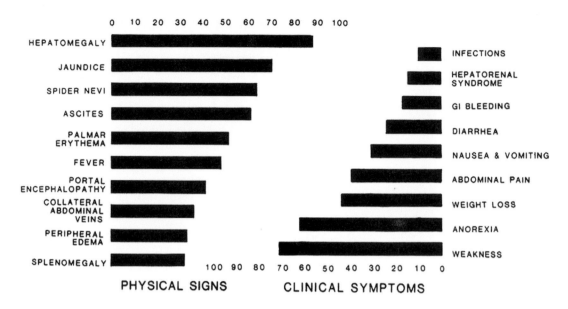

Fig. 3. Clinical features of alcoholic hepatitis. Clinical symptoms of alcoholic hepatitis are often nonspecific and include weakness, anorexia, and abdominal pain. In more severe cases, complications of portal hypertension predominate, including gastrointestinal (GI) tract bleeding and renal dysfunction. Physical examination findings are most notable for hepatomegaly and jaundice. Additional findings are dependent on the presence of portal hypertension or liver cirrhosis (or both), including stigmata of chronic liver disease and collateral vessels. Numbers refer to percentage of patients with the feature. (From Mendenhall CL. Alcoholic hepatitis. In: Schiff L, Schiff ER, editors. Diseases of the Liver. Vol 2. 7th ed. Philadelphia: JB Lippincott Company; 1993. p. 862. Used with permission.)

triglycerides and uric acid also are frequently increased. Patients are prone to ketoacidosis. Peripheral polymorphonuclear leukocytosis is prominent, and in some cases, a leukemoid reaction also may be observed. Aminotransferase levels usually are increased less than 5 to 10 times normal, but they may be higher with concomitant acetaminophen toxicity. Also, the level of AST almost always is higher than that of ALT, which is opposite to that in nonalcoholic steatohepatitis, in which the ALT level is often higher than the AST level. Both the modest increase in aminotransferase levels and the greater increase in AST than in ALT help to differentiate alcoholic hepatitis from alternative diagnoses. Some laboratory abnormalities reflect the severity of the alcohol-induced liver injury and are prognostically useful, including prothrombin time and bilirubin concentration. In moderate to severe cases of alcoholic hepatitis, prothrombin time and bilirubin concentration are increased, and in contrast to aminotransferase levels, prothrombin time and bilirubin concentration have prognostic utility. Several groups have attempted to use bilirubin concentration and prothrombin time as well as other laboratory variables to assess the prognosis of patients with alcoholic hepatitis. The most widely used of these assessments is the Maddrey discriminant function analysis:

Discriminant function = 4.6 (prothrombin time – control) + serum bilirubin concentration (mg/dL)

A discriminant function greater than 32 effectively identifies patients whose risk of death is higher than 50%. Other frequently observed laboratory abnormalities that may cause diagnostic confusion or suggest multifactorial liver disease include increases in iron saturation indices and ferritin, hepatitis C virus (HCV) antibody positivity, and increased levels of autoimmune markers such as antinuclear antibody and anti-smooth muscle antibody. Rather than reflecting the concomitant presence of hereditary hemochromatosis or autoimmune hepatitis, increases in iron indices and autoimmune markers more commonly reflect the pathogenic role of iron deposition and autoimmunity in the development of alcoholic hepatitis. In cases in which the alcohol history is questionable, a Doppler study is useful to exclude alternative diagnoses such as cholecystitis, biliary obstruction, and hepatic vein thrombosis, which may present in a manner similar to alcoholic hepatitis. The false diagnosis of gallstone disease can be catastrophic because of the high surgical morbidity and mortality of patients with alcoholic hepatitis.

Because of the inherent difficulties in obtaining a reliable history of alcohol use, various biochemical markers have been evaluated for the detection of surreptitious alcohol abuse. Many of the traditional serologic tests of alcohol abuse are based on indirectly assessing alcohol abuse by examining such markers of liver injury as AST, ALT, the ratio of AST to ALT, and GGT. However, because these tests assess alcohol abuse

Table 1. Laboratory Abnormalities in Alcoholic Hepatitis

Hematology
    Macrocytic anemia (increased MCV)
    Leukocytosis
    Thrombocytopenia
General chemistry
    Hyperglycemia
    Hyperuricemia
    Hypertriglyceridemia
    Ketosis
Tests of liver function and injury
    Hypoalbuminemia
    Hyperbilirubinemia
    Increased prothrombin time
    Increased AST/ALT (ratio of 1.5 to 2.5 and total
      increase less than 10-fold)
    Increased GGT
    Increased alkaline phosphatase (mild)

ALT, alanine aminotransferase; AST, aspartate aminotransferase; GGT, γ-glutamyltransferase; MCV, mean corpuscular volume.

indirectly by detecting liver injury, their sensitivity and specificity generally are less than 70%. Mean corpuscular volume (MCV) also indirectly assesses alcohol abuse by evaluating bone marrow toxicity of alcohol; it can be helpful as an adjunctive test. Newer tests include carbohydrate-deficient transferrin and mitochondrial AST. Carbohydrate-deficient transferrin reflects the desialylation of transferrin that occurs in response to high alcohol use, and mitochondrial AST is a specific isoform of the enzyme that is released from hepatocytes injured by alcohol. However, these tests have not been shown universally to be more effective than the less expensive AST-to-ALT ratio, GGT, and MCV.

Histologic Features

With advances in noninvasive liver diagnostic capacities over the past decade, the diagnosis of alcoholic hepatitis often is made without liver biopsy. However, liver biopsy is indicated if the diagnosis is in question after noninvasive evaluation. In particular, histologic examination may be useful in distinguishing coexisting or alternative liver disorders such as hereditary hemochromatosis in persons with high iron saturation, Wilson's disease in younger persons with low to low-normal ceruloplasmin levels, autoimmune hepatitis in persons with high titers of autoimmune markers, and hepatitis C in persons with HCV antibody positivity. Depending on the degree of coagulopathy and thrombocytopenia, liver biopsy, if pursued, often requires a transjugular rather than a percutaneous route.

In alcoholic hepatitis, liver biopsy specimens demonstrate several characteristic features, including centrilobular and sometimes periportal polymorphonuclear infiltrates, centrilobular hepatocyte swelling, ballooning degeneration, macrovesicular steatosis, and Mallory bodies (Fig. 2). Often, pericentral and perisinusoidal fibrosis is detected and is most prominent with a trichrome or Klatskin stain. The terminal hepatic venules often are obliterated, and indeed the zone 3 region of the liver acinus demonstrates the most prominent injury. Mallory bodies, eosinophilic-staining condensed cytoskeletal structures, are not specific for alcoholic hepatitis. However, their presence in association with other salient biopsy features strongly suggests alcoholic hepatitis. Prominent neutrophilic infiltration of hepatocytes containing Mallory bodies is termed "satellitosis." Giant mitochondria ("megamitochondria") are another characteristic feature. In up to 50% of cases, concomitant cirrhosis may be observed. Importantly, nonalcoholic steatohepatitis cannot be differentiated reliably from alcoholic hepatitis with liver biopsy specimens because of the overlap of histologic features.

Prognosis and Treatment

Abstinence

Abstinence is an important factor in both short- and long-term survival of patients with alcoholic hepatitis. For patients who recover and remain abstinent, the disease may continue to improve (i.e., clinical sequelae and laboratory variables) for as long as 6 months. Although the condition of some patients continues to deteriorate even with abstinence, the 5-year survival rate for this group is greater than 60%. However, for patients who continue to drink, the 5-year survival rate is less than 30%.

Nutrition

Malnutrition is almost universal among patients with alcoholic hepatitis because of concomitant poor dietary habits, anorexia, and encephalopathy. Although malnutrition was once thought to cause alcoholic liver disease, it is no longer considered to have a major role in the pathogenesis of the disease. However, maintenance of a positive nitrogen balance and provision of adequate energy requirements through nutritional support is a vital supportive treatment approach. Patients with alcoholic hepatitis generally have greater protein and energy needs because of the stress of illness and underlying malnutrition. Recommendations include 30 to 40 kcal/kg ideal body weight of caloric supplementation and 1 to 1.5 g protein/kg ideal body weight. Provision of nutrients in excess of calculated requirements is unlikely to be of benefit. Every attempt should be made to provide adequate calories enterally. However, parenteral support may be necessary for some patients. Encephalopathy should not require protein restriction in most patients. For patients with severe encephalopathy that is exacerbated by dietary protein, branched chain amino acid supplements should be considered or protein intake should be decreased transiently. Increased use of dietary vegetable protein may be better tolerated than animal protein. Other than for this scenario, amino acid supplementation probably does not improve survival sufficiently for the added cost. The use of androgenic anabolic steroids such as oxandrolone needs further study.

Portal Hypertension

Patients with alcoholic hepatitis may develop complications of portal hypertension regardless of the presence or absence of underlying cirrhosis. This clinical observation is supported by studies demonstrating that alcohol directly increases portal pressure, and it emphasizes the importance of the vascular component of intrahepatic resistance and portal hypertension. Hepatic encephalopathy, bleeding esophageal varices, ascites, spontaneous bacterial peritonitis, and hepatorenal syndrome are complications of portal hypertension commonly encountered in patients with alcoholic hepatitis. The management of these complications is discussed elsewhere in this book.

Infection

Because of underlying malnutrition, liver cirrhosis, and iatrogenic complications, infection is one of the most common causes of death of patients with alcoholic hepatitis. The patients must be evaluated carefully for infections, including spontaneous bacterial peritonitis, aspiration pneumonia, and lower extremity cellulitis. These infections should be treated aggressively with antibiotics. However, fever and leukocytosis are common in patients with alcoholic hepatitis, even without infection.

Corticosteroids

Corticosteroids have been studied extensively for the treatment of alcoholic hepatitis. Although many of the initial controlled trials did not show a benefit, further analysis suggested that patients with encephalopathy and more severe disease may benefit. Therefore, follow-up studies focused on the role of corticosteroids in the treatment of patients who had a discriminant function greater than 32 or hepatic encephalopathy (or both) but not renal failure, infection, gastrointestinal tract bleeding, or, in some studies, severe diabetes mellitus. Some studies and meta-analyses that used these criteria showed that corticosteroid therapy had a survival benefit for patients with a discriminant function greater than 32 or hepatic encephalopathy (or both). Currently, the use of corticosteroid therapy for alcoholic hepatitis varies among experienced hepatologists.

Other Treatment Options

Alcohol induces oxidative stress in the liver, resulting in an imbalance between oxidants and antioxidants. To decrease oxygen consumption by the liver, investigators have studied the role of propylthiouracil in treating alcoholic hepatitis. Although a randomized controlled trial demonstrated clinical benefit, the results of follow-up studies have been inconclusive. Also, because of the inherent hepatotoxicity of propylthiouracil, this drug remains experimental. Another putative antifibrotic agent, colchicine, has been evaluated in treating alcoholic hepatitis. Although an initial trial suggested that the drug was beneficial for treating alcoholic liver cirrhosis, no clinical benefit has been demonstrated for hepatitis. Other hepatoprotective compounds, such as *S*-adenosyl-L-methionine and phosphatidylcholine, may have a small beneficial effect but are not widely used outside of research protocols. The results of a recent study have suggested that pentoxifylline, an inhibitor of tumor necrosis factor, is of clinical benefit. However, confirmatory studies are needed.

- Liver biopsy should be considered if the cause of hepatitis is questioned and specific treatments for alcoholic hepatitis other than supportive care are contemplated.
- Histologic features cannot reliably differentiate alcoholic hepatitis from nonalcoholic steatohepatitis. The distinction is made best on the basis of the clinical history and the pattern of aminotransferase (ALT, AST) increase.
- For most patients, the treatment of alcoholic hepatitis includes abstinence, supportive care, and management of malnutrition, infection, and complications of portal hypertension.

ALCOHOLIC CIRRHOSIS

Clinical Presentation

A 56-year-old salesman is admitted to the hospital with a 2-hour history of hematemesis and dizziness. His history is remarkable for symptoms of fatigue and lower extremity edema. His wife notes that his memory has been poor recently and he has been a "social drinker" for many years, having a few martinis with clients and during business trips. Physical examination findings are notable for orthostasis, temporal wasting, spider angiomas on the chest, and bilateral pitting edema of the lower extremities. His skin is jaundiced, and a liver edge is palpable and firm. The tip of the spleen is palpable upon inspiration. Rectal examination shows melena in the vault. There is prominent asterixis.

This patient has the clinical features typical of alcoholic cirrhosis. The diagnosis and treatment are discussed below.

History and Physical Examination

For persons with a clinical history of marked and prolonged alcohol abuse, only about 20% eventually develop liver cirrhosis. The presence or absence of symptoms is due largely to the presence or absence of liver decompensation. Patients with cirrhosis and compensated liver function who are abstinent may have minimal symptoms. Symptoms in patients with liver decompensation reflect the severity of portal hypertension, malnutrition, and degree of synthetic liver dysfunction, including nonspecific fatigue, weakness, and anorexia. More specific symptoms are related to the presence of specific complications of cirrhosis and portal hypertension, including gastrointestinal tract bleeding, ascites, encephalopathy, renal failure, and hepatoma. Physical examination may demonstrate stigmata of chronic liver disease (spider angiomas, palmar erythema), complications of portal hypertension (ascites, splenomegaly, asterixis, pedal edema), excess estrogen (gynecomastia, hypogonadism), and systemic alcohol toxicity (peripheral neuropathy, dementia, Dupuytren's contracture).

Laboratory and Radiographic Features

Prominent laboratory abnormalities include an increase in prothrombin time and bilirubin and a decrease in albumin, as reflected in the Child-Pugh score. Radiographic imaging may be suggestive of cirrhosis and ensuing portal hypertension, as indicated by heterogeneic liver echotexture, splenomegaly, collateralization, and ascites on ultrasonography and colloid shift to spleen and bone marrow on liver and spleen scanning. Dynamic triple-phase computed tomography may show changes in liver contour, splenomegaly, collateralization, or ascites. Patients are at risk for hepatocellular carcinoma and should be evaluated biannually with ultrasonography and the serum alpha fetoprotein test, particularly patients who have had recent clinical decompensation.

Histologic Features

Traditionally, alcoholic cirrhosis is classified as a micronodular cirrhosis (Fig. 2). However, in many cases, larger nodules also develop, leading to mixed micro-macronodular cirrhosis. The earliest collagen deposition occurs around the terminal hepatic venules, and progression to pericentral fibrosis portends irreversible architectural changes. Hemosiderin deposition is often prominent. In patients with alcoholic cirrhosis who continue to drink actively, many of the aforementioned histologic features of alcoholic hepatitis also are present. Patients are at risk for hepatocellular carcinoma, particularly those with coexisting chronic viral hepatitis.

Prognosis and Treatment

A good prognosis depends on the absence of liver decompensation and complications of portal hypertension and the ability to maintain abstinence. The prognosis for patients with cirrhosis who are well compensated and able to maintain abstinence is reasonably good, with a 5-year survival rate greater than 80%. Even for patients with decompensation, the 5-year survival rate with abstinence is greater than 50%. However, patients who continue to drink have a much worse prognosis, with a 5-year survival rate less than 30%.

The only established effective treatment for alcoholic cirrhosis is liver transplantation. Currently, alcoholic liver disease is the second most common indication for liver transplantation in adults in the United States. However, fewer than 20% of patients with end-stage alcoholic liver disease have transplantation. Despite perceptions to the contrary, patients who have liver transplantation for alcoholic liver disease have high survival rates after transplantation, second only to those of patients who have transplantation for chronic cholestatic liver disease. Indeed, the risk of cellular rejection is lower in persons undergoing transplantation for alcoholic liver disease than for those with other conditions.

A major issue in maintaining excellent outcome for this population focuses on identifying candidates with a low risk of recidivism after transplantation. Alcohol relapse after transplantation varies among centers, but it is probably about 15% to 30%. Although detecting surreptitious alcohol use after transplantation is often difficult, the low incidence of graft loss from recurrent alcoholic liver disease suggests that most patients who return to drinking after transplantation do not drink to the point of damaging the graft. However, it must be considered that alcohol abuse after liver transplantation can cause rapid development of cirrhosis in the graft, interfere with compliance in taking immunosuppressive medications, and alter the perception of the general public of liver transplantation, thus adversely affecting potential organ donors. Therefore, selecting patients who are appropriate for liver transplantation requires a team involving a hepatologist, surgeon, addiction specialist, psychiatrist, and social worker. Currently, most transplant centers require 6 months of abstinence and appropriate addiction treatment before performing a liver transplant. Appropriate family and social support is also important. Generally, patients with active alcoholic hepatitis are not candidates for liver transplantation because they have not been abstinent for 6 months and they have high perioperative mortality. Also, many of these patients will have evidence of marked clinical improvement after 6 months of abstinence, thereby delaying or obviating liver transplantation.

- Alcohol is a cause of micronodular cirrhosis, but often mixed micro-macronodular cirrhosis is observed histologically.
- The only curative treatment for alcoholic cirrhosis is liver transplantation; however, only a small proportion of patients undergo transplantation, partly because of their inability to maintain prolonged abstinence.
- Transplantation outcomes for alcoholic liver disease are comparable to or better than those for most other indicators.

SPECIAL CLINICAL SITUATIONS

Alcohol and Hepatitis C

The increase in prevalence of HCV infection among alcoholic persons is 10 times that of the population at large. Although this may be explained partly by increased risk factors of HCV transmission in some alcoholic patients, a large proportion of these patients have no identifiable risk factors. Also, patients with HCV infection who are alcoholic or drink in excess have more aggressive disease, often at a younger age, and have a worse prognosis than patients who have only HCV infection. Furthermore, HCV RNA levels are higher, the histologic features of the liver appear more progressive, and the response to interferon therapy is worse for patients with HCV infection who drink alcohol in excess. Whether alcohol synergistically damages the liver in patients with HCV infection or, alternatively, facilitates progression of HCV disease through increased susceptibility by host immune factors is unclear. Patients with alcoholic liver disease who have concomitant viral hepatitis have a risk almost fivefold greater for the development of hepatocellular carcinoma than patients without concomitant viral hepatitis. Identifying which process is causative in liver injury in patients with both conditions can be difficult; however, assessing liver biopsy findings and aminotransferase patterns can be useful because both of these are different in HCV infection and alcoholic liver injury. Because the alcohol threshold necessary to exacerbate the course of HCV infection has not been determined, patients with HCV infection should be advised against any alcohol use.

Alcohol and Acetaminophen

Alcoholic persons are at increased risk for acetaminophen-induced hepatotoxicity. As little as 2.5 to 3 g per day of acetaminophen may result in pronounced toxicity. The reason for this is that both alcohol and acetaminophen are metabolized in part by cytochrome P-450 2E1, an enzyme in MEOS. With the induction of this enzyme by alcohol, a greater proportion of acetaminophen is metabolized by this pathway than by the sulfation and glucuronidation detoxification pathways. The byproduct of acetaminophen metabolism by CYP2E1 is *N*-acetyl-*p*-benzoquinoneimine (NApQI), which is toxic to the liver. The accumulation of this compound in conjunction with diminished antioxidant defenses in the liver (glutathione) lowers the threshold of acetaminophen toxicity in alcoholic persons. Thus, in this population, the clinical presentation of acetaminophen toxicity is distinct from that of alcoholic hepatitis. Aminotransferase levels are markedly increased, often more than 1,000 U/L, which is distinctly unusual for alcoholic hepatitis.

RECOMMENDED READING

Degos F. Hepatitis C and alcohol. J Hepatol. 1999;31 Suppl 1:113-8.

Imperiale TF, McCullough AJ. Do corticosteroids reduce mortality from alcoholic hepatitis? A meta-analysis of the randomized trials. Ann Intern Med. 1990;113:299-307.

Maddrey WC, Boitnott JK, Bedine MS, Weber FL Jr, Mezey E, White RI Jr. Corticosteroid therapy of alcoholic hepatitis. Gastroenterology. 1978;75:193-9.

McCullough AJ, O'Connor JF. Alcoholic liver disease: proposed recommendations for the American College of Gastroenterology. Am J Gastroenterol. 1998;93:2022-36.

Menon KV, Gores GJ, Shah VH. Pathogenesis, diagnosis, and treatment of alcoholic liver disease. Mayo Clin Proc. 2001;76:1021-9.

Morgan MY. The treatment of alcoholic hepatitis. Alcohol Alcohol. 1996;31:117-34.

Seeff LB, Cuccherini BA, Zimmerman HJ, Adler E, Benjamin SB. Acetaminophen hepatotoxicity in alcoholics: a therapeutic misadventure. Ann Intern Med. 1986;104:399-404.

CHAPTER 31

Vascular Diseases of the Liver

Patrick S. Kamath, M.D.

Vascular diseases of the liver can be divided into disorders of hepatic inflow (i.e., diseases of the portal venous and hepatic arterial inflow) and disorders of hepatic venous outflow (Table 1).

For a better understanding of the vascular diseases of the liver, a concise review of the vascular anatomy of the liver is important.

ANATOMY OF THE SPLANCHNIC CIRCULATION

The splanchnic circulation comprises the arterial blood supply and venous drainage of the entire gastrointestinal tract from the distal esophagus to the mid rectum and includes the spleen, pancreas, gallbladder, and liver. The arterial system is derived from the celiac artery and the superior and inferior mesenteric arteries. The superior mesenteric artery arises from the abdominal aorta just distal to the celiac trunk. For most of its course, this artery lies in the mesentery, with the ileocolic artery being the terminal branch. The superior mesenteric artery gives off three sets of branches: 1) several small branches to the pancreas and duodenum before entering the mesentery, 2) three large arteries that supply the proximal two-thirds of the large bowel, and 3) during its course through the mesenteric root, an arcade of arterial branches to supply the jejunum and ileum. The branches given off in the mesentery form a row of arterial arcades that terminate in the arteriae rectae of the wall of the small bowel. The venous drainage has a similar pattern, with the venae rectae forming a venous arcade that drains the small bowel. These join with the ileocolic, middle colic, and right colic veins to form the superior mesenteric vein.

The arterial routes of the splanchnic circulation, except for the hepatic artery, eventually empty into the portal venous system through the splenic vein and superior and inferior mesenteric veins. The portal vein, formed by the convergence of the splenic and superior mesenteric veins, constitutes the primary blood supply to the liver. After perfusing the liver, venous blood reenters the systemic circulation through the hepatic veins and suprahepatic inferior vena cava.

Reminiscent of the lungs, the liver receives a dual blood supply. The two sources are portal venous blood (derived from the mesenteric venous circulation including the digestive tract, spleen, and pancreas) and hepatic arterial blood (usually from the celiac artery). Total hepatic blood flow constitutes nearly 30% of total cardiac output. The portal venous inflow comprises 65% to 75% of hepatic blood inflow and the hepatic artery supplies approximately 25% to 35%. However, approximately 50% of the liver's oxygen requirements is delivered by hepatic arterial blood.

Table 1. Vascular Diseases of the Liver

Disorders of portal venous inflow
Acute mesenteric venous thrombosis
Chronic mesenteric venous thrombosis
Disorders of hepatic arterial inflow
Hepatic artery thrombosis
Hepatic arteriovenous fistula
Ischemic hepatitis
Disorders of hepatic venous outflow
Veno-occlusive disease
Budd-Chiari syndrome

The hepatic vascular bed is a low-pressure system that can maintain a large volume of blood. Sinusoidal blood collects within terminal hepatic venules and reenters the systemic circulation through the hepatic veins and inferior vena cava. The caudate lobe of the liver maintains a separate drainage of blood, accounting for the compensatory hypertrophy of this lobe often observed in chronic liver disease associated with outflow obstruction of the major hepatic veins (Budd-Chiari syndrome).

DISORDERS OF PORTAL VENOUS INFLOW

Acute Mesenteric Venous Thrombosis
Acute mesenteric venous thrombosis is discussed in the chapter on "Vascular Disorders of the Gastrointestinal Tract."

Chronic Mesenteric Venous Thrombosis
Chronic mesenteric venous thrombosis is very different from the acute form. Lack of visualization of the superior mesenteric vein on computed tomography (CT) or duplex ultrasonography in conjunction with extensive collateral venous drainage suggests the diagnosis of chronic mesenteric venous thrombosis. Angiography can help confirm the diagnosis but rarely is required. Although many patients present with nonspecific symptoms of several months' duration, an increasing proportion are being identified through imaging studies performed for unrelated reasons. These patients may be asymptomatic with respect to the primary event; hence, the time of the thrombotic event often is unclear. Patients in whom the thrombosis extends to involve the portal vein or splenic vein (or both) may experience portal hypertension and esophageal varices, with the attendant complications of variceal bleeding. They also may have splenomegaly and hypersplenism. Chronic mesenteric venous thrombosis should be differentiated from isolated splenic vein thrombosis due to pancreatic neoplasm or chronic pancreatitis. The latter, often called "sinistral (or left-sided) portal hypertension," is related to a local effect on the splenic vein and is not usually a disorder of the thrombotic pathway. Thus, anticoagulation for sinistral portal hypertension is not warranted. Patients with isolated chronic mesenteric venous thrombosis often remain asymptomatic because of extensive collateral venous drainage. Occasionally, some patients have gastrointestinal tract hemorrhage, and the use of pharmacologic agents such as propranolol to prevent variceal bleeding is recommended. Endoscopic therapy is used both to control active bleeding and to prevent rebleeding. Surgical intervention, such as portosystemic shunts, is restricted to patients whose bleeding cannot be controlled by conservative measures and who have a patent central vein for shunting. When thrombosis is extensive and no large vein is suitable for anastomosis, nonconventional shunts may be considered, such as anastomosing a large collateral vein with a systemic vein. Gastroesophageal devascularization also may be considered. For patients with thrombophilia, anticoagulation may be initiated after the risk of bleeding has been decreased with surgical stents.

DISORDERS OF HEPATIC ARTERIAL INFLOW

Hepatic Artery Thrombosis
Aside from patients who have had liver transplantation, the prevalence of hepatic artery thrombosis is not certain. Hepatic artery thrombosis is the cause of considerable morbidity and mortality in approximately 7% of adults and in perhaps as many as 40% of pediatric patients undergoing orthotopic liver transplantation. The problem is more extensive in the pediatric age group because of the small caliber of the vessels involved and the probable greater fluctuation in the concentration of coagulation factors.

Several risk factors are related to the development of hepatic artery thrombosis in adults, with technical aspects of the arterial anastomosis being the most important risk of early thrombosis. Other risk factors are older recipients, clotting abnormalities, tobacco use, and infections by agents such as cytomegalovirus. Late hepatic artery thrombosis has been associated with chronic rejection and blood-type–incompatible grafts.

The clinical presentation of hepatic artery thrombosis can vary from a mild increase in the serum level of aminotransferases to fulminant hepatic necrosis. The acute presentation, or early hepatic artery thrombosis, has a more severe clinical course and late hepatic artery thrombosis generally has a milder course. There is no agreement about the time point between early and late hepatic artery thrombosis. However, the later hepatic artery thrombosis develops after liver transplantation, the less severe the clinical presentation.

Early hepatic artery thrombosis results in massive injury to hepatocytes and bile duct epithelial cells. Ischemic damage to the bile ducts leads to dehiscence of the biliary anastomosis, resulting in bile duct strictures and intrahepatic abscesses. Thus, biliary sepsis may be a common presentation of early hepatic artery thrombosis. However, one-third of episodes of early hepatic artery thrombosis may be asymptomatic.

Hepatic artery thrombosis can be diagnosed with duplex ultrasonography, but visceral angiography may be necessary to confirm the diagnosis. When hepatic artery thrombosis is detected early after liver transplantation, surgical correction usually is recommended.

Hepatic Artery Aneurysm
Although aneurysm of the hepatic artery (Fig. 1) is rare, it is the fourth most common abdominal aneurysm. The aneurysms

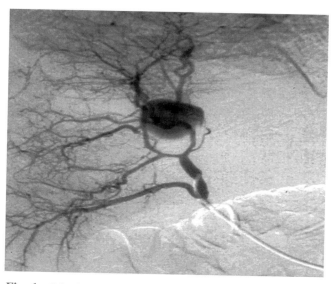

Fig. 1. Selective hepatic angiogram showing an aneurysm of the intrahepatic portion of the hepatic artery.

are usually small (<2 cm in diameter) and involve the main hepatic artery. Causes of hepatic artery aneurysms include atherosclerotic vascular diseases, infections such as bacterial endocarditis, liver abscess, syphilis, tuberculosis, and trauma from liver biopsy. The hepatic artery commonly is involved in polyarteritis nodosa, manifested as symptoms related to thrombosis, rupture, or dissection of the aneurysm.

Most hepatic artery aneurysms are discovered incidentally. If symptomatic, the first and dominating symptom is severe abdominal pain, suggesting dissection. Vague abdominal pain in these patients is related to compression of surrounding structures. Rupture of a hepatic artery aneurysm causes massive intraperitoneal hemorrhage or hemobilia manifested as abdominal pain, jaundice, and gastrointestinal tract bleeding. Hemobilia is usually a manifestation of an intrahepatic aneurysm.

Ruptured hepatic artery aneurysms are associated with a high mortality rate because, in most patients, the diagnosis is made only after rupture. Treatment of a ruptured aneurysm is emergency surgery or embolization of the aneurysm in patients who are not optimal candidates for surgery. For asymptomatic patients, the treatment of a hepatic artery aneurysm is debated. Clearly, aneurysms larger than 2 cm in diameter require treatment, and those between 1 and 2 cm in diameter may be treated. For aneurysms less than 1 cm in diameter, follow-up at 6-month intervals is reasonable. Treatment includes interventional radiologic approaches to embolize and occlude the aneurysm, ligation at surgery, or excision and reconstruction of the aneurysm. Intrahepatic aneurysms may be treated also by liver resection.

Hepatic Artery–Portal Vein Fistulas

Hepatic artery–portal vein fistulas are rare causes of portal hypertension. Although fistulas within the liver usually are iatrogenic, the result of liver biopsy, they may be related to neoplasms or Osler-Weber-Rendu syndrome. A hepatic artery–portal vein fistula should be suspected in a patient who has acute onset of abdominal pain and ascites, especially if associated with gastrointestinal tract bleeding, because rupture of the artery into the portal vein causes an acute increase in portal pressure. These fistulas may be accompanied by abdominal bruits in most patients. If untreated, the fistulas may result in cardiac failure. The best treatment is embolization and occlusion of the fistula. The usual result is complete cure of the portal hypertension.

Ischemic Hepatitis

In patients with congestive heart failure, portal blood flow is minimal and, thus, the major contribution of oxygenated blood to the liver is from the hepatic artery. In congestive heart failure, episodes of hypotension, as associated with arrhythmias, diminish hepatic arterial input, resulting in ischemic necrosis of the liver. Typical manifestations of ischemic hepatitis are a rapid increase over 24 to 48 hours in the serum level of aminotransferases (aspartate aminotransferase, alanine aminotransferase), to several thousand units, sometimes more than 10,000 U/L. This value rapidly returns to less than 100 U/L in 3 to 5 days. No specific treatment is required other than control of the cardiac condition. Extensive ischemic hepatitis may result in fulminant liver failure.

Other causes of ischemic hepatitis are hypovolemic shock of any cause and obstructive sleep apnea. Postoperative patients are particularly prone to ischemic liver damage because they often have coexisting arterial hypotension and hypoxemia. Furthermore, hepatic blood flow may be reduced by anesthetic agents. This problem may be of particular concern in patients who have open heart surgery. The typical histologic finding in these patients with ischemic liver damage is centrilobular hepatic necrosis (zone 3). The severity of liver damage is related to the duration of hypotension and the degree of hypoxemia.

DISORDERS OF HEPATIC VENOUS OUTFLOW

Veno-occlusive Disease

Veno-occlusive disease results from occlusion of the central and sublobular hepatic veins. Within the United States, the most common cause of veno-occlusive disease is preconditioning for bone marrow transplantation. Other causes include radiation to the liver, antineoplastic drugs such as azathioprine and 6-mercaptopurine, and ingestion of alkaloids containing pyrrolizidine.

The following discussion is predominantly on veno-occlusive disease of the liver in relation to patients undergoing bone marrow transplantation. In these patients, the incidence of veno-occlusive disease is approximately 50%, with a mortality rate of 20% to 40%. Early changes are related to hemorrhage in zone 3, as seen in transjugular liver biopsy specimens. Diagnostic criteria include subendothelial thickening of at least one terminal hepatic venule in association with luminal narrowing.

The pathogenesis of veno-occlusive disease is not well defined. It probably results from a combination of endothelial injury and activation of clotting mechanisms. It has been hypothesized that the depletion of glutathione in zone 3 hepatocytes makes them more prone to damage by antineoplastic agents such as busulfan. The resulting accumulation of oxygen free radicals leads to zone 3 necrosis and subsequent endothelial damage.

Clinical criteria for diagnosing veno-occlusive disease are either the Seattle or the Baltimore criteria. The Baltimore criteria reflect more severe veno-occlusive disease and require a weight gain of more than 5% in association with hepatomegaly and ascites. The Seattle criteria require a bilirubin level greater than 2 mg/dL in association with hepatomegaly, right upper quadrant pain, and a weight gain of more than 2%. According to both the Baltimore and Seattle criteria, the criteria should be met within 3 weeks after bone marrow transplantation. Bilirubin levels greater than 15 mg/dL are associated with a poor outcome.

Treatment of veno-occlusive disease is difficult and often unrewarding. Prophylactic strategies have included administration of heparin, prostaglandins, or ursodeoxycholic acid. Because of the lack of large randomized studies, it is difficult to determine the benefits of any of these therapies. The treatment of established veno-occlusive disease also is debated. Tissue plasminogen activator and heparin have been used in patients at high risk of dying from complications of veno-occlusive disease. If there is no response to thrombolytic therapy, either a surgical shunt or transjugular intrahepatic portosystemic shunt (TIPS) may be used. Although the initial results with portosystemic shunts may be beneficial, the long-term outcome for patients who require shunts is poor because they usually have severe veno-occlusive disease and intervention generally delays but does not prevent a fatal outcome.

Budd-Chiari Syndrome

Budd-Chiari syndrome is a heterogenous group of disorders characterized by obstruction of hepatic venous outflow. The site of obstruction may be at the level of small hepatic venules, large hepatic veins, inferior vena cava, or the right atrium. Obstruction at the level of the central and sublobular hepatic venules traditionally has been called "hepatic veno-occlusive disease." In countries such as Japan and India, obstruction of the inferior vena cava by membranes or webs or segmental narrowing of the vessel also may obstruct hepatic venous outflow.

Etiology

The main causes predisposing to Budd-Chiari syndrome include a hypercoagulable state, tumor invasion of the hepatic venous outflow tract, and miscellaneous causes. In some patients, no clear etiologic factor is discernible. Increasingly, the presence of multiple underlying disorders that cause Budd-Chiari syndrome is being recognized.

Hematologic abnormalities are detected in up to 87.5% of patients with Budd-Chiari syndrome, particularly myeloproliferative disorders. Overt polycythemia vera is the most common disorder encountered. Erythroid cell cultures and erythropoietin levels have been used to diagnose occult primary myeloproliferative disorders in patients originally thought to have idiopathic Budd-Chiari syndrome. Both fulminant and chronic forms of the syndrome have been described in patients with nocturnal hemoglobinuria. Inherited deficiencies of protein C, protein S, and antithrombin III are increasingly being reported in association with the syndrome. Protein C and protein S are vitamin K-dependent proteins that are synthesized in the liver and endothelial cells and act as fibrinolytic agents. Antithrombin III is a vitamin K-independent protease inhibitor that is synthesized in the liver and neutralizes activated clotting factors by forming a complex with a specific serine protease. Deficiencies of any of these proteins can result in both arterial and venous thrombosis, but the correlation between protein C and protein S levels and the risk of thrombosis is not precise. In several patients with Budd-Chiari syndrome, protein C deficiency has also been associated with an underlying myeloproliferative disorder. The diagnosis is not certain if these proteins become deficient in a patient with chronic liver disease. The presence of normal levels of factors II and VII in patients with Budd-Chiari syndrome or deficiencies of protein C and protein S in family members may point toward a congenital disorder.

The factor V Leiden mutation has been reported in approximately 23% of patients with Budd-Chiari syndrome. The mutation, caused by the substitution of an arginine residue by glutamine at position 506 in the factor V molecule, abolishes a protein C cleavage site in factor V and prolongs the thrombogenic effect of factor V activation. The term "resistance to activated protein C" is another name for this condition. Although about 2.9% to 6% of people of European descent are believed to be heterozygous for this mutation, the relative risk of thrombosis is thought to be low. In addition to being the sole cause of Budd-Chiari syndrome, this mutation also has been reported to occur in combination with other prothrombotic disorders.

Clinical Manifestations

The underlying pathophysiologic abnormality in Budd-Chiari syndrome is an increase in sinusoidal pressure caused by obstruction of hepatic venous outflow. This results in hypoxic damage to the hepatocytes and increased portal venous pressure.

Continued obstruction of hepatic venous outflow leads to further hepatic necrosis, ultimately resulting in cirrhosis. Because the caudate lobe drains directly into the inferior vena cava, it is not damaged. In fact, the caudate lobe hypertrophies, and this may, to various degrees, obstruct the inferior vena cava. The clinical presentation of Budd-Chiari syndrome depends on the extent and rapidity of hepatic vein occlusion and whether collateral circulation has developed to decompress the liver. Vague abdominal pain is the most common presenting symptom of the syndrome, and ascites is the most common abnormality noted on physical examination. Some patients with hepatic vein thrombosis are asymptomatic, presumably as a result of decompression of the portal system through the development of large intrahepatic and portosystemic collaterals.

Investigations

Doppler ultrasonography of the liver is the initial investigation of choice in patients with suspected Budd-Chiari syndrome. It demonstrates the hepatic veins, splenic vein, portal vein, and inferior vena cava. Necrotic areas are seen better on contrast-enhanced CT. The value of magnetic resonance imaging in diagnosing the syndrome has not been established.

Venography, with pressure measurements in hepatic veins and inferior vena cava, is necessary after the diagnosis of Budd-Chiari syndrome has been suggested by noninvasive studies. However, if the clinical suspicion of Budd-Chiari syndrome is high, especially in a patient with a fulminant or acute presentation, contrast venography may be necessary even though the ultrasonographic examination is negative. The characteristic appearance of the hepatic veins in Budd-Chiari syndrome is that of a spider's web with an extensive collateral circulation. Also, the inferior vena cava may be compressed by an enlarged caudate lobe or it may demonstrate thrombus. A transjugular liver biopsy of both the right and left lobes should be performed at the time of the angiographic investigation, if possible.

In addition to establishing the diagnosis of hepatic vein thrombosis, it is important to identify an underlying cause to determine management strategies. An appropriate hematologic work-up should be done to exclude the various disorders outlined in Table 2, including a bone marrow examination to determine if the patient has a myeloproliferative disorder.

Management

The aims of treatment of Budd-Chiari syndrome are to relieve obstruction of the hepatic outflow tract, to identify and treat the underlying cause, and to relieve symptoms. Treatment options include medical management, surgical portosystemic shunting, TIPS, and liver transplantation (Table 3). Although most patients who have Budd-Chiari syndrome can be offered some form of definitive therapy, those in whom the syndrome

Table 2.   Causes of Budd-Chiari Syndrome

Common causes
  Hypercoagulable states
    Inherited
      Antithrombin III deficiency
      Protein C deficiency
      Protein S deficiency
      Factor V Leiden mutation
      Prothrombin mutation
    Acquired
      Myeloproliferative disorders
      Paroxysmal nocturnal hemoglobinuria
      Antiphospholipid syndrome
      Cancer
      Pregnancy
      Oral contraceptive use
Uncommon causes
  Tumor invasion
    Hepatocellular carcinoma
    Renal cell carcinoma
    Adrenal carcinoma
  Miscellaneous
    Aspergillosis
    Behçet's syndrome
    Inferior vena cava webs
    Trauma
    Inflammatory bowel disease
    Dacarbazine therapy
  Idiopathic

From Menon KV, Shah V, Kamath PS. The Budd-Chiari syndrome. N Engl J Med. 2004;350:578-85. Used with permission.

is due to malignant disease are offered only palliative care because of the extremely poor prognosis of this condition.

Medical management consists of diuretic therapy for the treatment of ascites, anticoagulation to prevent extension of venous thrombosis, and treatment of the underlying cause. Ideal candidates for angioplasty include patients with inferior vena cava webs or focal hepatic vein stenosis; thrombolytic therapy is delivered best by a transfemoral or transjugular route, with infusion of either urokinase or tissue plasminogen activator directly into the thrombosed vein for about 24 hours.

The aim of portosystemic shunting is to use the portal vein to provide a venous outflow tract for the liver to reverse hepatic necrosis and to prevent chronic sequelae of hepatic venous outflow obstruction. The optimal candidates for surgical shunting are patients with a subacute presentation in whom ascites is not extensive, liver function is preserved, and the disease course is smoldering. Patients with fulminant or acute Budd-Chiari syndrome may need a less invasive procedure, such as TIPS, for the acute crisis before definitive therapy is planned. If liver biopsy findings show cirrhosis, the patient should be evaluated for liver transplantation. Indications for liver transplantation in Budd-Chiari syndrome include 1) end-stage chronic liver disease, 2) fulminant liver failure, and 3) deterioration of liver function after portosystemic shunting.

Table 3. Management of Budd-Chiari Syndrome (BCS)

Treatment	Indication	Advantages	Disadvantages
Thrombolytic therapy	Acute thrombosis	Reverses hepatic necrosis No long-term sequelae	Risk of bleeding Limited success
Angioplasty with and without stenting	IVC webs IVC stenosis Focal hepatic vein stenosis	Averts need for surgery	High rate of restenosis or shunt occlusion
TIPS	Possible bridge to transplantation in fulminant BCS Acute BCS Subacute BCS if portacaval pressure gradient < 10 mm Hg or occluded IVC	Low mortality Useful even with compression of IVC by caudate lobe	High rate of shunt stenosis Extended stents may interfere with liver transplantation
Surgical shunt	Subacute BCS Portacaval pressure gradient > 10 mm Hg	Definitive procedure for many patients Low rate of shunt dysfunction with portacaval shunt	Risk of procedure-related death Limited applicability
Liver transplantation	Fulminant BCS Presence of cirrhosis Failure of portosystemic shunt	Reverses liver disease May reverse underlying thrombophilia	Risk of procedure-related death Need for long-term immunosuppression

IVC, inferior vena cava; TIPS, transjugular intrahepatic portosystemic shunt.
From Menon KV, Shah V, Kamath PS. The Budd-Chiari syndrome. N Engl J Med. 2004;350:578-85. Used with permission.

RECOMMENDED READING

Chronic Mesenteric Venous Thrombosis

D'Cruz AJ, Kamath PS, Ramachandra C, Jalihal A. Non-conventional portosystemic shunts in children with extra-hepatic portal vein obstruction. Acta Paediatr Jpn. 1995;37:17-20.

Kumar S, Sarr MG, Kamath PS. Mesenteric venous thrombosis. N Engl J Med. 2001;345:1683-8.

Norton ID, Andrews JC, Kamath PS. Management of ectopic varices. Hepatology. 1998;28:1154-8.

Hepatic Artery Thrombosis

Pastacaldi S, Teixeira R, Montalto P, Rolles K, Burroughs AK. Hepatic artery thrombosis after orthotopic liver transplantation: a review of nonsurgical causes. Liver Transpl. 2001;7:75-81.

Sieders E, Peeters PM, TenVergert FM, de Jong KP, Porte RJ, Zwaveling JH, et al. Early vascular complications after pediatric liver transplantation. Liver Transpl. 2000;6:326-32.

Hepatic Artery Aneurysms

Baker KS, Tisnado J, Cho SR, Beachley MC. Splanchnic artery aneurysms and pseudoaneurysms: transcatheter embolization. Radiology 1987;163:135-9.

Busuttil RW, Brin BJ. The diagnosis and management of visceral artery aneurysms. Surgery. 1980;88:619-24.

Cooper SG, Richman AH. Spontaneous rupture of a congenital hepatic artery aneurysm. J Clin Gastroenterol. 1988;10:104-7.

Ischemic Hepatitis

Seeto RK, Fenn B, Rockey DC. Ischemic hepatitis: clinical presentation and pathogenesis. Am J Med. 2000;109:109-13.

Veno-occlusive Disease and Budd-Chiari Syndrome

Bearman SI. Veno-occlusive disease of the liver. Curr Opin Oncol. 2000;12:103-9.

Ganguli SC, Ramzan NN, McKusick MA, Andrews JC, Phyliky RL, Kamath PS. Budd-Chiari syndrome in patients with hematological disease: a therapeutic challenge. Hepatology. 1998;27:1157-61.

Menon KV, Shah V, Kamath PS. The Budd-Chiari syndrome. N Engl J Med. 2004;350:578-85.

CHAPTER 32

Portal Hypertension-Related Bleeding

Patrick S. Kamath, M.D.

INTRODUCTION

Portal hypertensive bleeding encompasses a spectrum of conditions that include esophageal, gastric, and ectopic varices and portal hypertensive gastrointestinal enteropathy. Esophageal variceal hemorrhage occurs through a combination of increased portal pressure and local factors within the varix itself. Management of esophageal varices includes primary prophylaxis of variceal hemorrhage, treatment of actively bleeding varices, and prevention of variceal rebleeding (secondary prophylaxis). Primary prophylaxis is pharmacologic therapy with β-blockers or variceal band ligation if β-blocker therapy fails or the therapy is not tolerated by the patient. Active bleeding is best treated endoscopically. Either pharmacologic or endoscopic therapy is appropriate for secondary prophylaxis. Surgical shunts or transjugular intrahepatic portosystemic shunts (TIPS) are second-line therapy.

PATHOGENESIS OF PORTAL HYPERTENSION

An increase in the hepatic venous pressure gradient—the difference between the wedged hepatic venous pressure and the free hepatic venous pressure of at least 10 mm Hg—is required for the development of esophageal varices, and a hepatic venous pressure gradient of 12 mm Hg or more is required for the rupture of esophageal varices.

In cirrhosis, portal hypertension occurs through an increase in resistance to portal venous outflow early in the disease process. This increase is due to mechanical factors related to distortion of liver architecture. However, approximately 30% of the increase in resistance occurs through potentially reversible vascular factors and is the target of pharmacotherapy.

Portal hypertension is maintained through the development of a systemic hyperdynamic circulation and peripheral vasodilation. The hyperdynamic circulation is characterized in the splanchnic circulation by vasodilation and increased flow at the level of the splanchnic arterioles. This leads to increased portal venous inflow and exacerbates the existing portal hypertension. Drugs such as octreotide and vasopressin reduce splanchnic hyperemia and portal venous inflow. Portal hypertension results in the development of collateral circulation which may decrease portal pressure. In addition to gastric and intestinal vascular ectasia, esophageal and gastric varices and portal hypertensive gastropathy are manifestations of portal hypertension.

ESOPHAGEAL VARICES

Pathogenesis

Local factors that determine risk of hemorrhage from esophageal varices include the radius of the varix, the thickness of the varix wall, and the pressure gradient between the varix and the esophageal lumen. Factors that determine the severity of bleeding are the degree of liver dysfunction and defective coagulation, portal pressure, and the size of the rent in the varix. Endoscopic sclerotherapy or band ligation attempts to decrease flow through the varix by inducing thrombosis and, ultimately, obliteration of varices.

Therapy

The current recommendations for treatment are summarized in Table 1.

Table 1. Recommendations for Treatment of Esophageal Varices

	First-line therapy	Second-line therapy	Other
Primary prophylaxis	β-Blockers	Endoscopic variceal ligation	
Control of bleeding	Endoscopy + pharmacologic treatment	TIPS	
Secondary prophylaxis	Endoscopy β-Blockers	TIPS	Transplantation

TIPS, transjugular intrahepatic portosystemic shunt.

Primary Prophylaxis

All patients with cirrhosis should have endoscopy to screen for the presence and size of esophageal varices. In approximately 25% of patients, varices bleed, usually within the ensuing 2 years. For patients with large varices and advanced liver disease, the risk of hemorrhage can be as high as 75%. Thus, prophylactic therapy is indicated for patients with large varices (> 5 mm in diameter). The presence or absence of high-risk endoscopic signs such as red wales does not influence the decision to initiate therapy. If no varices are detected at endoscopy, the procedure should be repeated in 2 or 3 years.

The established primary prophylaxis is treatment with nonselective β-adrenergic blocking agents (β-blockers) such as propranolol and nadolol. It is important to use only nonselective agents rather than β$_1$-selective agents. β$_1$-Blockade decreases cardiac output and splanchnic blood flow, whereas the additional β$_2$-blockade allows unopposed α$_1$-adrenergic constriction in the splanchnic circulation. This decreases portal blood flow and, consequently, portal pressure. Therapy is started at a low dose, with slow upward titration of the dose until a resting pulse rate of 55 to 60 beats/min is achieved or hypotension develops (systolic blood pressure < 90 mm Hg). A long-acting preparation of propranolol administered as a single dose in the early evening is preferred. This allows adequate β-blockade at night, when the risk of bleeding is high. With the long-acting preparation administered in the evening, β-blockade is less during the following day, thus decreasing the side effect of fatigue. At the same time, the risk of bleeding is lower during the day, and the lesser degree of β-blockade is not deleterious to the patient. Whenever possible, the hemodynamic response to pharmacologic therapy should be measured. The goal of therapy is to decrease the hepatic venous pressure gradient to less than 12 mm Hg or by 20% when compared with baseline.

Although sclerotherapy as a form of primary prophylaxis is no longer used, variceal band ligation may be an alternative approach to primary prophylaxis because of the lower rate of esophageal ulceration and more effective obliteration of variceal structures. Currently, esophageal variceal ligation is recommended for patients who have contraindications to therapy with β-blockers, who have not had a decrease in the hepatic vein pressure gradient, or who have experienced side effects from β-blocker therapy.

Control of Esophageal Variceal Hemorrhage

Active esophageal variceal bleeding is best managed through endoscopic means, preferably variceal band ligation. Immediate initiation of pharmacologic therapy after gastrointestinal tract bleeding has been detected in patients with cirrhosis is beneficial—even before endoscopy has demonstrated variceal bleeding. Pharmacologic therapy is continued for up to 5 days after endoscopic treatment of varices to reduce the risk of immediate rebleeding. Vasopressin is a potent splanchnic vasoconstrictor that decreases portal venous inflow, thereby decreasing portal pressure, but it is seldom used. Nitroglycerin is used in conjunction with vasopressin to further decrease portal pressure and reduce the ischemic side effects of vasopressin, which are pronounced and limit therapy in up to 30% of patients. Octreotide, a long-acting synthetic somatostatin analogue, is the pharmacologic agent most commonly used. It appears to decrease portal pressure by inhibiting glucagon release and the ensuing postprandial hyperemia and by a direct vasoconstrictive effect on splanchnic arteriolar smooth muscle. Although octreotide is safer than vasopressin, the efficacy of the compound has not been well established. However, a recent meta-analysis has suggested that octreotide is beneficial for acute bleeding. Octreotide is administered as an initial bolus of 50 μg, followed by an infusion at 50 μg/h for 5 days in conjunction with endoscopic variceal band ligation.

For treating active bleeding, the use of surgical shunts and TIPS is limited to patients with refractory bleeding or immediate rebleeding after two separate unsuccessful attempts at endoscopic intervention performed within 24 hours. Frequently, TIPS is preferred to surgical intervention, particularly in patients with Child-Pugh class B or C status. Therapy for the varices can also be administered concomitantly through the injection of gel foam or coils into the gastroesophageal collateral vessels at the time of TIPS. A surgical shunt should be considered in patients with Child-Pugh class A status and in patients for whom continued medical surveillance will be unlikely because TIPS requires close ultrasonographic follow-up of the shunt to evaluate for restenosis. The type of surgical shunt used depends on institutional expertise and the patient's potential as a candidate for liver transplantation.

Supportive and resuscitative care includes airway protection, volume replacement, treatment of coagulopathy, and vigorous surveillance and treatment of concomitant infection. Maintenance of a hematocrit of 25% to 30% is appropriate because aggressive transfusion of blood products may precipitate further bleeding by increasing portal pressure. Antibiotic prophylaxis for 7 days with norfloxacin is recommended to decrease the incidence of bacteremia and spontaneous bacterial peritonitis, which commonly accompany variceal hemorrhage. Antibiotic therapy is probably the most important reason why the mortality of variceal bleeding has decreased from 50% to about 20%. Lactulose therapy may be instituted to prevent and treat hepatic encephalopathy.

Secondary Prophylaxis

Secondary prophylaxis involves therapies to prevent rebleeding in patients who have already bled from esophageal varices. Intervention is essential because up to 80% of patients who have already bled from varices will bleed again within 2 years. Treatments include pharmacotherapy with β-blockers, either alone or in combination with oral nitrates, endoscopic sclerotherapy or band ligation, TIPS, and surgical shunts. Either β-blockers or endoscopic therapy are appropriate treatment options for patients who did not receive β-blockers for primary prophylaxis. Band ligation is the preferred endoscopic treatment because of the lower incidence of esophageal ulceration and ease of therapy. After controlling acute bleeding with variceal ligation, the next ligation session is scheduled in approximately 10 to 14 days. Subsequent sessions are scheduled every 3 or 4 weeks. Varices usually can be obliterated over several weekly sessions. Also, combination therapy of band ligation and β-blockers is administered to some patients, although the risk-benefit ratio of this approach is debated.

For patients in whom primary prophylaxis with β-blockers failed, the addition of oral nitrates to the pharmacologic regimen will further decrease portal pressure and the incidence of rebleeding. However, concern remains about the long-term effects of oral nitrates on patient survival; therefore, endoscopic obliteration is currently the preferred approach for secondary prophylaxis for patients in whom primary prophylaxis with β-blockers failed. TIPS should be used only in patients with recurrent or refractory bleeding despite pharmacologic and endoscopic therapies, especially if they are candidates for liver transplantation. There is hesitation in recommending widespread use of TIPS because of the risk of worsening encephalopathy, the potential for liver deterioration, and uncertain effects on long-term survival, particularly of patients with advanced

dysfunction of liver synthesis. Surgical shunts are recommended for patients with excellent liver synthetic function who are unlikely to require transplantation in the near future. All appropriate patients who have variceal hemorrhage should be evaluated for liver transplantation.

PORTAL HYPERTENSIVE LESIONS IN THE STOMACH

Gastric lesions that cause portal hypertensive bleeding include gastric varices, portal hypertensive gastropathy, and gastric vascular ectasia. Because no evidence-based management strategies are available for gastric sources of portal hypertensive bleeding, therapy often requires an empiric approach.

Gastric Varices

The most common type of gastric varices are esophageal varices that extend into the cardia of the stomach and are readily treated with endoscopic techniques such as sclerotherapy or band ligation. Varices in the fundus of the stomach, either as an extension of esophageal varices or as isolated gastric fundal varices, are the most common source of gastric variceal bleeding. Recent data have suggested that the frequency of bleeding from gastric varices is similar to that from large esophageal varices. Gastric varices are more likely to be found in patients who have bled from esophageal varices than in those who have not bled. The risk of bleeding from gastric varices is related to the size of the varix, liver function as determined by the Child-Pugh class, and the presence of red signs on the varix.

Currently, no data support the use of prophylactic treatment of gastric varices, even if they are in the fundus. Acute gastric variceal bleeding is best treated endoscopically with injection of cyanoacrylate glue. However, currently, this is not easily available in the United States. Other options include sclerotherapy with ethanolamine oleate or thrombin, but the success rate has been variable. Gastric variceal ligation should be limited to varices in the cardia.

Although pharmacologic therapy, for example, β-blockers, may be used for the prevention of gastric variceal rebleeding, no studies support this practice. Our policy generally has been to recommend a portosystemic shunt for the prevention of rebleeding in patients with documented gastric fundal variceal bleeding. TIPS is reserved for patients with poor liver function, and patients of Child-Pugh class A should be considered for portosystemic shunt surgery.

Portal Hypertensive Gastropathy

Portal hypertensive gastropathy is a source of gastrointestinal tract bleeding in some patients with cirrhosis and portal hypertension. The elementary lesion is a mosaic-like pattern of the gastric mucosa, but this is not specific. The more specific lesion is the red marking, which may be either a red point lesion less than 1 mm in diameter or a cherry red spot more than 2 mm in diameter. The presence of a mosaic-like pattern alone designates *mild* portal hypertensive gastropathy, whereas red markings superimposed on the mosaic pattern suggest *severe* portal hypertensive gastropathy. Lesions of portal hypertensive gastropathy tend to be more common in the proximal stomach, in patients with advanced stages of liver disease as noted by the Child-Pugh classification, in patients with esophageal varices, and in patients who have previously had esophageal variceal therapy. These lesions also are more common in patients with gastric varices. Approximately 3% of patients with severe gastropathy may present with acute upper gastrointestinal tract bleeding, and approximately 15% have chronic bleeding.

Anecdotally, acute bleeding from portal hypertensive gastropathy has been treated, with a high success rate, with vasoactive drugs such as vasopressin, somatostatin, and octreotide. Portosystemic shunts should be considered as rescue treatments if vasoactive drug therapy fails. Patients presenting with chronic bleeding may be treated with iron supplementation and β-blockers. For these patients, treatment should be continued indefinitely or until liver transplantation. Portosystemic shunts may be used as rescue treatment in patients who continue to be transfusion-dependent in spite of adequate β-blocker therapy.

Gastric Vascular Ectasia

A less common gastric mucosal lesion in portal hypertension is gastric vascular ectasia. This is characterized by red markings in the *absence* of a mosaic-like pattern, unlike in portal hypertensive gastropathy. These lesions may be difficult to differentiate from those of severe portal hypertensive gastropathy. Features that favor the diagnosis of gastric vascular ectasia are the dominant involvement of the gastric antrum and the absence of an underlying mosaic-like pattern. The red markings may be arranged in linear aggregates in the antrum, for which the term "gastric antral vascular ectasia" or "watermelon stomach" is used (Fig. 1). If the red markings do not have a typical linear arrangement, the lesion is designated "diffuse gastric vascular ectasia." The diffuse lesions also may involve the proximal stomach, sometimes making differentiation from severe portal hypertensive gastropathy difficult. When the diagnosis is uncertain, gastric mucosal biopsy, which usually is safe, may be helpful. Liver dysfunction seems to be necessary for the pathogenesis of vascular ectasia because these lesions may resolve with liver transplantation.

Treatment of gastric vascular ectasia is difficult. Some patients may be managed only with iron replacement therapy. β-Blockers do not seem to be effective for these lesions, although control trials have not been conducted because of the rarity of gastric vascular ectasia. Thermoablative therapies, such as

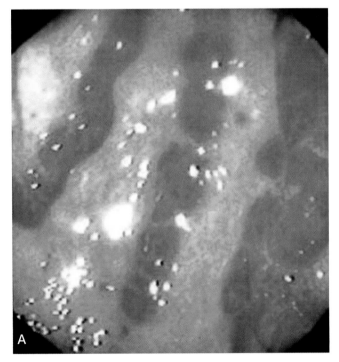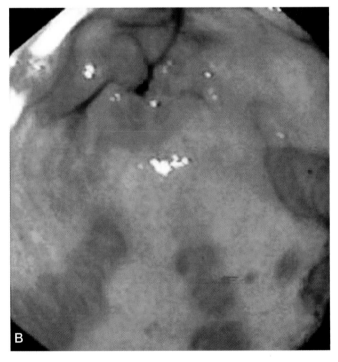

Fig. 1. *A* and *B*, Gastric antral vascular ectasia. Note the linear aggregates of red markings in the antrum and the absence of an underlying mosaic-like pattern.

argon plasma coagulation or laser therapy, may be tried, but the results, especially in the diffuse form, are poor. Antrectomy is effective, but the mortality and morbidity related to the operation can be substantial for patients with cirrhosis. These lesions do not respond to portosystemic shunts, either surgical or TIPS, but occasionally may respond to estrogen-progesterone combinations. We typically prescribe a combination of mestranol (50 mg) with norethindrone (1 mg daily) for these patients.

RECOMMENDED READING

Bosch J, Abraldes JG, Groszmann R. Current management of portal hypertension. J Hepatol. 2003:38 Suppl 1:S54-68.

D'Amico G, Morabito A. Noninvasive markers of esophageal varices: another round, not the last. Hepatology. 2004;39:30-4.

De Franchis R. Portal hypertension III: proceedings of the Third Baverno International Consensus Workshop on Definitions, Methodology, and Therapeutic Strategies. Oxford: Blackwell Science; 2001.

Garcia-Tsao G. Current management of the complications of cirrhosis and portal hypertension: variceal hemorrhage, ascites, and spontaneous bacterial peritonitis. Gastroenterology. 2001;120:726-48.

Grace ND, Groszmann RJ, Garcia-Tsao G, Burroughs AK, Pagliaro L, Makuch RW, et al. Portal hypertension and variceal bleeding: an AASLD single topic symposium. Hepatology. 1998;28:868-80.

Groszmann RJ, Wongcharatrawee S. The hepatic venous pressure gradient: anything worth doing should be done right. Hepatology. 2004;39:280-2.

Kamath PS, Lacerda M, Ahlquist DA, McKusick MA, Andrews JC, Nagorney DA. Gastric mucosal responses to intrahepatic portosystemic shunting in patients with cirrhosis. Gastroenterology. 2000;118:905-911.

Primignani M, Carpinelli L, Preatoni P, Battaglia G, Carta A, Prada A, et al. Natural history of portal hypertensive gastropathy in patients with liver cirrhosis: the New Italian Endoscopic Club for the study and treatment of esophageal varices (NIEC). Gastroenterology. 2000;119:181-7.

Schepke M. Kleber G, Nurnberg D, Willert J, Koch L, Veltzke-Schlieker W, et al, German Study Group for the Primary Prophylaxis of Variceal Bleeding. Ligation versus propranolol for the primary prophylaxis of variceal bleeding in cirrhosis. Hepatology. 2004;40:65-72.

Shah V. Cellular and molecular basis of portal hypertension. Clin Liver Dis. 2001;5:629-44.

CHAPTER 33

Ascites, Hepatorenal Syndrome, and Encephalopathy

Patrick S. Kamath, M.D.

Gastroesophageal variceal bleeding, ascites, and hepatic encephalopathy, the major and life-threatening complications of cirrhosis of the liver, are all related to portal hypertension.

ASCITES

Ascites is the most common major complication of cirrhosis of the liver. The complications of spontaneous bacterial peritonitis and hepatorenal syndrome increase the morbidity associated with ascites. Median survival is 2 to 5 years for patients with ascites, 6 months for patients with refractory ascites, and approximately 2 weeks for those with type 1 hepatorenal syndrome.

Pathogenesis of Ascites

Ascites results from a combination of two factors. The first factor involves renal retention of sodium, which leads to an increase in plasma volume. The second factor involves the movement of this extra fluid into the peritoneal space.

Patients with cirrhosis of the liver have increased hepatic sinusoidal pressure, which ultimately causes splanchnic and systemic vasodilatation. The systemic vasodilatation is sensed by the kidney as a decrease in effective arterial blood volume. This activates the renin-angiotensin-aldosterone system and sympathetic nervous system and stimulates the release of antidiuretic hormone. Activation of the renin-angiotensin-aldosterone system results in sodium and water retention and renal vasoconstriction; activation of the sympathetic nervous system results in renal vasoconstriction and a small amount of sodium and water retention; and the nonosmotic release of antidiuretic hormone results in water retention. Thus, the net effect of compensating for the decreased effect of arterial blood volume is an increase in sodium and water retention.

The excess fluid becomes localized in the peritoneal space because of portal hypertension. Normally, fluid is maintained in the hepatic vascular space by very low hydrostatic pressure. The hepatic sinusoids are freely permeable to albumin, and this produces an extremely low oncotic pressure gradient. Therefore, for fluid to remain within the vascular space, the hydrostatic pressure gradient has to be very low; that is, hepatic sinusoidal pressure has to be low. In cirrhosis of the liver, sinusoidal obstruction due to fibrosis and nodule formation and vasoactive factors, such as endothelial-derived vasoactive factor (i.e., endothelins), increase hepatic sinusoidal pressure. This leads to fluid "weeping" from the liver into the peritoneal space, causing ascites.

Evaluation of a Patient With Ascites

Cirrhosis of the liver is the most common cause of ascites. Almost 80% of patients with ascites have cirrhosis of the liver, about 10% have malignant ascites, and 5% have heart disease (Table 1). Approximately 4% of patients have a mixed form of ascites that is a combination of two of the following three: liver disease, heart disease, malignancy. Approximately only 1% of patients have ascites related to conditions such as tuberculosis, pancreatic ascites, or chylous ascites.

Diagnostic Testing for Ascites

A diagnostic paracentesis is essential in all patients who present with ascites. The most important investigation performed on ascitic fluid is the measurement of albumin. The difference between serum albumin and ascitic fluid albumin, preferably

Table 1. Causes of Ascites

Liver
    Cirrhosis
    Budd-Chiari syndrome
    Liver metastases
    Alcoholic hepatitis
    Veno-occlusive disease
    Portal vein thrombosis (rare)
Heart
    Congestive heart failure
    Constrictive pericarditis
    Right atrial myxoma
Malignant
    Peritoneal carcinomatosis
Infectious
    Tuberculous peritonitis
Kidney
    Nephrotic syndrome
    Continuous ambulatory peritoneal dialysis
Other
    Pancreatitis
    Myxedema
    Meig's syndrome
    Chylous ascites
    Collagen vascular diseases
    Protein-losing enteropathy

measured in samples obtained simultaneously, is the "serum-ascites albumin gradient." A gradient of 1.1 g/dL or more indicates portal hypertension due to either heart or liver disease, and a gradient less than 1.1 g/dL usually indicates a peritoneal process. A total protein less than 2.5 g/dL in ascitic fluid usually favors liver disease, and a total protein of 2.5 g/dL or more favors heart disease (Table 2).

Other investigations include cell count (normal, < 150 cells/mm^3). If the cell count is more than 250 neutrophils/mm^3, the diagnosis is spontaneous bacterial peritonitis. The amylase level is less in ascitic fluid than in serum. An amylase level that is higher in ascitic fluid than in serum, especially if it is more than 1,000 U/L, suggests pancreatic ascites. Also, the triglyceride level is less in ascitic fluid than in serum. A triglyceride level that is higher in ascitic fluid than in serum or the presence of chylomicrons suggests chylous ascites.

Ascitic fluid should be examined cytologically for malignant cells only if the serum-ascites albumin gradient is less than 1.1 g/dL. Also, culture studies for mycobacteria are performed only if tuberculosis is strongly suspected. Ascitic fluid glucose and pH are rarely measured except when secondary peritonitis (e.g., perforation of a viscus) is a consideration.

Management of Cirrhotic Ascites

Ascites results from renal retention of sodium and water. Therefore, treatment is aimed at achieving a negative sodium balance. This may be achieved with a low sodium diet, fluid restriction, and diuretic therapy, as follows:

Low Sodium Diet

The dietary intake of sodium should be restricted to 2 g/d (88 mEq/d). One teaspoon of salt has 5.2 g of sodium chloride or 2 g of sodium. However, total sodium intake, which includes any sodium that may be present in food, should not be more than 2 g/d. Therefore, the usual recommendation is that patients not add sodium to their food.

Fluid Restriction

Fluid restriction is not usually recommended for patients with cirrhosis. However, when they have dilutional hyponatremia (typically when serum sodium is < 125 mEq/L), fluid restriction is recommended. In this situation, fluid restriction does not normalize the serum sodium level. In fact, a further decrease in the serum sodium level is avoided.

Diuretic Therapy

Diuretic therapy usually consists of spironolactone and furosemide. Urinary sodium excretion is used to determine the efficacy of diuretic therapy (also, to monitor compliance with sodium restriction). If urinary sodium excretion is more than 30 mEq/d, spironolactone alone may be used for treatment. However, if urinary sodium excretion is between 10 and 30 mEq/d, a combination of spironolactone and furosemide is usually required. If urinary sodium excretion is less than 10 mEq/d, large-volume paracentesis is usually required in addition to spironolactone and furosemide.

Table 2. Serum-Ascites Albumin Gradient (SAAG)

	Ascitic fluid total protein	
	< 2.5 g/dL	≥ 2.5 g/dL
SAAG		
≥1.1 g/dL	Cirrhosis	Congestive heart disease
	Fulminant liver disease	Constrictive pericarditis
		Budd-Chiari syndrome
		Veno-occlusive disease
< 1.1 g/dL	Nephrotic syndrome	Peritoneal carcinomatosis
	Myxedema	Tuberculous peritonitis
		Pancreatic ascites
		Chylous ascites

Spironolactone

It is recommended that patients initially be treated with spironolactone. It can be given in a once-daily dose, with the dose adjusted at about 5-day intervals. The recommended initial dose is 100 mg/d; this is increased by 100 mg/d about every 5 days until a clinical response is achieved. A daily weight loss between 250 and 500 g is considered optimal fluid loss. If daily weight loss is not more than 200 g despite a spironolactone dose of 400 mg/d, treatment with furosemide may be started.

Furosemide

Furosemide is usually started at a dose of 40 mg/d, which is increased gradually to 160 mg/d. The ratio generally maintained between spironolactone and furosemide is 100:40, that is, 100 mg of spironolactone and 40 mg of furosemide, 200 mg of spironolactone and 80 mg of furosemide, and so forth. With this combination, the serum level of potassium usually remains normal.

Complications of diuretic therapy include worsening renal function, encephalopathy, and orthostatic hypotension.

Therapeutic Paracentesis

Large-volume paracentesis, or total-volume paracentesis, is safe and effective treatment for patients with ascites. This procedure is performed in patients who have tense ascites. Therapeutic paracentesis is especially recommended if abdominal discomfort causes decreased nutrient intake and increased cardiorespiratory compromise. It also is required when patients have an umbilical hernia with impending rupture. Usually 6 to 8 g of albumin is given intravenously for each liter of ascitic fluid removed. Removal of ascitic fluid without replacement of albumin can result in postparacentesis circulatory dysfunction. In this condition, ascites accumulates rapidly and renal dysfunction worsens.

Other plasma expanders, such as polygeline, dextran 70, or hetastarch, have been used, but the only volume expander associated with increased survival is albumin.

Complications of large-volume paracentesis, including abdominal wall hematomas, hemoperitoneum, and bowel perforation, are unusual and occur in fewer than 1 in 1,000 paracenteses.

Refractory Ascites

Most patients who have ascites that is difficult to control are noncompliant with sodium restriction. This can be confirmed by measuring 24-hour urine sodium excretion. A 24-hour urine sodium excretion in excess of the daily intake of sodium (88 mEq/d) indicates noncompliance with sodium restriction. "Refractory ascites" is defined as low urine sodium excretion, difficult-to-manage ascites, and maximal tolerated dose of diuretics. Refractory ascites includes both diuretic-resistant ascites and diuretic-intractable ascites. "Diuretic-resistant ascites" is defined as daily weight loss less than 200 mg in spite of dietary sodium restriction and intensive diuretic therapy up to 400 mg/d spironolactone and 160 mg/d furosemide. In comparison, "diuretic-intractable ascites" is defined as ascites that cannot be treated adequately because of diuretic-induced complications. Most patients with refractory ascites have advanced liver disease. It is important to rule out the use of nonsteroidal anti-inflammatory drugs and other nephrotoxic agents. Refractory ascites usually is treated with large-volume paracentesis. However, because this does not prevent the recurrence of ascites, diuretic therapy and sodium restriction need to be continued.

HEPATORENAL SYNDROME

Hepatorenal syndrome is divided into type 1 and type 2. Patients with ascites initially progress to type 2 hepatorenal syndrome, which is a decrease in the glomerulofiltration rate to less than 40 mL/min or an increase in the serum level of creatinine to more than 1.5 mg/dL in the presence of advanced liver disease and portal hypertension. Before hepatorenal syndrome is diagnosed, the following should be excluded: shock, bacterial sepsis, use of nephrotoxic agents, hypovolemia related to excessive diuretic use, or dehydration from diarrhea. Moreover, urinary protein excretion should be less than 500 mg/d, with a normal urinary sediment. The usual manifestation of type 2 hepatorenal syndrome is refractory ascites.

In type 1 hepatorenal syndrome, the progression in renal dysfunction is more rapid than in type 2. Creatinine clearance decreases to less than 20 mL/min or the serum level of creatinine increases to more than 2.5 mg/dL in less than 2 weeks. Type 1 hepatorenal syndrome is diagnosed mainly in patients with superimposed alcoholic hepatitis, spontaneous bacterial peritonitis, or other infections.

The initial step in the evaluation of a patient with hepatorenal syndrome is to measure the fractional excretion of sodium. If the value is less than 1, the patient has prerenal azotemia, hepatorenal syndrome, or glomerulonephritis. If the value is greater than 1, consider acute tubular necrosis and urinary obstruction. In prerenal azotemia, renal function rapidly improves with volume expansion. With glomerulonephritis, the urinary sediment is abnormal. After prerenal azotemia and glomerulonephritis have been ruled out, the diagnosis is hepatorenal syndrome.

Management of Refractory Ascites and Hepatorenal Syndrome

Large-volume Paracentesis

Refractory ascites, a manifestation of type 2 hepatorenal syndrome, is managed with repeated large-volume paracentesis. It is important that 6 to 8 g of albumin be infused for every liter of ascitic fluid removed. Albumin should be replaced within a few hours, certainly within 6 hours, after completion of large-volume paracentesis.

Peritoneovenous Shunt

A peritoneovenous shunt, rarely used to treat refractory ascites, involves placing a subcutaneous tube between the peritoneal space and superior vena cava via the internal jugular vein. A peritoneovenous shunt is not superior to repeated large-volume paracentesis for the treatment of refractory ascites. Complications include catheter infection, occlusion or thrombosis, and low-grade disseminated intravascular coagulation. In patients with liver cirrhosis, these shunts are indicated only if paracentesis has failed to treat refractory ascites and a transjugular intrahepatic portosystemic shunt (TIPS) cannot be placed.

Transjugular Intrahepatic Portosystemic Shunts

TIPS functions like a side-to-side portocaval shunt and decreases hepatic sinusoidal pressure. This shunt reduces renin-angiotensin-aldosterone levels, leading to diuresis and natriuresis. TIPS is more effective than paracentesis in treating refractory ascites, but without any notable survival benefit and at increased cost. There is suggestion that type 1 hepatorenal syndrome may respond to TIPS, but this procedure should still be considered experimental. Important predictors of survival after TIPS include the cause of liver disease, prothrombin time, and the serum levels of bilirubin and creatinine. Long-term complications of TIPS include shunt stenosis and hepatic encephalopathy.

Systemic Vasoconstrictors

Patients with hepatorenal syndrome have splanchnic vasodilatation and renal vasoconstriction. Splanchnic vasoconstrictors such as terlipressin have been administered in combination with albumin replacement for 2 to 4 weeks to treat type 1 hepatorenal syndrome. Splanchnic vasoconstriction results in the redistribution of blood to the renal circulation. Other agents used to treat hepatorenal syndrome include midodrine (can be given orally) in combination with octreotide. Treatment with these agents is not recommended outside treatment trials.

Orthotopic Liver Transplantation

Liver transplantation is the only therapy for refractory ascites and hepatorenal syndrome that is effective and increases long-term survival. The outcome for patients who have hepatorenal syndrome is poorer than for those without the syndrome. Moreover, up to one-third of patients with type 1 hepatorenal syndrome may require dialysis after liver transplantation.

SPONTANEOUS BACTERIAL PERITONITIS

Spontaneous bacterial peritonitis is diagnosed when the ascitic fluid neutrophil count is more than 250 cells/mm^3 (neutrocytic ascites). It occurs in 10% to 30% of inpatients who have cirrhotic ascites and in fewer than 4% of outpatients. The organisms that usually have been associated with spontaneous bacterial peritonitis include the gram-negative bacilli *Escherichia coli* and *Klebsiella pneumoniae*; however, there is increasing risk of infection with gram-positive organisms, mainly *Streptococcus* and *Enterococcus*. Most infections are monomicrobial. The trend toward infection with gram-positive organisms is probably related to prophylactic antibiotic therapy, especially with norfloxacin.

Spontaneous bacterial peritonitis occurs because of the translocation of bacteria from the intestinal lumen to mesenteric lymph nodes. This translocation is more likely to occur in patients with advanced cirrhosis of the liver and in those who have had gastrointestinal tract bleeding.

Patients with spontaneous bacterial peritonitis may be asymptomatic, may have unexplained deterioration of liver function, or have new-onset hepatic encephalopathy. Other features that lead one to suspect spontaneous bacterial peritonitis include fever, abdominal pain, hypothermia, diarrhea, and deterioration of renal function.

Neutrocytic ascites suggests the diagnosis of spontaneous bacterial peritonitis. The diagnosis is confirmed if cultures of the ascitic fluid are positive for bacteria. However, the treatment is similar for culture-positive neutrocytic ascites and culture-negative neutrocytic ascites. Moreover, the response to treatment and outcome are identical for the two conditions. Bacterial ascites is defined by a positive bacterial culture and neutrophil count less than 250 cells/mm^3. Bacterial ascites usually resolves spontaneously without antibiotic therapy.

Secondary bacterial peritonitis is differentiated from spontaneous bacterial peritonitis by a higher leukocyte count, the presence of multiple organisms, the presence of fungi or anaerobes in culture, ascitic fluid glucose level less than 50 mg/dL, and lactate dehydrogenase level higher than in the serum. Secondary bacterial peritonitis is suspected if the response to antibiotic therapy is inadequate for presumed spontaneous bacterial peritonitis. If secondary bacterial peritonitis is a consideration, computed tomography of the abdomen with an oral contrast agent is recommended.

Management of Spontaneous Bacterial Peritonitis

Antibiotic therapy is recommended with cefotaxime, 2 g given intravenously every 12 hours for at least 5 days. Forty-eight hours after cefotaxime therapy is initiated, repeat paracentesis should be considered. If the neutrophil count decreases more than 25%, the patient is having a response to treatment and antibiotic therapy is continued for a total of 5 days. However, if the neutrophil count does not decrease, secondary bacterial peritonitis should be suspected and computed tomography, with an oral contrast agent, should be performed. In addition to antibiotics, albumin is administered at a dose of 1.5 g/kg body weight on day 1 and at a dose of 1 g/kg body weight on day 3. This is associated with improved survival.

Patients who have had spontaneous bacterial peritonitis should receive antibiotic prophylaxis long-term or until liver transplantation. The antibiotic usually recommended is norfloxacin, 400 mg/d. The only other indication for antibiotic prophylaxis against spontaneous bacterial peritonitis is gastrointestinal tract bleeding in a patient with cirrhosis. In these patients, norfloxacin, 400 mg, is given once daily for 7 days, but intravenous antibiotics such as ceftriaxone may be preferable.

HEPATIC ENCEPHALOPATHY

Hepatic encephalopathy is the neuropsychiatric manifestation of liver failure and is associated with shunting of blood from the portovenous system into the systemic circulation. Currently, hepatic encephalopathy is classified on the basis of type, duration, and characteristics. In addition, a separate category of "minimal hepatic encephalopathy" has been proposed for patients who do not have overt hepatic encephalopathy but have abnormalities on neuropsychologic testing. The types of hepatic encephalopathy are as follows: type A, occurs in acute liver failure; type B or bypass encephalopathy, occurs in patients with portosystemic shunts even in the absence of chronic liver disease; and type C, occurs with cirrhosis of the liver. If hepatic encephalopathy occurs intermittently, it is called "episodic hepatic encephalopathy." If a precipitating cause is identified, it is called "precipitated hepatic encephalopathy." If a precipitating factor is not identified, then it is "spontaneous hepatic encephalopathy." "Persistent hepatic encephalopathy" refers to patients who continue to have cognitive impairment despite therapy.

Pathogenesis of Hepatic Encephalopathy Associated With Cirrhosis of the Liver

Ammonia is considered the major etiologic factor for hepatic encephalopathy. Ammonia enters the brain and stimulates peripheral benzodiazepine-type receptors, which are located primarily on astrocytes. Stimulation of these receptors increases neurosteroid synthesis, which in turn stimulates γ-aminobutyric acid (GABA) neurotransmission. GABA is the predominant depressant in the central nervous system.

Manganese is also considered by some to be pathogenic in hepatic encephalopathy. In fact, high levels of manganese have been noted on magnetic resonance imaging as hyperintense signals in the globus pallidus.

Clinical Features

Patients with overt hepatic encephalopathy present with alteration in alertness and consciousness. However, no specific manifestations suggest hepatic encephalopathy because all the manifestations can occur in other metabolic encephalopathies. According to the West Haven criteria, hepatic encephalopathy is graded from 0 to IV, with 0 indicating no overt encephalopathy and IV indicating a patient in coma. Hepatic encephalopathy has no localizing signs on neurologic examination, although motor slowing, ataxia, and bilateral deep tendon hyperreflexia may be noted and asterixis may be present.

Precipitating Factors

Precipitating factors of hepatic encephalopathy include gastrointestinal tract bleeding, a large protein meal, use of sedatives or tranquilizers, electrolyte abnormalities or hypoxia, constipation, and hypoglycemia.

Management of Hepatic Encephalopathy

The three steps in the management of hepatic encephalopathy include treating the precipitating cause, reducing the production and absorption of ammonia, and reversing the underlying liver disease if possible. The following discussion focuses on reducing the production and absorption of ammonia.

Dietary Measures

Patients receiving lactulose therapy usually can tolerate dietary protein up to 1.0 to 1.5 g/kg body weight daily. For patients with grade IV hepatic encephalopathy, protein restriction can be complete. However, as the level of consciousness improves, protein intake is increased by 10 g every 2 to 3 days as tolerated. Long-term restriction of dietary protein to less than 1 g/kg daily should be avoided. If animal protein precipitates encephalopathy in a patient, vegetable or dairy proteins may be used. Most patients can tolerate a diet of vegetable protein up to 120 g daily, although sodium restriction may make this diet unpalatable.

Nonabsorbable Disaccharides

Lactulose (β-galactosidofructose) or lactitol (β-galactosidosorbitol) may help remove dietary and endogenous ammonia, although this treatment is not supported by controlled trials. Lactulose acidifies the colonic contents, thus trapping ammonia, which is then excreted as ammonium. Lactulose is given at a dose sufficient to produce two or three semiformed stools daily. If patients are comatose, lactulose enemas may be given.

Antibiotics

Antibiotics such as neomycin, metronidazole, and rifaximin have been used in the treatment of hepatic encephalopathy. However, no benefit has been shown for long-term treatment with these antibiotics.

Portosystemic Shunt Obliteration

If hepatic encephalopathy develops after placement of a TIPS, the diameter of the shunt can be reduced by interventional radiologic techniques. Transhepatic or transvenous embolization may be performed in patients in whom a spontaneous portosystemic shunt has developed.

Liver Transplantation

Liver transplantation is the only effective long-term treatment for patients who have intractable hepatic encephalopathy and cirrhosis of the liver.

RECOMMENDED READING

Ahboucha S, Butterworth RF. Pathophysiology of hepatic encephalopathy: a new look at GABA from the molecular standpoint. Metab Brain Dis. 2004;19:331-43.

Evans LT, Kim WR, Poterucha JJ, Kamath PS. Spontaneous bacterial peritonitis in asymptomatic outpatients with cirrhotic ascites. Hepatology. 2003;37:897-901.

Ferenci P, Lockwood A, Mullen K, Tarter R, Weissenborn K, Blei AT. Hepatic encephalopathy: definition, nomenclature, diagnosis, and quantification: final report of the working party at the 11th World Congresses of Gastroenterology, Vienna, 1998. Hepatology. 2002;35:716-21.

Grabau CM, Crago SF, Hoff LK, Simon JA, Melton CA, Ott BJ, et al. Performance standards for therapeutic abdominal paracentesis. Hepatology. 2004;40:484-8.

Menon KVN, Kamath PS. Hepatic encephalopathy: diagnosis and management. In: Noseworthy JH, editor. Neurological therapeutics: principles and practice. London: Martin Dunitz; 2003. p. 1294-1301.

Runyon BA, Practice Guidelines Committee, American Association for the Study of Liver Diseases (AASLD). Management of adult patients with ascites due to cirrhosis. Hepatology. 2004;39:841-56.

SECTION VII

Liver II

CHAPTER 34

Metabolic Liver Disease

David J. Brandhagen, M.D.
John B. Gross, Jr., M.D.

Metabolic liver disease encompasses a diverse group of disorders that can cause liver damage through various mechanisms. Many are due to inborn errors of metabolism that are relatively uncommon. However, metabolic liver disease accounts for 30% of all liver transplants performed in children. The various metabolic liver diseases are listed in Table 1. This chapter reviews hereditary hemochromatosis, Wilson's disease, and alpha₁-antitrypsin deficiency because they are the metabolic liver diseases most gastroenterologists are likely to encounter. These three disorders are compared in Table 2.

HEREDITARY HEMOCHROMATOSIS

Hereditary hemochromatosis is an autosomal recessive disorder associated with increased intestinal absorption of iron and the deposition of excessive amounts of iron in the liver, pancreas, and other organs. It is the most common single-gene, inherited disorder in the U.S. white population. Approximately 1 in every 200 to 300 white persons in the United States is homozygous for the hemochromatosis mutation, and at least 1 in every 10 is a heterozygous carrier.

Not all iron overload is due to hereditary hemochromatosis, which should be distinguished from iron overload caused by other conditions. Secondary iron overload should be suspected in patients with chronic anemias who have ineffective erythropoiesis or have had multiple blood transfusions, prolonged iron supplementation, and chronic liver disease. In secondary iron overload, iron often accumulates in Kupffer cells rather than hepatocytes, as typical of hereditary hemochromatosis. However, severe iron overload from hereditary hemochromatosis may be indistinguishable from that due to secondary causes.

Table 1. Metabolic Liver Diseases

Inborn errors of carbohydrate metabolism
    Glycogen storage disease
Inborn errors of protein metabolism
    Tyrosinemia
    Urea cycle defects
Inborn errors of lipid metabolism
    Gaucher's disease
    Niemann-Pick disease
Inborn errors of bile acid metabolism
    Byler disease
    Benign recurrent cholestasis
Inborn errors of copper metabolism
    Wilson's disease
Inborn errors of iron metabolism
    Hereditary hemochromatosis
Unclassified
    Alpha₁-antitrypsin deficiency
    Cystic fibrosis

Modified from Ghishan FK. Inborn errors of metabolism that lead to permanent hepatic injury. In: Zakim D, Boyer TD, editors. Hepatology: a textbook of liver disease. 4th ed. Philadelphia: Saunders; 2003. p. 1397-1459. Used with permission.

The *HFE* Gene

The gene associated with hereditary hemochromatosis was initially named *HLA-H* but has been renamed *HFE*. It is located on the short arm of chromosome 6. Two point mutations have been designated "C282Y" and "H63D." More recently, other

Table 2. Comparison of Hemochromatosis, Wilson's Disease, and Alpha₁-Antitrypsin Deficiency

	Hemochromatosis	Wilson's disease	Alpha₁-antitrypsin deficiency
Inheritance	Autosomal recessive	Autosomal recessive	Autosomal codominant
Homozygote frequency	1:200-300	1:30,000	1:2,000
Heterozygote frequency	1:10	1:100	1:30
Gene	*HFE*	*ATP7B*	
Number of mutations*	2 (C282Y, H63D)	>100	
Chromosome	6	13	14
Diagnosis	Transferrin saturation, ferritin, liver iron concentration, *HFE* gene test	Ceruloplasmin, slit-lamp exam for Kayser-Fleischer rings, urine and liver copper quantification	Alpha₁-antitrypsin phenotype
Treatment	Phlebotomy	Penicillamine, trientine, or zinc	None/orthotopic liver transplantation

Clinically significant.

mutations have been described, but these are rare and not likely to be of major clinical importance. In the initial study and several other studies in the United States and Europe, from 60% to 93% of patients with iron overload were homozygous for C282Y. The wide range in the prevalence of C282Y homozygotes may be due partly to different diagnostic criteria for hereditary hemochromatosis and to geographic differences in the prevalence of *HFE* mutations.

The greatest risk for iron overload exists in persons homozygous for the C282Y mutation. Iron overload also occurs in a small proportion of persons with other *HFE* mutations (especially compound heterozygotes who have one copy of C282Y and one copy of H63D and occasionally H63D homozygotes), but it is usually of lesser severity. Approximately 1% to 2% of the white population are compound heterozygotes or H63D homozygotes and only a small percentage of these persons develop problems with iron overload. In addition, 20% of the U.S. population is heterozygous for H63D. A single copy of H63D does not appear to be a risk factor for the development of iron overload. It also is important to remember that clinically important iron overload can occur in the absence of *HFE* gene mutations. Therefore, a negative *HFE* gene test does not exclude iron overload.

Novel Genes and Proteins

Several other genes and proteins of iron metabolism have been discovered recently, including ferroportin, transferrin receptor 2, hemojuvelin, and hepcidin. Ferroportin is an iron exporter located on enterocytes, macrophages, and hepatocytes basolateral, and mutations in its gene have been associated with an autosomal dominant form of iron overload. Transferrin receptor 2 is located mainly on hepatocytes, and mutations in its gene *TFR2* have led to a rare autosomal recessive form of iron overload. Hemojuvelin (*HJV*) is the recently discovered gene for juvenile hemochromatosis located on chromosome 1q.

Of all the proteins, the one that has generated the most interest is hepcidin, a small polypeptide produced in the liver. Hepcidin inhibits iron absorption in the small intestine and prevents the release of iron from macrophages. It may function as a regulator of iron stores. Hepcidin levels are markedly increased in infectious and inflammatory conditions. It may be responsible for the development of anemia of inflammation (anemia of chronic disease). Hepcidin levels are inappropriately low in hereditary hemochromatosis, and hepcidin knockout mice develop iron overload in a pattern similar to human hereditary hemochromatosis. Preliminary studies have found that mutations in hepcidin may influence disease expression in hereditary hemochromatosis. This has led to reconsideration of the pathophysiology of iron metabolism. Previous models emphasized the role of enterocyte crypt cells in sensing body iron stores. It may be that the liver is the primary site for sensing the body iron stores, and it responds by increasing or decreasing the production of hepcidin. Future studies of hepcidin and other proteins of iron metabolism will undoubtedly clarify the pathophysiology of iron metabolism and hereditary hemochromatosis.

Clinical Features

Persons with hereditary hemochromatosis absorb only a few milligrams of iron each day in excess of the amount needed. Therefore, clinical manifestations often occur after the fifth decade, when 15 to 40 g of iron have accumulated (normal body iron stores are approximately 4 g). Disease expression may occur earlier in some persons and may not occur at all in others. Clinical expression is influenced by age, sex, iron content of the diet, blood loss as occurs in menstruation and pregnancy, and unknown factors, including mutations in genes other than *HFE*.

Thus women, despite an equal frequency of homozygosity, express the disease less frequently than men. Other factors such as alcohol and hepatitis C may accelerate disease expression.

The classic description of hereditary hemochromatosis is cutaneous hyperpigmentation, diabetes mellitus, and cirrhosis ("bronze diabetes"). Other clinical manifestations include fatigue, abdominal pain, hepatomegaly, abnormal liver enzyme levels, hepatocellular carcinoma, cardiomyopathy, cardiac conduction disorders, hypothyroidism, hypogonadism, impotence, and arthropathy. An example of hemochromatosis arthropathy is shown in Figure 1.

In the past, hereditary hemochromatosis usually was diagnosed at an advanced stage. Currently, most patients with newly diagnosed hereditary hemochromatosis are asymptomatic. This shift toward earlier diagnosis probably is due partly to increased physician awareness and, until recently, the inclusion of serum iron studies on many multichannel chemistry panels. The most common symptoms are fatigue, arthralgias, and impotence. Most, if not all, clinical manifestations are preventable if the disease is diagnosed early and treated appropriately. Some of its manifestations, such as skin bronzing, cardiomyopathy, cardiac conduction disorders, hepatomegaly, and abnormal liver tests, frequently are reversible after excess iron stores have been removed. Most of the other clinical manifestations are not reversible.

Diagnosis

A diagnosis of hereditary hemochromatosis is made on the basis of a combination of clinical, laboratory, and pathologic criteria, including an increase in serum transferrin saturation [100 × (serum iron concentration ÷ total iron binding capacity)] and an increase in the serum concentration of ferritin. There is diurnal variation in serum iron values, and measurements may be affected by the ingestion of food; therefore, if transferrin saturation is increased, the measurement should be repeated in the early morning with the patient fasting. A transferrin saturation more than 45% is the earliest phenotype abnormality in hereditary hemochromatosis.

Although serum transferrin saturation is the best initial screening test, the results may be normal early in the course of the disease. Also, the serum concentration of ferritin may be increased in 30% to 50% of patients with viral hepatitis, nonalcoholic fatty liver disease, or alcoholic liver disease. The serum concentration of ferritin usually provides a reasonable estimate of total body iron stores, but it is also an acute phase reactant and is increased in various infectious and inflammatory conditions in the absence of iron overload. For this reason, it should not be used as the initial screening test to detect hereditary hemochromatosis.

A diagnostic algorithm for hereditary hemochromatosis is provided in Figure 2. The *HFE* gene test is most useful for

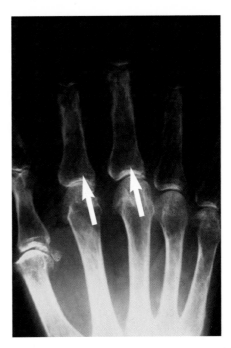

Fig. 1. Hemochromatosis arthropathy. A radiograph of the hand shows cartilage loss, marginal sclerosis, and osteophyte formation in the second and third metacarpophalangeal joints (*arrows*) without involvement of the fourth and fifth joints. Involvement of the second and third metacarpophalangeal joints is characteristic of hemochromatosis arthropathy. Occasionally, calcium pyrophosphate dihydrate crystals may be present (chondrocalcinosis). (Modified from Riely CA, Vera SR, Burrell MI, Koff RS. The gastroenterology teaching project, unit 8—inherited liver disease. Used with permission.)

surveillance of adult first-degree relatives of an identified proband. Screening for the disease in family members is crucial because 25% of siblings and 5% of children of a proband will have the disease. *HFE* gene testing should replace the more cumbersome and expensive HLA typing previously used to screen for hereditary hemochromatosis in siblings. Also, *HFE* gene testing is often useful in helping to resolve ambiguous cases, such as iron overload associated with hepatitis C, alcoholic liver disease, or other causes of end-stage liver disease. Before the *HFE* gene test is performed, the person should be counseled by a qualified professional about the risks, benefits, and alternatives of genetic testing. Although rare, the possibility of insurance, employment, or other discrimination based on *HFE* test results is a concern. For this reason, *HFE* gene testing usually is not recommended for anyone younger than 18 years.

Before the availability of the *HFE* gene test, liver biopsy often was used to confirm the diagnosis of hereditary hemochromatosis. Hepatic iron may be assessed with an iron stain such as Perls' Prussian blue. In hereditary hemochromatosis, iron initially accumulates in periportal hepatocytes, but eventually it is distributed throughout the liver. In secondary iron overload,

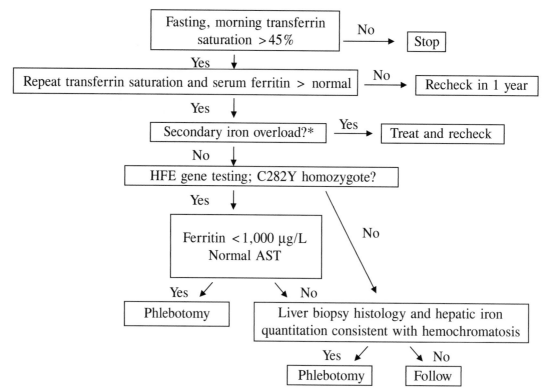

Fig. 2. Diagnostic algorithm for hereditary hemochromatosis. AST, aspartate aminotransferase. *Anemias with ineffective erythropoiesis, multiple blood transfusions, oral/parenteral iron supplements. (Modified from Brandhagen DJ, Fairbanks VF, Batts KP, Thibodeau SN. Update on hereditary hemochromatosis and the *HFE* gene. Mayo Clin Proc. 1999;74:917-21. By permission of Mayo Foundation for Medical Education and Research.)

iron often is present predominantly in Kupffer cells, which may help distinguish it from hereditary hemochromatosis. In severe iron overload, this distinction cannot be made. The histologic features of the liver in hereditary hemochromatosis and secondary iron overload are demonstrated in Figure 3.

In hereditary hemochromatosis, iron stores in the liver progressively increase with age. This has led to the development of the hepatic iron index, which is the hepatic iron concentration in micromoles/gram dry weight liver divided by the patient's age in years. Originally, this index was intended to distinguish between hereditary hemochromatosis homozygotes and heterozygotes and persons with alcoholic liver disease. In the initial study, the hepatic iron index was greater than 1.9 for all homozygotes and less than 1.9 for all heterozygotes or patients with alcoholic liver disease. A hepatic iron index greater than 1.9 is not diagnostic of hereditary hemochromatosis because patients with severe iron overload of any cause may have an index greater than 1.9. Also, because hereditary hemochromatosis is increasingly diagnosed at an earlier stage, not all homozygotes will have a hepatic iron index greater than 1.9.

Treatment

The treatment of hereditary hemochromatosis usually is reserved for patients with evidence of iron overload as indicated by an increase in the serum concentration of ferritin. Therapeutic phlebotomy is the preferred treatment because it is simple, relatively inexpensive, and effective. It begins with removal of 500 mL of blood weekly. The hemoglobin concentration should be measured just before each phlebotomy. Weekly phlebotomy should continue as long as the hemoglobin concentration is above a preselected value (usually 12-13 g/dL). If the concentration is below the preselected value, phlebotomy should not be performed. Once the hemoglobin concentration remains below the preselected value for three consecutive weeks without phlebotomy, the serum concentration of ferritin and transferrin saturation should be determined again. Iron depletion is confirmed if the ferritin level is not greater than 50 μg/L, with a transferrin saturation in the low-normal range. Once iron depletion has been accomplished, most patients require four to eight "maintenance" phlebotomies annually to keep the ferritin level lower than 50 μg/L.

Generally, iron chelators such as desferoxamine are not used to treat iron overload in hereditary hemochromatosis. Iron chelators are expensive and must be given by subcutaneous infusion. Also, they are much less effective than phlebotomy in removing excess iron. Currently, an effective oral iron chelator is not available in the United States.

Patients with hereditary hemochromatosis should refrain from taking iron supplements, including multivitamins with

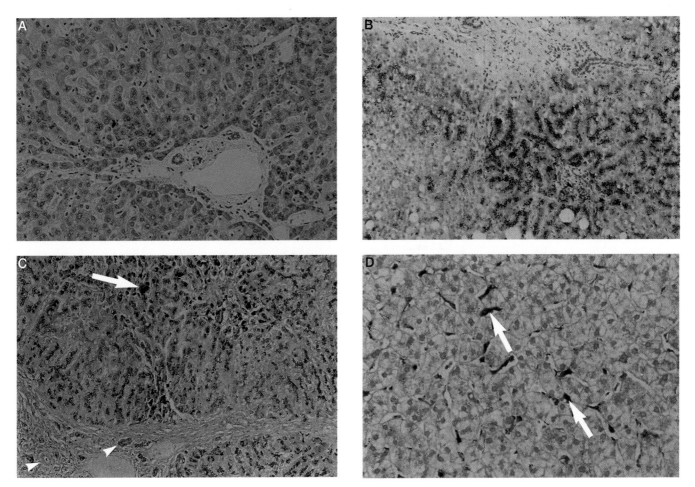

Fig. 3. Iron deposition in the liver. *A*, Mild (grade 1 of 4) iron deposition in hepatocytes. *B*, Moderate hemosiderin deposition in precirrhotic homozygous hemochromatosis. Zone 1 hepatocytes are predominantly involved, biliary hemosiderin is not evident, and fibrosis has not yet occurred—all indicating relatively early precirrhotic disease (liver iron concentration, 10,307 μg Fe/g dry weight; iron index, 3.2). (Original magnification x133.) *C*, Marked hemosiderosis and cirrhosis in homozygous hemochromatosis. Although most iron is in hepatocytes, some Kupffer cells (*arrow*) and biliary iron (*arrowheads*) are also present. (Original magnification x133.) *D*, Kupffer cell hemosiderosis. The presence of hemosiderin in Kupffer cells alone (*arrows*) is typical of mild transfusion hemosiderosis, is nonspecific, and should not prompt further consideration of hemochromatosis. (Original magnification x240.) *A-D*, Perls' Prussian blue stain. (*A* from Brandhagen DJ. Liver transplantation for hereditary hemochromatosis. Liver Transpl. 2001;7:663-72. Used with permission. *B-D* from Baldus WP, Batts KP, Brandhagen DJ. Liver biopsy in hemochromatosis. In: Barton JC, Edwards CQ, editors. Hemochromatosis: genetics, pathophysiology, diagnosis, and treatment. Cambridge: Cambridge University Press; 2000. p. 187-99. Used with permission.)

iron, and high-dose vitamin C supplements. A "low iron diet" is not necessary, but red meat should be consumed in moderation. Patients also should avoid consuming raw seafood because of an increased risk of *Vibrio vulnificus* infection. Also, poorly cooked meat should be avoided, and patients should avoid alcohol or minimize its intake because iron and alcohol are synergistic hepatotoxins.

Despite being common, hereditary hemochromatosis is an uncommon indication for orthotopic liver transplantation (OLT), accounting for fewer than 1% of all liver transplants performed in the United States. Of note, the survival rate of patients with hereditary hemochromatosis undergoing OLT is worse than that of those undergoing OLT for most other indications. The 1-year survival rate for patients with hereditary hemochromatosis is approximately 50%, compared with more than 90% for most other indications. Most deaths of liver transplant recipients who have hereditary hemochromatosis are caused by cardiac or infectious complications.

Prognosis

For patients in whom hereditary hemochromatosis is diagnosed and treated before diabetes mellitus and cirrhosis develop, the age- and sex-adjusted survival rate is normal. However, when cirrhosis or diabetes develops, survival decreases markedly.

Up to one-third of patients with hereditary hemochromatosis and cirrhosis develop hepatocellular carcinoma, which often is the cause of death. This represents a 200-fold increased risk for the development of liver cancer. Patients with cirrhosis due to hereditary hemochromatosis usually do not develop decompensated liver disease characterized by ascites, hepatic encephalopathy, or gastroesophageal varices.

The Role of Liver Biopsy

HFE gene testing may eliminate the need for liver biopsy in many patients. Traditionally, liver biopsy was performed in patients with iron overload to confirm the diagnosis of hereditary hemochromatosis and to exclude cirrhosis. In patients with iron overload who are C282Y homozygotes, liver biopsy is not necessary to confirm the diagnosis. However, liver biopsy is still the "gold standard" for assessing the degree of fibrosis. Definitively excluding cirrhosis is important because of the increased risk of the development of hepatocellular carcinoma. The risk for cancer persists even after excess iron stores have been depleted. For these patients, screening with ultrasonography and alpha fetoprotein every 6 months may be appropriate.

There may be a subset of patients with hereditary hemochromatosis whose risk of cirrhosis is minimal, and liver biopsy would be unnecessary. Several recent studies have confirmed that certain noninvasive predictors are accurate in excluding cirrhosis in C282Y homozygotes. In these studies, there were virtually no cases of cirrhosis in C282Y homozygotes who had a serum concentration of ferritin less than 1,000 µg/L and a normal aspartate aminotransferase value. A serum concentration of ferritin less than 1,000 µg/L seems to be the best predictor of the absence of cirrhosis in C282Y homozygotes. However, the positive predictive value of a serum concentration greater than 1,000 µg/L is poor because only about 50% of those with this value had cirrhosis. Liver biopsy is advisable for this group of patients to definitely assess for the presence of cirrhosis. Similar information is not available for non-C282Y homozygotes. Liver biopsy may be necessary for this group of patients to confirm the diagnosis and to exclude cirrhosis.

Screening for Hemochromatosis

Currently, experts disagree about the utility of screening for the general population. Despite the disease fulfilling many of the criteria of a condition appropriate for population screening, some public health experts do not advocate screening. They cite lack of information about the burden of disease and disease expression in those with *HFE* mutations as reasons for not endorsing population screening. However, the natural history of the disease in an asymptomatic patient identified by population screening may never be known because many would consider it unethical to withhold treatment once iron overload develops.

A recent study screened for hereditary hemochromatosis in more than 41,000 patients attending a health appraisal clinic. All subjects underwent a history and physical examination and completed a detailed symptom questionnaire. Also, serum iron studies and the *HFE* gene test were performed. Although the majority of C282Y homozygotes had increased serum transferrin saturation and ferritin, symptoms did not differ among the 152 C282Y homozygotes and non-C282Y homozygotes. The authors concluded that less than 1% of C282Y homozygotes develop clinical evidence of hereditary hemochromatosis. However, the study had several potential problems. The study population may have been biased toward a less symptomatic group because patients attending a "health appraisal clinic" might be expected to be healthier. Also, many patients who already had the diagnosis of hereditary hemochromatosis were excluded, thereby potentially selecting out a less symptomatic group. Finally, liver biopsies were not performed. Plasma collagen IV, a surrogate marker of fibrosis, was measured. Of interest, the median levels of plasma collagen IV were statistically higher in the hereditary hemochromatosis group than in the group without the disease. Although the majority of C282Y homozygotes probably will not develop serious problems with iron overload, the true prevalence of clinically relevant disease manifestations in hereditary hemochromatosis remains unknown. With the information currently available, it seems reasonable to screen for iron overload in persons with a family history of hereditary hemochromatosis symptoms or signs suggestive of the disease or chronic liver disease.

WILSON'S DISEASE

Wilson's disease is an autosomal recessive disorder characterized by abnormal intrahepatic copper metabolism and deposition of excess copper in the liver, brain, cornea, and other organs. Approximately 1/30,000 persons are homozygous and 1/100 are heterozygous carriers of a Wilson's disease gene mutation. It is likely that only about half of all persons with the disease have come to medical attention. Not all cases of copper excess in the liver are due to Wilson's disease. Patients with chronic cholestatic biliary disorders such as primary biliary cirrhosis, primary sclerosing cholangitis, or biliary atresia often have excess copper levels in the liver, although usually not to the degree seen in Wilson's disease.

Copper Metabolism and Pathogenesis

Body copper homeostasis is achieved through biliary excretion. In Wilson's disease, intestinal copper absorption is normal but biliary excretion of copper is decreased. Copper toxicity has a major role in the pathogenesis of the disease. Copper accumulates in the liver as a result of an abnormal copper transport protein and eventually appears in other organs, particularly the brain. Excess copper exerts its toxic effect by the generation of free radicals that result in lipid peroxidation, similar to the mechanism proposed for iron-induced damage in hereditary hemochromatosis. Deficiency of ceruloplasmin is not the cause of Wilson's disease; rather, it is an effect of the abnormal cellular trafficking of copper.

Genetics

The gene for Wilson's disease (*ATP7B*) was isolated in 1993. Located on chromosome 13, it codes for a copper-transporting P-type adenosine triphosphatase (ATPase) that is located in the endoplasmic reticulum and possibly the biliary canalicular membrane. Thus far, more than 100 mutations have been described. Attempts to correlate genotype with phenotype have not shown a consistent pattern. From 30% to 40% of North American and European patients have the H1069Q mutation. Unlike hereditary hemochromatosis, in which approximately 85% of cases are homozygous for the C282Y mutation, the majority of cases of Wilson's disease are compound heterozygotes (one copy of two different mutations). The number of clinically important mutations makes genetic testing less useful in this disease than in hereditary hemochromatosis.

Clinical Features

The variation in clinical presentation is tremendous, ranging from asymptomatic patients to those with crippling neurologic symptoms. The median age at presentation is 12 to 23 years, with the oldest age being 58 years. The five main categories of clinical presentation include hepatic, neurologic, psychiatric, hematologic, and ophthalmologic. In one large clinical series, the initial clinical manifestations were hepatic in 42% of patients, neurologic in 34%, psychiatric in 10%, and hematologic in 12%. Wilson's disease can simulate any syndrome of liver disease, including fulminant liver failure, chronic hepatitis, and cirrhosis. Liver manifestations tend to be more common in childhood, whereas neurologic symptoms tend to appear in the second and third decades. Although Wilson's disease should be considered in all young patients with liver disease, it is responsible for fewer than 5% of cases of chronic hepatitis in persons younger than 35 years. Fulminant liver failure due to Wilson's disease is four times more common in females than males. Reports of hepatocellular cancer in Wilson's disease are rare, even though many patients have advanced fibrosis at a young age.

Neurologic syndromes are dominated by extrapyramidal motor symptoms, including rigidity or spasticity, tremor, ataxia, dysarthria, drooling, and involuntary movements. Dementia and seizures are rare. Psychiatric problems may be dramatic, with psychosis or depression, or they may be subtle and manifested as behavioral problems or declining performance in school. Unfortunately, children are often classified as having behavioral problems until progressive and sometimes irreversible neurologic

symptoms begin to develop.

Patients may first present with hemolytic anemia, frequently seen in association with acute, severe, or fulminant hepatitis. The constellation of young age, severe liver dysfunction, and hemolytic anemia should be assumed to be Wilson's disease until proved otherwise. Occasionally, the disease is identified because of incidental eye findings, either brown Kayser-Fleischer rings, representing copper deposition in the periphery of the cornea, or sunflower cataracts. The cataracts are seen only with a slit lamp and do not interfere with vision. The eye findings in Wilson's disease are shown in Figure 4. Renal manifestations include proximal or distal renal tubular acidosis and nephrolithiasis. Another manifestation is azure lunulae, a blue discoloration of the base of the fingernails that is an uncommon but characteristic finding.

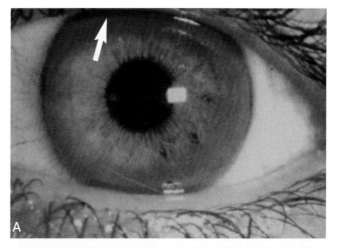

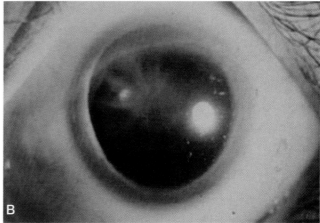

Fig. 4. *A*, Kayser-Fleischer ring (*arrow*). *B*, Sunflower cataract. (From Zucker SD, Gollan JL: Wilson's disease and hepatic copper toxicosis. In: Zakim D, Boyer TD, editors. Hepatology: a textbook of liver disease. 3rd ed. Philadelphia: WB Saunders; 1996. p. 1405-39. Used with permission.)

Diagnosis

The differential diagnosis of Wilson's disease is large and depends on the presenting clinical syndrome. The disease should be considered in any person younger than 30 years who has liver disease. Autoimmune hepatitis and chronic viral hepatitis are the most frequently considered alternative diagnoses. The combination of liver disease and extrapyramidal motor abnormalities should strongly suggest Wilson's disease. The combination of severe liver disease and hemolytic anemia should never be missed. Traditionally, the diagnosis requires at least two of the following: 1) Kayser-Fleischer rings, 2) low level of ceruloplasmin, 3) typical neurologic symptoms, and 4) liver copper concentration greater than 250 µg/g dry weight.

Kayser-Fleischer rings are seen in many patients with neurologic symptoms but are not found frequently in patients with liver disease. These rings also have been detected by slit lamp in conditions associated with chronic cholestasis, such as primary biliary cirrhosis and sclerosing cholangitis. The serum level of ceruloplasmin (oxidase assay) is less than 20 mg/dL in 95% of patients with Wilson's disease. Even though the level of ceruloplasmin may be nonspecifically increased as an acute phase reactant or as a result of estrogen administration, a level higher than 30 mg/dL essentially excludes the diagnosis of Wilson's disease except in rare patients presenting with fulminant hepatitis. Twenty percent of Wilson's disease heterozygotes have a ceruloplasmin level less than 20 mg/dL but do not develop clinical disease. Almost any chronic liver disease in which liver synthetic function is decreased may be associated with a ceruloplasmin level that is lower than normal. The serum concentration of copper may be low, normal, or increased and thus is not particularly helpful. However, it is useful for calculating the free (nonceruloplasmin) copper level, which is often increased in severe acute Wilson's disease. Although urinary copper excretion may be increased in other liver diseases, a value less than 100 µg/24 hours in a patient with clinical disease would be very unusual in symptomatic Wilson's disease. A low urinary copper excretion rate may indicate acquired copper deficiency. This may be confusing because cases of severe copper deficiency may be associated with neurologic symptoms. The neurologic syndrome in these cases is myelopathy with weakness and ataxia.

In most cases, liver biopsy is necessary to confirm the diagnosis, particularly in those with a normal level of ceruloplasmin or without Kayser-Fleischer rings or neurologic symptoms. Steatosis often is present, and glycogenated nuclei often are seen. Tissue analysis for copper is the "gold standard" for confirming the diagnosis of Wilson's disease. A normal liver concentration of copper (< 35 µg/g dry weight) excludes the diagnosis. Most patients with the disease have liver copper concentrations greater than 250 µg/g dry weight, but this is not a specific finding and may occur in chronic cholestatic conditions or, rarely, in autoimmune hepatitis. Unlike hereditary hemochromatosis, children with Wilson's disease may already have marked liver fibrosis; thus, liver biopsy should be strongly considered in children to stage the liver disease.

Biochemical tests often show characteristic patterns, but these are not consistent enough to be confirmatory. The alkaline phosphatase level may be low, and the aminotransferase levels tend to be increased less than would be expected from other signs of liver necrosis. In fulminant Wilson's disease, the uric acid level usually is low or undetectable, often because of concomitant proximal renal tubular acidosis. In fulminant liver failure, a marked increase in the serum level of copper strongly suggests the diagnosis of Wilson's disease, although a normal level does not exclude fulminant Wilson's disease. A diagnostic algorithm for Wilson's disease is provided in Figure 5. Complete gene sequencing is available at a few referral centers; this may disclose a functionally significant mutation in a case in which the results of standard tests are equivocal.

Family Screening

As in hereditary hemochromatosis, screening should be directed at siblings because each has about a 25% chance of having Wilson's disease. If treatment is begun in the presymptomatic phase of the disease before cirrhosis is established, it is essentially curative. Because copper metabolism in infancy and early childhood may simulate Wilson's disease, children should not be tested before age 5. Screening should include aminotransferase and ceruloplasmin levels and a slit-lamp examination for Kayser-Fleischer rings. If the results are normal, screening should be repeated every 5 years until age 20. If the ceruloplasmin level is less than 20 mg/dL but there are no Kayser-Fleischer rings or convincing neurologic symptoms, liver biopsy is necessary. Currently, the role of genetic testing is limited. Direct testing for gene mutations is not likely to be helpful in screening because of the multiplicity of mutations. However, either gene sequencing or linkage analysis studies can be used for screening once the pattern in the index case is known. This may be of value if standard copper test results are equivocal.

Treatment

"Decoppering" Agents

Penicillamine and trientine were developed as metal chelators and are approved for the treatment of Wilson's disease. Tetrathiomolybdate is another copper-binding agent that may be approved soon. Penicillamine is an effective first-line treatment, but up to 20% of patients experience drug toxicity, including hypersensitivity reactions, bone marrow suppression, proteinuria, autoimmune disorders, and dermatologic conditions. A starting dose of 250 to 500 mg/d is gradually increased to 1 to

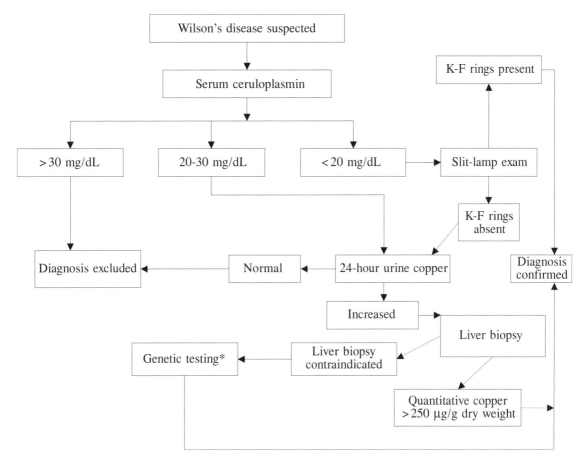

Fig. 5. Diagnostic algorithm for Wilson's disease. K-F, Kayser-Fleischer. *Genetic testing is performed within families when diagnosis is already established in one family member using the index patient DNA as a reference. (Modified from Zakko WF, Gollan JL. Wilson's disease and related disorders. In: Friedman LS, Keeffe EB, editors. Handbook of liver disease. Edinburgh: Churchill Livingstone; 1998. p. 239-54. Used with permission.)

2 g/d divided into two to four doses. The drug should be given with small doses of pyridoxine because it can deplete vitamin B_6 levels. Treatment response is demonstrated by an acute increase in urinary copper excretion that gradually plateaus at a lower level over 6 to 12 months. Initially, urinary copper output is often more than 2,000 µg daily, decreasing to 400 to 500 µg daily in the maintenance phase. The urine and serum levels of copper and the ceruloplasmin level should be measured and a complete blood count should be performed weekly during the first month, then every 1 or 2 months during the first 6 months. Patients whose condition is stable can then be followed annually. The slit-lamp examination should be repeated annually to document the disappearance of Kayser-Fleischer rings (if present). As many as 20% of patients with neurologic symptoms may experience worsening of their symptoms during the first month of treatment. This deterioration has been irreversible in some patients.

Trientine was introduced as an alternative to penicillamine and should be the first choice for treatment. It is given in similar doses and also has satisfactory long-term efficacy. The cupriuresis is less pronounced than with penicillamine, but an initial increase is expected. Trientine has a lower incidence of adverse effects and a lower rate of neurologic worsening at the start of treatment. Occasionally, iron deficiency may develop because of sideroblastic anemia.

Tetrathiomolybdate has shown promise as an effective decoppering agent, with approval still pending.

Inhibition of Copper Absorption

Zinc acetate, 50 mg three times daily, is effective therapy for presymptomatic patients and pregnant women. It also is an alternative maintenance therapy for patients presenting with symptomatic disease after 6 to 12 months of standard treatment for removal of copper. Zinc acetate induces synthesis of metallothionein in the intestinal epithelium, which then preferentially binds copper and prevents its absorption. Treatment is monitored by checking urinary levels of zinc and copper. The urinary zinc excretion should be at least 2,000 µg/day.

For pregnancy, penicillamine is probably safe, but zinc is a better choice for patients whose condition is stable. The teratogenicity of trientine is unknown, and it should not be given during pregnancy.

A problem with medical therapy for patients with Wilson's disease is compliance. It is hard to convince young people, many of whom feel well, of the need to take medicine two to four times daily for the rest of their lives. The tragedy is that if a patient stops treatment, the probability of death from fulminant liver failure within 1 to 2 years is very high, even if the patient was initially asymptomatic.

Transplantation

The indications for liver transplantation include fulminant liver failure, end-stage liver disease unresponsive to medical therapy, and chronic deterioration of liver function despite long-term therapy. Liver transplantation is curative because it corrects the metabolic defect in Wilson's disease. Transplantation is the treatment of choice for fulminant liver failure because of the low probability that medical therapy will be effective. Nevertheless, medical therapy should be started because occasionally patients recover. A prognostic index based on the serum levels of bilirubin, aspartate aminotransferase, and prothrombin time can help predict the risk of death of patients with fulminant liver failure. Postdilution hemofiltration has been used temporarily to remove large amounts of free copper and has produced temporary improvement in hemolysis and encephalopathy. Patients who received a liver transplant for fulminant hepatic failure have a 1-year survival rate of 73%; among those with chronic liver failure, the rate is about 90%. There are anecdotal reports of marked neurologic improvement after liver transplantation, but transplantation performed solely for refractory neurologic symptoms is considered experimental because of the limited experience and uncertain outcome.

ALPHA₁-ANTITRYPSIN DEFICIENCY

Genetics and Function

Alpha₁-antitrypsin (AAT) deficiency is an autosomal codominant disorder characterized by lung and liver injury. AAT is a member of the serine protease supergene family. It functions to protect tissues from proteases such as neutrophil elastase. AAT is encoded by a gene on the long arm of chromosome 14. The phenotype Pi*MM (Pi, protease inhibitor) is present in 95% of the population and is associated with normal serum levels of AAT. For liver disease, the Z allele is the most clinically relevant. The homozygote frequency of the Z allele is 1:2,000, with a heterozygote frequency of 1:30. The Pi*ZZ phenotype is accompanied by a severe deficiency in AAT, and the Pi*MZ phenotype leads to intermediate deficiency.

Pathogenesis

The pathogenesis of liver disease associated with AAT deficiency likely is due to the accumulation of the mutant AAT protein in the endoplasmic reticulum. The abnormally folded protein is unable to exit the endoplasmic reticulum. Unlike the lungs, the liver is not damaged by the uninhibited effects of elastases and other proteolytic enzymes. This is supported by the observation that patients with two copies of the rare AAT null allele may develop lung disease but do not develop liver disease.

Clinical Features

AAT deficiency may cause premature emphysema and liver disease. In the only population-based study performed, the Swedish neonatal screening study identified 127 AAT-deficient children who were followed prospectively through age 18 years. Neonatal cholestasis developed in 11%, and 6% had other liver disease without jaundice. Liver test abnormalities developed 1 to 2 months after birth and usually normalized by 6 months. A small proportion of children developed end-stage liver disease or presented with fulminant hepatic failure in infancy. Most (83%) AAT-deficient children were healthy throughout childhood, although most had liver test abnormalities in early life. In adolescents and adults, AAT deficiency may cause hepatitis or cirrhosis. It has been estimated that 2% of adults between 20 and 50 years old with the Pi*ZZ phenotype will develop cirrhosis, compared with 19% of those older than 50. In adults, hereditary hemochromatosis is the most common inherited cause of cirrhosis, but AAT deficiency is the most common metabolic indication for OLT. It is debated whether persons with the Pi*MZ phenotype are at risk for the development of chronic liver disease. Several studies have noted an increased prevalence of the Pi*MZ phenotype among those undergoing OLT for cryptogenic cirrhosis compared with those having OLT for other indications. The risk of cirrhosis in Pi*Z heterozygotes is estimated at approximately 3%. Patients with cirrhosis due to AAT deficiency have a greatly increased risk of hepatocellular carcinoma, with some studies reporting a prevalence of primary liver cancer of up to 30%.

Diagnosis

The diagnosis of AAT deficiency is made by AAT phenotyping. Serum levels of AAT should not be used to diagnose AAT deficiency because they may be falsely increased in inflammatory conditions, malignancies, pregnancy, and with estrogen supplementation. Unlike lung disease, liver damage does not correlate with serum levels of AAT. The diagnosis is confirmed by liver biopsy. The characteristic finding is the presence of eosinophilic, periodic acid-Schiff–positive, diastase-resistant globules in the endoplasmic reticulum of periportal hepatocytes. Because these globules may be present also in heterozygotes and in homozygotes without liver disease, their presence does not imply liver disease. Furthermore, because the globules may be variably distributed throughout the liver, their absence does not exclude the diagnosis of AAT deficiency. The histologic features of the liver in AAT deficiency are shown in Figure 6.

Treatment

No effective medical treatment is available for the liver manifestations of AAT deficiency. Patients should refrain from using tobacco in an attempt to decrease the risk of emphysema developing. They also should minimize alcohol consumption.

In some cases of lung disease, AAT has been infused, but it is not helpful for liver disease. AAT deficiency may be amenable to somatic gene therapy. Gene therapy probably would be beneficial only for the lung disease unless a method of delivering the corrected gene product to the endoplasmic reticulum of hepatocytes was available.

OLT is the only definitive treatment for AAT deficiency. It cures the liver disease because the recipient assumes the Pi phenotype of the donor. In contrast to hereditary hemochromatosis, survival after OLT for AAT deficiency is excellent. However, OLT must be performed before advanced lung disease develops.

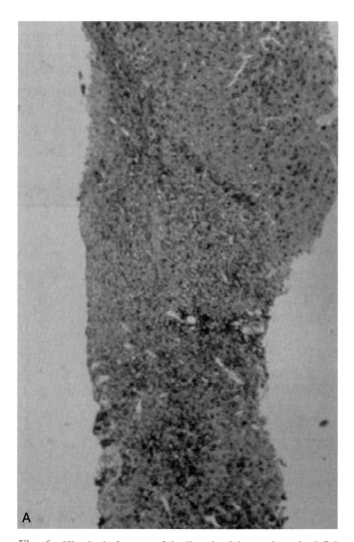 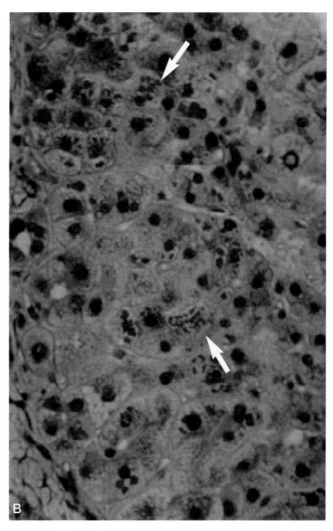

Fig. 6. Histologic features of the liver in alpha₁-antitrypsin deficiency. *A*, Chronic hepatitis with cirrhosis due to alpha₁-antitrypsin deficiency. *B*, Characteristic periodic acid-Schiff–positive diastase-resistant globules (*arrows*) have accumulated in hepatocytes. (Modified from Riely CA, Vera SR, Burrell MI, Koff RS. The gastroenterology teaching project, unit 8—inherited liver disease. Used with permission.)

RECOMMENDED READING

Hereditary Hemochromatosis

Beutler E, Felitti VJ, Koziol JA, Ho NJ, Gelbart T. Penetrance of 845G→A (C282Y) *HFE* hereditary haemochromatosis mutation in the USA. Lancet. 2002;359:211-8.

Frazer DM, Anderson GJ. The orchestration of body iron intake: how and where do enterocytes receive their cues? Blood Cells Mol Dis. 2003;30:288-97.

Ganz T. Hepcidin, a key regulator of iron metabolism and mediator of anemia of inflammation. Blood. 2003 Aug 1;102:783-8. Epub 2003 Mar 27.

Morrison ED, Brandhagen DJ, Phatak PD, Barton JC, Krawitt EL, El-Serag HB, et al. Serum ferritin level predicts advanced hepatic fibrosis among U.S. patients with phenotypic hemochromatosis. Ann Intern Med. 2003;138:627-33. Erratum in: Ann Intern Med. 2003;139:235.

Pietrangelo A. Hereditary hemochromatosis: a new look at an old disease. N Engl J Med. 2004;350:2383-97.

Pietrangelo A. Non-*HFE* hemochromatosis. Hepatology. 2004;39:21-9.

Tavill AS, American Association for the Study of Liver Diseases, American College of Gastroenterology, American Gastroenterological Association. Diagnosis and management of hemochromatosis. Hepatology. 2001;33:1321-8.

Wilson's Disease

El-Youssef M. Wilson disease. Mayo Clin Proc. 2003;78:1126-36.

Alpha$_1$-Antitrypsin Deficiency

American Thoracic Society/European Respiratory Society Statement. Standards for the diagnosis and management of individuals with alpha-1 antitrypsin deficiency. Am J Respir Crit Care Med. 2003;168:818-900.

Ghishan FK. α_1-antitrypsin deficiency. In: Zakim D, Boyer TD, editors. Hepatology: a textbook of liver disease. Vol 2. 4th ed. Philadelphia: Saunders; 2003. p. 1385-95.

Sveger T. Liver disease in alpha$_1$-antitrypsin deficiency detected by screening of 200,000 infants. N Engl J Med. 1976;294:1316-21.

CHAPTER 35

Cholestatic Liver Disease:
Primary Biliary Cirrhosis, Primary Sclerosing Cholangitis, and Drug-Induced Cholestasis

Keith D. Lindor, M.D.

Cholestatic liver disease in adults without biliary obstruction encompasses a broad differential diagnosis. However, drug-induced cholestasis may be the most common explanation for cholestasis in these patients. Primary biliary cirrhosis is the most common cholestatic liver disease in adults. Primary sclerosing cholangitis is about half as common as primary biliary cirrhosis. Other cholestatic conditions in adults include autoimmune cholangitis (sometimes known as "antimitochondrial antibody [AMA]-negative primary biliary cirrhosis") and miscellaneous conditions.

DIFFERENTIAL DIAGNOSIS

The differential diagnosis for cholestasis in adults without biliary obstruction is listed in Table 1.

Primary Biliary Cirrhosis

Primary biliary cirrhosis has a prevalence of about 150 to 300 per million persons, involves women in 90% of cases, and is characterized by AMAs in 95% of patients. These patients present with biochemical features of cholestasis and may be symptomatic. Fatigue is the most common symptom, but it is nonspecific and not useful in establishing the diagnosis. Pruritus is less common but may occur in 30% to 50% of patients. Increasingly, primary biliary cirrhosis is being recognized in asymptomatic patients on the basis of abnormal liver test results. The alkaline phosphatase level is prominently increased, but serum levels of cholesterol and IgM can also be abnormally high. The most characteristic finding is AMAs, which recognize the lipoic acid binding site on an enzyme in the pyruvate dehydrogenase complex. The diagnosis often is established

Table 1. **Differential Diagnosis for Cholestasis in Adults Without Biliary Obstruction**

Drug-induced cholestasis
Primary biliary cirrhosis
Autoimmune cholangitis
Primary sclerosing cholangitis
Small-duct primary sclerosing cholangitis
Idiopathic adulthood ductopenia
Idiopathic biliary ductopenia
Cholestasis of pregnancy
Cystic fibrosis
HIV-associated cholestasis
Sarcoidosis
Granulomatous hepatitis

HIV, human immunodeficiency virus.

by the finding of high-titer AMA in the appropriate clinical setting. Although liver biopsy helps confirm the diagnosis and provides information about histologic staging, it may not be required in most cases. Cross-sectional imaging studies such as ultrasonography, computed tomography, or magnetic resonance imaging can help exclude biliary obstruction. Direct cholangiography is not needed to establish this diagnosis.

Autoimmune Cholangitis

Autoimmune cholangitis, or AMA-negative primary biliary cirrhosis, is characterized by clinical and histologic features identical to those of primary biliary cirrhosis. However, the patients do not have AMAs, but 95% have either antinuclear or anti-smooth muscle antibodies. Occasionally, these patients are confused with those who have overlapping autoimmune hepatitis and primary biliary cirrhosis, but the histologic features and biochemical profile generally help differentiate autoimmune cholangitis from the overlap between primary biliary cirrhosis and autoimmune hepatitis.

Primary Sclerosing Cholangitis

Primary sclerosing cholangitis is the next most common cholestatic condition in adults. About 70% of the patients have inflammatory bowel disease, and unlike primary biliary cirrhosis, primary sclerosing cholangitis is more common in men than in women. The age at onset tends to be younger, around 40 years for primary sclerosing cholangitis compared with 50 years for primary biliary cirrhosis. AMAs are rarely present (≤2% of patients). Liver biopsy can help confirm the diagnosis. Biopsy specimens may show more fibrosis surrounding the bile ducts and less inflammation than seen in primary biliary cirrhosis, although these characteristic findings are not generally apparent. Unlike primary biliary cirrhosis, direct cholangiography is necessary to establish the diagnosis of primary sclerosing cholangitis. Occasionally, patients have normal cholangiographic findings, but the histologic and clinical features (history of inflammatory bowel disease) suggest primary sclerosing cholangitis. These patients are considered to have small-duct primary sclerosing cholangitis.

Drug-Induced Cholestasis

Drug-induced cholestasis can take several forms: 1) canalicular (bland), 2) hepatocanalicular, 3) cholangiolar, or 4) vanishing bile ducts. In most patients, the condition subsides promptly, but in some, it can lead to prolonged cholestasis and, occasionally, biliary cirrhosis. Examples of the causes of these forms of injury are listed in Table 2.

In most cases, the cholestasis resolves over 2 to 4 weeks after cessation of the drug, but in some cases, it may persist for several months. Rarely, in cases of vanishing bile duct injuries, cholestasis may be permanent. Ursodiol is prescribed by some physicians to speed resolution, but no controlled data are available to support this practice.

TREATMENT OF SPECIFIC CONDITIONS

Primary Biliary Cirrhosis

Currently, we prescribe ursodiol at a dose of 13 to 15 mg/kg daily, in divided doses, for patients with any stage of primary biliary cirrhosis who have abnormal findings on liver tests. Patients who meet minimal listing criteria for liver transplantation should be referred for evaluation, but there is no harm

Table 2. Forms of Drug-Induced Cholestasis and the Drugs Responsible

Form	Drugs responsible
Canalicular	Anabolic steroids
	Estrogen
	Rifampin
Hepatocanalicular	Chlorpromazine
	Erythromycin
	Amoxicillin-clavulanate
Cholangiolar	Benoxaprofen
Vanishing bile duct	Paraquat
	Chlorpromazine

in initiating ursodiol treatment while awaiting a donor organ. Ursodiol treatment should be approached gradually over 2 to 3 weeks to avoid precipitating pruritus, which can occur if the full dose is given initially. Ursodiol improves survival free of transplantation, decreases the risk of cirrhosis and varices developing, and lowers lipid levels. Prognostic models valid in the absence of therapy remain valid when scores are recalculated after 6 months of therapy and can provide useful information. However, not all patients have a response to ursodiol therapy. Approximately 35% of patients have complete biochemical normalization, with an excellent clinical response. Once ursodiol treatment is begun, it appears to be a lifelong need, and patients should be instructed accordingly. Side effects are minimal.

Autoimmune Cholangitis

Patients with autoimmune cholangitis typically have a response to ursodiol therapy, showing the usual response of patients with primary biliary cirrhosis. Occasionally, these patients have a response to corticosteroids or the combination of ursodiol and corticosteroids. This is particularly likely in patients with overlap of primary biliary cirrhosis and autoimmune cholangitis. Most clinicians would begin treatment with ursodiol alone and add corticosteroids if the results of liver biochemistry tests did not improve after 3 to 6 months.

Primary Sclerosing Cholangitis

Primary sclerosing cholangitis is the most troublesome of the more common adult cholestatic liver diseases because no effective therapy is available. Ursodiol in standard doses has inconsistent effects. Patients may have evidence of rapidly progressive jaundice, may suddenly develop pruritus, or may have fever with right upper quadrant pain. When any of these occur, cholangiography (usually endoscopic retrograde cholangiopancreatography [ERCP]) should be considered, although magnetic resonance cholangiography is also an alternative (Fig. 1). Cholangiocarcinoma, a biliary stone in the common bile duct, or a dominant stricture all can be responsible for these manifestations and can be differentiated best with ERCP. The endoscopic approach allows biopsy with brushing for suspected malignancy, extrication of biliary stones, or dilatation of dominant strictures. The role of stenting after dilatation has not been defined clearly.

MANAGEMENT OF COMPLICATIONS OF CHOLESTASIS

Complications of cholestasis require management. Malabsorption and deficiency of fat-soluble vitamins may occur, especially if cholestasis is severe. These patients require periodic monitoring. Levels of vitamins A, E, and D can be measured in serum directly, and the level of vitamin K can be inferred from the prothrombin time. Replacement with water-soluble forms of the vitamins can be offered (vitamin A, 50,000 units twice weekly; vitamin E, 200 units twice daily; vitamin D, 50,000 units twice weekly; and vitamin K, 5 mg daily). Adequacy of replacement can be reassessed by measuring levels after 6 to 12 months of therapy. Hypercholesterolemia, common in patients with cholestasis, does not appear to be frequently associated with atherosclerosis. We have not been aggressive in prescribing antihyperlipidemic therapy for these patients because some of these agents may be hepatotoxic; instead, we have usually settled for the antihypercholesterolemic effects of ursodiol when given for primary biliary cirrhosis.

Pruritus

Pruritus can be one of the most troublesome symptoms of patients with cholestasis. The severity of the pruritus is not closely correlated with the severity of the underlying liver disease, and pruritus may resolve as the disease progresses. Ursodiol reduces pruritus in some patients with primary biliary cirrhosis, but for those who remain symptomatic, antihistamines (i.e., diphenhydramine 25-30 mg by mouth at bedtime) may relieve the pruritus and permit sleep. Cholestyramine (4-g packets three or four times daily) may help relieve itching, but it can be unpleasant to use. Rifampin (150-300 mg twice daily) has a rapid onset of action and may be useful long-term, although liver toxicity may develop in 15% of patients. Naltrexone (50 mg daily) may be useful for some patients, although there is less experience with this drug than the others. Liver transplantation is available for patients who have severe, intolerable pruritus.

Bone Disease

Although the insufficient delivery of bile acids to the gut lumen in advanced cholestasis may lead to fat-soluble vitamin deficiency, osteomalacia due to vitamin D deficiency occurs in fewer than 5% of patients with osteopenic bone disease and cholestasis. Almost all bone disease evaluated in North America in this setting is due to osteoporosis, which is the result of insufficient bone matrix rather than a mineralization defect as found in osteomalacia. The cause of the osteoporosis is uncertain. The patients lose bone at a rate about twice that of the normal population. About 33% of patients with primary biliary cirrhosis and about 20% of those with primary sclerosing cholangitis are osteopenic at the time of diagnosis, and about 10% of them

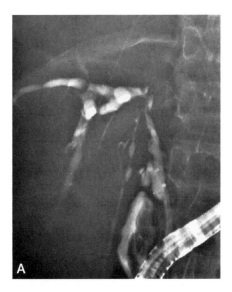
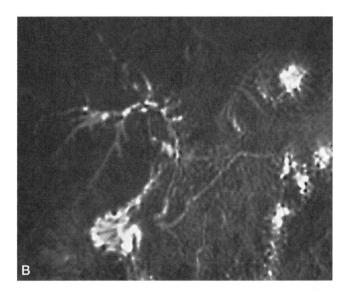

Fig. 1. Comparison of the findings of, *A*, endoscopic retrograde cholangiopancreatography and, *B*, magnetic resonance cholangiography in the same patient with primary sclerosing cholangitis.

experience vertebral fractures within a few years after diagnosis. The management of the bone disease includes exercise and adequate calcium intake with 1.5 g of elemental calcium daily along with vitamin D supplementation, if deficient. Postmenopausal women may have a response to hormone replacement therapy, usually given as patch therapy. Calcitonin therapy does not appear to be effective, and treatment with bisphosphonates has been suggested to be more effective.

RECOMMENDED READING

Angulo P, Lindor KD, Therneau TM, Jorgensen RA, Malinchoc M, Kamath PS, et al. Utilization of the Mayo risk score in patients with primary biliary cirrhosis receiving ursodeoxycholic acid. Liver. 1999;19:115-21.

Balan V, Dickson ER, Jorgensen RA, Lindor KD. Effect of ursodeoxycholic acid on serum lipids of patients with primary biliary cirrhosis. Mayo Clin Proc. 1994;69:923-9.

Crippin JS, Lindor KD, Jorgensen R, Kottke BA, Harrison JM, Murtaugh PA, et al. Hypercholesterolemia and atherosclerosis in primary biliary cirrhosis: What is the risk? Hepatology. 1992;15:858-62.

Corpechot C, Carrat F, Bahr A, Chretien Y, Poupon RE, Poupon R. The effect of ursodeoxycholic acid therapy on the natural course of primary biliary cirrhosis. Gastroenterology. 2005;128:297-303.

Guañabens N, Parés A, Monegal A, Peris P, Pons F, Alvarez L, et al. Etidronate versus fluoride for treatment of osteopenia in primary biliary cirrhosis: preliminary results after 2 years. Gastroenterology. 1997;113:219-24.

Jorgensen RA, Dickson ER, Hofmann AF, Rossi SS, Lindor KD. Characterisation of patients with a complete biochemical response to ursodeoxycholic acid. Gut. 1995;36:935-8.

Lacerda MA, Ludwig J, Dickson ER, Jorgensen RA, Lindor KD. Antimitochondrial antibody-negative primary biliary cirrhosis. Am J Gastroenterol. 1995;90:247-9.

Lewis JH. Drug-induced liver disease. Med Clin North Am. 2000;84:1275-311.

Lindor KD, Mayo Primary Sclerosing Cholangitis-Ursodeoxycholic Acid Study Group. Ursodiol for primary sclerosing cholangitis. N Engl J Med. 1997;336:691-5.

Lindor KD, Jorgensen RA, Therneau TM, Malinchoc M, Dickson ER. Ursodeoxycholic acid delays the onset of esophageal varices in primary biliary cirrhosis. Mayo Clin Proc. 1997;72:1137-40.

Lindor KD, Jorgensen RA, Tiegs RD, Khosla S, Dickson ER. Etidronate for osteoporosis in primary biliary cirrhosis: a randomized trial. J Hepatol. 2000;33:878-882.

Menon KV, Angulo P, Weston S, Dickson ER, Lindor KD. Bone disease in primary biliary cirrhosis: independent indicators and rate of progression. J Hepatol. 2001;35:316-23.

Michieletti P, Wanless IR, Katz A, Scheuer PJ, Yeaman SJ, Bassendine MF, et al. Antimitochondrial antibody negative primary biliary cirrhosis: a distinct syndrome of autoimmune cholangitis. Gut. 1994;35:260-5.

Olsson RG, Boberg KM, Schaffalitzky de Muckadel O, Lindgren S, Hultcrantz R, Folvik G, et al. Five-year treatment with high-dose UDCA in PSC [abstract]. J Hepatol. 2004;40 Suppl 1:161.

Poupon RE, Lindor KD, Cauch-Dudek K, Dickson ER, Poupon R, Heathcote EJ. Combined analysis of randomized controlled trials of ursodeoxycholic acid in primary biliary cirrhosis. Gastroenterology. 1997;113:884-90.

Poupon RE, Lindor KD, Parés A, Chazouilleres O, Poupon R, Heathcote EJ. Combined analysis of the effect of treatment with ursodeoxycholic acid on histologic progression in primary biliary cirrhosis. J Hepatol. 2003;39:12-6.

Rost D, Rudolph G, Kloeters-Plachky P, Stiehl A. Effect of high-dose ursodeoxycholic acid on its biliary enrichment in primary sclerosing cholangitis. Hepatology. 2004;40:693-8.

Rouillard S, Lane NE. Hepatic osteodystrophy. Hepatology. 2001;33:301-7.

Talwalkar JA, Angulo P, Johnson CD, Petersen BT, Lindor KD. Cost-minimization analysis of MRC versus ERCP for the diagnosis of primary sclerosing cholangitis. Hepatology. 2004;40:39-45.

Talwalkar JA, Lindor KD. Primary biliary cirrhosis. Lancet. 2003;362:53-61.

Talwalkar JA, Lindor KD. Primary sclerosing cholangitis. Inflamm Bowel Dis. 2005;11:62-72.

Talwalkar JA, Souto E, Jorgensen RA, Lindor KD. Natural history of pruritus in primary biliary cirrhosis. Clin Gastroenterol Hepatol. 2003;1:297-302.

Wolfhagen FH, Sternieri E, Hop WC, Vitale G, Bertolotti M, Van Buuren HR. Oral naltrexone treatment for cholestatic pruritus: a double-blind, placebo-controlled study. Gastroenterology. 1997;113:1264-9.

Zein CO, Angulo P, Lindor KD. When is liver biopsy needed in the diagnosis of primary biliary cirrhosis? Clin Gastroenterol Hepatol. 2003;1:89-95.

CHAPTER 36

Autoimmune Hepatitis

Albert J. Czaja, M.D.

DIAGNOSIS

Autoimmune hepatitis is an unresolving inflammation of the liver of unknown cause that is associated with interface hepatitis on histologic examination, hypergammaglobulinemia, and autoantibodies. An international panel has codified the diagnostic criteria, and the definite diagnosis requires exclusion of hereditary (Wilson's disease, genetic hemochromatosis, and alpha$_1$-antitrypsin deficiency), viral (hepatitis A, B, or C virus infection), and drug-induced (minocycline, isoniazid, propylthiouracil, α-methyldopa, and nitrofurantoin) conditions (Table 1). The 6-month requirement to establish chronicity has been waived, and an acute, even fulminant, presentation has been recognized that may resemble acute viral or toxic hepatitis. A cholestatic form of autoimmune hepatitis is not recognized, and a marked increase (more than twofold the upper limit of normal) in the serum level of alkaline phosphatase or the presence of pruritus suggests another diagnosis. Celiac disease can be associated with a liver disease that resembles autoimmune hepatitis, and it should be excluded in patients with cryptogenic chronic hepatitis by screening for IgA antibodies to endomysium. Endomysial antibodies are more specific for celiac disease in autoimmune hepatitis than IgA antibodies to tissue transglutaminase which can be stimulated by hepatic inflammation and fibrogenesis.

Interface hepatitis (periportal hepatitis or "piecemeal necrosis") is the histologic hallmark of the disease (Fig. 1). The morphologic pattern is nonspecific, and it occurs in acute and chronic liver disease of diverse causes. Portal plasma cell infiltration enhances specificity for autoimmune hepatitis, but its presence does not establish the diagnosis, nor does its absence discount the disease (Fig. 2). A lobular or panacinar hepatitis frequently accompanies interface hepatitis (Fig. 3). Multinucleated hepatocytes ("giant cell hepatitis") are rare manifestations of autoimmune hepatitis, whereas "rosettes" of hepatocytes are typical of the syndrome. Acinar zone 3 perivenular necrosis with and without sparing of the portal tracts has been reported, and it may be an early or acute form of autoimmune hepatitis before the classic changes of interface hepatitis occur within the portal tracts.

A scoring system that grades individual components of the syndrome provides an objective method for assessing the strength of the diagnosis, evaluating variant syndromes, and comparing populations in different geographical regions and treatment trials (Table 2). The recently revised system is not necessary for a confident diagnosis in most instances.

FREQUENCY AND ETHNIC DISTRIBUTION

Autoimmune hepatitis afflicts 100,000 to 200,000 persons in the United States, and it accounts for 2.6% of the liver transplants in Europe and 5.9% in the United States. Among Caucasoid northern Europeans, its mean annual incidence is 1.9 per 100,000 and its point prevalence is 16.9 per 100,000. Its occurrence is similar to that of primary biliary cirrhosis and primary sclerosing cholangitis and less than that of chronic viral hepatitis and alcoholic liver disease. Autoimmune hepatitis occurs mainly in women (female-to-male ratio is 3.6:1), and it affects all ages, including infants. Originally described in Caucasoid northern Europeans and North Americans, autoimmune hepatitis has also been recognized in black, Hispanic, Arab, subcontinental Indian, Turkish, Alaskan native, and Japanese populations. Distribution of the disease is worldwide.

Table 1.   Criteria for Diagnosis of Autoimmune
Hepatitis (AIH)

Diagnostic criteria	
Definite AIH	**Probable AIH**
Normal alpha$_1$-antitrypsin phenotype	Partial alpha$_1$-antitrypsin deficiency
Normal ceruloplasmin level	Abnormal copper or ceruloplasmin level but Wilson's disease excluded
Normal iron and ferritin levels	Nonspecific iron or ferritin abnormalities
No active hepatitis A, B, or C infection	No active hepatitis A, B, or C infection
Daily alcohol < 25 g	Daily alcohol < 50 g
No recent hepatotoxic drugs	No recent hepatotoxic drugs
Predominant serum aminotransferase abnormality	Predominant serum aminotransferase abnormality
Globulin, γ-globulin, or IgG level ≥1.5 times normal	Hypergammaglobulinemia of any degree
ANA, SMA, or anti-LKM1 ≥1:80 in adults and ≥1:20 in children; no AMA	ANA, SMA, or anti-LKM1 ≥1:40 in adults; other autoantibodies
Interface hepatitis—moderate to severe	Interface hepatitis—moderate to severe
No biliary lesions, granulomas, or prominent changes suggestive of another disease	No biliary lesions, granulomas, or prominent changes suggestive of another disease

AMA, antimitochondrial antibodies; ANA, antinuclear antibodies; anti-LKM1, antibodies to liver/kidney microsome type 1; IgG, serum immunoglobulin G level; SMA, smooth muscle antibodies. Modified from Czaja AJ. Autoimmune liver disease. In: Zakim D, Boyer TD, editors. Hepatology: a textbook of liver disease. Vol 2. 4th ed. Philadelphia: Saunders; 2003. p. 1163-1202. Used with permission.

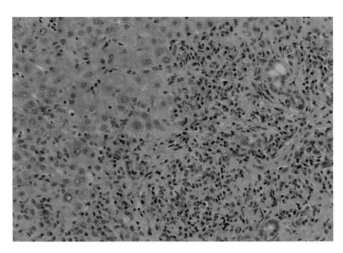

Fig. 1. Interface hepatitis. The limiting plate of the portal tract is disrupted by an inflammatory infiltrate that extends into the acinus. Interface hepatitis is a prerequisite for the diagnosis of autoimmune hepatitis, but it is not specific for the diagnosis. (Hematoxylin and eosin; x200.)

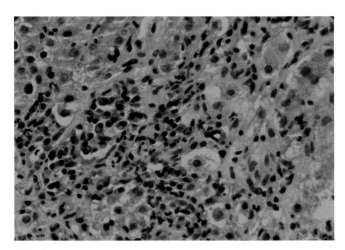

Fig. 2. Portal plasma cell infiltration. Plasma cells are characterized by a cytoplasmic halo adjacent to a deeply basophilic nucleus. Plasma cells are typically abundant at the interface and throughout the acinus, but they do not have diagnostic specificity. (Hematoxylin and eosin; x400.)

ETIOLOGY

The cause of autoimmune hepatitis is unknown. Multiple agents have been implicated as triggers of the disease, including certain viruses (hepatitis A, hepatitis B, hepatitis C, and measles viruses) and drugs (α-methyldopa, propylthiouracil, isoniazid, nitrofurantoin, and minocycline). Hepatitis A virus infection and minocycline have been implicated most commonly worldwide. Most cases have no identifiable trigger.

Triggers may share epitopes that resemble self-antigens, and they may break self-tolerance by overcoming antigenic ignorance, mimicking sequestered epitopes, or generating neoepitopes. Molecular mimicry between foreign antigens and self-antigens is the most frequently proposed initiating mechanism. A long lag time between exposure and expression and the possibility of persistent disease in the absence of a trigger complicate efforts to define an etiologic basis. The target autoantigen responsible for autoimmune hepatitis may have a short epitope that is easily mimicked.

CLINICAL FEATURES

Women constitute at least 70% of cases, and 50% are younger than 40 years (Table 3). Onset is usually between the third and

Table 2. Revised Scoring System of the International Autoimmune Hepatitis Group for the Diagnosis of Autoimmune Hepatitis*

Factors	Score	Factors	Score
Female sex	+2	Hepatotoxic drugs	
ALP:AST		Yes	−4
(ALT) ratio		No	+1
>3	−2	Alcohol use	
<1.5	+2	<25 g/d	+2
γ-Globulin or		>60 g/d	−2
IgG levels		HLA-DR3 or HLA-DR4	+1
>2 nL	+3	Concurrent immune	
1.5-2 nL	+2	disease	+2
1-1.4 nL	+1	Other liver-related	
ANA, SMA, or		autoantibody	+2
anti-LKM1		Interface hepatitis	+3
>1:80	+3	Plasmacytic infiltrate	+1
1:80	+2	Rosettes	+1
1:40	+1	No characteristic features	−5
<1:40	0	Biliary changes	−3
Antimitochon-		Other features (fat,	
drial antibodies	−4	granulomas)	−3
Viral markers		Treatment response	
Seropositive	−3	Complete	+2
Seronegative	+3	Relapse	+3

ALP:AST, ratio of serum alkaline phosphatase to aspartate aminotransferase level; ALT, serum alanine aminotransferase level; ANA, antinuclear antibodies; anti-LKM1, antibodies to liver/kidney microsome type 1; IgG, serum immunoglobulin G; SMA, smooth muscle antibodies.
**Pretreatment score: definite diagnosis, >15; probable diagnosis, 10-15. Post-treatment score: definite diagnosis, >17; probable diagnosis, 12-17.*
Modified from Czaja AJ: Autoimmune hepatitis. In: Feldman M, Friedman LS, Sleisenger MH, editors. Sleisenger & Fordtran's gastrointestinal and liver disease: pathophysiology/diagnosis/ management. Vol 2. 7th ed. Philadelphia: Saunders; 2002. p. 1462-73. Used with permission.

fifth decades, but patients may range in age from 9 months to 77 years. The bimodal age distribution that was proposed originally is probably an artifact of referral patterns to tertiary medical centers. Forty percent of patients have an abrupt onset of symptoms, and a fulminant presentation is possible, especially in the young. Features of chronic liver disease, including hyper-gammaglobulinemia and histologic cirrhosis, are commonly present, suggesting exacerbation of a preexistent, subclinical disease. In other patients, the presentation is indistinguishable from that of severe acute hepatitis, and the histologic features

include interface and lobular hepatitis without fibrosis or cirrhosis.

Familial occurrences are rare, but the disease has been reported in siblings, parents, and grandparents of afflicted persons. First-degree relatives may have abnormal serum immunoglobulin levels (47%), autoantibodies (42%), and hypergammaglobulinemia (34%). In one series, 3 of 55 families (5%) had more than one family member with chronic liver disease. The rarity of familial clustering, the uncertain pathogenesis of the disease, and the multifactorial nature of the illness do not justify family screening.

Easy fatigability is the most common symptom at presentation (85% of patients) (Table 3). Other symptoms include jaundice (46% of patients), polymyalgias (30%), anorexia (30%), diarrhea (28%), cosmetic changes such as facial rounding, hirsutism, or acne (19%), and, less commonly, delayed menarche or amenorrhea, obscure fever (rarely as high as 40°C), and right upper quadrant discomfort. Pruritus and weight loss are unusual, and they suggest an alternative diagnosis or a disease complicated by biliary obstruction or hepatocellular cancer. At initial consultation, 34% of patients may be asymptomatic, but they have the same histologic features and need for treatment as symptomatic patients. Most asymptomatic patients become symptomatic.

PHYSICAL FINDINGS

Hepatomegaly is the most common physical finding at presentation (78% of patients) (Table 3). Ascites (20% of patients) and hepatic encephalopathy (14%) are infrequent and connote advanced liver disease and cirrhosis. Hyperpigmentation and xanthelasmas are rare. The original clinical description of

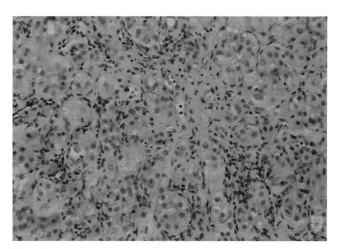

Fig. 3. Panacinar hepatitis. Cellular infiltrates line sinusoidal spaces in association with liver cell degenerative and regenerative changes. Rosettes of hepatocytes are also present. (Hematoxylin and eosin; x200.)

Table 3. Typical Features of Autoimmune Hepatitis

	Patients, %
Clinical features	
Female sex	70
Younger than 40 years	50
Acute onset	40
Common symptoms	
Fatigue	85
Jaundice	46
Myalgias	30
Frequent physical finding	
Hepatomegaly	78
Typical laboratory findings	
Increased serum levels of AST and ALT	100
Increased serum levels of γ-globulin and IgG	90
Mild hyperbilirubinemia (bilirubin <3 mg/dL)	83
Serum level of alkaline phosphatase increased <2× normal	67
ANA, SMA, or anti-LKM1	87

ALT, alanine aminotransferase level; ANA, antinuclear antibodies; anti-LKM1, antibodies to liver/kidney microsome type 1; AST, aspartate aminotransferase; IgG, immunoglobulin G; SMA, smooth muscle antibodies.

"lupoid hepatitis" that included acne, hirsutism, obesity, amenorrhea, and cirrhosis in young women ("Kunkel's girls") rarely is encountered. Twenty-six percent of patients with autoimmune hepatitis have normal physical examination findings despite severe inflammatory activity.

LABORATORY FEATURES

Abnormalities in serum aminotransferase levels are essential for the diagnosis (Table 3). The serum γ-globulin level is typically, but not invariably, increased, and the diagnosis is suspect without this finding. In most instances, the serum aminotransferase level at presentation does not exceed 500 U/L (range, 150 U/L to >1,000 U/L), and the γ-globulin level ranges from 2 to 3 g/dL. A polyclonal increase in serum immunoglobulin concentrations is typical, and the IgG fraction predominates. Hyperbilirubinemia is present in 83% of patients with severe inflammatory activity, but the serum bilirubin level exceeds 3 mg/dL in only 46%. Similarly, an abnormal increase in the serum alkaline phosphatase level can be demonstrated in 81% of patients, but it is more than twofold the upper limit of normal in only 33% and more than fourfold the upper limit of normal in only 10%.

CONCURRENT IMMUNE DISEASES

Immune diseases are commonly associated with autoimmune hepatitis (30%-48% frequency) (Table 4). Their presence does not establish the diagnosis or affect prognosis. Adults have mainly autoimmune thyroiditis, Graves' disease, ulcerative colitis, or synovitis, and children have mainly vitiligo or insulin-dependent diabetes mellitus. Celiac sprue may be asymptomatic and present in 3% of patients. Multiple immune diseases occur in 6% of patients. Ulcerative colitis does not compel the diagnosis of primary sclerosing cholangitis, but it does justify cholangiography. Fifty-nine percent of patients with autoimmune hepatitis and ulcerative colitis have normal cholangiograms, and they respond well to corticosteroid treatment.

AUTOANTIBODIES

Autoantibodies are markers of autoimmune hepatitis (Table 5). They are not pathogenic, and their behavior does not have important clinical implications. Serum titers do not have prognostic significance, and low titers should not dissuade the diagnosis if other features implicate the disease. Autoantibodies may be absent in some patients at presentation; serum titers can fluctuate during the course of illness; and the same autoantibodies at presentation may not be expressed later. As floating variables, their major clinical value is to support the diagnosis.

Table 4. Immune Diseases Associated With Autoimmune Hepatitis

Autoimmune thyroiditis*	Iritis
Celiac sprue	Lichen planus
Coomb's-positive hemolytic anemia	Myasthenia gravis
	Neutropenia
Cryoglobulinemia	Pericarditis
Dermatitis herpetiformis	Peripheral neuropathy
Erythema nodosum	Pernicious anemia
Fibrosing alveolitis	Pleuritis
Focal myositis	Pyoderma gangrenosum
Gingivitis	Rheumatoid arthritis*
Glomerulonephritis	Sjögren's syndrome
Graves' disease*	Synovitis*
Idiopathic thrombocytopenic purpura	Systemic lupus erythematosus
	Ulcerative colitis*
Insulin-dependent diabetes†	Urticaria
Intestinal villous atrophy	Vitiligo†

Most common associations.
†*Mainly in children.*
Modified from Czaja AJ. Autoimmune liver disease. In: Zakim D, Boyer TD, editors. Hepatology: a textbook of liver disease. Vol 2. 4th ed. Philadelphia: Saunders; 2003. p. 1163-1202. Used with permission.

The repertoire of conventional autoantibodies that should be measured in all patients being evaluated for the disease are antinuclear antibodies (ANA), smooth muscle antibodies (SMA), and antibodies to liver/kidney microsome type 1 (anti-LKM1) (Table 5). Other autoantibodies that support the diagnosis and whose assay is generally available in clinical laboratories are perinuclear antineutrophil cytoplasmic antibodies (pANCA). These occur in 50% to 90% of patients with type 1 autoimmune hepatitis and purportedly are useful in the evaluation of seronegative ("cryptogenic") chronic hepatitis. In this same fashion, IgA antibodies to endomysium are useful for excluding the liver disease associated with celiac disease.

Investigational antibodies that are likely to enhance diagnosis and prognosis but are not yet generally available include antibodies to the following: actin (anti-actin), soluble liver antigen/liver pancreas (anti-SLA/LP), asialoglycoprotein receptor (anti-ASGPR), chromatin, and liver cytosol type 1 (anti-LC1) (Table 5). Anti-ASGPR, anti-SLA/LP, and anti-chromatin are associated with relapse after treatment withdrawal, and anti-actin and anti-LC1 are associated with aggressive disease in young patients. The investigational antibodies may emerge as prognostic indices. Anti-SLA/LP hold the most promise because they are associated with relapse after corticosteroid withdrawal, severe disease activity, and HLA-DR3.

Cryptogenic chronic hepatitis may be reclassifiable as autoimmune hepatitis by repeat testing for the conventional autoantibodies or testing for pANCA or anti-SLA/LP. Determination of IgA antibodies to endomysium may indicate celiac disease in patients with cryptogenic chronic hepatitis. The clinical utility of testing for the investigational autoantibodies anti-ASGPR, anti-actin, anti-chromatin, and anti-LC1 has not been fully defined.

Antimitochondrial antibodies (AMA), including those against the M2 antigens associated with primary biliary cirrhosis, occur in 8% to 20% of patients with autoimmune hepatitis. Assays based on indirect immunofluorescence may mistake anti-LKM1 for AMA because the diagnostic patterns of indirect immunofluorescence on the murine kidney tubule can be confused. Other patients may have an overlap syndrome with primary biliary cirrhosis, early-stage primary biliary cirrhosis, or coincidental collateral autoantibody production.

The typical autoantibodies of autoimmune hepatitis can occur also in chronic hepatitis B and C. They are usually low-titer, background reactivities that should not alter diagnosis or management. Anti-LKM1 have been found in as many as 10% of patients with chronic hepatitis C. These antibodies are different from the anti-LMK1 found in classic autoimmune hepatitis. Homologies have been described between the antigenic target

Table 5. Autoantibodies Associated With Autoimmune Hepatitis (AIH)

	Target	Clinical value
Standard repertoire		
Antinuclear antibodies	Centromere Ribonucleoproteins	Diagnosis of type 1 AIH
Smooth muscle antibodies	Actin, tubulin, vimentin, desmin, skeletin CYP2D6	Diagnosis of type 1 AIH
Anti-LKM1		Diagnosis of type 2 AIH
Supplemental repertoire		
pANCA	Possible nuclear membrane lamina	Diagnosis of type 1 AIH Reclassification of cryptogenic hepatitis
IgA antibodies to endomysium	Endomysium monkey esophagus	Celiac disease and cryptogenic hepatitis
Investigational repertoire		
Antibodies to actin	Microfilaments	Diagnosis of type 1 AIH
Anti-SLA/LP	Cytosolic transfer Ribonucleoprotein complex	Associated with relapse and HLA-DR3 Reclassification of cryptogenic hepatitis
Anti-ASGPR	Asialoglycoprotein receptor	Histologic activity and relapse
Antibodies to chromatin	Octomeric chromatin molecule with multiple epitopes	ANA-positive disease associated with relapse
Anti-LC1	Formiminotransferase cyclodeaminase	Diagnosis of type 2 AIH Prognostic value

ANA, antinuclear antibodies; anti-ASGPR, antibodies to asialoglycoprotein receptor; anti-LC1, antibodies to liver cytosol type 1; anti-LKM1, antibodies to liver/kidney microsome type 1; anti-SLA/LP, antibodies to soluble liver antigen/liver-pancreas; pANCA, perinuclear antineutrophil cytoplasmic antibodies.

of anti-LKM1 and the genome of the hepatitis C virus (HCV), and this molecular mimicry may result in cross-reacting antibodies in some patients.

SUBCLASSIFICATIONS

Three types of autoimmune hepatitis have been proposed on the basis of serologic markers, but only two types have distinctive profiles (Table 6). None has been ascribed a unique cause, individual management strategy, or special type of behavior. The International Autoimmune Hepatitis Group has not endorsed subclassification of autoimmune hepatitis, but the designations have become clinical jargon. Type 1 and type 2 autoimmune hepatitis have different clinical features; however, type 3 is similar to type 1 and has no justification.

Type 1 Autoimmune Hepatitis

Type 1 autoimmune hepatitis is characterized by the presence of ANA or SMA or both (Table 6). It is the most common form of the disease worldwide, especially in Caucasoid northern Europeans and North Americans. Seventy percent of patients are women younger than 40 years and more than 30% have concurrent immune diseases, especially autoimmune thyroiditis, synovitis, or ulcerative colitis. Symptoms have acute onset in 40% of patients, and, rarely, the disease may have a fulminant presentation. At presentation, 25% of patients have cirrhosis, indicating that type 1 autoimmune hepatitis has an indolent, subclinical stage that is aggressive. The target autoantigen of type 1 autoimmune hepatitis is unknown.

Type 2 Autoimmune Hepatitis

Type 2 autoimmune hepatitis is characterized by the presence of anti-LKM1 (Table 6). It is predominantly a disease of children (2-14 years). Among Caucasoid North American adults with autoimmune hepatitis, only 4% have anti-LKM1. In contrast, 20% of patients in Europe are adults. The target autoantigen is the cytochrome monooxygenase CYP2D6, which is an important drug-metabolizing enzyme. Patients with type 2 autoimmune hepatitis have a high frequency of concurrent autoimmune diseases, especially insulin-dependent (type 1)

Table 6. Types of Autoimmune Hepatitis

| Feature | Autoimmune hepatitis | | |
	Type 1	Type 2	"Type 3"*
Characteristic autoantibodies	ANA, SMA	Anti-LKM1	Anti-SLA/LP
Associated autoantibodies	pANCA	Anti-LC1	ANA, SMA
	Anti-actin	Anti-ASGPR	Anti-ASGPR
	Anti-ASGPR		
Age at onset	All ages	Mainly pediatric (2-14 y)	All ages
Common concurrent immune diseases	Autoimmune thyroiditis	Vitiligo	Same as type 1
	Ulcerative colitis	Type 1 diabetes	
	Synovitis	Autoimmune thyroiditis	
		APECED	
Implicated genetic factors	*DRB1*0301* (N. Europe)	HLA-B14	HLA-DR3
	*DRB1*0401* (N. Europe)	HLA-DR3	
	*DRB1*1501* (protective)	*C4A-QO*	
		*DRB1*07*	
Autoantigen	Uncertain	CYP2D6	tRNP(Ser)Sec
		CYPIA2 (APECED)	
		CYPIA6 (APECED)	
Treatment	Corticosteroids	Corticosteroids	Corticosteroids

ANA, antinuclear antibodies; anti-ASGPR, antibodies to asialoglycoprotein receptor; anti-LC1, antibodies to liver cytosol type 1; anti-LKM1, antibodies to liver/kidney microsome type 1; anti-SLA/LP, antibodies to soluble liver antigen/liver pancreas; APECED, autoimmune polyendocrinopathy-candidiasis-ectodermal dystrophy; pANCA, perinuclear antineutrophil cytoplasmic antibodies; SMA, smooth muscle antibodies; tRNP(Ser)Sec, transfer ribonucleic acid protein complex for selenoprotein.
*Controversial and unjustified.
Modified from Czaja AJ. Autoimmune liver disease. In: Zakim D, Boyer TD, editors. Hepatology: a textbook of liver disease. Vol 2. 4th ed. Philadelphia: Saunders; 2003. p. 1163-1202. Used with permission.

diabetes mellitus, vitiligo, and autoimmune thyroiditis (Table 6). They also commonly have organ-specific autoantibodies, such as antibodies to parietal cells, islets of Langerhans, and thyroid, but they lack pANCA. Type 2 autoimmune hepatitis responds as well to corticosteroid therapy as does type 1 disease, and it may also have an acute, occasionally fulminant, presentation that must be recognized and treated promptly.

Type 2 autoimmune hepatitis is present in 15% of patients with autoimmune polyendocrinopathy-candidiasis-ectodermal dystrophy (APECED). This syndrome is characterized by ectodermal dysplasia, mucocutaneous candidiasis, and multiple endocrine organ failure (parathyroid, ovarian, and adrenal). A single gene defect on chromosome band 21q22.3 has been identified as the basis of the syndrome, and the disease is inherited in mendelian fashion. The *APECED* gene encodes for a transcription factor called the autoimmune regulator (AIRE), which modulates clonal deletion of autoreactive T cells. Unlike other autoimmune diseases, APECED does not have HLA-DR associations or female predominance.

Type 3 Autoimmune Hepatitis

Type 3 autoimmune hepatitis is characterized by the presence of anti-SLA/LP, but this finding does not justify its designation as a separate clinical entity (Table 6). Anti-SLA/LP are common in type 1 autoimmune hepatitis, and patients with these markers are indistinguishable from those with type 1 autoimmune hepatitis by age, sex distribution, frequency and nature of other autoantibodies, and responsiveness to corticosteroid therapy. Patients with anti-SLA/LP typically have HLA-DR3 and a propensity for relapse after withdrawal of corticosteroid therapy. The target autoantigen of anti-SLA/LP is a 50-kDa cytosolic protein that is probably a transfer RNA complex responsible for incorporating selenocysteine into peptide chains. The most important clinical applications of the assay for anti-SLA/LP may be the identification of patients who need treatment for an indefinite period and the assessment of cryptogenic chronic hepatitis. The antibodies have 99% specificity for the diagnosis of autoimmune hepatitis but only 16% sensitivity.

GENETIC PREDISPOSITIONS

Type 1 autoimmune hepatitis has a strong genetic predisposition, and 85% of Caucasoid northern European and North American patients have HLA-DR3, HLA-DR4, or both DR3 and DR4 (Table 7). Susceptibility resides within the *DRB1* gene. *DRB1*0301* is the principal susceptibility allele, and *DRB1*0401* is a secondary, but independent, risk factor. HLA-DR3 and HLA-DR4 are associated with different clinical expressions and treatment outcomes. Patients with HLA-DR3 (*DRB1*0301*) are younger, and respond less well to corticosteroid therapy than patients with HLA-DR4 (*DRB1*0401*).

For patients with HLA-DR3 (*DRB1*0301*), remission occurs less frequently, treatment failure occurs more often, and death from liver failure or requirement for liver transplantation is more common. In contrast, patients with HLA-DR4 (*DRB1*0401*) are older, more commonly women, have a greater occurrence of other immune diseases, and have a higher frequency of remission during corticosteroid treatment. HLA-DR15 (*DRB1*1501*) protects against type 1 autoimmune hepatitis in Caucasoid patients. Different ethnic groups have different susceptibility alleles.

TREATMENT REGIMENS

Prednisone alone or a lower dose of prednisone in combination with azathioprine is effective in the treatment of all forms of autoimmune hepatitis. Each regimen induces clinical, laboratory, and histologic remission in 65% of patients within 18 months and in 80% within 3 years. Each schedule also enhances survival expectations. The life expectancy of treated patients exceeds 80% after 20 years of observation, and it is no different from that of age- and sex-matched normal persons from the same geographical region. Treatment with corticosteroids also may reduce hepatic fibrosis. Improvement in hepatic fibrosis occurs in conjunction with a decrease in liver inflammation, and corticosteroids may facilitate the disappearance of fibrosis by suppressing inflammatory activity. Small case studies have suggested that cirrhosis also can disappear during treatment, but this needs to be confirmed with assays that reflect cirrhosis more reliably than conventional needle biopsy of the liver.

The absolute and relative indications for treatment are based on degrees of severity as assessed by clinical, laboratory, and histologic findings (Table 8). Patients with inactive cirrhosis, portal or mild interface hepatitis and no symptoms, or decompensated inactive cirrhosis with ascites, encephalopathy, or gastrointestinal bleeding, or a combination of these, do not warrant immunosuppressive therapy. The diagnosis of autoimmune hepatitis does not compel that treatment be initiated.

The preferred treatment schedule is prednisone in combination with azathioprine (Table 9). The combination schedule uses a lower dose of prednisone and is associated with fewer corticosteroid-related side effects. It is especially useful for patients with obesity, acne, menopause, labile hypertension, brittle diabetes, emotional lability, or osteopenia, or a combination of these. The prednisone-alone schedule is useful for patients with severe, preexistent cytopenia, pregnancy or contemplation of pregnancy, or active malignancy. Both regimens are similarly effective and differ only in the frequency of side effects. The regimen of alternate-day corticosteroid in titrated doses has not improved histologic features and has been abandoned in adults.

Table 7.   Genetic Predispositions for Type 1 Autoimmune Hepatitis and Clinical Associations

Genetic risk factor	Pertinence	Associations
HLA-DR3	Principal risk factor in Caucasoid North Americans and northern Europeans	Type 1 autoimmune hepatitis Young age at onset Treatment failure more common Liver transplant more often
HLA-DR4	Secondary risk factor in Caucasoid North Americans and northern Europeans	Type 1 autoimmune hepatitis Older patients Women Frequent immune disease Good response to treatment
DRB1*0301	Principal susceptibility allele in Caucasoid North Americans and northern Europeans	Same as HLA-DR3
DRB1*0401	Secondary susceptibility allele in Caucasoid North Americans and northern Europeans	Same as HLA-DR4
DRB1*1501	Protective allele in Caucasoid North Americans and northern Europeans	Low frequency of type 1 autoimmune hepatitis

Table 8.   Treatment Indications for Autoimmune Hepatitis

Absolute	Relative	None
Serum AST level > tenfold upper limit of normal	Symptoms (fatigue, arthralgia, jaundice)	No symptoms and mild interface or portal hepatitis
Serum AST level > fivefold upper limit of normal and γ-globulin level > twice normal	Serum AST and/or γ-globulin less than absolute criteria	Inactive cirrhosis
Bridging necrosis or multilobular necrosis in liver tissue	Interface hepatitis	Decompensated inactive cirrhosis

AST, aspartate aminotransferase.

LIVER TRANSPLANTATION

Liver transplantation is effective for the treatment of decompensated disease unresponsive to conventional therapies. Five-year survival rates for patients and grafts range from 83% to 92%, and the actuarial 10-year survival after transplantation is 75%. Disease recurrence is common (17% of patients), but it typically is mild and managed by adjustments in the immunosuppressive regimen. Progression to cirrhosis and graft failure is possible, and patients should be monitored closely for this possibility, especially if corticosteroid treatment is discontinued after transplantation. Patients with recurrent disease typically have HLA-DR3 or HLA-DR4 (or both), but recurrence is not related to a mismatch of these markers between donor and recipient. No findings at presentation predict prognosis and need for transplantation, and the decision to perform liver transplantation should be made after a trial of corticosteroid treatment.

Autoimmune hepatitis can develop de novo in recipients who receive a liver transplant for nonautoimmune liver disease.

Children seem to have a predilection for de novo autoimmune hepatitis. Immunosuppression with cyclosporine is a common feature, and the drug may affect thymic-negative selection of autoreactive immunocytes. Treatment with prednisone and azathioprine usually is effective. De novo autoimmune hepatitis after transplantation is rare, occurring in 2.5% to 3.4% of allografts, but it can result in graft loss if not treated with corticosteroids.

RELAPSE

Relapse connotes recrudescence of disease activity after drug withdrawal. It is characterized by an increase in the serum aspartate aminotransferase (AST) level to at least threefold normal. From 50% to 86% of patients have relapse after remission, most commonly during the first 6 months after the termination of therapy (50% of patients). The high frequency of relapse does not dissuade an attempt at drug withdrawal if

Table 9. Conventional Treatment Schedules

Weeks administered	Combination therapy		Prednisone therapy, mg daily
	Prednisone, mg daily	Azathioprine, mg daily	
1	30	50	60
1	20	50	40
2	15	50	30
Maintenance until end point	10	50	20

remission is achieved. Therapy should not be instituted with the preconception that it will be indefinite.

Relapse justifies re-treatment with the original drug schedule, and patients typically enter another remission. The major consequence of relapse and re-treatment is the development of drug-related complications (59% vs. 29%, $P < .05$). Benefit-risk analyses justify alternative management strategies after two relapses.

Patients who have multiple relapses warrant long-term, low-dose prednisone or azathioprine therapy for an indefinite period. The low-dose prednisone strategy requires a careful reduction in the daily maintenance dose until the lowest level is achieved to prevent symptoms and maintain serum AST levels less than fivefold the upper limit of normal. Azathioprine therapy for an indefinite period requires induction of clinical and laboratory remission by conventional treatments and then gradual corticosteroid withdrawal as the dose of azathioprine is increased to 2 mg/kg daily.

Relapse does not preclude permanent discontinuation of medication late in the course of the disease. Twenty-eight percent of patients who have relapse and receive re-treatment ultimately develop inactive disease and medication can be withdrawn. The possibility of permanent withdrawal of drug therapy justifies periodic attempts at dose reduction.

SUBOPTIMAL RESPONSES

Nine percent of patients have deterioration despite compliance with the drug regimen ("treatment failure"); 13% develop intolerable side effects and must prematurely discontinue medication ("drug toxicity"); and 13% have improvement but not to a degree that satisfies remission criteria ("incomplete response"). High-dose prednisone (60 mg daily) or prednisone (30 mg daily) in conjunction with azathioprine (150 mg daily) is the treatment failure regimen that induces laboratory remission in 75% of patients within 2 years. Only 20% achieve histologic

remission, and patients remain at risk for progression of the disease and the development of treatment-related complications.

OTHER TREATMENTS

Mycophenolate mofetil, mercaptopurine, tacrolimus, cyclosporine, cyclophosphamide, methotrexate, budesonide, and ursodeoxycholic acid are empiric therapies that have been used successfully in a small number of patients who cannot tolerate conventional regimens or whose disease is recalcitrant to them (Table 10). Cyclosporine has been administered as initial therapy, especially in children, but its advantage over standard regimens as first-line treatment has not been established. Most new immunosuppressive agents have emerged from the transplantation arena, and they are available for empiric use in highly selected patients. Mercaptopurine (1.5 mg/kg daily) is a standard drug with a new application. Limited clinical experience has indicated it has value in treating patients whose condition has deteriorated with conventional corticosteroid regimens.

LONG-TERM SURVEILLANCE

Follow-up must be life-long to assess progression to cirrhosis, late relapse after remission, treatment failure during indefinite

Table 10. Promising New Immunosuppressive Drugs for Autoimmune Hepatitis

Drug	Dose	Empiric uses
Cyclosporine	5-6 mg/kg daily	First-line therapy for children and adults Corticosteroid failure Corticosteroid intolerance
Tacrolimus	4 mg twice daily	Corticosteroid failure
Mycophenolate mofetil	2 g daily	Treatment failure Corticosteroid intolerance
Ursodeoxycholic acid	13-15 mg/kg daily	First-line therapy for mild disease Corticosteroid intolerance Incomplete response to standard therapy
Budesonide	3 mg twice daily	First-line therapy for mild disease Incomplete response to standard therapy
Mercaptopurine	1.5 mg/kg daily	Treatment failure

therapy, or malignant transformation. The prognosis is excellent despite histologic cirrhosis, probably because the synthetic function of the liver is preserved and complications of portal hypertension are rare. Hepatocellular cancer can develop in patients who have had cirrhosis for at least 5 years, but it is rare (1 per 965 patient-years of observation). Recommendations for cancer screening have not been codified. The risk of extrahepatic malignancy is 1.5 times normal, and tumors have diverse cell types. Standard health maintenance screening protocols should be applied.

VARIANT SYNDROMES

Disease that has features of autoimmune hepatitis and another liver disease ("overlap syndrome") or features similar to but atypical of classic disease ("outlier syndrome") comprises the variant syndromes (Table 11). Retrospective analyses have suggested that autoimmune liver disease can be reclassified as a variant form in 18% of patients. Standardized diagnostic criteria are lacking; the natural history is uncertain; and treatment algorithms have not been validated. The three principal variant syndromes are autoimmune hepatitis and primary biliary cirrhosis, autoimmune hepatitis and primary sclerosing cholangitis, and autoimmune hepatitis and cholangitis. Autoimmune hepatitis and cholangitis is probably a heterogeneous disorder that includes AMA-negative primary biliary cirrhosis, small-duct primary sclerosing cholangitis, and classic autoimmune hepatitis with incidental collateral bile duct injury.

Mixed hepatitic and cholestatic features are the most important clues to the presence of a variant form. AMAs, serum level of alkaline phosphatase increased to more than twofold normal, concurrent inflammatory bowel disease, histologic evidence of destructive cholangitis or ductopenia, and recalcitrance to corticosteroid therapy justify considering a variant form. Cholangiography is indicated if primary sclerosing cholangitis is possible and should be performed in all adults with autoimmune hepatitis and ulcerative colitis.

Treatment is empiric and includes prednisone, prednisone in combination with azathioprine, ursodeoxycholic acid, or prednisone and ursodeoxycholic acid (Table 11). The serum alkaline phosphatase level at presentation identifies patients with variant syndromes who may have a response to corticosteroid therapy. If the serum alkaline phosphatase level is less than twice the upper limit of normal, patients can show improvement with corticosteroid therapy; they usually have disease with overlapping features of autoimmune hepatitis and primary biliary cirrhosis (AMA-positivity). Treatment is based on the predominant manifestations of the disease, and regimens appropriate for hepatitic, cholestatic, or equally mixed hepatitic and cholestatic features are administered. Histologic improvement is unusual in autoimmune hepatitis and cholangitis or autoimmune hepatitis and primary sclerosing cholangitis. In these cases, the indications for therapy and the type of treatment are directed mainly by the symptoms.

Features of autoimmune hepatitis can be present in chronic hepatitis C, and HCV viremia can be present in autoimmune

Table 11. Variant Syndromes of Autoimmune Hepatitis (AIH) and Empiric Treatments

Variant syndrome	Salient features	Empiric treatment strategies
AIH and primary biliary cirrhosis	AMA positivity Cholestatic and hepatitic tests Increased serum IgM and IgG levels	Corticosteroids if serum ALP is ≤ twice normal Ursodeoxycholic acid if serum ALP is > twice normal and/or florid duct lesions found on biopsy
AIH and primary sclerosing cholangitis	Ulcerative colitis Pruritus Cholestatic and hepatitic tests ALP:AST >1.5 Abnormal cholangiogram	Corticosteroids and ursodeoxycholic acid
AIH and cholangitis	Fatigue Pruritus Cholestatic and hepatitic tests AMA negative ANA and/or SMA positive Normal cholangiogram	Prednisone, ursodeoxycholic acid, or both, depending on hepatitic and cholestatic components

ALP, serum alkaline phosphatase; AMA, antimitochondrial antibodies; ANA, antinuclear antibodies; AST, serum aspartate aminotransferase; SMA, smooth muscle antibodies.

hepatitis. In patients with autoimmune hepatitis, interferon therapy can exacerbate the autoimmune manifestations, and in patients with chronic hepatitis C, corticosteroid therapy increases the viral load. Most patients have chronic hepatitis C and autoimmune features, and treatment should be as for chronic viral hepatitis. Rare patients have classic autoimmune hepatitis, including the characteristic histologic changes and coincidental HCV infection. Chronic hepatitis C in these patients is probably a background finding; corticosteroid therapy can improve the predominant autoimmune disease.

SUMMARY

Autoimmune hepatitis has a global distribution and affects all age groups. The diagnosis has been codified by an international panel. The ability of autoimmune hepatitis to present as acute or fulminant disease is recognized. Subclassifications by serologic markers do not connote different causes or outcome, and the designations are controversial. Autoantibodies are diverse and nonpathogenic. The implicated autoantigens are cytosolic enzymes capable of transforming self- or foreign proteins into antigenic peptides. The disease has a strong genetic predisposition and is closely associated with HLA-DR3 and HLA-DR4 in Caucasoid North Americans and northern Europeans. These risk factors affect susceptibility, clinical expression, and treatment outcome. Patients with HLA-DR3 are young, and therapy fails or liver transplantation is required more often than for patients with HLA-DR4. Corticosteroid therapy is effective for all forms of the disease, and liver transplantation is the salvage procedure for decompensated disease.

RECOMMENDED READING

Alvarez F, Berg PA, Bianchi FB, Bianchi L, Burroughs AK, Cancado EL, et al, International Autoimmune Hepatitis Group. International Autoimmune Hepatitis Group report: review of criteria for diagnosis of autoimmune hepatitis. J Hepatol. 1999;31:929-38.
Codified criteria by an international panel for the diagnosis of autoimmune hepatitis, including a revised scoring system to quantify the strength of diagnosis.

Czaja AJ: Frequency and nature of the variant syndromes of autoimmune liver disease. Hepatology. 1998;28:360-5.
Determination of the frequency of the variant syndromes in autoimmune liver disease and their responsiveness to corticosteroid therapy.

Czaja AJ. Understanding the pathogenesis of autoimmune hepatitis. Am J Gastroenterol. 2001;96:1224-31.
Review of the theories of pathogenesis, including trigger factors, genetic predispositions, putative mechanisms of hepatocyte destruction, and defects in immunomodulation.

Czaja AJ. Autoimmune hepatitis after liver transplantation and other lessons of self-intolerance. Liver Transpl. 2002;8:505-13.
Concise presentation of the consequences of liver transplantation in autoimmune hepatitis, including recurrent and de novo disease, and speculations about possible mechanisms for loss of self-tolerance.

Czaja AJ. Treatment of autoimmune hepatitis. Semin Liver Dis. 2002;22:365-78.
Review of current treatment strategies and emerging therapies that promise greater blanket immunosuppression than conventional corticosteroid regimens and site-specific interventions directed at pertinent pathogenic mechanisms.

Czaja AJ. The autoimmune hepatitis/hepatitis C overlap syndrome: does it exist? In: Leuschner U, Broome U, Stiehl A, editors. Cholestatic liver disease: therapeutic options and perspectives. Lancaster, UK: Lancaster Publishing Services; 2004. p. 132-46.
Review of the concepts of overlap syndromes and criteria for diagnosis illustrated by assessing autoimmune features in chronic hepatitis C.

Czaja AJ, Carpenter HA. Decreased fibrosis during corticosteroid therapy of autoimmune hepatitis. J Hepatol. 2004;40:646-52.
Important study indicating that fibrosis can decrease with corticosteroid treatment.

Czaja AJ, Carpenter HA. Progressive fibrosis during corticosteroid therapy of autoimmune hepatitis. Hepatology. 2004;39:1631-8.
Demonstration that progressive fibrosis is associated with persistent histologic activity and HLA DR3-DR4 heterozygosity.

Czaja AJ, Doherty DG, Donaldson PT. Genetic bases of autoimmune hepatitis. Dig Dis Sci. 2002;47:2139-50.
Review of the effects of sex, HLA phenotype, and polymorphisms of key autoimmune promoters on occurrence, clinical expression, and treatment outcome.

Czaja AJ, Freese DK. Diagnosis and treatment of autoimmune hepatitis. Hepatology. 2002;36:479-97.
Diagnostic and management guidelines that are evidence-based and current.

Czaja AJ, Norman GL. Autoantibodies in the diagnosis and management of liver disease. J Clin Gastroenterol. 2003;37:315-29.
Comprehensive review of the conventional and investigational autoantibodies used in the diagnosis of autoimmune liver diseases.

Gonzalez-Koch A, Czaja AJ, Carpenter HA, Roberts SK, Charlton MR, Porayko MK, et al. Recurrent autoimmune hepatitis after orthotopic liver transplantation. Liver Transpl. 2001;7:302-10.
Determination of the frequency of recurrent autoimmune hepatitis after liver transplantation, predisposing factors, and outcome.

CHAPTER 37

Nonalcoholic Fatty Liver Disease

Albert J. Czaja, M.D.

DIAGNOSIS

Nonalcoholic fatty liver disease (NAFLD) is a chronic disease, usually mild and commonly asymptomatic, characterized by the histologic features of macrovesicular steatosis with or without lobular (acinar) hepatitis in the absence of excess alcohol consumption (Fig. 1). NAFLD is a designation that encompasses patients with bland steatosis, active inflammation, or cirrhosis (Fig. 2). Nonalcoholic steatohepatitis (NASH) is within the spectrum of NAFLD and is associated with histologic activity. Transitions between NASH and bland steatosis probably occur. NASH may also result in cirrhosis (Fig. 3). Steatosis can diminish as patients progress to cirrhosis, and in some patients cryptogenic cirrhosis may have evolved from NAFLD.

NAFLD is commonly associated with obesity, hyperlipidemia, or diabetes mellitus, but the absence of these risk factors does not preclude the diagnosis. Drugs (corticosteroids, amiodarone, perhexilene maleate, methotrexate, nucleoside analogues, and tamoxifen), clinical conditions (total parenteral nutrition, protein-calorie malnutrition, jejunoileal bypass), and disorders (abetalipoproteinemia, bulimia, celiac disease, Wilson's disease, chronic hepatitis C, Weber-Christian disease, or limb lipodystrophy) can be associated with fatty liver, and these considerations should be excluded by appropriate clinical history and laboratory testing (Table 1).

The diagnosis of NAFLD requires liver biopsy evaluation, but the clinical history, laboratory findings, and features seen on liver ultrasonography are usually sufficient to exclude other similar conditions and to implicate the disease. NAFLD should be considered in all asymptomatic patients with chronic hepatitis of undetermined nature, and it is not excluded by normal body weight or the absence of risk factors.

DIFFERENTIAL DIAGNOSIS

Alcohol-induced and drug-related liver diseases are the other main diagnostic considerations (Table 2). Threshold levels of alcohol consumption that support the diagnosis of alcoholic liver disease are 20 g daily for women and 80 g daily for men. Other discriminatory features between NAFLD and alcoholic hepatitis are the higher frequencies of NAFLD in women and patients with diabetes mellitus, obesity, dyslipidemia (20%-81%), body mass index (BMI) of 25 kg/m^2 or more (39%-100%), and serum aspartate aminotransferase (AST):alanine aminotransferase (ALT) ratio less than 1 (65%-90%). Patients

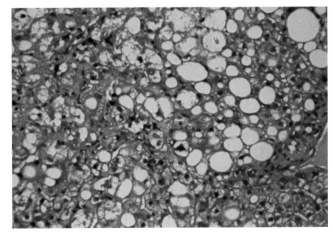

Fig. 1. Histologic features of nonalcoholic steatohepatitis. Macrovesicular steatosis is present, with inflammatory infiltrates within the lobule (acinus). Steatosis in the absence of lobular (acinar) inflammation is still within the histologic spectrum of nonalcoholic fatty liver disease. (Hematoxylin-eosin; ×200.)

Table 1. Risk Factors Associated With Nonalcoholic Fatty Liver Disease

Metabolic
  Obesity
  Diabetes mellitus
  Dyslipidemia
Drug-associated
  Corticosteroids
  Amiodarone
  Perhexilene maleate
  Methotrexate
  Nucleoside analogues
  Tamoxifen
Disease-related
  Abetalipoproteinemia
  Celiac disease
  Wilson's disease
  Chronic hepatitis C
  Weber-Christian disease
  Limb lipodystrophy
  Bulimia
Condition-related (archaic)
  Jejunoileal bypass
  Total parenteral nutrition

with alcoholic hepatitis are more commonly symptomatic than those with NAFLD and more frequently have a serum AST:ALT ratio greater than 1 (average ratio, 2.6), cirrhosis, hyperbilirubinemia, hypoalbuminemia, and hypoprothrombinemia (Table 2). Drug-induced liver disease requires the exclusion of drugs such as corticosteroids, amiodarone, perhexilene maleate, methotrexate, and tamoxifen by careful clinical history.

PREVALENCE

NAFLD occurs in 9% of overweight patients and 21% to 33% of those with morbid obesity. Postmortem studies have reported NAFLD in 3% of subjects with lean body weight, and it is recognized in 6% to 21% of patients with diabetes mellitus. Twenty-one percent of patients with an asymptomatic increase in serum AST level have NAFLD. Ultrasonographic surveys of the general population indicate the presence of fatty liver in 16% to 25% of adults in the United States, and it is the most common cause of increased serum levels of ALT in blood donors. NAFLD is more common than chronic hepatitis C in the United States, and its prevalence, especially in the pediatric and adolescent groups, will increase as the epidemic of obesity worsens. Of adolescents with abnormal liver tests, 60% are obese or overweight; 1% to 2% of adolescents have NAFLD.

PATHOGENESIS

The pathogenic mechanisms of NAFLD are unknown. The multiple hypotheses that have been advanced are not mutually exclusive. The prevailing hypothesis is that NAFLD reflects insulin resistance and increased oxidative stress on the

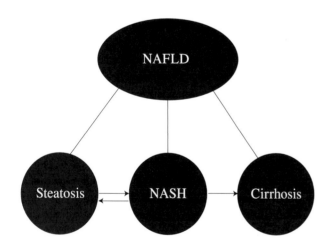

Fig. 2. Components of nonalcoholic fatty liver disease (NAFLD). The designation of NAFLD encompasses patients with steatosis, nonalcoholic steatohepatitis (NASH), and cirrhosis. Transitions are possible between steatosis and NASH, and NASH may progress to cirrhosis. A direct transition between steatosis and cirrhosis is uncertain.

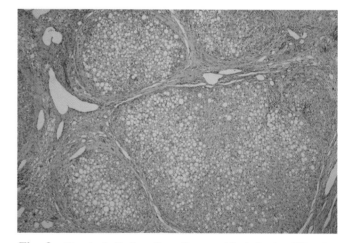

Fig. 3. Nonalcoholic fatty liver disease with cirrhosis. Fibrosis bands and regenerative nodules connote cirrhosis. Macrovesicular steatosis is also present, with minimal inflammatory infiltrate. Steatosis can diminish or disappear as cirrhosis develops. (Hematoxylin-eosin; ×100.)

Table 2. Distinctions Between Alcoholic and Nonalcoholic Fatty Liver Disease

Feature	Alcoholic hepatitis, % of patients	Nonalcoholic steatohepatitis, % of patients
Women	42	81
Diabetes mellitus	23	75
Obesity	29	71
Symptomatic	88	23
Serum AST:ALT >3	86	32
Bilirubin >3 mg/dL	55	17
Increased γ-glutamyl transpeptidase	69	55
Prolonged prothrombin time	10	0
Mallory bodies	16	3
Fibrosis or cirrhosis	63	38

ALT, alanine aminotransferase; AST, aspartate aminotransferase.

hepatocytes. Obesity and diabetes mellitus are associated with increased tissue resistance to insulin, and hyperinsulinemia, in turn, impairs mitochondrial β-oxidation of free fatty acids. Because of this block in fatty acid catabolism, fat accumulates in zone 3 hepatocytes, which in turn increases their susceptibility to injury by lipid peroxidation.

Oxidative stress is created by the formation of reactive oxygen species such as hydrogen peroxide, malondialdehyde, and 4-hydroxynonenal, and these compounds activate liver stellate cells to produce collagen and attract neutrophils that generate an inflammatory reaction. Increased cytochrome CYP2E1 activity in animal models of NASH has been associated with oxidative stress. Lipid peroxidation that follows hepatic steatosis results in hepatocyte inflammation, liver fibrosis, and cell death.

Insulin resistance also alters the production of very-low-density lipoproteins (VLDLs), which are important in the disposal of free fatty acids from the liver as triglycerides. VLDL synthesis is impaired in NASH, and intracellular degradation of VLDL may be increased. Leptin is a mediator in insulin signaling, obesity, and hepatic steatosis, and it may have a role in the production of NASH by affecting the partitioning of fat between mitochondrial β-oxidation and triglyceride synthesis. Derangements in leptin signaling can result in fat accumulation within the liver and liver fibrosis.

Endotoxemia from intestinal overgrowth or altered mucosal permeability has been proposed as a basis for fatty liver in alcoholic liver disease, and in genetically obese mice with hepatic steatosis, low levels of endotoxin produce NASH, when compared with control animals. In patients with bacterial overgrowth, endotoxemia can result in peroxisomal dysfunction, glutathione depletion, and the release of tumor necrosis factor-α from monocytes. This milieu, in turn, favors superoxide production, with the generation of toxic aldehydes and the release of free fatty acids that cause fat accumulation and hepatocyte injury. Tumor necrosis factor-α has been implicated as a prime mediator in the fatty liver associated with endotoxemia. Elemental iron also promotes insulin resistance and oxidative stress, and hepatic iron overload may contribute to liver cell injury in genetic hemochromatosis and NASH.

Multiple interactive processes stimulate lipogenesis and inhibit lipolysis, and the final common pathway may relate to cytokine imbalances that modulate oxidative stress and the various factors that counterbalance lipogenesis and lipolysis. Endogenously produced alcohol by gastrointestinal flora in aging laboratory mice and patients with morbid obesity and jejunoileal bypass have generated hypotheses about an alcohol component of NAFLD. Breath ethanol content increases with BMI, and it is independent of liver test abnormalities or histologic changes. Hepatitis C virus does not cause NAFLD, but fatty liver may coexist with chronic hepatitis C and increase its severity through lipid peroxidation.

CLINICAL FEATURES

NAFLD occurs mainly in women (77%-100% of cases) (Table 3). Common risk factors are BMI of 25 kg/m² or more (50%-95% of patients) and diabetes (27%-75% of patients), and as many as 92% of patients have obesity or diabetes (or both). The mean age at diagnosis is 50 years (range, 16-80 years) and most patients (77%) are asymptomatic. Right upper quadrant pain, which typically is mild, is the most common symptom, and fatigue or malaise may also occur. The absence of risk factors does not exclude the diagnosis, and 3% to 42% of patients have normal blood glucose and lipid levels and lean body weight. Patients frequently have other medical conditions, including heart disease, hypertension, or hypothyroidism, and they often are taking multiple medications. Fulminant liver necrosis or rapid progression to cirrhosis suggests a drug-induced steatosis (nucleoside analogues, antimitotic agents, or tetracycline), an inborn error of metabolism (tyrosinemia), or Wilson's disease.

The BMI is determined by dividing the weight in kilograms (kg) by the height in meters squared (m²). This index is useful in defining obesity. Overweight (excess weight for height) requires a BMI of 25 kg/m² or more and obesity (excess fat), a BMI of 30 kg/m² or more. For 46% of patients with NAFLD, the BMI is 31 kg/m² or more (average BMI, 32±1 kg/m²). Older age, obesity, diabetes mellitus, and an AST:ALT ratio greater than 1 identify a subset of patients with severe fibrosis, and these patients may warrant liver biopsy examination to con-

Table 3. Typical Features of Nonalcoholic Steatohepatitis

Feature	Patients, %
Clinical	
Female	77-100
Obesity	50-95
Diabetes mellitus	27-75
Obesity and/or diabetes mellitus	92
Common symptoms	
None	77
Right upper quadrant pain	10
Fatigue	10
Frequent physical findings	
Hepatomegaly	90
Lean body weight	3-42
Typical laboratory findings	
Increased serum AST and ALT	70
Serum AST:ALT < 1	60
Increased serum γ-globulin	30
Hyperbilirubinemia (>2 mg/dL)	17
Hyperlipidemia	12-54
Smooth muscle antibodies	3
Antinuclear antibodies	20

ALT, alanine aminotransferase; AST, aspartate aminotransferase.

firm the diagnosis and stage the disease. Autopsy studies have indicated that 20% of markedly obese subjects have NAFLD and 14% have liver fibrosis. The importance of obesity as a risk factor for NAFLD is underscored by the presence of NASH in 24% to 36% of patients undergoing bariatric surgery and liver fibrosis in 8% to 26%.

PHYSICAL FINDINGS

The most common physical finding is obesity (Table 2). Manifestations of conditions predisposing to NAFLD may also be present, such as cushingoid features or diabetic neuropathy. Hepatomegaly may occur in 12% to 75% of patients, but features of severe or advanced liver disease such as jaundice, spider angiomas, splenomegaly, or ascites are rare.

LABORATORY FINDINGS

Increased serum levels of AST and ALT typify the disease, but the increase is more than threefold the upper limit of normal in only 30% of patients (range, two- to fivefold the upper limit of normal) (Table 2). The serum AST:ALT ratio is less than 1 in 65% to 90% of patients, and a serum AST:ALT ratio of 2 or more strongly suggests alcoholic liver disease. Although the serum AST:ALT ratio is useful in distinguishing NAFLD

from alcoholic liver disease, other liver conditions can be associated with similar perturbations in the ratio and the findings lack diagnostic specificity.

Serum levels of bilirubin exceed 3 mg/dL in only 17% of patients, and hypergammaglobulinemia occurs in 30%. Serum levels of alkaline phosphatase may be increased to threefold the upper limit of normal in 50% of patients, and γ-glutamyl transpeptidase concentrations also may be increased. Indices of the synthetic function of the liver, including serum albumin levels and prothrombin time, are normal unless there is cirrhosis with decompensation.

Serum levels of transferrin and ferritin are increased in 20% to 50% of patients, and the mutations of genetic hemochromatosis have been demonstrated in 30%. The low frequency of iron overload in patients with NAFLD and abnormal iron indices and the lack of correlation between the iron studies and the gene mutations of hemochromatosis do not justify routine genetic testing or phlebotomy. Heterozygous phenotypes for alpha$_1$-antitrypsin deficiency occur more commonly in patients with NAFLD than in those with chronic hepatitis C and fatty liver, but the clinical significance of this association is not clear.

Autoantibodies, including antinuclear antibodies (20% of patients) and smooth muscle antibodies (3% of patients), occur commonly in NASH (23% of patients), and they have been associated with an increased histologic activity index, higher stage of fibrosis, greater insulin resistance, and greater serum levels of γ-globulin than in patients seronegative for autoantibodies. The serologic markers and hypergammaglobulinemia can be confused with autoimmune hepatitis, and assessment of liver biopsy specimens is required to establish the diagnosis. High (fivefold or more of the upper limit of normal) serum levels of AST and ALT are typical of autoimmune hepatitis and unusual in NAFLD. Similarly, NAFLD may emerge in corticosteroid-treated patients who have autoimmune hepatitis, and examination of liver tissue is required to develop the most appropriate treatment strategy. Corticosteroid therapy may be misapplied in these situations and potentially may aggravate the condition.

Hypertriglyceridemia, hypercholesterolemia, or hyperglycemia occur in 20% to 81% of patients. Fifty-four percent of patients with NAFLD who weigh 50% more than their ideal body weight have type IV hyperlipidemia.

HISTOLOGIC FEATURES

Macrovesicular steatosis is the hallmark of NAFLD (Fig. 1). The fat is distributed throughout the lobule, but as in alcoholic liver disease, changes are most prominent in the perivenular area (zone 3). The presence of a lobular (acinar) hepatitis justifies the designation of NASH. Focal necroses, ballooning degeneration of hepatocytes, hyalin bodies (Mallory bodies, or "alcoholic hyalin"), and fibrosis, including cirrhosis, may also be present (Fig. 4). Perivenular and sinusoidal fibrosis can develop, and the histologic pattern may be indistinguishable from that of alcoholic hepatitis. As many as 30% of patients have fibrosis or cirrhosis, according to liver biopsy examination findings, despite minimal enzyme changes. Features of steatosis and inflammatory activity may diminish or disappear as cirrhosis develops.

RADIOLOGIC TESTS

Liver ultrasonography is useful in supporting the clinical diagnosis of NAFLD, but it does not establish the diagnosis or indicate the cause of the steatosis. Diffuse fatty infiltration of the liver is characterized by a diffuse bright hyperechoic pattern (Fig. 5). Thirty percent of hepatocytes must be infiltrated with fat before detection, and negative ultrasonographic findings do not exclude NAFLD. The sensitivity of liver ultrasonography for steatosis is 94% and its specificity is 84%. The negative predictive value is 14% to 42%. The performance measures of liver ultrasonography apply only to comparisons between fatty and normal livers, and the ability of ultrasonography to differentiate fatty liver from other parenchymal liver diseases is less certain.

Computed tomograms suggest fatty infiltration when there is signal attenuation of the right lobe of the liver and a lower mean computed tomographic number for liver than for spleen (Fig. 6). Magnetic resonance imaging shows the entire spectrum of fatty infiltration and is useful in excluding fat. Focal fatty changes can mimic primary or metastatic liver disease because islands of normal liver tissue are accentuated by the fatty infiltration of adjacent hepatocytes. Computed tomography and magnetic resonance imaging are rarely required to supplement the ultrasonographic assessment.

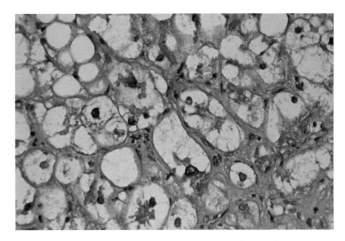

Fig. 4. Mallory bodies in nonalcoholic steatohepatitis. Mallory bodies, or "alcoholic hyalin," are visible as eosinophilic concretions in ballooned hepatocytes. (Hematoxylin-eosin; ×400.)

INVESTIGATIONAL TESTS

No laboratory tests establish the diagnosis of NAFLD or confidently distinguish between NAFLD and alcoholic liver disease. Desialylated (carbohydrate-deficient) transferrin is a marker of alcoholism, and the sensitivity and specificity of the test for alcohol consumption are 81% and 98%, respectively. Alcohol inhibits sialyltransferase and glycosylation of transferrin, and the carbohydrate-deficient molecule is detectable after 60 to 80 g of alcohol are consumed daily for 4 to 6 weeks. The performance measures of the test have not been corroborated, and determinations of the ratio of desialylated transferrin to total transferrin have not reliably differentiated NAFLD from alcoholic liver disease.

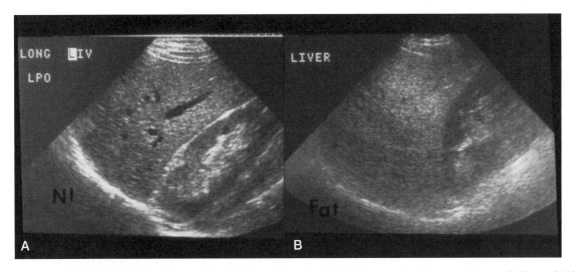

Fig. 5. Ultrasonographic findings in hepatic steatosis. *A*, Normal liver has distinctive vascular features, whereas, *B*, liver with fatty infiltration has a diffuse bright echotexture and blurring of hepatic vessels.

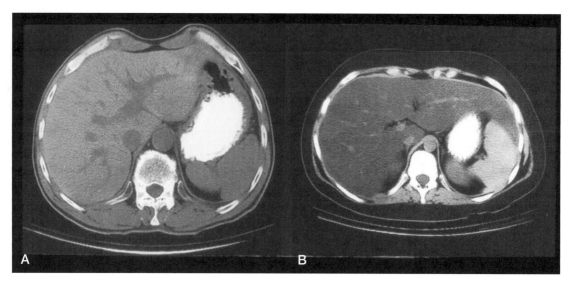

Fig. 6. Features of hepatic steatosis visualized with computed tomography. *A*, Normal liver has no attenuation of the signal compared with the spleen, whereas, *B*, liver with fatty infiltration has an attenuated signal compared with the spleen.

Mitochondrial AST increases after chronic alcohol use because of enzyme induction, impaired transfer of the enzyme from the cytosol to mitochondria, and increased efflux from hepatocytes. The ratio of mitochondrial AST to total AST has a sensitivity of 92% but a specificity of only 50% for chronic alcoholism. Also, it has not been incorporated into clinical practice as a discriminator between NAFLD and chronic alcoholic liver disease.

Cholinesterase hydrolyzes butyrylthiocholine, and it is stimulated by nonesterified fatty acids and butyrylthiocholine production. Blood cholinesterase levels are increased in NASH and NAFLD, but only high concentrations (≥9,000 IU/L) have specificity for NASH. The low sensitivity of the test (47%) has limited its clinical application.

Immunohistochemical techniques that stain for insulin receptors in liver tissue can suggest states of insulin resistance. Preliminary studies have suggested that these techniques may be useful in distinguishing between NAFLD and alcoholic liver disease.

NATURAL HISTORY

No prospective studies are available to establish the natural history and prognosis of NAFLD. After 6 years of follow-up, 54% of patients have no change in their liver tests and 12% have improvement (Table 4). Fibrosis develops in 23% of patients within 9 years after diagnosis, and cirrhosis has been described in 12% of patients within 8 years. Liver failure has been recognized in 3% of patients within 17 years. Studies that included mainly patients who had bland steatosis described

a benign long-term prognosis, whereas those that included mainly patients who had NASH suggested a more aggressive disorder. NASH and liver fibrosis have been associated with an 11% mortality rate after 10 years. The 5- and 10-year survival rates for patients with NASH may be as low as 67% and 59%, respectively, if deaths due to the comorbid conditions of obesity and diabetes are included. Liver transplantation has been required for some patients (1%-2%) with cirrhosis, and recurrence of NAFLD after transplantation has been described.

TREATMENT

The principal treatments are exercise, dieting, discontinuation of alcohol and hepatotoxic drugs, and management of diabetes and hyperlipidemia. Liver transplantation is warranted in patients with decompensated cirrhosis, but preoperative risk factors for NAFLD must be eliminated or reduced to prevent recurrence.

Exercise, dieting, and weight loss are cornerstones of therapy and can reverse the disease, especially in patients who are more than 50% above the ideal weight. Exercise can decrease hepatic steatosis even in the absence of weight loss because it can alter substrate use in skeletal muscle and increase insulin sensitivity. Weight loss must be gradual and conservative because rapid weight reduction can exacerbate the disease. Loss of the first 30 lb is the critical determinant of success.

Special diets are of uncertain benefit, and the practical approach is to recommend a low calorie, balanced diet. Polyunsaturated fats in fish and flax seed oils alter insulin sensitivity and prostaglandin metabolism, but their effects on NAFLD are uncertain.

Table 4. Outcome of Nonalcoholic Steatohepatitis*

Outcome	Patients, %	Follow-up, y
No change	54	6
Fibrosis	23	1-9
Cirrhosis	12	8
Improvement	12	1-9
Liver failure	3	17

*Extrapolations from retrospective studies.

Gastric bypass surgery has been associated with histologic improvement within 1 year and with an effective weight reduction of 12% to 42% in patients who are 75% or more overweight. Precipitous weight loss can exacerbate the disease, and liver failure and death have occurred after the procedure.

Cytoprotective agents, such as ursodeoxycholic acid, have not been effective in a randomized trial, but antioxidant agents, such as vitamin E, S-adenosylmethionine, betaine, and N-acetylcysteine, are still being studied. Betaine, which is a methyl donor in the remethylation of homocysteine to methionine, has shown promise in adults, as has vitamin E in children.

Antidiabetic and insulin-sensitizing agents can alter glucose uptake in skeletal muscle, decrease central adiposity, and affect mitochondrial mass. Metformin down-regulates liver gluconeogenesis and stimulates mitochondrial β-oxidation of fatty acids. When 500 mg was given three times daily for 4 months, it improved laboratory indices and insulin sensitivity in 14 patients. Troglitazone provided similar improvements in 10 patients treated for 3 to 6 months. In a small randomized trial, pioglitazone has also been shown to improve metabolic indices and histologic features in patients with NASH and glucose intolerance or type 2 diabetes mellitus.

Antilipidemic agents, such as bezafibrate, can improve steatosis associated with tamoxifen, and gemfibrozil can reduce the laboratory indices of liver inflammation. Hydroxymethylglutaryl-CoA reductase inhibitors, such as atorvastatin, have not induced histologic improvement. Also, statins have been associated with subclinical skeletal muscle toxicity due to mitochondrial injury that has dissuaded their use as a primary treatment. However, statins are generally safe for the treatment of hyperlipidemia in patients with NASH.

SUMMARY

NAFLD is a common cause of chronic hepatitis. Obesity, diabetes mellitus, and hyperlipidemia are risk factors for the disease, but the diagnosis must be considered for all patients, including those of lean body weight. Alcohol- and drug-induced injuries must be excluded. Treatment is based on diet, exercise, and control of risk factors. Liver ultrasonography is useful in supporting the diagnosis, but examination of liver tissue is the only way to establish the diagnosis and to assess disease activity and stage. The histologic changes may be identical to those of alcoholic liver disease. Clinical and laboratory features are remarkable because of their mild nature. Severe manifestations or findings of liver decompensation point to alternative diagnoses. Progression to cirrhosis and liver failure are possible, and liver transplantation may be necessary. Insulin-sensitizing agents have shown promise in improving laboratory and histologic findings.

RECOMMENDED READING

Adams LA, Lindor KD, Angulo P. The prevalence of autoantibodies and autoimmune hepatitis in patients with nonalcoholic fatty liver disease. Am J Gastroenterol. 2004;99:1316-20.
Emphasizes the frequency of autoantibodies and hypergammaglobulinemia in NASH, suggests that autoantibodies are markers of disease severity and propensity for liver fibrosis, and stresses the importance of liver biopsy assessment in distinguishing between NASH and autoimmune hepatitis in some cases.

Angulo P. Nonalcoholic fatty liver disease. N Engl J Med. 2002;346:1221-31.
Crisp description of the clinical entity.

Angulo P, Keach JC, Batts KP, Lindor KD. Independent predictors of liver fibrosis in patients with nonalcoholic steatohepatitis. Hepatology. 1999;30:1356-62.
Defines comorbid factors for fibrosis.

Angulo P, Lindor KD. Treatment of nonalcoholic fatty liver: present and emerging therapies. Semin Liver Dis. 2001;21:81-8.
Review of putative pathogenic mechanisms and rationale for new treatments.

Bacon BR, Farahvash MJ, Janney CG, Neuschwander-Tetri BA. Nonalcoholic steatohepatitis: an expanded clinical entity. Gastroenterology. 1994;107:1103-9.
Emphasizes the presence of nonalcoholic steatohepatitis in patients without risk factors. Indicates that the disease must be considered for all patients.

Czaja AJ, Carpenter HA, Santrach PJ, Moore SB. Host- and disease-specific factors affecting steatosis in chronic hepatitis C. J Hepatol. 1998;29:198-206.

Indicates that the steatosis of chronic hepatitis C is related more closely to the virus than host factors, whereas host factors are associated with NAFLD.

Hay JE, Czaja AJ, Rakela J, Ludwig J. The nature of unexplained chronic aminotransferase elevations of a mild to moderate degree in asymptomatic patients. Hepatology. 1989;9:193-7.
Indicates that nonalcoholic steatohepatitis is common in mild asymptomatic chronic hepatitis and may be associated with antinuclear antibodies.

Kim WR, Poterucha JJ, Porayko MK, Dickson ER, Steers JL, Wiesner RH. Recurrence of nonalcoholic steatohepatitis following liver transplantation. Transplantation. 1996;62:1802-5.
Indicates need for liver transplantation in some patients, especially those with jejunoileal bypass, and the possibility of recurrence with fibrosis.

Matteoni CA, Younossi ZM, Gramlich T, Boparai N, Liu YC, McCullough AJ. Nonalcoholic fatty liver disease: a spectrum of clinical and pathological severity. Gastroenterology. 1999;116:1413-9.
Demonstrates that fatty infiltration of the liver itself is not adequate to predict disease outcome. Prognosis relates to ballooning degeneration, Mallory bodies, or fibrosis (or a combination of these).

Neuschwander-Tetri BA, Caldwell SH. Nonalcoholic steatohepatitis: summary of an AASLD Single Topic Conference. Hepatology. 2003;37:1202-19. Erratum in: Hepatology. 2003;38:536.
Comprehensive current review of all aspects of the disease and investigational activities.

Powell EE, Cooksley WG, Hanson R, Searle J, Halliday JW, Powell LW. The natural history of nonalcoholic steatohepatitis: a follow-up study of forty-two patients for up to 21 years. Hepatology. 1990;11:74-80.
Describes low-grade severity, slow progression, and potential for cirrhosis in patients followed from 1.5 to 21.5 years.

Sanyal AJ, Campbell-Sargent C, Mirshahi F, Rizzo WB, Contos MJ, Sterling RK, et al. Nonalcoholic steatohepatitis: association of insulin resistance and mitochondrial abnormalities. Gastroenterology. 2001;120:1183-92.
Describes peripheral insulin resistance, increased fatty acid β-oxidation, and liver oxidative stress in NASH as well as unique mitochondrial changes, with the loss of cristae and paracrystalline inclusions.

Sheth SG, Gordon FD, Chopra S. Nonalcoholic steatohepatitis. Ann Intern Med. 1997;126:137-45.
Comprehensive practical review.

Sorbi D, Boynton J, Lindor KD. The ratio of aspartate aminotransferase to alanine aminotransferase: potential value in differentiating nonalcoholic steatohepatitis from alcoholic liver disease. Am J Gastroenterol. 1999;94:1018-22.
Clinically useful guidelines for distinguishing between alcoholic and nonalcoholic varieties.

CHAPTER 38

Liver Disease and Pregnancy

J. Eileen Hay, M.B.,Ch.B.

Most pregnant women are young and healthy, and liver disease is uncommon in this patient population. Also, the presence of liver disease must not be confused with some of the physiologic changes of pregnancy that mimic features commonly associated with liver dysfunction, including spider nevi and palmar erythema in 50% of pregnant women, increased alkaline phosphatase levels from placental production, and decreased serum concentrations of albumin and hemoglobin with expanded blood volume (Table 1). Changes in bilirubin and aminotransferase concentrations, hepatomegaly, splenomegaly, liver tenderness, or bruits do not occur in normal pregnancy, and the clinical finding of jaundice is always abnormal. Abnormalities in liver enzyme levels occur in 5% of pregnancies and jaundice in 0.1%, with a clinical significance that is highly variable from a self-limiting to a rapidly fatal condition.

For diagnostic purposes, it is useful to divide liver diseases in pregnant women into three main categories (Table 2):

1. Liver diseases occurring coincidentally in a pregnant patient (viral hepatitis is the most common cause of jaundice in a pregnant woman)
2. Pregnancy occurring in women with chronic liver disease
3. Liver diseases unique to pregnancy, including hyperemesis gravidarum, intrahepatic cholestasis of pregnancy (ICP), preeclampsia, HELLP (hemolysis, elevated liver enzymes, low platelet count) syndrome, and acute fatty liver of pregnancy (AFLP)

These liver diseases, unique to pregnancy, can be considered liver complications of pregnancy itself, and they have a characteristic timing in relation to the trimesters of pregnancy. Hepatitis E and herpes hepatitis, although not related etiologically to pregnancy, characteristically produce a fulminant and often deadly disease in the third trimester of pregnancy.

DIAGNOSTIC STRATEGY IN A PREGNANT PATIENT

The clinical presentation and trimester of pregnancy are of vital diagnostic importance (Table 2). Answers to the following questions help formulate a rational approach to these patients:

Table 1. Physiologic Changes in Liver Tests During Pregnancy

Test	Change
Bilirubin	Unchanged
AST, ALT	Unchanged
Prothrombin time	Unchanged
Alkaline phosphatase	Increases 2- to 4-fold
Fibrinogen	Increases 50%
Globulin	Increases in α- and β-globulins
	Decreases in γ-globulin
Alpha fetoprotein	Moderate increase, especially with twins
Leukocytes	Increase
Ceruloplasmin	Increase
Cholesterol	Increases 2-fold
Triglycerides	Increase

ALT, alanine aminotransferase; AST, aspartate aminotransferase.

1. Are there any features of underlying chronic liver disease (including liver transplantation) or risk factors for viral disease?
2. Is the presentation compatible with acute viral hepatitis?
3. Are there any features to suggest biliary disease?
4. Is there any history of drugs or toxins?
5. Are there any features of Budd-Chiari syndrome?
6. Is there any evidence or risk factors for sepsis?
7. Does the presentation fit one of the liver diseases unique to pregnancy?

Clinical features and laboratory testing, including serologic testing for hepatitis, will easily decrease the large number of diagnostic possibilities and, in many patients, allow a diagnosis. For some patients, imaging of the liver, endoscopic retrograde cholangiopancreatography (ERCP), or liver biopsy is necessary. Ultrasonography of the liver and abdomen is safe during all three trimesters of pregnancy and is helpful in the evaluation of biliary tract disease, patency of hepatic and portal veins, AFLP, hematomas, and rupture. In ICP, liver ultrasonographic features are usually normal, although gallstones and biliary sludge can be seen. To confirm the diagnosis of choledocholithiasis, ERCP can be performed safely in pregnant women. Radiation exposure for fluoroscopy is well below the fetal safety level. Midazolam, meperidine, and glucagon can be given with safety. If indicated, sphincterotomy and stone extraction should be performed at the same time. Hepatic venography is necessary to confirm Budd-Chiari syndrome in a patient with compatible clinical and ultrasonographic features.

LIVER DISEASES OCCURRING COINCIDENTALLY IN A PREGNANT PATIENT

Viral Hepatitis

Jaundice in pregnancy may be due to any of the many causes of jaundice in a nonpregnant patient. Viral hepatitis, due to hepatitis A, B, C, D, or E virus; herpes simplex virus; cytomegalovirus, or Epstein-Barr virus, accounts for 40% of cases of jaundice in pregnant women in the United States. Hepatitis A, B, and C have the same frequency in pregnant and nonpregnant populations and during each of the three trimesters of pregnancy. Acute hepatitis A occurs in 1 per 1,000 pregnant women and acute hepatitis B in 2 per 1,000; hepatitis D is rare. Hepatitis E is extremely rare in the United States but is endemic to large areas of Asia, Africa, and Central America, where, in the third trimester of pregnancy, it becomes fulminant, with a high mortality rate, probably influenced by malnutrition. In India, 25% of women with fulminant liver failure are pregnant, and in almost all of them, liver failure is due to acute viral hepatitis. Herpes simplex hepatitis is rare.

Apart from hepatitis E and herpes simplex hepatitis, the clinical and serologic course of acute hepatitis is the same as for nonpregnant patients; also, the hepatitis does not appear to affect the pregnant state adversely. Although rare, herpes simplex hepatitis must be diagnosed because specific therapy is life-saving; in pregnant women, it typically occurs as a primary infection in the third trimester and has systemic features, with a prodrome and fever, diffuse vesicular rash and leukopenia,

Table 2.   Causes and Timing of Liver Disease During Pregnancy

Disease category	Specific disease	Trimester of pregnancy
Chronic liver disease/portal hypertension	Chronic hepatitis B	1-3
	Hepatitis C	1-3
	Autoimmune disease	1-3
	Wilson's disease	1-3
	Cirrhosis of any cause	1-3
	Extrahepatic portal hypertension	1-3
Liver disease coincidental with pregnancy	Acute viral hepatitis	1-3
	Budd-Chiari syndrome	Postpartum
	Gallstones	1-3
	Drug-induced	1-3
Liver disease unique to pregnancy	Intrahepatic cholestasis of pregnancy	2-3
	Hyperemesis gravidarum	1
	Preeclampsia	3, late 2
	HELLP syndrome	3, late 2
	Acute fatty liver of pregnancy	3

HELLP, hemolysis, elevated liver enzymes, low platelets.

vulvar or oropharyngeal vesicular lesions and coagulopathy. Usually, these patients are anicteric even with liver failure.

Serologic testing for hepatitis A, B, and C viruses and for Epstein-Barr virus and cytomegalovirus should be performed in all cases of acute jaundice in pregnancy. Antibody to hepatitis E virus should be assayed if the patient is from, or has been a recent traveler to, an endemic area. Testing for hepatitis C virus RNA in the absence of antibody to hepatitis C virus has been positive in several pregnant patients who subsequently developed hepatitis C. Serologic testing, liver biopsy, and culture may be necessary to diagnose herpes simplex hepatitis.

Management of patients with acute viral hepatitis is supportive, except for herpes simplex infection in which prompt therapy with acyclovir or vidarabine is life-saving and without which 50% of mothers die. Acute or chronic viral hepatitis is not an indication for termination of pregnancy except in herpes infection that does not respond to antiviral therapy. Congenital malformations in the fetus occur only with early cytomegalovirus infection. Viral hepatitis is not an indication for cesarean section, and breast-feeding should not be discouraged.

Perinatal transmission of hepatitis B is highest in those with acute hepatitis, especially with hepatitis B e antigen–positivity or a high hepatitis B virus DNA level in the third trimester (50%-80%), lower in mothers with hepatitis B e antibodies (25%), and lowest in inactive carriers (5%). Without therapy, 80% to 90% of these babies become chronically infected. Transmission of hepatitis B is not transplacental but occurs at delivery and is preventable in more than 95% of cases by passive-active immunoprophylaxis of the babies at birth (Table 3). Breastfeeding is not contraindicated even if the mother has active hepatitis B. Vertical transmission of hepatitis A and D is rare. The frequency of mother-to-infant transmission of hepatitis C is 1% to 5%, with maternal risk factors being coinfection with human immunodeficiency virus, history of intravenous drug abuse, and maternal viremia of more than 10^6 copies/mL. Transmission is not affected by mode of delivery or breastfeeding. There is no effective therapy to prevent hepatitis C. Hepatitis A vaccine and postexposure immunoglobulin prophylaxis can be given safely to the mother during pregnancy. Newborns of mothers with hepatitis A in the third trimester should be given passive immunoprophylaxis with immune globulin within 48 hours after birth.

Gallstones and Biliary Disease

Increased lithogenicity of bile and biliary stasis during pregnancy predispose pregnant women to enhanced formation of biliary sludge and stones. A recent natural history study showed that stones or sludge developed by the postpartum period in 10% of patients with no stones before pregnancy. Despite this prevalence, symptomatic gallstones occur in only 0.1% to 0.3% of pregnancies and symptoms usually occur after multiple pregnancies rather than during gestation. The most common clinical presentations are biliary colic (5% jaundice in pregnancy), gallstone pancreatitis (50% of women younger than 30 years with pancreatitis are pregnant), and, least common, acute cholecystitis. The clinical features of biliary disease and pancreatitis are the same as in nonpregnant patients, can occur at any time of gestation, and may recur during pregnancy.

For acute biliary colic or acute cholecystitis, conservative therapy with bed rest, intravenous fluids, and antibiotics is instituted initially and is successful in more than 80% of patients, with no fetal or maternal mortality, although symptoms are likely to recur. An impacted common bile duct stone and worsening gallstone pancreatitis are indications to proceed with ERCP, sphincterotomy, and stone extraction under antibiotic coverage. Indications for cholecystectomy in pregnancy are generally considered to be very limited—intractable biliary colic, severe acute cholecystitis not responding to conservative measures, acute gallstone pancreatitis—with a widely variable reported incidence of 0.005% to 0.1% of pregnancies. The second trimester is the safest period, with fetal morbidity less than 1%. Surgery should be avoided during the first 10 weeks of pregnancy because of the risk of abortion with anesthesia and the potential teratogenic effect of carbon dioxide. In the third trimester, the uterus may impinge on the surgical field. Also, there is an increased risk of premature labor. More recent studies have suggested that, because of the frequent recurrence of biliary symptoms in pregnancy, surgical intervention is indicated for all symptomatic patients who present in the second trimester and has little morbidity or mortality.

If needed, what type of cholecystectomy should be performed? The laparoscopic technique is less invasive, with reduced pain, shorter recovery time, and fewer complications. However, the increased abdominal pressure and, more particularly, increased arterial $PaCO_2$ and the relative acidosis that occur with carbon dioxide capnoperitoneum may confer a risk to the fetus. With standard precautions for obstetric anesthesia and with relative maternal hyperventilation and minimal intra-abdominal carbon

Table 3. Prophylaxis Regimen for Babies of HBsAg-Positive Mothers

Preparation	Dose	Route of administration
HBIG	0.5 mL	IM at birth
HBV vaccine*	0.5 mL (10 µg)	IM at birth (2 days)
		IM at 1 mo
		IM at 6 mo

HBIG, hepatitis B immunoglobulin; HBsAg, hepatitis B surface antigen; HBV, hepatitis B virus; IM, intramuscularly.
*Recombinant vaccine.

dioxide pressure to minimize changes in maternal $PaCO_2$ and pH, there have been many reports of successful laparoscopic cholecystectomy during the second trimester, with no adverse outcome. Whether maternal arterial monitoring or transvaginal fetal monitoring is beneficial is not known. Operative cholangiography is performed as needed during either operative or laparoscopic cholecystectomy, with fetal shielding to reduce radiation exposure.

Other Diseases

Budd-Chiari syndrome is rare, and when it occurs in the setting of pregnancy, it is usually in the postpartum period and has been associated with antiphospholipid syndrome, thrombotic thrombocytopenic purpura, preeclampsia, and septic abortion. Sepsis associated with pyelonephritis or abortion can cause jaundice in early pregnancy, and severe gram-negative sepsis with jaundice has been described in the third trimester.

PREGNANT PATIENTS WITH CHRONIC LIVER DISEASE

Many women with chronic viral or autoimmune hepatitis or Wilson's disease are of childbearing age. Chronic hepatitis B is present in 0.5% to 1.5% of pregnancies and chronic hepatitis C in 2.3% of some indigent populations. An uncomplicated pregnancy with no disease flare is expected in women with mild disease or disease in remission. Patients with Dubin-Johnson syndrome or benign recurrent intrahepatic cholestasis may become more jaundiced during pregnancy, especially in the second and third trimesters, but the only significance of such jaundice is the necessity to rule out other possible causes. Gilbert syndrome and Rotor's syndrome are unaffected by pregnancy.

Autoimmune disease is not expected to flare in pregnancy but is treated with increased doses of corticosteroids as necessary; azathioprine therapy in pregnancy has not been associated with increased fetal risk. Patients with Wilson's disease must be treated adequately before pregnancy and continue receiving therapy throughout the pregnancy. Discontinuation of therapy results in the risk of fulminant Wilson's disease. Penicillamine is the best therapy, but rarely, it has been associated with congenital defects; trientine is a safe alternative for fetal health but of less proven efficacy for the mother.

Most patients with advanced cirrhosis are amenorrheic and infertile, but if pregnancy occurs, increased maternal and fetal problems can be expected. Little is known about the optimal management of pregnant patients who have cirrhosis and portal hypertension. The main risk to the mother is massive gastrointestinal tract bleeding (20%-25% of cases), a risk that has been decreased by shunt surgery. Patients with known esophageal varices should be considered for β-blocker therapy,

endoscopic therapy, shunt surgery, or even liver transplantation before pregnancy. Whether prophylactic therapy for esophageal varices in early pregnancy is beneficial has not been tested. In most patients, vaginal deliveries should be performed wherever possible with early forceps or vacuum suction to avoid lengthy labor, while avoiding abdominal surgery. In patients with known large varices, avoidance of labor by cesarean section is recommended because vaginal delivery is thought to greatly increase portal pressure; however, some studies have suggested that variceal bleeding does not increase with vaginal delivery. Postpartum hemorrhage occurs in 15% to 30% of these patients and is reduced by correction of coagulopathy. Other maternal risks are liver decompensation, jaundice, thrombocytopenia, and rupture of splenic aneurysms. Postpartum bacterial infections are more common in patients with cirrhosis and warrant prophylactic treatment with antibiotics. The complications of portal hypertension need to be managed the same way as in nonpregnant patients; acute variceal bleeding is managed endoscopically, as in nonpregnant patients, although vasopressin is contraindicated. Also, ascites and hepatic encephalopathy are treated in the standard way.

The pregnant liver transplant recipient represents a unique clinical situation that requires specialized care. With the success of liver transplantation, more pregnancies are being reported in these patients, with excellent outcome for fetus, mother, and graft. However, there is some risk to the allograft from acute cellular rejection or recurrent viral hepatitis; consequently, it is imperative to closely monitor immunosuppression, regularly follow liver function tests, and adequately investigate all liver abnormalities during pregnancy. A liver biopsy specimen may be needed to diagnose rejection, which must be treated as it is in nonpregnant patients.

LIVER DISEASES UNIQUE TO PREGNANCY

The liver diseases unique to pregnancy have characteristic clinical features and timing of onset in relation to pregnancy (Table 2). Their causes are poorly understood, but they fall into two main categories depending on their association with or without preeclampsia. The most common of these disorders, and second only to viral hepatitis as a cause of jaundice in pregnant patients, is ICP, a disease of severe pruritus, mild jaundice, and biochemical cholestasis limited to the second half of pregnancy. Genetic, hormonal, and exogenous factors have been implicated in its cause. In the United States, ICP occurs in 0.1% of pregnancies, with jaundice in about 20% of cases. Hyperemesis gravidarum, with an incidence of 0.3%, is intractable nausea and vomiting that occur in the first trimester; high aminotransferase levels occur in 50% of patients and, occasionally, jaundice. ICP and hyperemesis gravidarum are not associated with preeclampsia.

The preeclampsia-associated liver diseases are preeclampsia itself, HELLP syndrome, and AFLP. Preeclampsia occurs in 5% to 10% of pregnancies, but the liver is involved in only a small proportion of patients. Preeclampsia is the most common cause of liver tenderness and abnormal liver tests in pregnant patients.

Hyperemesis Gravidarum

Hyperemesis gravidarum is intractable vomiting that occurs in the first trimester of pregnancy and is so severe that intravenous hydration is needed. It is a poorly understood neurohormonal disorder with hormonal (increased levels of estrogen and chorionic gonadotropin and transient hyperthyroidism) and immunologic abnormalities.

Clinical Features and Diagnosis

Vomiting must be severe and intractable to support the diagnosis of hyperemesis gravidarum. It occurs in the first trimester of pregnancy, typically between 4 and 10 weeks of gestation and may be complicated by liver dysfunction and, occasionally, jaundice. High aminotransferase levels occur in 50% of patients, up to 20-fold above the normal range. The diagnosis is made on clinical grounds and rests on the presence of intractable, dehydrating vomiting in the first trimester. Uncomplicated vomiting in pregnancy does not cause liver dysfunction. If the aminotransferase levels are high, serologic testing for viral hepatitis should be performed. In the rare case in which liver biopsy is required to exclude more serious disease, the histologic appearance of the liver is generally normal but may show cholestasis with rare cell dropout. Despite high aminotransferase levels, there is no inflammation or marked necrosis.

Management

Hospitalization is necessary for hydration and parenteral nutrition; otherwise, therapy is symptomatic, with antiemetics.

Intrahepatic Cholestasis of Pregnancy

ICP is a specific liver disease unique to pregnancy. It is characterized by severe pruritus, mild jaundice, and biochemical cholestasis, which appear in the second half of pregnancy and disappear after delivery, typically to recur in subsequent pregnancies. ICP is second only to viral hepatitis as a cause of jaundice in pregnant women.

Incidence and Cause

ICP is identified all over the world but has striking geographic, ethnic, temporal, and seasonal variations. In the United States, it occurs in 0.1% of pregnancies, with jaundice in 20% of cases, but it has a much higher incidence in other countries. Its cause is poorly understood but is probably multifactorial, with genetic, hormonal, and exogenous factors. The familial cases and high incidence in certain ethnic groups (Araucanian Indians of Chile) suggest a genetic predisposition to ICP, although dietary factors such as selenium deficiency may have a role. No HLA susceptibility has been found. ICP recurs in 45% to 70% of pregnancies and has a clear seasonal variability, suggesting that exogenous factors also have a role.

The pathogenesis is clearly related in some way to female sex hormones. Estrogens may cause cholestasis in nonpregnant women who develop ICP in pregnancy. These and other observations suggest that ICP is due to a genetically abnormal or exaggerated liver metabolic response to the physiologic increase in estrogens during pregnancy. Impaired sulfation (an important detoxification pathway) has been found in some patients with ICP. Abnormalities in progesterone metabolism have also been found, some probably genetic, some exogenous. Exogenous progesterone therapy given in the third trimester of pregnancy has been found to increase the serum levels of bile acid and alanine aminotransferase, and progesterone given to prevent premature delivery can precipitate ICP in some women. Progressive familial intrahepatic cholestasis is a group of inherited disorders with defects in bile formation. In progressive familial intrahepatic cholestasis 3, there is a defect in the multidrug resistance gene 3 (*MDR3*), a gene involved with transfer of phospholipids across the canalicular membrane. The heterozygous state of several different defects in this gene has been linked to ICP in some women.

The cause of sudden fetal death in ICP is unknown. Perhaps the high circulating level of bile acid causes vasospasm of the placental vessels, leading to fetal asphyxia. Abnormalities found in placental bile acid transport systems in ICP can be improved with ursodeoxycholic acid (UDCA) therapy.

Clinical Features and Diagnosis

The onset of pruritus around 25 to 32 weeks of gestation in a patient who has no other signs of liver disease is strongly suggestive of ICP; rarely, it occurs earlier in the pregnancy. The diagnosis is even more likely if the pruritus has been present in other pregnancies and then disappeared immediately after delivery. In a first pregnancy, the diagnosis generally is made on clinical grounds alone and can only be confirmed with the rapid postpartum disappearance of the pruritus. The pruritus affects all parts of the body, is worse at night, and may be so severe that the patient is suicidal. Excoriations are usually obvious, and occasionally the cholestasis is complicated by diarrhea or steatorrhea. Jaundice occurs in 10% to 25% of patients and usually follows the pruritus by 2 to 4 weeks. Jaundice without pruritus is rare. Occasionally, the patient will be receiving progesterone therapy.

Variable levels of aminotransferase are seen in ICP, from mild to 10- to 20-fold elevations; the increase in bilirubin concentration is usually less than 5 mg/dL. Determination of the alkaline phosphatase level is less helpful in pregnancy. The most specific and sensitive marker of ICP is the serum level of bile acid, which is always increased and can be 100 times more than normal and may correlate with fetal risk. Liver biopsy is needed only if the clinical suspicion of a more serious liver disease is strong. In ICP, the liver has a near-normal appearance, with mild cholestasis and minimal or no hepatocellular necrosis. The differential diagnosis of cholestasis in pregnancy includes coincidental cholestatic diseases (drugs, cholestatic viral hepatitis, sepsis, gallstones) and preexisting chronic biliary disease.

Management

With ICP, the main risk is to the fetus, with premature deliveries (up to 60% of cases), perinatal deaths, and fetal distress. Fetal monitoring for chronic placental insufficiency is essential but will not prevent all fetal deaths. Acute anoxic injury can be prevented only by delivery as soon as the fetus is mature. Pruritus and liver dysfunction resolve immediately after delivery, with no maternal mortality; however, some patients are severely distressed, even suicidal, with the pruritus. Management strategies for the mother have focused on symptomatic relief rather than early delivery of the baby. Withdrawal of exogenous progesterone has caused remission of the pruritus in some patients before delivery.

UDCA is the agent of choice for treatment of ICP. UDCA has been shown to be successful in producing relief from pruritus, with parallel improvement in liver tests and no adverse maternal or fetal effects. Three small double-blind trials randomly assigned 29 patients to UDCA (600-1,000 mg/d) and 27 to placebo, and the results consistently showed clinical and biochemical improvement with UDCA. Fetal outcome was improved, with less prematurity. High-dose UDCA (1.5-2.0 g/d) has recently been shown to relieve pruritus in most patients, to decrease abnormal maternal levels of bile acid, and to be completely safe for the fetus. Also, the babies born to these mothers had almost normal levels of bile acid compared with babies of untreated mothers.

Treatment with cholestyramine, 8 to 24 g/d, can sometimes relieve pruritus in 1 to 2 weeks, but biochemical measures, maternal malabsorption, and fetal prognosis are not improved. By suppressing fetoplacental estrogen production, dexamethasone treatment (12 mg/d for 7 days) improved symptoms, liver tests, and fetal lung maturity in 10 pregnant women and had no adverse effects. Intravenous S-adenosyl-L-methionine therapy is of unproven efficacy and is inferior to UDCA. Epomediol and silymarin have produced symptomatic but not biochemical relief in a few patients. Benzodiazepines, antihistamines, and phenobarbital have not been effective in providing relief.

ICP recurs in 45% to 70% of subsequent pregnancies and, occasionally, with the use of oral contraceptives. Patients with ICP are more likely to develop gallstones and gallbladder disease

than patients without ICP. Some rare familial cases of apparent ICP have persisted post partum, with progression to subsequent fibrosis and cirrhosis.

Preeclampsia

Preeclampsia-associated liver diseases include preeclampsia itself, HELLP syndrome, and AFLP. Preeclampsia is the triad of hypertension, edema, and proteinuria in the third trimester of pregnancy. It occurs in 5% to 10% of pregnancies, with the liver involved in only a small proportion of patients. It is the most common cause of liver tenderness and abnormal liver tests in pregnant patients. The cause of preeclampsia appears to involve defective placentation, leading to generalized endothelial dysfunction.

Clinical Features

Patients with preeclampsia may present with right upper quadrant pain, jaundice, and a tender, normal-size liver. The aminotransferase levels vary from mild to a 10- to 20-fold increase; the bilirubin concentration is usually less than 5 mg/dL. Involvement of the liver always indicates severe preeclampsia.

Management

No specific therapy is needed for liver involvement of preeclampsia, and its only significance is that it indicates severe disease and the need for immediate delivery to avoid eclampsia, liver rupture, or hepatic necrosis. HELLP and AFLP may complicate preeclampsia.

HELLP Syndrome

Severe preeclampsia is complicated in 2% to 12% of cases (0.2%-0.6% of all pregnancies) by *h*emolysis, *e*levated *l*iver tests, and *l*ow *p*latelet count: HELLP syndrome.

Clinical Features and Diagnosis

No diagnostic clinical features distinguish between HELLP syndrome and preeclampsia. Most patients with HELLP syndrome present with epigastric or right upper quadrant pain (65%-90% of patients), nausea and vomiting (35%-50%), "flu-like" illness (90%), and headache (30%). They usually have edema and weight gain (60% of patients), right upper quadrant tenderness (80%), and hypertension (80%). Jaundice is uncommon (5% of patients), and some patients have no obvious preeclampsia. Most patients (71%) present between 27 and 36 weeks of gestation, but it can be earlier or up to 48 hours after delivery. HELLP syndrome is more common in multiparous and older patients.

Because of microangiopathic hemolytic anemia, the characteristic histologic finding in both HELLP syndrome and preeclampsia is periportal hemorrhage and fibrin deposition; also, periportal hepatocytes are necrotic, and thrombi may form in small portal arterioles. In severe disease, areas of infarction may be multiple or diffuse; hemorrhage dissects through the portal connective tissue initially from zone 1 and then more diffusely to involve the entire lobule, leading to large hematomas, capsular tears, and intraperitoneal bleeding. Liver biopsy is rarely needed for diagnosis.

The diagnosis of HELLP syndrome must be established quickly because of the maternal and fetal risk and the necessity for immediate delivery. Its diagnosis requires the presence of all three criteria: 1) hemolysis with an abnormal blood smear and an increase in lactic dehydrogenase (>600 U/L) and indirect bilirubin, 2) aspartate aminotransferase more than 70 U/L, and 3) a platelet count of less than 100×10^9/L and, in severe cases, less than 50×10^9/L. Prothrombin time, activated partial thromboplastin time, and fibrinogen levels are usually normal, with no increase in fibrin-split products, but occasionally disseminated intravascular coagulation may be present. The increase in aminotransferase level can vary from mild to 10- to 20-fold, and serum bilirubin is usually less than 5 mg/dL. Computed tomography (limited views) is indicated in HELLP syndrome to detect liver rupture, subcapsular hematomas, and intraparenchymal hemorrhage or infarction (Fig. 1). These abnormalities may correlate with the decreased platelet count but not with liver test abnormalities.

Management

The priority in the management of patients with HELLP syndrome is antepartum stabilization of the mother, with treatment of hypertension and disseminated intravascular coagulation, and seizure prophylaxis. The patient should be transferred to

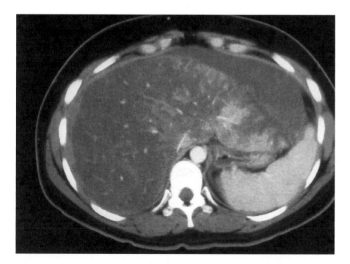

Fig. 1. Computed tomography of abdomen of 28-year-old woman with severe HELLP syndrome at 39 weeks' gestation. A large subcapsular hematoma extends over the left lobe; the right lobe has a heterogeneous, hypodense appearance because of widespread necrosis, with "sparing" of the areas of the left lobe (compare perfusion with the normal spleen).

a tertiary referral center if possible and computed tomography of the abdomen performed.

Delivery is the only definitive therapy; if the patient is near-term or the fetal lung is mature, immediate delivery should be performed, probably by cesarean section, although well-established labor should be allowed to proceed in the absence of obstetric complications or disseminated intravascular coagulation. Many patients (40%-50%) require cesarean section, especially primigravida remote from term in whom the cervix is unfavorable. Half the patients require blood or blood products to correct the hypovolemia, anemia, or coagulopathy. Management remote from term is controversial, and sometimes in milder cases at less than 34 weeks of gestation, a more conservative approach with high-dose glucocorticoids is taken in an attempt to prolong the pregnancy and improve fetal lung maturity. This therapy may also be of benefit in stabilizing the mother's condition during the time of transfer to a tertiary referral center.

Most patients have rapid, early resolution of HELLP syndrome after delivery, with normalization of the platelet count by 5 days; however, some have persisting thrombocytopenia, hemolysis, and progressive increase in bilirubin and creatinine levels. The persistence of signs for more than 72 hours, with no improvement or life-threatening complications, is usually an indication for plasmapheresis. Many different treatment modalities have been used, including plasma volume expansion, antithrombotic agents, corticosteroids, plasmapheresis, plasma exchange with fresh frozen plasma, and dialysis, but no clinical trials have been conducted. Serious maternal complications are common: disseminated intravascular coagulation in 20% of patients, abruptio placentae in 16%, acute renal failure in 8%, pulmonary edema in 8%, acute respiratory distress syndrome in 1%, severe ascites in 8%, or liver failure in 2%. Maternal mortality rates range from 1% to 25%. Once delivered, most babies do well.

Hemorrhage of the liver without rupture is generally managed conservatively in hemodynamically stable patients, but they need close hemodynamic monitoring in an intensive care unit, correction of coagulopathy, immediate availability of large-volume transfusion of blood and blood products, immediate intervention for rupture, and follow-up diagnostic computed tomographic studies as needed. Exogenous trauma must be avoided, including abdominal palpation, convulsions, emesis, and unnecessary transportation.

Liver rupture is a rare, life-threatening complication of HELLP syndrome. It is usually preceded by an intraparenchymal hemorrhage that progresses to a contained subcapsular hematoma in the right lobe; the capsule then ruptures, with hemorrhage into the peritoneum. Survival depends on rapid and aggressive medical treatment and immediate surgical management. However, the best surgical management is still debated, and evacuation of the hematoma with packing and drainage, hepatic artery ligation, partial hepatectomy, direct pressure, packing or hemostatic wrapping, application of topical hemostatic agents, oversewing of laceration, and angiographic embolization are all options. Aggressive supportive management of hypovolemia, thrombocytopenia, and coagulopathy are essential before surgery. Maternal mortality from liver rupture is high at 50%, and perinatal mortality rates are 10% to 60%, mostly from placental rupture, intrauterine asphyxia, or prematurity.

The risk of recurrence of HELLP syndrome in subsequent pregnancies is difficult to assess from the available data; the reported incidence ranges from 3% to 25%. Subsequent deliveries by these patients have an increased risk of preeclampsia, preterm delivery, intrauterine growth retardation, and abruptio placentae.

Acute Fatty Liver of Pregnancy

AFLP is a sudden catastrophic illness that occurs almost exclusively in the third trimester and in which microvesicular fatty infiltration results in encephalopathy and liver failure.

Incidence and Cause

The cause of AFLP may involve abnormalities in intramitochondrial fatty acid oxidation. Long-chain 3-hydroxyacyl-CoA dehydrogenase deficiency has been identified in some babies of mothers with AFLP, suggesting that AFLP may be due to heterozygosity in the mother and homozygosity in the fetus. This situation would overwhelm the increased demands of fatty acid metabolism in pregnancy, perhaps exacerbated by external factors. In its most severe form, AFLP is uncommon to rare (<0.005% of pregnancies), although milder cases are probably more common.

Clinical Features and Diagnosis

Unlike HELLP syndrome, 50% of patients with AFLP are nulliparous, with an increased incidence in twin pregnancies. AFLP occurs almost exclusively in the third trimester, from 28 to 40 weeks of gestation, most commonly at 36 weeks. In a few patients, the presentation is jaundice in the postpartum period. The presentation can vary from asymptomatic to fulminant liver failure; jaundice is present in most patients. The typical patient has 1 to 2 weeks of anorexia, nausea, vomiting, and right upper quadrant pain and is ill-looking, with jaundice, hypertension, edema, ascites, a small liver (but it may be enlarged initially), and a variable degree of hepatic encephalopathy. Intrauterine death may occur. About 50% of patients with AFLP have preeclampsia.

In AFLP, AST levels can vary from near-normal to 1,000 (usually about 300 U/L), and the bilirubin concentration is usually less than 5 mg/dL, but higher in severe or complicated disease. Other typical abnormalities are normochromic, normocytic anemia; high leukocyte count; normal-to-low platelet count; abnormal prothrombin time, activated partial thromboplastin time, and fibrinogen with or without disseminated intravascular coagulation; metabolic acidosis; renal dysfunction (often progressing to oliguric renal failure); hypoglycemia; high ammonia level; and often biochemical pancreatitis. Computed tomography is more sensitive than ultrasonography for detecting AFLP. Liver biopsy is rarely indicated for management but is essential for a definitive diagnosis of AFLP. Microvesicular, and infrequently macrovesicular, fatty infiltration is most prominent in zone 3; this fat consists of free fatty acids. Also, there is lobular disarray, with pleomorphism of hepatocytes and mild portal inflammation with cholestasis, an appearance similar to that of Reye's syndrome and tetracycline and valproic acid toxicity (Fig. 2). Although the histologic

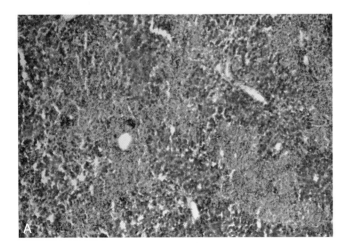
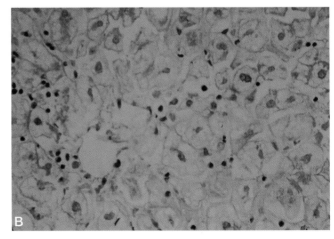

Fig. 2. Histologic appearance of the liver of a 32-year-old primigravida with acute fatty liver of pregnancy. *A*, Sudan stain (low power) shows diffuse fatty infiltration (red staining) involving predominantly zone 3, with relative sparing of periportal areas. *B*, Hematoxylin and eosin stain (high power) shows hepatocytes stuffed with microvesicular fat (free fatty acids) and centrally located nuclei.

features usually are diagnostic, they occasionally cannot be differentiated from those of viral hepatitis or preeclampsia.

For severely ill patients with liver failure in the third trimester, the differential diagnoses are AFLP, HELLP syndrome (Table 4), thrombotic thrombocytopenic purpura, hemolytic uremic syndrome, and fulminant viral hepatitis.

Management

Early recognition of AFLP, with immediate termination of pregnancy or delivery, and intensive supportive care are essential for the survival of both the mother and fetus. Recovery before delivery has not been reported. Although the inciting injury ceases with delivery, the patient requires support until liver function has time to recover. By 2 or 3 days after delivery, the aminotransferase levels and encephalopathy improve, but until this recovery occurs, intensive supportive care is needed to manage the many complications of liver failure. Patients who are critically ill at the time of presentation, who develop complications (encephalopathy, hypoglycemia, coagulopathy, bleeding), or whose condition continues to deteriorate despite emergency delivery, ideally should be transferred to a liver center.

Delivery is usually by cesarean section, but the necessity for this has not been tested in randomized trials. Rapid controlled vaginal delivery with fetal monitoring is probably safer if the cervix is favorable, and it will reduce the incidence of major intra-abdominal bleeding. It probably is best to maintain an international normalized ratio less than 1.5 and a platelet count more than 50×10^9/L during and after delivery and to provide antibiotic prophylaxis. With correction of the coagulopathy, epidural anesthesia is probably the best choice and will allow a better ongoing assessment of the patient's level of consciousness.

Intensive supportive care is the same as for any patient with fulminant liver failure. Plasmapheresis has been used in some cases, but its benefit is unproven. Corticosteroids are ineffective. Although liver function starts to improve within 3 days after delivery, the disease then enters a cholestatic phase, with increasing levels of bilirubin and alkaline phosphatase. Depending on the severity and complications, recovery can occur in days or be delayed for months. It is complete when no signs of chronic liver disease are present. With advances in supportive management of these patients, including early delivery, the maternal mortality rate is currently 10% to 18% and the fetal mortality rate is 9% to 23%. Infectious and bleeding complications remain the most life-threatening conditions. Liver transplantation has a limited role in these patients because of the great potential for recovery with delivery; however, it should be considered for patients whose clinical course continues to deteriorate with advancing fulminant liver failure after the first 1 or 2 days post partum without signs of liver regeneration.

Table 4.   Diagnostic Differences Between AFLP and HELLP Syndrome

	AFLP	HELLP
Parity	Nulliparous, twins	Multiparous, older
Jaundice	Common	Uncommon
Mean bilirubin, mg/dL	8	2
Encephalopathy	Present	Absent
Platelets	Low-normal	Low
Prothrombin time	Prolonged	Normal
APTT	Prolonged	Normal
Fibrinogen	Low	Normal-increased
Glucose	Low	Normal
Creatinine	High	High
Ammonia	High	Normal
Computed tomography	Fatty infiltration	Hemorrhage

AFLP, acute fatty liver of pregnancy; APTT, activated partial thromboplastin time; HELLP, hemolysis, elevated liver enzymes, low platelets.

Many patients do not become pregnant again after AFLP, either by choice, because of the devastating effect of the illness, or by necessity, from hysterectomy to control postpartum bleeding. However, AFLP does not tend to recur in subsequent pregnancies, although rare cases have been reported. Because long-chain 3-hydroxyacyl-CoA dehydrogenase deficiency may occur in up to 20% of these infants, babies must have screening tests for this deficiency, which needs to be diagnosed rapidly to allow early dietary intervention.

RECOMMENDED READING

Bacq Y, Sapey T, Brechot MC, Pierre F, Fignon A, Dubois F. Intrahepatic cholestasis of pregnancy: a French prospective study. Hepatology. 1997;26:358-64.

Ko CW, Beresford SA, Schulte SJ, Matsumoto AM, Lee SP. Incidence, natural history, and risk factors for biliary sludge and stones during pregnancy. Hepatology. 2005;41:359-65.

Mabie WC. Acute fatty liver of pregnancy. Gastroenterol Clin N Am. 1992;21:951-60.

Sibai BM, Ramadan MK, Usta I, Salama M, Mercer BM, Friedman SA. Maternal morbidity and mortality in 442 pregnancies with hemolysis, elevated liver enzymes, and low platelets (HELLP syndrome). Am J Obstet Gynecol. 1993;169:1000-6.

Steingrub JS. Pregnancy-associated severe liver dysfunction. Crit Care Clin. 2004;20:763-76.

Wolf JL. Liver disease in pregnancy. Med Clin North Am. 1996;80:1167-87.

CHAPTER 39

Liver Manifestations of Human Immunodeficiency Virus Infection

J. Eileen Hay, M.B., Ch.B.

INTRODUCTION

Only a few years ago, liver complications of human immunodeficiency virus (HIV) infection were almost incidental to patient survival. Now, with potent antiretroviral regimens and better prevention and treatment of opportunistic infections, HIV-infected patients are living longer and liver-related complications have become a major source of morbidity and mortality. Because hepatocytes are CD4-negative, primary HIV infection has little effect on the liver, but the shared risk factors of homosexuality and parenteral drug use make viral hepatitis B and C common in this patient population. Highly active antiretroviral therapy (HAART) has become standard care for HIV-infected patients; it has important hepatotoxicity in addition to all the other potential hepatotoxins to which these patients are exposed. Chronic viral hepatitis and drug hepatotoxicity are now the major liver complications in these patients.

As acquired immunodeficiency syndrome (AIDS) develops, the resulting immunosuppression renders the liver and bile ducts susceptible to various pathologic processes, including infections, malignancies, and a unique type of cholangiopathy (Table 1). At this stage, diagnostic efforts directed toward hepatobiliary problems in AIDS patients will depend on the overall clinical picture, the degree of immunosuppression, other complications of AIDS, and the severity and acuity of the liver problem. Several concepts must be kept in mind: 1) in late disease, liver abnormalities are ubiquitous and rarely responsible for morbidity or death, 2) liver involvement is often part of an already diagnosed disseminated opportunistic infection or malignancy, 3) treatment for liver disorders is often unsatisfactory, and 4) biliary lesions may be amenable to therapy.

COINFECTION WITH CHRONIC VIRAL HEPATITIS

HIV can modify and be modified by the presence of other viruses, especially hepatitis viruses. Chronic viral hepatitis due to hepatitis B or hepatitis C has a higher prevalence among HIV-infected patients than among the general population, due at least partly to shared risk factors of homosexuality and intravenous drug use. With the efficacy of HAART in prolonging the survival of these patients, chronic viral hepatitis is now a major cause of morbidity in these patients and a leading cause of non-AIDS–related death.

Hepatitis B

The hepatitis B virus (HBV) is a parenterally transmitted virus, particularly by sexual exposure. Its high-risk groups of homosexual men and intravenous drug abusers is a population similar to that of HIV infection. Almost all HIV-infected patients have serologic evidence of HBV, some of which is the result of past infection or vaccination. In a recent study of 16,000 patients, 7.6% of unvaccinated HIV patients had chronic hepatitis B.

HBV and HIV appear to interact, both directly and indirectly, in infected cells. Although considered predominantly hepatotropic, HBV DNA has been identified in lymphoid cells (the site of HIV-1), and expression of its X gene is capable of upregulating genes under the control of the HIV long-terminal repeat (the part of the HIV genome that controls viral replication). HIV replication may be enhanced in cells containing both HIV and HBV; also, the presence of HBV in HIV-infected cells may decrease endogenous interferons, which have a role in controlling at least the early stages of HIV infection. Cell-mediated immunity, through the action of cytotoxic T lymphocytes, is

Table 1. **Hepatobiliary Abnormalities in AIDS**

Liver/parenchymal	Biliary
Opportunistic infections	AIDS cholangiopathy
Bacterial	Papillary stenosis
Bartonella henselae	Sclerosing cholangitis
Coxiella burnetii	Extrahepatic
Listeria	strictures
Staphylococcus	Tumors
Streptococcus	Lymphoma
Salmonella	Kaposi's sarcoma
Mycobacterial	Acalculous cholecystitis
Mycobacterium avium-	Non-AIDS–related
intracellulare	disorders
Mycobacterium	
tuberculosis	
Other atypical myco-	
bacteria	
Viral	
Cytomegalovirus	
Epstein-Barr virus	
Adenovirus	
Herpes simplex virus	
Fungal	
Cryptococcus	
Histoplasma	
Coccidioides	
Nocardia	
Candida	
Protozoan	
Microsporida	
Pneumocystis jiroveci	
Hepatitis viruses A, B, C, D, E	
Drugs	
Sulfonamides	
HAART	
Peliosis hepatis (*Bartonella*	
henselae)	
Tumors	
Lymphoma	
Kaposi's sarcoma	
Steatosis	
Nonspecific hepatitis	

AIDS, acquired immunodeficiency syndrome; HAART, highly active antiretroviral therapy.

responsible for the clearance of HBV-infected hepatocytes from the body. Because HIV infection leads to a progressive decline in cell-mediated immunity, the presence of HIV allows greater replication of HBV, thereby promoting the carrier state and making reactivation and chronic infection more likely. In the pre-HAART era, reduced immunity also reduced inflammation,

but even then the beneficial effect of reduced hepatocellular damage was eventually overwhelmed by the greater viral load. In the HAART era, disease progression is more rapid, with increasing cirrhosis and increasing mortality of coinfected patients.

Data are available to define the clinical course of HIV and HBV coinfection. In most patients, the relative timing of HBV and HIV infections cannot be determined. However, the major HBV epidemic predated the outbreak of HIV. Large epidemiologic studies have not shown accelerated progression to AIDS in HBV-infected patients. Following HBV infection, the risk of chronic carriage of HBV is much higher in HIV-positive (21%) than in HIV-negative (4%-7%) patients. Those who do clear HBV tend to have higher CD4 counts. During acute hepatitis, the peak transaminase values are similar to those of HIV-negative patients, but the duration of hepatitis is prolonged. In chronic infection, the transaminase levels are lower, but viral replication is increased. Histologically, the liver disease is less severe, with reduced fibrosis, but there is a greater presence of hepatitis B core antigen (HBcAg) in hepatocytes and increased levels of circulating HBV DNA in HIV-positive patients.

Several agents are effective for treating HBV in coinfected patients, and treatment for both viruses is needed. Lamivudine is highly effective against both HIV and HBV, and generally 150 mg of lamivudine twice daily is added to the HAART regimen, with excellent tolerance. However, resistant strains emerge at a rate of about 15% to 20% per year, and the hepatitis B e antigen (HBeAg) seroconversion rate is low (~10%). Adefovir is excellent for lamivudine-resistant strains but has no effect on HIV. Tenofovir has been studied less well, but a single dose of 300 mg daily is excellent against both HIV and HBV, with perhaps higher seroconversion rates. No data are available about the use of pegylated interferons in patients with HBV and HIV coinfection.

All seronegative patients should be vaccinated against HBV. However, the response to vaccination against HBV was often suboptimal in HIV-positive patients in the pre-HAART era, and in one study, only 50% of patients had a response. Currently, the rates of seroconversion are better. Determination of antibody status after vaccination may be warranted. In AIDS, there may be a decline in antibody to hepatitis B surface (anti-HBs), either with naturally acquired immunity or from the vaccine. A very high chronic carriage rate has been reported in patients who acquired hepatitis B about the time of vaccination, but this has not been confirmed in other studies.

Reactivation of HBV may occur in HIV infection. HBV reactivation can occur without circulating HBeAg, and HBV DNA must be sought to make the diagnosis. Although liver inflammation tends to decrease with immunosuppression, in the later stages of AIDS, unchecked HBV replication results in high levels of virus in the hepatocytes and may lead to the fibrosing cholestatic variant of HBV and, eventually, liver failure.

Hepatitis C

The prevalence of hepatitis C virus (HCV) positivity in HIV-infected patients is less than for HBV, and coinfection with HCV occurs in about 30% of HIV-positive patients. Acquisition of HCV and HIV appear to be independent of each other; because HIV and HCV have a common means of transmission (especially parenteral), the rate of HCV infection is high in some populations of HIV-infected patients. In the United States, the Adult AIDS Clinical Trials Group (ACTG) has reported on 7,000 HIV-infected patients, and hemophiliacs and patients with intravenous drug use were the high-risk group for coinfection with HCV (73%). Only 3.5% of low-risk patients (heterosexual contact, health care workers) were HCV-positive. The two viruses cause a synergistic increase in the vertical transmission of both, probably from higher viral loads in coinfected patients. Sexual and perinatal viral transmission correlates with viral load and the degree of immunosuppression. Vertical transmission of HCV from mother to child is more common in the presence of HIV infection.

HCV testing can be a problem in HIV-infected patients. The hypergammaglobulinemia of AIDS can lead to a false-positive enzyme-linked immunosorbent assay, and confirmation with the recombinant immunoblot assay is essential. Conversely, antibody production can be impaired with false-negative results.

The presence of HIV affects the course of HCV infection. HCV is directly cytopathic rather than immunopathic; therefore, the immunosuppression of HIV infection does not decrease liver inflammation. Furthermore, HIV coinfection results in an increased HCV viral load, presumably from unopposed HCV replication. This results in a more rapidly progressive clinical course and increased sexual and vertical transmission. Data from hemophiliac and intravenous drug abuser studies suggest that HIV promotes faster progression of fibrosis in HCV infection. Cirrhosis occurs earlier in HIV coinfection (average, 7 years, but as early as 3 years) than in hepatitis C alone (average, 23 years). More coinfected patients have progression to cirrhosis (15%-20%) than those with HCV infection alone (2%-6%), and the risk of hepatocellular carcinoma is probably increased. Very rapid progression to the fibrosing cholestatic variant of hepatitis C is uncommon.

There is still controversy about whether HCV affects outcome of HIV infection. In a large Swiss study of 3,000 patients, mortality was increased for HIV patients with coinfection, but a much smaller U.S. study did not confirm this. A more recent cohort study of 18,000 hospitalized U.S. veterans with HIV infection (12,761 with HIV alone and 5,320 with HIV and HCV coinfection) showed a decrease in the mortality rate for coinfected patients, but this effect was much less in the HAART era.

Initiation of HAART may transiently exacerbate HCV infection (increase alanine aminotransferase [ALT] level and viral load), but the introduction of HAART is overall beneficial. In patients with newly diagnosed HIV and HCV, HAART is generally started first because it may decrease HCV load and hepatic fibrosis. Therapy for hepatitis C is considered after 1 to 2 months. However, coinfection causes increased HAART hepatotoxicity and decreased efficacy of HAART; therefore, initiation of HCV therapy can be given first if the CD4 count is more than $500/mm^3$ and there have not been any opportunistic infections. In a patient with cirrhosis, however, it may be safer to start with HCV therapy to prevent flares associated with immune reconstitution.

The optimal treatment of HCV infection in HIV-positive patients has been a problem, with lower response rates to interferon and ribavirin, more contraindications to therapy, and higher toxicity rates than in the HIV-negative population. Combination therapy with pegylated interferon and ribavirin has the best response rate, although it is still lower than with hepatitis C alone. The AIDS Pegasys Ribavirin International Coinfection Trial randomized 868 patients to peginterferon alone, peginterferon with ribavirin, or standard interferon with ribavirin and reported a sustained virologic response (SVR) of 40% with peginterferon plus ribavirin, which was better than the 12% with standard interferon and ribavirin or with peginterferon alone. The SVR with combination therapy for patients with genotype 1 disease was less at 29%, especially for those with a high viral load. Virologic response of a twofold log reduction in viral levels at 12 weeks predicted an SVR, as in non-HIV patients. The ACTG treatment trial in the United States enrolled 133 patients, with an SVR of 27%. The SVR was better for patients with non-genotype 1 HCV, no intravenous drug use, and low baseline HIV RNA. In both trials, the side-effect profile was reasonable, with 12% of patients discontinuing drug therapy because of adverse events. Of some concern, however, is the potential inactivation of thymidine analogues by ribavirin; theoretically, this can result in the loss of HIV virologic control. Careful HIV virologic evaluation is necessary as HCV therapy is introduced. The decision to treat hepatitis C in coinfected patients is still made on a case-by-case basis (Table 2).

OTHER VIRAL HEPATITIS

Hepatitis A

The hepatitis A virus (HAV) is excreted in high concentration in stool, and frequent oroanal sexual activity correlates well with the risk of HAV acquisition in homosexual men. The

Table 2.   Antiretroviral Therapy for HCV in HIV-
          coinfected Patients

Consider therapy	Defer therapy
Stable HIV disease	Recent change in HAART
Higher CD4 count	HAART side effects exacer-
Stable HAART regimen	bated by HCV therapy
No active opportunistic	Inability to comply with
infections	therapy (social or psychiatric
Advanced fibrosis found	problems)
on biopsy	No fibrosis found on liver
Compensated liver disease	biopsy
Genotypes 2 and 3	
Inability to tolerate HAART	
because of HCV	

*HAART, highly active antiretroviral therapy; HCV, hepatitis C
virus; HIV, human immunodeficiency virus.*

clinical and virologic course does not appear to be altered in HIV-infected patients. HAV vaccine is safe in HIV-infected patients and is recommended particularly for those coinfected with HBV or HCV.

Hepatitis D

Hepatitis D virus (HDV) is a cytopathic virus, and HIV infection leads to worsening of the liver disease, with more inflammation of the liver. HIV appears to decrease the inhibitory effect of HDV on HBV. In HIV-infected patients, HDV antigen is more likely to be detectable in serum, and anti-HDV, less likely.

HAART HEPATOTOXICITY

Hepatotoxicity occurs with all three classes of antiretroviral therapy: nucleoside analogue reverse transcriptase inhibitors (NRTIs), protease inhibitors, and non-NRTIs (NNRTIs). Chronic viral hepatitis B or C coinfection increases the hepatotoxicity of antiretroviral therapy. Currently, HAART is the standard care for HIV infection and requires a minimum of three antiretroviral agents from two or more classes of antiretroviral therapy. Each combination has its drug interactions and toxicities. Overall, up to 14% of patients have liver test abnormalities after starting HAART, especially in the presence of HCV coinfection.

The protease inhibitors are associated with liver test abnormalities in 3% to 10% of HIV-infected patients and in as many as 20% of coinfected patients. Many of the newer antiretroviral regimens are protease inhibitor–sparing, although some data suggest that treatment with protease inhbitors may

be beneficial in patients with HCV and HIV coinfection. Ritonavir is particularly associated with severe hepatotoxicity due to acute hepatitis. Although this is independent of hepatitis C status, ritonavir generally is not used to treat coinfected patients.

The toxic effects of NRTIs on the liver include mitochondrial injury with hyperlipidemia, hepatic steatosis, lactic acidosis, or fulminant liver failure (or a combination). This typically occurs after 3 months or more of therapy. In a recent series of 12 cases of symptomatic lactic acidosis in hospitalized patients with HIV infection receiving antiretroviral therapy, all 12 patients were receiving NRTIs, especially stavudine plus didanosine, and only four patients were receiving protease inhibitors. Transient, reversible liver test abnormalities have been reported since the introduction of zidovudine (AZT) therapy; although severe hepatotoxicity from zidovudine has been uncommon, reactions as severe as acute cholestatic hepatitis have been well documented, necessitating the discontinuation of therapy. Didanosine and stavudine are the NRTIs most likely to produce increased aspartate aminotransferase (AST) and ALT levels (11%-16% of patients), and lamivudine, abacavir, and tenofovir less so (<1% of patients). There is some concern about the interaction between ribavirin and this group of drugs.

NNRTIs have been associated with severe hepatotoxicity that usually occurs in the first 2 weeks of therapy (in 15% of patients treated with nevirapine and in 8% treated with efavirenz). The risk was greatest in those with chronic viral hepatitis and those concurrently prescribed protease inhibitors. Both protease inhibitors and NNRTIs are metabolized extensively in the liver by the P-450 system and can act as inhibitors or inducers (or both) of that system, a situation made more complex by the multitude of concurrent medications used to treat HIV infection.

For HIV-infected patients who are just starting HAART, liver function must be tested regularly, at 1 month and then every 3 months. Mild liver function abnormalities during HAART (i.e., aminotransferase levels less than 10 times the upper limit of normal and without clinical evidence of acute hepatitis, a hypersensitivity reaction [first 2 weeks of therapy], or lactic acidosis [typically after 3 months of therapy]) are generally observed without discontinuing therapy. Liver tests are repeated every 2 weeks until the results are stable or improved. When aminotransferase levels are more than 10 times the upper limit of normal or acute hepatitis, hypersensitivity reaction, or lactic acidosis develops, antiretroviral therapy must be stopped and the cause of the abnormality established.

There are some implications for HAART in HIV-infected patients with chronic hepatitis B or C coinfection. Drug hepatotoxicity occurs in up to 20% of coinfected patients, but it is rarely severe. If ribavirin is used to treat hepatitis C, didanosine should not be used. Protease inhibitors (especially high-dose ritonavir) and stavudine, didanosine, and nevirapine are generally avoided in patients who have cirrhosis or hepatic decompensation.

In addition to HAART, patients with HIV infection are exposed iatrogenically to numerous other potential hepatotoxins and most hospitalized AIDS patients are taking drugs with potential to affect the liver. The concomitant protein-calorie malnutrition in these patients may predispose them to the toxic effects of certain drugs by influencing plasma binding and liver metabolism. AIDS patients with fever and increasing liver test abnormalities who are already taking multiple medications represent a difficult diagnostic problem. It may be necessary to discontinue nonessential or suspect medications to detect a drug-induced effect. Compared with the general population, AIDS patients appear to be at higher risk for adverse reactions to sulfonamides, such as trimethoprim-sulfamethoxazole.

LIVER COMPLICATIONS OF HIV INFECTION ASSOCIATED WITH IMMUNOSUPPRESSION

Opportunistic Infections

Mycobacterium avium-intracellulare

In AIDS patients, *Mycobacterium avium-intracellulare* (MAI) infection is the most common cause of systemic bacterial infection and is found in 50% of cases at autopsy. MAI is generally a late opportunistic infection that has prominent gastrointestinal tract and liver involvement as part of the disseminated process. Clinically, it is a "wasting" syndrome, with fever, malaise, anorexia, night sweats, diarrhea, and abdominal pain.

The liver is affected in 80% of patients with MAI infection. Hepatosplenomegaly and a marked increase in the alkaline phosphatase level are the typical clinical features. Enlarged lymph nodes may be present in the retroperitoneum, peripancreatic area, or in the porta hepatis and may cause biliary obstruction and jaundice. Histologic examination of the liver shows poorly formed granulomas and positive staining (Ziehl-Neelsen, auramine-rhodamine) of smears for the organism. Because bacteremia is usually sustained, the organism can be detected within 5 days to 3 weeks in blood cultures in almost all patients who have disseminated disease, obviating the need for a liver biopsy in most patients. The mean survival of patients with disseminated MAI infection is 4 months, although some show improvement with multidrug regimens.

Mycobacterium tuberculosis

Tuberculosis (TB) is especially common in AIDS patients from Haiti or Africa, in intravenous drug abusers, and in economically disadvantaged people. When TB is diagnosed after the onset of AIDS, it is extrapulmonary in 75% of patients. Liver involvement results in miliary granulomas and, rarely, abscess.

Blood cultures are often positive for *M. tuberculosis*, although less often than for MAI. Histologic examination and culture of liver biopsy tissue confirm the diagnosis, although granulomas may be scanty in comparison with those in MAI infection. *M. kansasii* may also cause disseminated disease with liver involvement.

Cytomegalovirus

Cytomegalovirus (CMV) infection is extremely common in AIDS: 100% of HIV-positive homosexual males are seropositive, 90% of AIDS patients have CMV infection at autopsy, and 50% of AIDS patients have CMV viremia. With gastrointestinal tract involvement (which is common), 30% to 50% of AIDS patients have hepatobiliary disease manifested by a moderately increased alkaline phosphatase level, mildly increased transaminase levels, and a normal bilirubin concentration. CMV hepatitis always occurs when there is widespread multiorgan involvement, with patients presenting with malaise, fever, and weight loss. The diagnosis is made by culturing tissue or blood or by histologic examination of tissue (or both). In CMV hepatitis, staining with hematoxylin and eosin shows characteristic large intranuclear and multiple small cytoplasmic inclusions in Kupffer cells, bile duct epithelial cells, and, occasionally, hepatocytes and is as good as in situ hybridization or immunohistochemistry. Therapy is with ganciclovir, 10 mg/kg daily intravenously for 14 to 21 days. For relapses, a maintenance dose of 5 mg/kg daily may be necessary. Foscarnet can be used for resistant strains.

Other Viral Infections

Herpes simplex virus, human herpesvirus 6, adenovirus, and Epstein-Barr virus have all been reported as possible liver pathogens in AIDS, usually occurring in disseminated disease. Herpes simplex virus may present as fulminant hepatitis, with very high transaminase levels and with necrotic, hemorrhagic foci in the liver and typical Cowdry type A intranuclear eosinophilic inclusions surrounded by a halo. Herpes simplex virus hepatitis is treated with acyclovir, 15 to 30 mg/kg daily intravenously in three divided doses. If the infection is resistant, foscarnet or vidarabine can be prescribed. Disseminated adenovirus produces liver necrosis with massive hemorrhagic foci; adjacent areas may have "smokey" intranuclear inclusions. In children with AIDS, Epstein-Barr virus has been reported to cause chronic active hepatitis, but this has not been seen in adults.

Cryptococcus, Histoplasma, and *Coccidioides*

Cryptococcosis is common in AIDS patients and may be the first manifestation. The disease may be limited to the central nervous system and skin, but the disseminated form involves the liver, with poorly formed granulomas. The diagnosis is made by culturing the blood, cerebrospinal fluid, or tissue (liver, bone marrow); cryptococcal antigen is present in serum. Therapy is with amphotericin B plus flucytosine.

Histoplasmosis is a pulmonary infection endemic in the Ohio, Mississippi, and Missouri River valleys; Caribbean; and Central and South America. AIDS patients are susceptible to a disseminated form, either after primary exposure or as a manifestation of reactivated infection. This results in poorly formed granulomas spread diffusely in the liver (with hepatomegaly), spleen, lungs, bone marrow, and gastrointestinal tract (Table 3). The diagnosis is usually made by culturing and staining the bone marrow. Therapy is with amphotericin B.

Coccidioidomycosis, also a pulmonary infection, is endemic in the southwest United States. Disseminated disease has been reported in about a third of AIDS patients in Tucson, Arizona. All the patients have pulmonary disease as well as widespread dissemination to multiple organs, including the liver, with resulting liver test abnormalities.

Pneumocystis jiroveci (formerly, *carinii*)

This is the most common cause of pneumonia in AIDS patients. Rarely in very severe pneumonitis or in patients receiving aerosolized pentamidine, extrapulmonary involvement occurs with widespread dissemination. In this setting, hepatitis can occur; treatment is with trimethoprim-sulfamethoxazole.

Table 3. Differential Diagnosis of Intrahepatic Granulomas in Persons Infected With Human Immunodeficiency Virus

Mycobacteria
    Mycobacterium avium-intracellulare
    Mycobacterium tuberculosis
Fungi
    Histoplasma capsulatum
    Cryptococcus neoformans
    Coccidioides immitis
    Candida albicans
Other infections
    Cytomegalovirus
    Toxoplasma gondii
    Cat-scratch fever
Drugs
    Sulfonamides (eosinophils)
    Isoniazid
Neoplasm
    Lymphoma

Microsporidium

Encephalitozoon cuniculi has been reported to cause fulminant hepatitis with a marked increase in transaminase and alkaline phosphatase levels and suppurative necrosis of the liver, with granulomas in the portal tracts. Giemsa staining of the tissue affected establishes the diagnosis. Metronidazole therapy may be effective.

Toxoplasma gondii

Increasingly, toxoplasmosis is being recognized in immuno-compromised hosts, and disseminated disease, including severe hepatitis, has been described in AIDS patients. In one case, autopsy showed severe focal hepatocellular necrosis, with numerous foci of cells containing the organism.

Leishmania

Visceral leishmaniasis has been reported in HIV-positive patients who live in or travel to areas where the disease is endemic. Patients with HIV infection can have an atypical course of leish-maniasis that often precedes the onset of AIDS. The clinical features include fever, weight loss, anemia, lymphadenopathy, hepatosplenomegaly, and, occasionally, jaundice. The disease is usually refractory to therapy, with progressive involvement of the liver and bone marrow.

Entamoeba

Entamoeba histolytica is the most important protozoan parasite of the gastrointestinal tract in humans. The organism is frequently found in the stools of homosexual men in the United States and United Kingdom, presumably through oroanal or genitoanal transmission. Invasive amebiasis generally is not considered a hallmark of HIV infection, but in the Far East, amebic liver abscesses and colitis have been described as the presenting features of HIV infection.

Peliosis Hepatis

Peliosis hepatis is a rare condition characterized by small cystic blood-filled spaces in the liver parenchyma. Similar lesions can occur in the spleen, lymph nodes, bone marrow, and lungs. Early associations of peliosis hepatis were with wasting conditions such as cancer and TB; more recently, it has been associated with anabolic steroids and other drugs. The association of peliosis hepatis and HIV infection has now been established. In addition, cutaneous bacillary angiomatosis has been found in some of these patients and this has led to the morphologic finding of an identical bacterium in both liver and skin lesions. The lesions of peliosis hepatis in HIV-infected patients contain Warthin-Starry–positive bacilli, but lesions of peliosis hepatis due to other causes do not. Studies suggest that this fastidious, gram-negative bacillus is *Bartonella henselae*, an agent closely related to the rickettsial pathogen, *Rochalimaea quintana*.

The peliotic spaces of bacillary peliosis hepatis are often associated with a fibromyxoid stroma that contains a few inflammatory cells, capillaries, and clumps of granular material that correspond to clusters of bacilli seen with electron microscopy. Clinically, most patients present with weight loss, fever, anorexia, nausea, and abdominal pain. Rupture with hemoperitoneum has been reported. Hepatomegaly is present in most, if not all, patients. Liver tests show a moderate-to-severe increase in the alkaline phosphatase level, mild-to-moderate increase in aminotransferase levels, and a near-normal bilirubin concentration. Computed tomography (CT) shows abdominal lymphadenopathy and heterogeneous parenchyma in the liver or spleen.

Treatment with erythromycin, 2 g daily, has clinical efficacy, and doxycycline and antituberculous drugs may also be effective. Without treatment, bacillary peliosis hepatis in HIV-infected patients is progressive and may be fatal.

Tumors

Lymphomas

High- or intermediate-grade non-Hodgkin's lymphomas of B-cell origin occur in approximately 3% of AIDS patients, and their presence is a diagnostic criterion for the diagnosis of AIDS in an HIV-positive person. The prevalence of lymphoma may be increasing, perhaps because of longer survival times with anti-HIV drugs and prophylactic antibiotic therapy. Virtually all lymphomas in HIV infection have a diffuse, nonfollicular architecture. The three basic subtypes are Burkitt's lymphoma, large cell lymphoma, and immunoblastic lymphoma; however, T-cell, "biphenotypic," and atypical Hodgkin's lymphomas also occur. Patients with monoclonal tumors typically have low CD4 cell counts and a particularly poor prognosis. Also, polyclonal tumors behave in an aggressive, malignant fashion. The majority of these lymphomas are negative for Epstein-Barr virus.

In AIDS patients, lymphomas are typically extranodal (90% of patients), and they may develop as the first manifestation of AIDS, they may develop in patients with established AIDS, or they may be found at autopsy. Most patients present with B symptoms of weight loss, fevers, and night sweats. Parenchymal organ involvement is the rule, especially the central nervous system (20%-40% of patients) and the gastrointestinal tract (15%-30% of patients), with lesions occurring in the liver (15% of patients), gallbladder, and bile ducts. In one-third of patients with involvement of the gut, the liver is affected either microscopically or macroscopically (solid or cystic lesions). Although liver involvement is commonly metastatic, primary hepatic lymphoma has been reported. Liver masses are often asymptomatic, but if bulky or strategically situated in the porta hepatis, they may produce right upper quadrant pain, fever, and jaundice, particularly in association with an increased level of alkaline phosphatase. Cystic lesions may become secondarily infected. Gallbladder lesions usually are clinically silent.

The diagnosis is made initially with ultrasonographic (US) or CT imaging of the liver, which may show large, often multifocal, solid intrahepatic space-occupying lesions. Histologic confirmation of the diagnosis with fine-needle aspiration of a liver mass or enlarged lymph nodes has been found to be a useful, cost-effective, and well-tolerated diagnostic procedure for lymphomas. Aggressive chemotherapy has achieved remission rates of 50%, but relapses occur relatively soon after chemotherapy, often in the central nervous system, and survival may be shortened by worsening opportunistic infections. Chemotherapy is most appropriate and efficacious for patients with a high CD4 cell count, no previous diagnosis of AIDS, and a good performance score. Most lymphomas are radioresistant. Surgery may be required for intestinal involvement. The prognosis is poor, with median survival of 5 to 6 months, especially with monoclonal tumors and preexisting AIDS.

Kaposi's Sarcoma

An aggressive variant of Kaposi's sarcoma, with prominent skin lesions on the upper extremities and early involvement of lymph nodes, is found throughout the AIDS population, although its prevalence is highest among homosexual men. Like non-Hodgkin's lymphomas, Kaposi's sarcoma in an HIV-positive patient establishes the diagnosis of AIDS. In developed countries, the frequency of Kaposi's sarcoma is decreasing among AIDS patients. This, together with its prevalence in patients affected by AIDS from sexual exposure and its occurrence in HIV-negative persons within the HIV risk groups, suggest that Kaposi's sarcoma may be caused by a separate sexually transmitted agent or agents, probably a virus. There is evidence that a viral product of HIV infection may directly stimulate the growth of Kaposi's sarcoma. The basic elements of Kaposi's sarcoma are spindle cells (derived from malignant proliferation of lymphatic endothelial cells) and vascular clefts with extravasated erythrocytes. Hemorrhage and central necrosis are common.

Unlike lymphomas, Kaposi's sarcoma is an early manifestation of AIDS (the initial sign in 30% of patients), and patients almost always present with cutaneous lesions, which can be single or few in number for years before worsening. Visceral involvement is rarely diagnosed before skin lesions appear, but its occurrence may be frequent (the gut is involved in 40% of cases) but asymptomatic. Kaposi's sarcoma may involve the liver (50% of patients), spleen (40%), or biliary tree, but in almost all instances, intrahepatic involvement is found only at autopsy. The liver is studded with characteristic purplish brown nodules distributed diffusely over the surface and in the subcapsular regions. Intrahepatic Kaposi's sarcoma rarely produces clinical symptoms.

Visceral Kaposi's sarcoma requires therapy only if it is symptomatic (e.g., type B symptoms). Lesions respond to alpha interferon, radiotherapy, or cytotoxic chemotherapy. Lesions that bleed may require endoscopic or surgical treatment.

Other Tumors

Fibrosarcomas of the liver have been reported in HIV-positive children in Africa.

Steatosis and Nonspecific Hepatitis

Macrovesicular steatosis is the most common abnormality seen in biopsy specimens and may be present in as many as 40% of AIDS patients. It may be diffuse, centrilobular, or periportal. Hepatomegaly is common with steatosis, and the serum level of alkaline phosphatase is often increased one to two times. The most likely causes of steatosis are poor nutritional status (severe protein malnutrition), weight loss, chronic illness, and parenteral nutrition.

Nonspecific portal inflammation is common (found in 35% of biopsy specimens) and is of little use diagnostically. These changes are seen less frequently in autopsy specimens, suggesting a possible correlation with the immune response. Chronic active hepatitis is rare except in children with AIDS, in whom lobular and portal lymphocytic infiltrate with T8-positive lymphocytes and endotheliitis can develop, suggesting an autoimmune process similar to graft-versus-host disease.

BILIARY TRACT DISEASE IN HIV INFECTION

Increasingly, typical and atypical biliary infection and malignancies are being recognized in patients with AIDS, although non-AIDS–related biliary problems must be kept in mind. In the clinical assessment and management of these patients, the search for treatable conditions, especially those amenable to minimal intervention, must be emphasized.

AIDS Cholangiopathy

A cholestatic syndrome with typical cholangiographic features has been well described in AIDS patients. This cholangiopathy has four related but different forms, as follows:

1. Papillary stenosis—defined as a common bile duct dilated to more than 8 mm, distal tapering with marked proximal dilatation (Fig. 1 A)
2. Sclerosing cholangitis—characterized by focal strictures and dilatation of intrahepatic and extrahepatic bile ducts (Fig. 1 B)
3. Combined papillary stenosis and sclerosing cholangitis—the most common form (50% of cases)
4. Long extrahepatic bile duct strictures—longer than 1 to 2 cm in patients with no previous biliary surgery and no chronic pancreatitis

The common bile duct often has a beaded mucosal pattern suggestive of mucosal edema. The intrahepatic ducts are markedly irregular, especially in the left system, with sacculations containing intraductal debris or sloughed mucosa—cholangiographic features that are not usually seen in primary sclerosing cholangitis.

The definitive cause of AIDS cholangiopathy is elusive. HIV may infect and destroy bile duct cells directly or this lesion may represent the stereotypic pattern of injury in AIDS from a large number of pathogens and tumors. In biopsy samples obtained at endoscopic retrograde cholangiopancreatography (ERCP), surgery, or autopsy, the most common specific

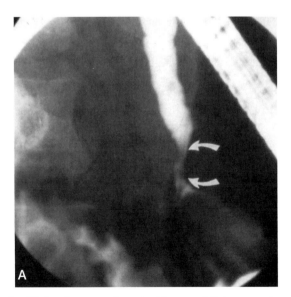

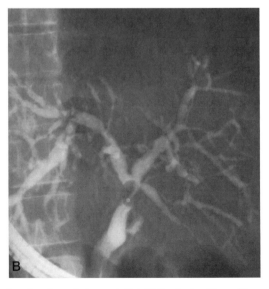

Fig. 1. Cholangiograms of acquired immunodeficiency syndrome cholangiopathy showing, *A*, tapered distal bile duct with papillary stenosis (*arrows*) and proximal common bile duct dilatation and, *B*, changes typical of sclerosing cholangitis.

pathologic feature is CMV or *Cryptosporidium* (occasionally both). MAI, malignancies, several microsporidial species, including *Enterocytozoon bieneusi* and *Septata intestinalis*, also have been identified occasionally. However, no definitive etiologic agent is identified in 40% to 50% of patients. Many other unproven possibilities have been suggested, from diarrhea-associated ("colitis-like"), unidentified viral or microsporidial infection, enhanced class II antigens on bile duct cells, and circulating immune complexes to copper hepatotoxicity.

The clinical presentation is that of a patient with known AIDS (on average, for about 1 year) who has a subacute or chronic course of right upper quadrant pain, fever, nausea, vomiting, and, often, diarrhea. Jaundice is rare because the biliary obstruction is incomplete. Acute bacterial cholangitis is uncommon before any invasive procedures have been performed. A cholestatic liver profile is the rule: a marked increase in the alkaline phosphatase level to five times normal, only a moderate increase in transaminase levels, and a near-normal bilirubin concentration. US and CT of the liver show abnormality in only 70% of patients: dilated intrahepatic and extrahepatic bile ducts, thickened bile duct wall, and distal tapering. Extrinsic compression of the biliary tree from enlarged lymph nodes or Kaposi's sarcoma is best excluded with multiple transverse CT scans through the common bile duct. Cholangiography, usually by ERCP, best defines the biliary irregularities described above. The papilla of Vater may appear indurated. Endoscopic biopsy samples or bile aspirates (or both) should be obtained for culture, smears, and histologic examination. In one series, the microbiologic yield was highest for patients who underwent biopsy (duodenal and papillary) and bile sampling on multiple occasions. *Cryptosporidium* was identified in 57% of the patients, CMV in 28%, and Microsporida in 7%. In about 40% of patients, no definitive cause is identified. In all patients with biliary cryptosporidiosis, *Cryptosporidium* is identified in stool, which should also be examined for microsporidia. Pancreatic abnormalities also may be present.

Endoscopic sphincterotomy is performed for AIDS-related papillary stenosis. This relieves pain dramatically (in 86% of patients in one series) but has little effect on biochemical indices; progressive intrahepatic sclerosing cholangitis may develop. Occasionally, surgical sphincterotomy is necessary if ERCP is not successful. Balloon dilatation or endoscopic or percutaneous stent placement may be considered for bile duct obstruction. Chemotherapy is indicated for lymphoma or Kaposi's sarcoma

of the bile duct (see below). The use of ursodeoxycholic acid or antiviral agents (e.g., ganciclovir), is unproven. Parenteral metronidazole for biliary microsporidiosis has had no effect in the few cases reported. The 1-year survival rate after the diagnosis of AIDS cholangiopathy is poor (14%) and related to progression of AIDS itself. Currently, all specific therapy for *Cryptosporidium* infection is experimental.

Tumors

Lymphomas

As in the liver parenchyma, AIDS-associated lymphomas may occur primarily in the bile ducts. In this location, lymphomas are likely to present, even as small intramural lesions, with symptomatic jaundice and a cholestatic profile. Although US and CT studies of the liver may be abnormal, especially if multiple transverse sections are taken through the porta hepatis, the diagnosis is usually made with ERCP, with brushings and biopsy specimens. Occasionally, a bile cytology study is useful.

Kaposi's Sarcoma

Kaposi's sarcoma can cause obstruction of the common bile duct, resulting in jaundice and cholangitis.

Acalculous Cholecystitis

Acalculous cholecystitis has been well described in AIDS patients and has been associated with infection due to CMV, *Cryptosporidium*, *Campylobacter*, *Serratia*, and *Candida* organisms. Grossly, the gallbladder wall is indurated, hemorrhagic, and necrotic. Histologically, the mucosa is diffusely ulcerated with areas of necrosis, and either intranuclear inclusions of CMV or coccidial forms of cryptosporidia are seen within or adherent to the mucosal surface. Most patients present with an acute or subacute illness lasting days or weeks and consisting of fever, fatigue, and right upper quadrant pain (crampy, constant, or dull) and tenderness. Murphy's sign is usually present. Patients are not jaundiced.

Liver tests are unhelpful, but US shows the absence of stones, thickened gallbladder wall, and pericholecystic fluid. Air in the gallbladder wall suggests necrosis. Radionuclide scintigraphy generally shows a nonfunctioning gallbladder, despite a patent cystic duct. Most patients respond well to cholecystectomy.

RECOMMENDED READING

Benhamou Y, Di Martino V, Bochet M, Colombet G, Thibault V, Liou A, et al. Factors affecting liver fibrosis in human immunodeficiency virus—and hepatitis C virus—coinfected patients: impact of protease inhibitor therapy. Hepatology. 2001;34:283-7.

Bruno R, Sacchi P, Puoti M, Soriano V, Filice G. HCV chronic hepatitis in patients with HIV: clinical management issues. Am J Gastroenterol. 2002;97:1598-606.

Kottilil S, Polis MA, Kovacs JA. HIV infection, hepatitis C infection, and HAART: hard clinical choices. JAMA. 2004;292:243-50.

Martinez EH. Hepatitis B and hepatitis C co-infection in patients with HIV. Rev Med Virol. 2001;11:253-70.

Ogedegbe AO, Sulkowski MS. Antiretroviral-associated liver injury. Clin Liver Dis. 2003;7:475-99.

Sasadeusz J. Human immunodeficiency virus-hepatitis C coinfection: swapping new problems for newer ones. Intern Med J. 2001;31:418-21.

Shukla NB, Poles MA. Hepatitis B virus infection: co-infection with hepatitis C virus, hepatitis D virus, and human immunodeficiency virus. Clin Liver Dis. 2004;8:445-60.

Spengler U, Lichterfeld M, Rockstroh JK. Antiretroviral drug toxicity: a challenge for the hepatologist? J Hepatol. 2002;36:283-94.

CHAPTER 40

Liver Transplantation

Michael R. Charlton, M.B.B.S.

INTRODUCTION

Since 1963, when Starzl performed the first liver transplant in a human, the procedure has become a standard of care in the management not only of decompensated acute and chronic liver disease but also of some tumors and metabolic disorders. The increasing acceptance of liver transplantation as a therapy reflects the dramatic improvement in outcomes following this procedure. In the last 20 years, the 1-year patient survival rate has improved from approximately 30% to 86%. Currently, the 5-year patient survival rate is 72%. Graft survival rates are generally about 10% less than patient survival rates (rates are from the United Network of Organ Sharing [UNOS], http://www.optn.org). The basis for the increase in patient and graft survival rates is complex but undoubtedly includes improved 1) patient selection (most early recipients had metastatic liver disease), 2) immunosuppression (<2% of livers are currently lost to chronic rejection), 3) surgical technique, and 4) expertise in related fields (e.g., intensive care, anesthesia, infectious diseases).

In 2004, 6,167 liver transplantation procedures were performed in the United States (compared with 4,987 in 2000), and 10% of these were performed in children. Thus, the total number of transplants has increased 23.7% in less than 5 years despite a decrease in the number of living donors during the same period. Most (95%) transplanted organs originated from deceased donors. Currently, more than 17,000 patients are listed for liver transplantation. Both the waiting list and the median waiting time have increased more than 10-fold since 1990.

INDICATIONS

Acute Liver Disease

Patients with acute liver failure are assigned the highest priority (status 1) for organ allocation on liver transplant waiting lists. The four broad indications for listing a patient with acute liver disease for liver transplantation include the following:

1. Fulminant liver failure (must have at least stage II encephalopathy)
2. Primary nonfunction of a transplanted liver within 7 days after the original liver transplant
3. Hepatic artery thrombosis within 7 days after the original liver transplant
4. Acute decompensated Wilson's disease (even if not encephalopathic)

Chronic Liver Disease

Under the current organ allocation system, any patient with cirrhosis who has 7 Child-Turcotte-Pugh points can, and probably should, be listed for liver transplantation. A Child-Turcotte-Pugh score of 7 or higher is referred to as the "minimal listing criterion"—no clinical events or complications are required.

Patients who meet the minimal listing criterion are prioritized according to their model for end-stage liver disease (MELD) score. MELD scores replaced the Child-Turcotte-Pugh classification as a scoring system for prioritizing potential liver transplant recipients in February 2002. This change was made because MELD scores were shown to be highly predictive of mortality while patients waited for liver transplantation. MELD scores are calculated with a formula incorporating three easily measured laboratory variables: serum total bilirubin concentration, serum creatinine level, and international normalized ratio (INR) for prothrombin time. Preordained MELD scores are assigned to patients with hepatocellular carcinoma. Indications for liver transplantation other than chronic or acute liver diseases for which MELD scores can be assigned (rather than calculated) include familial amyloidosis, primary hyperoxaluria, hepatopulmonary syndrome, and severe familial hypercholesterolemia. Patients with cholangiocarcinoma or tumors that are metastatic to the liver can only be listed for liver transplantation under exceptional circumstances after appealing to the appropriate regional review board and these transplantations are generally performed only under specific study protocols. Extra MELD points are assigned every 3 months to candidates assigned MELD scores under exceptional circumstances.

In liver transplantation, donor and recipient need only have compatible blood groups; no HLA matching is required. Time on the waiting list is no longer a factor for organ allocation other than for status-1 patients and as a tiebreaker for patients with identical MELD scores.

Liver failure associated with hepatitis C is the most common indication for liver transplantation worldwide, accounting for more than 30% of liver transplantations. Alcoholic liver disease is the second most common indication, followed by cholestatic and cryptogenic liver diseases. Fulminant liver failure accounts for approximately 5% of liver transplantations.

Patient and graft survival rates after liver transplantation is highest for patients with primary biliary cirrhosis. Patients with malignancy or fulminant liver failure have relatively poorer patient and graft survival rates. All other indications for primary transplantation, including hepatitis B and C, have comparable patient and graft survival rates. All nonviral chronic liver diseases can recur after transplantation, including primary sclerosing cholangitis, primary biliary cirrhosis, and autoimmune liver disease. Recurrence of nonviral liver diseases rarely affects graft survival.

Recurrence of hepatitis B can be prevented in more than 90% of recipients infected with hepatitis B virus by the administration of hepatitis B immunoglobulin, usually with lamivudine or adefovir, indefinitely. The first dose is given during the anhepatic phase of the operation.

In contrast to nonviral causes of decompensated liver disease, which recur in less than 20% of recipients, posttransplant recurrence of hepatitis C virus (HCV) infection, as defined by detection of HCV RNA, is nearly universal. Almost half of HCV-infected liver transplant recipients develop histologic evidence of recurrence (defined by histologic activity index ≥3 and/or fibrosis stage ≥2) within the first postoperative year. In the National Institutes of Health–sponsored Liver Transplant Database, one in five recipients who developed histologic evidence of recurrent hepatitis C either died or required retransplantation because of

hepatitis C–induced allograft failure within the first 5 years postoperatively. Thus, in the medium term, approximately 10% of patients who received a liver transplant for hepatitis C will die or lose the allograft because of recurrent disease. Factors known to be associated with diminished patient and graft survival in HCV-infected recipients include donor older than 50 years, higher average daily corticosteroid doses, treatment for acute rejection, use of OKT3 (a murine monoclonal antibody to CD3-bearing T cells), higher Child-Turcotte-Pugh score at time of transplantation, and nonwhite recipient race. Treatment of hepatitis C with interferon and ribavirin has an end-of-treatment response rate of about 25% in transplant recipients and is tolerated relatively poorly by this group of patients. The risk of rejection during interferon therapy appears to be small.

CONTRAINDICATIONS

To be candidates for single-organ liver transplantation, potential recipients should have robust cardiovascular, pulmonary, and renal function. Absolute contraindications and relative contraindications are listed in Table 1.

IMMUNOSUPPRESSION

The most common immunosuppression regimens include a calcineurin inhibitor (cyclosporine or tacrolimus) plus corticosteroids plus an antiproliferative agent (mycophenolate mofetil or azathioprine). Treatment with corticosteroids and antiproliferative agents is often withdrawn gradually during the first year after transplantation. The characteristics of these agents are summarized in Table 2.

Table 1. Contraindications to Liver Transplantation

Absolute contraindications
    Severe pulmonary hypertension (mean systolic
        pulmonary artery pressure > 35 mm Hg)
    Uncontrolled systemic sepsis
    Extrahepatic malignancy unless tumor-free for ≥2 years
        and recurrence probability < 10%
    Alcoholic hepatitis, untreated alcoholism, chemical
        dependency
    Severe psychologic disease likely to affect compliance
    Extensive portal and mesenteric vein thrombosis
Relative contraindications
    Portal vein thrombosis
    HIV infection
    Extensive previous abdominal surgery
    Social isolation

HIV, human immunodeficiency virus.

Table 2.   Characteristics of Agents Used for Immunosuppression in Liver Transplant Recipients

Corticosteroids
    Broad immunosuppressive properties
    Inhibits interleukin-2 release from macrophages
    Suppresses antibody production
    Decreases ability of antibody to recognize antigen
    Effective as induction and maintenance therapy & treatment of rejection
    Usual dose varies widely
    Side effects: hypertension, osteopenia, glucose intolerance, dyslipidemia
Azathioprine
    Metabolized in liver to 6-mercaptopurine
    Parent drug & metabolite have immunosuppressive properties
    Interferes with DNA synthesis (nonspecific actions)
    Effective only as induction therapy, not rejection treatment
    Usual maintenance therapy dose: 2 mg/kg daily (intravenously or orally)
    Side effects: bone marrow suppression, increased tumorigenesis
Mycophenolate mofetil
    Ester of mycophenolic acid (active metabolite of mycophenolate mofetil)
    Mycophenolic acid is inosine monophosphate dehydrogenase inhibitor, inhibiting de novo pathway of guanosine
     nucleotide synthesis
    Mycophenolic acid inhibits proliferative responses of T and B lymphocytes
    Effective only as maintenance therapy, not rejection treatment
    Usual maintenance dose: 1 g orally twice daily
    Side effects: diarrhea, leucopenia, opportunistic infections
    Does not cause renal impairment
Cyclosporine
    Binds with cyclophilin to inhibit calcineurin phosphatase, preventing interleukin-2 production (cyclosporine & tacrolimus:
     broadly referred to as "calcineurin inhibitors")
    Useful for maintenance immunosuppression
    Initial dosing: 8 mg/kg daily orally in 2 divided doses
    Side effects: hypertension, nephrotoxicity, neurotoxicity, dyslipidemia, hypertrichosis
    Multiple drug interactions because it is metabolized by cytochrome P-450 (P-450 inhibitors increase and inducers
     decrease cyclosporine levels)
Tacrolimus
    Binds with immunophilin
    Inhibits calcineurin phosphatase to inhibit interleukin-2 production, T-cell proliferation, & generation of cytotoxic T cells
    Useful for maintenance immunosuppression
    In contrast to cyclosporine, can be used to treat acute cellular rejection
    Initial dosing: 0.1 mg/kg daily orally in 2 divided doses
    Side effects: similar to cyclosporine but less hypertrichosis
OKT3
    Murine monoclonal anti-CD3
    Binds & destroys CD3-bearing T cells
    Dosing: variable, usually 5 mg/d intravenously for 10 days
    Side effects: anaphylaxis & capillary leak, long-term risk of lymphoproliferative disease after transplant
Sirolimus
    Induces cell cycle arrest by interrupting interleukin-2 receptor signaling pathways
    Useful alternative to calcineurin inhibitors
    Maintenance dose: 2-10 g/d
    Less renal toxicity than tacrolimus or cyclosporine
    Possible antitumor properties
    Side effects: hyperlipidemia, anemia, edema, oral ulcers, possibly hepatic artery thrombosis when used early

COMPLICATIONS

The more common complications that occur after liver transplantation are discussed below.

Primary Non-Function

Clinically, primary non-function is like fulminant liver failure, with onset immediately after transplantation. It occurs in less than 4% of recipients. A failure to produce bile, or the production of clear bile, is the hallmark of this condition. Aminotransferase levels are characteristically increased. Although primary non-function is more common in grafts with steatosis that affects more than 50% of the liver, it can also occur idiopathically. No therapy has proved effective other than retransplantation.

Hepatic Artery Thrombosis

This complication is more common in children and in size-mismatched grafts. Onset is usually within the first postoperative week. Clinical manifestations are usually subtle, with mild-to-moderate biochemical abnormalities that are usually asymptomatic. In adults, hepatic artery thrombosis is associated with subsequent graft failure, with hepatic abscess formation or diffuse biliary stricturing (or both) despite early repair or revision of the hepatic artery. Repeat liver transplantation may be required.

Biliary Stricture Formation

The most common site for formation of a biliary stricture is at the surgical anastomosis. Two-thirds of strictures respond to endoscopic therapy and one-third ultimately require surgical revision of the anastomosis or conversion to a Roux-en-Y bilioenterostomy. Nonanastomotic strictures are more likely 1) with longer cold and warm ischemia times, 2) after ABO incompatible liver transplantation, 3) after hepatic artery thrombosis, and 4) in patients whose original liver disease was primary sclerosing cholangitis. The median time for development of nonanastomotic strictures is 11 weeks posttransplantation (compared with 2 weeks for anastomotic strictures). Stenting and external biliary drainage are performed as needed. Approximately one-half of the patients with nonanastomotic biliary strictures either die or undergo retransplantation because of stricture-associated complications.

Acute Cellular Rejection

Acute cellular rejection occurs in 15% to 50% of liver transplant recipients (most common in recipients with fulminant liver failure, least common in recipients with alcoholic liver disease). Acute cellular rejection is characterized by mild-to-moderate biochemical abnormalities and, occasionally, fever. It is most common in patients undergoing liver transplantation for fulminant liver failure. Acute cellular rejection is a *histologic* diagnosis; thus, liver biopsy is required to confirm the diagnosis. Histologically, acute cellular rejection is characterized by portal lymphocytic infiltrates, cholangitis, and endotheliitis. No ultrasonographic or serologic indices can definitively confirm or exclude acute cellular rejection. The peak incidence is on postoperative day 7, with more than 90% of cases occurring in the first 2 months postoperatively. Treatment is usually corticosteroid boluses, to which 85% of patients have a response. Patients who do not have a response to corticosteroid treatment are usually given OKT3, which has a response rate of approximately 90%. Single episodes of acute cellular rejection do not affect patient and graft survival for recipients except those infected with HCV.

Infections

Approximately one in five liver transplant recipients develops a systemic fungal, viral, or bacterial infection in the first postoperative month. Cytomegalovirus (CMV) is the most common nonhepatotropic viral infection and is most common in CMV IgG-negative recipients who receive an organ from a CMV IgG-positive donor. The incidence of CMV infection peaks with the first two postoperative months and is rare after the first 12 months. Candidiasis is the most common systemic fungal infection. Opportunistic infections can also be seen with *Aspergillus*, *Nocardia*, *Cryptococcus*, and *Pneumocystis*.

Tumors

Only three types of tumors are more prevalent in liver transplant recipients than in the U.S. population as a whole: skin cancer (squamous and basal cell), carcinoma of the cervix, and lymphoma. More than 40% of liver transplant recipients eventually develop skin cancer and approximately 10% develop posttransplant lymphoproliferative disease or lymphoma. Posttransplant lymphoproliferative disease is associated with Epstein-Barr virus infection and administration of OKT3.

A Few Salient Facts About Liver Transplantation

- Recipients who have received a transplant previously (i.e., those undergoing retransplantation) have much lower graft and patient survival rates at all time points than those undergoing primary transplantation.
- Graft and patient survival rates are lowest at all time points for patients who were on life support just before transplantation.
- Transplant recipients with a medical urgency status of 1 have the lowest graft and patient survival rates at nearly all time points.
- The median waiting time for registrants with blood type O is much longer than for those with other blood types.

RECOMMENDED READING

Charlton M, Ruppert K, Belle SH, Bass N, Schafer D, Wiesner RH, et al. Long-term results and modeling to predict outcomes in recipients with HCV infection: results of the NIDDK liver transplantation database. Liver Transpl. 2004;10:1120-30.

Wiesner RH, Demetris AJ, Belle SH, Seaberg EC, Lake JR, Zetterman RK, et al. Acute hepatic allograft rejection: incidence, risk factors, and impact on outcome. Hepatology. 1998;28:638-45.

Yu AS, Keeffe EB. Liver transplantation. In: Zakim D, Boyer T, editors. Hepatology: a textbook of liver disease. Vol 2. 4th ed. Philadelphia: Saunders; 2003. p. 1617-56.

Liver I and II

Questions and Answers

QUESTIONS

Multiple Choice (choose the one best answer)

1. A 43-year-old woman presents with a 2-year history of daily right upper quadrant discomfort that is dull and intermittent. She has a body mass index of 38 and no constitutional symptoms. She has been taking oral contraceptives for 15 years. Her only other medication is atorvastatin. Physical examination findings are remarkable for right upper quadrant tenderness which persists and is slightly accentuated when she raises her head off the examination table. A complete blood count and electrolyte studies are normal. A liver panel is remarkable for alanine aminotransferase (ALT) that is 1.5 times the upper limit of normal. The bilirubin and alkaline phosphatase levels are normal. Ultrasonography shows a 0.5-cm nonmobile gallbladder mass that does not shadow. Doppler studies of the gallbladder mass are negative. The liver displays an increase in echotexture. A 5-cm echogenic mass is present. Computed tomography of the right lobe (Figure) demonstrates decreased density of the liver relative to the spleen and a 6-cm mass in segment 6. Nodular peripheral enhancement is noted on the arterial phase study, with delayed filling of the lesions during the venous phase examination. The most appropriate management of this patient is:

a. Referral to a surgeon
b. Ultrasonographically guided biopsy of the mass
c. Discontinuation of the oral contraceptives, and imaging studies repeated in 3 months
d. Reassurance
e. Magnetic resonance imaging of the liver

Precontrast

Arterial Phase

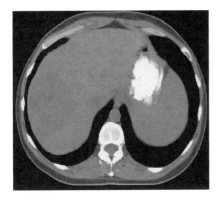
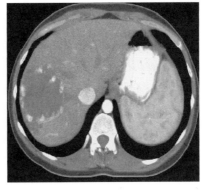

Question 1

2. A 54-year-old, asymptomatic man is referred for evaluation of a liver mass. At age 50, he had right hemicolectomy for colon cancer. He states that no lymph nodes were involved. No adjuvant chemotherapy was given. He has hypertension and is taking enalapril. Aside from a midline abdominal scar, physical examination findings are unremarkable. A complete blood count, liver panel, and electrolyte study are all normal. Colonoscopy shows a 7-mm polyp in the sigmoid colon; it is removed. Ultrasonography of the liver shows a 3-cm isoechoic mass in the right lobe. You order a magnetic resonance imaging study. The mass is isointense on both T1 and T2 studies. Following gadolinium administration, prominent arterial enhancement is observed during the arterial phase studies, with a rapid washout on the venous phase studies. No central scar is present. The appropriate management of this patient is:
   a. Referral to an oncologist for chemotherapy
   b. Reassurance
   c. Fine-needle aspiration of the lesion
   d. Referral to a radiologist for a radiofrequency ablation procedure
   e. Biopsy of the liver away from the mass

3. A 64-year-old woman is referred for evaluation of a liver mass. She has developed progressive anorexia and has lost 15 lb. Her history is remarkable for hypertension, hypothyroidism, and coronary artery disease. Her medications include thyroid hormone and metoprolol. On examination, the left lobe of the liver is palpable. Laboratory studies demonstrated the following: hemoglobin 11.1 g/dL, leukocytes 5.4×10^9/L, and platelets 554×10^9/L. The alkaline phosphatase level is increased 2.5-fold, alanine aminotransferase is 1.5 times the upper limit of normal, and total bilirubin is 0.8 mg/dL. Carcinoembryonic antigen and alpha fetoprotein values are normal, but CA 19-9 is 864 U/L (normal <80). Ultrasonography shows a 7-cm mixed echogenic mass in the left lobe of the liver. On computed tomography, the mass has no arterial enhancement but displays venous phase enhancement. Chest radiography does not show any lung metastases. The best management of this lesion is:
   a. Referral to a surgeon
   b. Chemoembolization
   c. Observation, with repeat imaging in 2 months
   d. Colonoscopy and endoscopy of the upper gastrointestinal tract
   e. Endoscopic ultrasonography

4. A 51-year-old man with hepatitis C and a history of alcohol abuse comes for his semiannual evaluation. Two years

ago, combination therapy with pegylated interferon and ribavirin failed. He has been abstinent from alcohol for 4 years. He is fatigued and has noted peripheral edema. His current medications include propranolol for prophylaxis of variceal bleeding (larger varices on endoscopy 2 months ago) and furosemide. Physical examination shows muscle wasting, spider angiomas, splenomegaly, and peripheral edema. The following were reported on laboratory evaluation: albumin 2.9 g/dL, total bilirubin 2.1 mg/dL, international normalized ratio 1.0, hemoglobin 12.1 g/dL, leukocytes 3.1×10^9/L, and platelets 56×10^9/L. Alpha fetoprotein is normal. Ultrasonography of the liver shows a 4-cm mass in the right lobe. No Doppler signal is detected in the right portal vein. Ascites is also noted on ultrasonography. Magnetic resonance imaging demonstrates enhancement in the mass, worrisome for hepatocellular carcinoma. The mass involves the right portal vein. What is the appropriate next step?
   a. Repeat imaging studies in 2 months, reassure the patient that he likely has macroregenerative nodules, and see him back in 6 months
   b. Reassure the patient that he likely has macroregenerative nodules, and see him back in 6 months
   c. Perform endoscopy of the upper gastrointestinal tract and colonoscopy to exclude a source for potential hepatic metastases
   d. Make a clinical diagnosis of hepatocellular carcinoma, and refer the patient to a tertiary care center
   e. Biopsy the left lobe of the liver

5. A 65-year-old man is referred for evaluation of a liver mass. He has a low-grade fever to 101.3°F, night sweats, and a 12-lb weight loss. He has been ill for 3 weeks. There is no antecedent history of liver disease. He has urinary outflow obstructive symptoms and has been treated in the past for prostatitis. On physical examination, his temperature is 100.5°F, pulse rate 105 beats/min, and blood pressure 128/83 mm Hg. He has tenderness of the right upper quadrant. The prostate is enlarged and soft. Laboratory values include the following: leukocytes 11.5×10^9/L, alkaline phosphatase increased 3-fold, alanine aminotransferase increased 2-fold, and prostate-specific antigen 8 ng/mL (normal, <4.5). Microscopic examination of a urine specimen shows pyuria and bacteria. Computed tomography shows a heterogenous 4-cm mass in the right lobe of the liver. It has peripheral enhancement following intravenous administration of contrast. The next management step should be:
   a. Prostate biopsy
   b. Magnetic resonance imaging of the liver to further define the lesion

c. Ultrasonographically guided aspiration of the lesion

d. Further staging studies, including bone marrow examination to exclude lymphoma

6. A 60-year-old man is brought to the emergency department by his wife, who comments that the patient has a drinking problem and has been complaining of back pain for the past several days. Physical examination findings are notable for spider angiomas and palmar erythema. The liver edge is firm and the span is increased. The spleen is palpable. No ascites or lower extremity edema is appreciated. Laboratory studies demonstrate the following: hemoglobin 11.9 g/dL, leukocytes 12.1×10^9/L, platelets 130×10^9/L, blood urea nitrogen 50 mg/dL, creatinine 2.3 mg/dL, aspartate aminotransferase 4,200 U/L, alanine aminotransferase 5,193 U/L, total bilirubin 3.1 mg/dL, alkaline phosphatase 70 U/L, and international normalized ratio 1.6. Which of the following is the *most* likely cause of this patient's liver disease?

a. Pancreatic cancer

b. Acute hepatitis A

c. Acetaminophen toxicity

d. Ischemic hepatitis

e. Alcoholic hepatitis

7. A 40-year-old man comes to the emergency department complaining of several days of fatigue and abdominal pain. The pain is described as dull, achy, and in the right upper quadrant. He says he does not use intravenous drugs but has infrequently used intranasal cocaine. He notes occasionally having sex with prostitutes, but none in the recent past. He states he does not take any regular medications except 4 to 6 tablets of acetaminophen (Extra-Strength Tylenol) daily because of abdominal pain. He describes himself as a social drinker but denies any problems of alcohol abuse. His wife nods in agreement. On physical examination, he appears fatigued. Temperature is 100.9°F, pulse rate 100 beats/min, and blood pressure 100/65 mm Hg. The sclerae are mildly icteric. Cardiac examination reveals a systolic flow murmur. Abdominal examination is notable for an enlarged, tender liver. There is no asterixis. Laboratory findings are as follows: hemoglobin 12.5 g/dL, mean corpuscular volume 108 fL, platelets 120×10^9/L, leukocytes 15.9×10^9/L with a left shift, blood urea nitrogen 29 mg/dL, creatinine 1.9 mg/dL, aspartate aminotransferase 96 U/L, alanine aminotransferase 60 U/L, γ-glutamyltransferase 430 U/L, alkaline phosphatase 220 U/L, total bilirubin 2.5 mg/dL, and ceruloplasmin 26 mg/dL. Ultrasonography of the liver demonstrates heterogenous echotexture without ascites. Which of the following is the most appropriate treatment option?

a. *N*-acetylcysteine 140 mg/kg orally

b. 40 mg of methylprednisolone daily

c. Chemical addiction counseling

d. Colchicine

e. Propylthiouracil

8. A 24-year-old man with a seizure disorder has liver biopsy because increased levels of liver enzymes have been observed for 6 months. A biopsy specimen shows prominent microvesicular steatosis. No inflammation or fibrosis is noted. Which of the following is *most* likely to contribute to this histologic finding?

a. Excess copper accumulation in the liver

b. Excess consumption of alcohol

c. Obesity

d. Diabetes mellitus

e. Valproic acid

9. A 31-year-old well driller has had abnormal liver function tests for 1 to 2 years. He complains of fatigue, pedal edema, and jaundice. He has drunk 1/3 of a bottle of brandy daily for about 10 years. He states he does not take recreational drugs or have a family history of liver problems. He has been taking chlordiazepoxide (Librium) and atenolol for 2 weeks. Physical examination findings are notable for tachycardia and low-grade fever. Scleral icterus is prominent. Abdominal examination shows shifting dullness. The liver span is increased to percussion. Laboratory values are as follows: hemoglobin 10.7 g/dL, mean corpuscular volume 105 fL, platelets 71×10^9/L, international normalized ratio 1.7, aspartate aminotransferase (AST) 130 U/L, alanine aminotransferase (ALT) 59 U/L, γ-glutamyltransferase (GGT) 587 U/L, alkaline phosphatase 279 U/L, total bilirubin 6.3 mg/dL, ceruloplasmin 19 mg/dL, creatinine 1.8 mg/dL, alpha$_1$-antitrypsin 228 mg/dL, iron 118 μg/dL, iron binding capacity 120 μg/dL, antinuclear antibody 2.7 U (mildly positive), smooth muscle antibody 1:20, and hepatitis serologic test negative. Ultrasonography of the liver demonstrates diffusely increased parenchymal echogenicity and splenomegaly. Which laboratory value is most predictive of the patient's survival?

a. Serum creatinine

b. ALT

c. AST

d. GGT

e. Alkaline phosphatase

10. A 30-year-old woman has vague right upper quadrant pain that increases after fatty meals. She does not have features typical of biliary colic, nor does she have features of cholangitis. She takes oral contraceptives. Physical examination

findings are unremarkable. Computed tomography of the abdomen is performed and the results are shown in the Figure. What would you recommend at this time?

a. Biopsy of the mass
b. Resect the mass
c. Angiography
d. Continue oral contraceptives
e. Radiofrequency tumor ablation

11. In Budd-Chiari syndrome, transjugular intrahepatic porto-systemic shunt is preferred to surgical shunts in all the following situations *except*:

a. Portal vein pressure 10 mm Hg less than infrahepatic inferior vena cava pressure
b. Myeloproliferative disorders with excellent long-term outcome
c. Patients with acute Budd-Chiari syndrome
d. Patients with pronounced ascites
e. Patients with Child-Pugh class C liver disease

12. A definite indication for antibiotic prophylaxis with norfloxacin for spontaneous bacterial peritonitis in patients with cirrhosis is:

a. Patients with ascites who are undergoing endoscopic sclerotherapy
b. Gastrointestinal tract bleeding without ascites
c. Ascites with gram-negative urinary infection
d. Ascites with albumin concentration < 1 g/dL
e. Patients with ascites who are undergoing esophageal dilatation

13. A patient with cirrhotic ascites has a daily dose of 100 mg spironolactone plus 40 mg furosemide. In spite of this, he is gaining approximately 500 g of weight daily. Laboratory values are as follows: bilirubin 2.8 mg/dL, creatinine 1.4 mg/dL, and serum sodium 129 mEq/L. Urinary sodium is 80 mEq/L, and daily urine output is 1.5 L. The most appropriate management should be:

a. Increase spironolactone to 200 mg
b. Increase furosemide to 80 mg
c. Increase both furosemide to 80 mg and spironolactone to 200 mg
d. Ensure sodium restriction to 90 mEq/d
e. Add torsemide (Demadex) 5 mg daily

14. You are asked to evaluate a 35-year-old man because of a family history of hereditary hemochromatosis. The patient's brother has the diagnosis of C282Y homozygous hereditary hemochromatosis. Your patient is completely asymptomatic and has no important medical problems. He does not take iron supplements and has no other risk factors

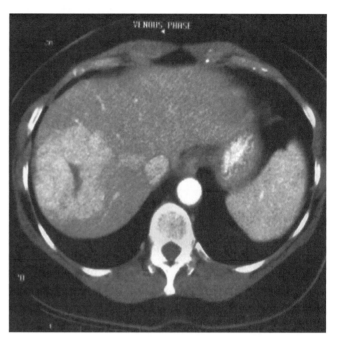

Question 10

for iron overload. Physical examination findings are entirely normal. Serum iron studies are noteworthy for the following: iron 180 µg/dL (normal, 50-150), transferrin saturation 78% (normal, 14%-50%), and serum ferritin 575 µg/L (normal, 20-300). A complete blood count and values for aspartate and alanine aminotransferases, alkaline phosphatase, and bilirubin are normal. *HFE* gene testing confirms the presence of two copies of the C282Y mutation. The most appropriate next step would be to:

a. Perform liver biopsy to confirm the diagnosis and exclude cirrhosis
b. Initiate therapeutic phlebotomy without liver biopsy
c. Do not prescribe phlebotomy because ferritin is increased only mildly
d. Initiate treatment with deferoxamine
e. Order magnetic resonance imaging of the liver, and if iron stores are increased, initiate therapeutic phlebotomy

15. You are asked to evaluate a 49-year-old man with increased serum iron values. Diabetes was recently diagnosed. His primary care physician checked serum transferrin saturation and ferritin to exclude hereditary hemochromatosis. His serum iron level was increased at 210 µg/dL (normal, 50-150) and transferrin saturation was 90% (normal, 14%-50%), with a serum ferritin level of 1,714 µg/L (normal, 20-300). The patient also has arthritis, mild impotence, and atrial fibrillation. He consumes 2 or 3 alcoholic beverages weekly and has done so for 30 years. Physical examination findings are noteworthy for a 2/6

systolic ejection murmur at the right upper sternal border, with an irregular heart rhythm. The rest of the examination findings are unremarkable. The levels of aspartate aminotransferase, alanine aminotransferase, alkaline phosphatase, and bilirubin are normal, as are the results of abdominal ultrasonography with Doppler examination of liver vasculature. *HFE* gene testing did not detect evidence of the C282Y or H63D mutations. What would you recommend next?

a. No additional evaluation

b. Initiate therapeutic phlebotomy

c. Liver biopsy

d. Magnetic resonance imaging (MRI) of the liver to look for iron deposition

16. A 28-year-old woman is referred to you because of a recently detected increase in transferrin saturation. As part of a routine health evaluation, serum iron studies were noteworthy for the following: iron 180 µg/dL (normal, 35-145), transferrin saturation of 80% (normal, 14%-50%), and ferritin 80 µg/L (normal, 20-200). The patient is healthy, with no important medical problems. She is completely asymptomatic. She does not take iron supplements and does not have other risk factors for secondary iron overload. Physical examination findings are completely normal. A fasting, morning transferrin saturation test is repeated, and transferrin saturation is increased to a similar degree. The most appropriate next step is:

a. Liver biopsy with quantification of hepatic iron

b. Abdominal ultrasonography with Doppler evaluation of liver vasculature

c. *HFE* gene testing

d. Screening for iron overload in patient's blood relatives

e. Therapeutic phlebotomy

17. A 21-year-old man has fulminant liver failure. He was well until 2 weeks before admission, when jaundice developed. One week later, he was hospitalized because of gradually progressive confusion. The patient is well, without other known medical problems. He does not drink alcohol. He denies risk factors for viral hepatitis. Physical examination findings are noteworthy for a somnolent patient who is arousable to voice. He has slight asterixis, scleral icterus, and deep jaundice. The physical findings are otherwise unremarkable. Laboratory tests show the following: hemoglobin 9.8 g/dL, uric acid 1.1 mg/dL (normal, 4.3-8.0), alkaline phosphatase 60 U/L (normal, 98-250), aspartate aminotransferase 300 U/L (normal, 12-31), alanine aminotransferase 70 U/L (normal, 10-45), total bilirubin 40.0 mg/dL (normal, 0.1-1.1), direct bilirubin 12 mg/dL (normal, 0-0.3), and international normalized

ratio 2.5. Serologic tests for hepatitis A, B, and C are negative, as are tests for antinuclear and smooth muscle antibodies. Serum ceruloplasmin level is 23.5 mg/dL (normal, 22.9-43.1). The alpha₁-antitrypsin phenotype is MM. Which of the following statements is true?

a. The normal value for ceruloplasmin essentially excludes the diagnosis of Wilson's disease

b. A slit-lamp examination should be performed to look for Kayser-Fleischer rings

c. The patient is too ill to be considered for liver transplantation

d. Liver biopsy should be the next diagnostic study

18. As part of a routine health evaluation, a 26-year-old man recently had liver tests and the results were noteworthy for aspartate aminotransferase 45 U/L (normal, 12-31) and alanine aminotransferase 68 U/L (normal, 10-45). The values for alkaline phosphatase, bilirubin, albumin, and prothrombin time are normal. A complete blood count was normal except for a slightly low platelet count of 120×10^9/L. His medical history is noteworthy for jaundice as an infant. This resolved after a few months, and he had no further problems with liver disease until recently. He is healthy, with no other medical problems. He does not take any medications. He drinks minimal alcohol. Relevant family history is cirrhosis in his brother. Abdominal ultrasonography demonstrates mildly coarsened hepatic echotexture, but the findings are otherwise unremarkable. Tests to exclude chronic causes of liver disease are noteworthy for an alpha₁-antitrypsin ZZ phenotype. You recommend the following:

a. *HFE* gene test

b. No further evaluation

c. Liver biopsy

d. Administration of alpha₁-antitrypsin

19. A 49-year-old woman was admitted to the hospital for "liver transplantation." She had been well until 3 months ago when she began gaining weight (16 lb). Two months ago, she recognized dark urine and yellow skin. Over the last month, fatigue developed and her "color worsened." She started spironolactone (Aldactone) therapy but gained another 12 lb. She received a blood transfusion in 1980. The family history is negative for liver disease, and she says she has not had exposure to hepatotoxic medications or chemicals. Tests for the following were negative: hepatitis B surface antigen, antibody to hepatitis B core, IgM antibody to hepatitis A virus, antibody to hepatitis C virus, antibody to human immunodeficiency virus, IgM antibody to cytomegalovirus, and IgM antibody to viral capsid antigen for Epstein-Barr virus. Physical examination

disclosed deep jaundice, protuberant abdomen, shifting dullness, hepatomegaly, moderate pitting leg edema to mid calves, and no asterixis. Paracentesis results were unremarkable. The rest of the evaluation showed the following: serum aspartate aminotransferase 624 U/L, bilirubin 11.9 mg/dL, γ-globulin 3.05 g/dL, albumin 2.01 g/dL, international normalized ratio 1.5, and antinuclear antibody 1:40. Tests for smooth muscle antibody and antibody to liver/kidney microsomes (anti-LKM)1 were negative. A liver biopsy specimen showed multilobular necrosis. What is the most appropriate treatment strategy?

a. Liver transplantation
b. Observation for at least 3 more months
c. Interferon and ribavirin
d. Prednisone 60 mg daily
e. Cyclosporine 6 mg/kg daily

20. A 41-year-old woman was given the diagnosis of autoimmune hepatitis in 1978, when she became jaundiced 1 month after a normal delivery. She had no risk factors for viral infection, and she had not received a blood transfusion. Prednisone therapy was started and continued for 18 months. She recovered fully, and the laboratory abnormalities resolved. She remained asymptomatic for 17 years. Eighteen months ago, she noted fatigue and laboratory tests disclosed the following: serum aspartate aminotransferase 256 U/L, alanine aminotransferase 275 U/L, bilirubin 1.2 mg/dL, smooth muscle antibody 1:80, and antinuclear antibody 1:40. A liver biopsy specimen showed "portal and lobular hepatitis, portal lymphoid aggregates, portal plasma cells, macrovesicular fat, and septal fibrosis." She was treated with prednisone and azathioprine for 6 months, but without improvement. Mercaptopurine (100 mg daily) was substituted for the azathioprine, and treatment was continued for another 10 months, without biochemical resolution. She was gaining weight and disturbed by her cushingoid appearance. Hepatitis C virus RNA was demonstrated in her serum with the polymerase chain reaction. What is the appropriate next treatment strategy?

a. Liver transplantation
b. Discontinuation of medication and weight reduction
c. Interferon and ribavirin after discontinuation of current therapy
d. High-dose prednisone 60 mg daily
e. Cyclosporine 6 mg/kg daily

21. A 38-year-old man presented with "abnormal liver tests" discovered during a routine insurance physical examination 6 months ago. Retrospectively, he had "felt weird" for at least 4 years. Test findings did not improve during a 2-month period of observation, and serologic studies were negative for hepatitis A, B, and C. Four months ago, a liver biopsy specimen showed "chronic hepatitis," and therapy was started with prednisone 15 mg daily. Treatment continued for the next 4 months, and laboratory test results improved, but the abnormalities did not resolve. There were no epidemiologic risk factors for viral infection, exposure to hepatotoxic medication or chemicals, or family history of liver disease. He had a past history of Graves' disease, and he had undergone thyroidectomy 16 years ago. Physical examination findings were normal. Laboratory evaluation disclosed increased serum levels of aspartate aminotransferase (146 U/L), bilirubin (1.1 mg/dL), γ-globulin (2.3 g/dL), immunoglobulin G (2260 mg/dL), and alkaline phosphatase (959 U/L). Serum titers of smooth muscle antibody (1:1,280) and antinuclear antibody (1:1,280) were increased, and antimitochondrial antibody was undetectable. A liver biopsy specimen showed periportal fibrosis, mild ductopenia, and mild interface hepatitis. Results of endoscopic retrograde cholangiopancreatography were negative. What is the best diagnosis?

a. Autoimmune hepatitis
b. Primary sclerosing cholangitis
c. Non-A, non-B, non-C hepatitis
d. Primary biliary cirrhosis
e. Autoimmune cholangitis

22. A 37-year-old woman with type 1 autoimmune hepatitis has been treated for 4 years with prednisone 20 mg daily. The laboratory indices of liver inflammation had improved to near normal, and she had been free of liver-related symptoms. She had gained 55 lb during the treatment interval and had developed insulin-requiring diabetes. During recent follow-up, her aspartate aminotransferase level had increased to 187 U/L. The alanine aminotransferase level was 205 U/L, bilirubin was 1.2 mg/dL, γ-globulin was 1.6 g/dL, and the antinuclear antibody titer was 1:40. Smooth muscle antibody, antibody to liver/kidney microsomes (anti-LKM)1, hepatitis B surface antigen, and antibodies to hepatitis A virus and hepatitis C virus were negative. What is the next course of action?

a. Liver biopsy
b. High-dose prednisone 60 mg daily
c. Azathioprine 150 mg daily, then prednisone withdrawal
d. Gastric bypass
e. Cyclosporine 6 mg/kg daily

23. A 28-year-old man was rejected as a blood donor because his serum level of aspartate aminotransferase was 123 U/L. He had quiescent chronic ulcerative colitis and no risk factors for alcohol-, viral- or drug-induced liver injury. Physical examination disclosed a slender habitus and no

icterus or hepatomegaly. Laboratory values included the following: alanine aminotransferase 102 U/L, alkaline phosphatase 221 U/L, γ-globulin 1.8 g/dL, and antinuclear antibody titer 1:80. Hepatitis B surface antigen and antibodies to hepatitis A virus, hepatitis C virus, and human immunodeficiency virus were undetectable. Ultrasonography of the liver was normal. Which diagnosis is most confidently excluded?

a. Autoimmune hepatitis
b. Chronic hepatitis C
c. Wilson's disease
d. Nonalcoholic steatohepatitis
e. Primary sclerosing cholangitis

24. A 70-year-old man developed osteomyelitis of the left tibia after a motor vehicle accident. His infectious disease consultant recommended long-term amoxicillin-clavulanate therapy. Four weeks after he started this treatment, his wife noticed he had yellow eyes. He also had dark urine and some mild pruritus but no other complaints. He was evaluated by his family physician, who noted the following: total bilirubin 7.2 mg/dL, bilirubin 5.3 mg/dL, alkaline phosphatase 852 U/L (upper limit of normal, 125), and mild absolute eosinophilia 7%. Serologic tests for hepatitis A, B, and C were negative, and ultrasonographic findings were unremarkable, with bile ducts of normal size. A liver biopsy specimen showed central zonal cholestasis, bile duct proliferation, and moderate portal inflammation with a high number of eosinophils. Drug hepatotoxicity was diagnosed, and he was sent home to be followed up on a weekly basis. Three weeks later, he returned to his local physician. Bilirubin was now 9.5 mg/dL, alkaline phosphatase 919 U/L, and alanine aminotransferase 70 U/L. Which of the following is true about this patient?

a. He is likely to develop biliary cirrhosis
b. A course of corticosteroids should be started at this time
c. Another biopsy should be performed to rule out acute hepatic necrosis
d. Observation alone should be continued
e. Start treatment with ursodiol to prevent progression of cholestatic disease

25. A 48-year-old woman presents with a 6-month history of gastroesophageal reflux and a 3-month history of dysphagia for solid foods, particularly bread and meat. She has a 20-year history of Raynaud's phenomena and now has noted that the skin over her fingers has tightened and red spots have developed over the dorsum of the fingers. She has loose stools 2 or 3 times a week. She states she does not have any bloody or black tarry stools. On physical examination, she has slight hepatomegaly and telangiectasia

over the dorsum of her fingers and around her mouth. No other findings were noted. Laboratory tests showed the following: total bilirubin 1.5 mg/dL, direct bilirubin 0.6 mg/dL, alkaline phosphatase 621 U/L (upper limit of normal, 140), alanine aminotransferase 90 U/L, and albumin 3.2 g/dL. An ultrasonographic study was negative. Which of the following tests is likely to give the diagnosis of her liver disease?

a. Endoscopic retrograde cholangiopancreatography
b. Antinuclear antibody
c. Anticentromere antibody
d. Hepatitis C virus RNA
e. Antimitochondrial antibody

26. An 11-year-old boy with known cystic fibrosis and pancreatic insufficiency presents with an increased level of alkaline phosphatase (1,100 U/L). His mother gives a past history of neonatal jaundice, which gradually resolved. He has no other symptoms of cholestasis at this time, particularly no history of fever and chills, pruritus, or other symptoms related to cholestasis. He has been taking antibiotics regularly, usually a quinolone. Physical examination findings are unremarkable except for a moderately enlarged liver. Laboratory values include the following: bilirubin 0.8 mg/dL, aspartate aminotransferase 61 U/L, and alkaline phosphatase 930 U/L. Testing for antimitochondrial antibody was negative. Ultrasonographic findings were unremarkable; endoscopic retrograde cholangiopancreatography visualized only the extrahepatic bile ducts, which were said to be normal. What finding is *unlikely* to be present on liver biopsy?

a. Enlarged foamy hepatocytes
b. Focal biliary cirrhosis
c. Steatosis
d. Intralobular bile ducts filled with mucin
e. Centrilobular cholestasis

27. A 46-year-old man has a 9-month history of an increased alkaline phosphatase level. His only symptom is occasional pruritus. He gives a 19-year history of chronic ulcerative colitis diagnosed on the basis of colonoscopy and colon biopsy when he was 30 years old. He has occasional episodes of bloody stools. Physical examination showed occasional skin excoriations and a slightly enlarged liver. Laboratory values included the following: total bilirubin 1.3 mg/dL, alkaline phosphatase 437 U/L, aspartate aminotransferase 56 U/L; CA19-9 is normal. Colonoscopy showed diffused erythema of the entire colon. Colon biopsy specimens are negative for dysplasia. Endoscopic retrograde cholangiopancreatography showed narrowing and beading of the entire extra- and intrahepatic biliary system, without

evidence of a dominant structure. A liver biopsy specimen showed stage 3 disease, with fibrotic duct lesions appearing throughout the biopsy specimen. The patient has read about ursodiol in the treatment of cholestatic liver disease. Which is true about ursodiol in the treatment of primary sclerosing cholangitis?

a. Prevents histologic progression of disease
b. Prolongs survival free of liver transplant
c. May decrease risk of developing colon and bile duct neoplasia
d. Delays the development of portal hypertension
e. May improve the symptoms of chronic ulcerative colitis

28. Six months ago, a 43-year-old woman of Irish descent was given the diagnosis of primary biliary cirrhosis on the basis of a positive antimitochondrial antibody and stage 1 disease detected with liver biopsy. The patient now presents with a 3-month history of a 15-lb weight loss, anemia, foul-smelling diarrhea, and skin rash. Physical examination findings are unremarkable. The iron level is 11 µg/dL, and saturation is 7%. Other laboratory values include vitamin A 210 µg/L (upper limit of normal, 360), total bilirubin 0.7 mg/dL, alkaline phosphatase 310 U/L, aspartate aminotransferase 54 U/L, and albumin 3.5 g/dL. Ultrasonographic and colonoscopic findings are negative. Computed tomography of the abdomen does not show any abnormality. Stool ova and parasites and pathogens are negative. Stool fat is 26 g/d on a 100-g fat diet. Examination of the skin reveals a papular, vesicular eruption on the elbows, knees, and trunk associated with burning and itching. The next step in this evaluation should be which of the following?

a. Diagnosis of irritable bowel syndrome and treatment with increased fiber
b. Treat with a low fat diet and medium-chain triglycerides for bile acid deficiency associated with primary biliary cirrhosis
c. Start pancreatic enzyme replacement therapy
d. Check anti-endomysial antibody
e. Treatment trial with metronidazole for bacterial overgrowth

29. A 24-year-old is at 10 weeks' gestation in her first pregnancy. She has had 2 days of nausea, vomiting, and mild fever. She is jaundiced but looks well and has mild tender hepatomegaly. Liver tests show the following: aspartate aminotransferase 860 U/L, alanine aminotransferase 1,156 U/L, and bilirubin 4.5 mg/dL. The most likely diagnosis is:

a. Hyperemesis gravidarum

b. Acute viral hepatitis
c. Acute cholecystitis
d. Intrahepatic cholestasis of pregnancy
e. Urinary tract infection

30. A 32-year-old is at 18 weeks' gestation of her third pregnancy. She is a minimal social drinker and takes no medications (prescribed or over-the-counter). During her last pregnancy and the earlier part of this pregnancy, she has had four episodes of continuous epigastric and right upper quadrant pain, each lasting about 12 hours and then resolving spontaneously. She now has been admitted with an episode of more severe epigastric pain and vomiting. She is distressed but hemodynamically stable and afebrile; the abdomen is diffusely tender but soft. Tests show the following: bilirubin 2.5 mg/dL, aspartate aminotransferase 75 U/L, alanine aminotransferase 48 U/L, alkaline phosphatase 310 U/L (normal to 215), amylase 1,200 U/L, and lipase 5,000 U/L. Ultrasonography shows gallstones in the gallbladder, the common bile duct is 5 mm in diameter without evidence of stone, and liver echotexture is normal with no bile duct dilatation. The patient is kept NPO (nothing by mouth) and given intravenous hydration. By day 4, the pain is gone; liver tests are near normal; and she has resumed eating. Her pregnancy continues normally. Which of the following is the next best step?

a. Endoscopic retrograde cholangiopancreatography to exclude common duct stone
b. Elective cholecystectomy after delivery
c. Laparoscopic cholecystectomy
d. Therapy with ursodiol
e. No further therapy

31. Which of the following is one of the necessary criteria for the diagnosis of HELLP syndrome?

a. Presence of preeclampsia
b. Subcapsular hematoma or parenchymal necrosis visible on computed tomography
c. Bilirubin > 5 mg/dL
d. Platelet count < 50 × 10^9/L
e. Abnormal blood smear

32. A 37-year-old healthy primigravida delivered a healthy baby by cesarian section 6 days earlier. She now presents with a 3-day history of increasing pain, distension, and vomiting. On physical examination, she is mildly jaundiced, dyspneic, and tachycardic; blood pressure is 110/70 mm Hg. Abdominal examination demonstrates hepatomegaly and tense ascites. She is mentally alert. Tests show the following: aspartate aminotransferase 2,800 U/L, alanine aminotransferase 2,292 U/L, bilirubin 3.0

mg/dL, albumin 3.2 mg/dL, international normalized ratio 3.6, lactate 3.0 mmol/L, PaO_2 (room air) 84 mm Hg, $PaCO_2$ 27 mm Hg, pH 7.38, base excess −8, and bicarbonate 18 mmol/L. The most likely diagnosis is:

a. Fulminant liver failure

b. Pulmonary embolus

c. Septic shock

d. Budd-Chiari syndrome

e. Herpes hepatitis

33. In patients with intrahepatic cholestasis of pregnancy (ICP), which of the following applies?

a. Babies should have screening tests for long-chain 3-hydroxyacyl-CoA (LCHAD) deficiency

b. ICP produces maternal distress from pruritus but no maternal or fetal morbidity

c. The most specific biochemical test for ICP is increased alkaline phosphatase level

d. Ursodiol can improve symptoms and liver tests

e. ICP always recurs in subsequent pregnancies

34. A 36-year-old man with a history of intravenous drug abuse is found to be positive for human immunodeficiency virus (HIV) and hepatitis C virus (HCV) infection. The CD4 count is 200, and he is asymptomatic. The aspartate aminotransferase level is 65 U/L and alanine aminotransferase is 103 U/L, and liver synthetic function is normal. A liver biopsy specimen shows moderate inflammation with minimal fibrosis. The most suitable therapy at this point is:

a. Simultaneous introduction of highly active antiretroviral therapy (HAART) and combination antiviral therapy for HCV

b. Simultaneous introduction of HAART and interferon therapy for HCV

c. Combination therapy for HCV, with close follow-up of HIV RNA levels

d. HAART with consideration for antiviral therapy in 2 months

35. A 34-year-old male homosexual with known human immunodeficiency virus (HIV) infection and a CD4 count of 36/μL presents with a 1.5-year history of worsening right upper quadrant pain. He has stopped taking all his medications over the past few months. On examination, he is afebrile, hemodynamically stable, and has no jaundice or stigmata of liver disease. Mild tenderness is noted in the right upper quadrant. Aspartate aminotransferase and alanine aminotransferase are each 140 U/L, alkaline phosphatase 755 U/L, and bilirubin 0.3 mg/dL. Computed tomography (CT) of the abdomen shows no focal masses or bile duct dilatation in the liver, no stones in the gallbladder, or any notable lymphadenopathy. The following statement is true about this patient:

a. Bacterial cholangitis is a likely diagnosis

b. Acquired immunodeficiency syndrome (AIDS) cholangiopathy is unlikely because the patient is not jaundiced

c. In the absence of any biliary abnormality found on CT, endoscopic retrograde cholangiopancreatography (ERCP) is unlikely to be helpful

d. This patient's chronic course is typical of AIDS cholangiopathy

36. The following is true of viral hepatitis in a patient infected with the human immunodeficiency virus (HIV):

a. The risk of acquisition of hepatitis C correlates with homosexual activity in men

b. The risk of acquisition of hepatitis C increases with HIV viral load and increasing immunosuppression

c. Vaccination against hepatitis B virus is rarely successful and may be contraindicated

d. Not only does HIV worsen hepatitis C but hepatitis C virus (HCV) potentiates progression of HIV infection to acquired immunodeficiency syndrome (AIDS)

e. On introducing highly active antiretroviral therapy (HAART), most patients with HCV infection will have worsening liver tests because of the hepatotoxicity of HAART, and the combination of antiretroviral medications must be selected carefully

37. A 35-year-old woman with Child-Pugh-Turcotte class A cirrhosis (6 points) secondary to hepatitis C is debilitated by persistent fatigue. She has esophageal varices that have never bled. She has no history of encephalopathy, has no ascites, and has no evidence of hepatocellular carcinoma. She inquires whether she is a candidate for liver transplantation. The most appropriate response would be to:

a. Perform a cardiopulmonary evaluation to determine her suitability as a transplant candidate

b. Explain that she does not fulfill the minimal listing criterion for liver transplantation for which the risk would outweigh potential benefit

c. Tell her that although cadaveric liver transplantation is not appropriate, the possibility of a living donor could be explored

d. Offer to obtain psychologic evaluation before pursuing liver transplantation

38. A 47-year-old liver transplant recipient develops a low-grade fever and a moderate increase (2-4 times the previous day's values) in bilirubin, alkaline phosphatase, aspartate aminotransferase, and alanine aminotransferase on the seventh

postoperative day. Ultrasonography with Doppler examination of the portal and hepatic vasculature is normal. The most appropriate management would be:

a. Check the laboratory values again the following morning
b. Perform liver biopsy
c. Obtain bacterial, fungal, and viral cultures, and perform liver biopsy if cultures are negative after 48 hours
d. Add a new immunosuppression agent, and biopsy if laboratory values do not improve

39. Which one of the following statements is true about liver transplantation?

a. Patients receiving a liver transplant for fulminant liver failure have a survival rate superior to that of patients who have transplantation for decompensated chronic liver disease
b. HLA matching between donor and recipient improves graft survival
c. Hepatocellular carcinoma is a contraindication for liver transplantation
d. The calcineurin inhibitors, cyclosporine and tacrolimus, are both associated with nephrotoxicity

40. A 58-year-old asymptomatic diabetic woman is evaluated because of abnormal liver enzymes discovered 8 months ago. Her only medication is glyburide. She drinks one glass of wine monthly. Physical examination findings are notable for moderate obesity. Laboratory tests are notable for the following: alanine aminotransferase (ALT) 104 U/L and aspartate aminotransferase (AST) 95 U/L. Hepatitis C virus antibody (anti-HCV) and hepatitis B surface antigen (HBsAg) are negative. Ultrasonography of the liver shows changes in liver echotexture consistent with fat. Which of the following is true about the most likely diagnosis?

a. Liver biopsy will exclude alcohol as a cause
b. Ursodiol is beneficial
c. Strong association with increased serum level of γ-globulin
d. Progresses to cirrhosis in a small fraction of patients
e. Gluten-free diet will improve aminotransferase levels

41. A 30-year-old asymptomatic man is referred for evaluation of abnormal liver enzymes. He started isoniazid (INH) and pyridoxine therapy 6 weeks ago because of a positive tuberculin skin test. Evaluation before the introduction of therapy included normal liver enzymes and no evidence of active tuberculosis on chest radiography and sputum specimens. Laboratory tests show the following: aspartate aminotransferase (AST) 73 U/L, alanine aminotransferase (ALT) 87 U/L, and total bilirubin 0.7 mg/dL. Which of the following should you do now?

a. Continue INH and pyridoxine therapy
b. Check hepatitis B surface antigen (HBsAg), antibody to hepatitis C virus (anti-HCV), antinuclear antibody (ANA), ceruloplasmin, and serum iron tests
c. Perform liver ultrasonography
d. Stop INH and pyridoxine therapy
e. Perform liver biopsy

42. A 68-year-old man is referred because of an abnormal level of alanine aminotransferase. Two weeks ago, he presented to his primary care provider with upper abdominal discomfort. Laboratory tests at that time demonstrated the following: alanine aminotransferase 212 U/L, aspartate aminotransferase 200 U/L, alkaline phosphatase 110 U/L, total bilirubin 1.5 mg/dL, direct bilirubin 0.4 mg/dL, and amylase 184 U/L. The pain improved after 12 hours, and he was sent to you for further assessment. The pain was epigastric, moderately severe, and associated with nausea but no vomiting. He now feels well, with a good appetite and stable weight. Liver enzymes were normal 1 year ago. He drinks one alcoholic beverage per month and says he has no risk factors for viral hepatitis. Past history is notable for hypertension and hyperlipidemia, and he has been taking metoprolol and atorvastatin for 2 years. Physical examination findings are notable only for mild obesity. Laboratory studies now include normal complete blood count, liver biochemistry values, and amylase. Right upper quadrant ultrasonography shows multiple small gallbladder stones, change in liver echotexture consistent with fat, and no bile duct dilatation. Abdominal computed tomography is negative except for changes in liver density consistent with fat. Which of the following would you advise now?

a. Observation with repeat liver tests in 3 months
b. Liver biopsy
c. Stop atorvastatin
d. Cholecystectomy
e. Esophagogastroduodenoscopy

43. A 43-year-old woman is sent to you for evaluation because of abnormal liver tests and fatigue. She says she has no abdominal pain, fluid retention, gastrointestinal tract bleeding, or changes in mental status. She currently drinks one bottle of wine daily and has done so for the last 15 years. She also has a remote history of intravenous drug abuse. She takes acetaminophen 1 g/d for long-standing low back pain. Physical examination findings are notable for spider angiomas and splenomegaly; there is no ascites, peripheral edema, or asterixis. Laboratory studies are notable for the following: hemoglobin 12.5 g/dL, leukocytes 6.9×10^9/L, platelets 24×10^9/L, total bilirubin 3.4 mg/dL, direct bilirubin 1.9 mg/dL, aspartate aminotransferase 121

U/L, alanine aminotransferase 58 U/L, international normalized ratio 1.5, and hepatitis C virus (HCV) RNA positive. Right upper quadrant ultrasonography shows the following: gallbladder stones, liver echotexture consistent with fat, patent umbilical vein, and splenomegaly. In addition to cessation of alcohol, which of the following would you advise?

a. Pegylated interferon and ribavirin therapy
b. Liver biopsy
c. Splenectomy
d. Administration of *N*-acetylcysteine
e. Liver ultrasonography every 6 months

44. A 15-year-old girl is referred because of abnormal liver tests. Two weeks ago, she had a sore throat, which was followed a week later by headache, mild fever, nausea, and anorexia. She has taken 2 to 4 naproxen tablets for each of the last 7 days but says she has not taken any other medications or illicit drugs, has not had any sexual activity, and has not used alcohol. Physical examination findings are notable for mild jaundice, mild enlargement of posterior cervical lymph nodes, and mild splenomegaly. Liver size and consistency are normal. Laboratory studies are notable for the following: hemoglobin 13 g/dL, leukocytes 6.1×10^9/L (with an automated differential of 32% neutrophils, 65% lymphocytes, and 3% monocytes), platelets 112×10^9/L, alanine aminotransferase 458 U/L, aspartate aminotransferase 354 U/L, alkaline phosphatase 180 U/L, total bilirubin 3.8 mg/dL, direct bilirubin 2.2 mg/dL, and international normalized ratio 1.0. Which of the following is most likely to lead to the diagnosis?

a. IgM antibody to hepatitis A virus
b. Heterophile antibody test (mononucleosis screen)
c. IgM antibody to hepatitis B core
d. Hepatitis C virus RNA
e. Stop naproxen and observe

45. A 45-year-old woman is referred because of abnormal liver tests. Three months ago, she was seen by her local physician because of a 9-month history of fatigue and arthralgias. Laboratory studies at that time included the following: aspartate aminotransferase 104 U/L, alanine aminotransferase 132 U/L, alkaline phosphatase 256 U/L, and total bilirubin 1.3 mg/dL. The patient considers herself in excellent health. She eats a nutritious diet, takes multiple vitamin supplements, exercises daily, and says she has no alcohol intake. There is no history of intravenous drug use. Physical examination findings are normal. Repeat liver enzymes 2 months later are essentially unchanged. Hepatitis B surface antigen, antibody to hepatitis B core, antibody to hepatitis C virus (HCV), antinuclear antibody, ceruloplasmin, and iron studies are negative or normal. A liver biopsy specimen shows a prominence of lipid-filled stellate cells, with mild perisinusoidal fibrosis. Which of the following is most appropriate at this time?

a. Cessation of vitamin supplements
b. Give ursodiol
c. Serologic studies for celiac sprue
d. Doppler ultrasonography of the liver
e. HCV RNA by polymerase chain reaction (PCR)

46. A previously well 23-year-old woman was brought to the emergency department by her family with a 1-week history of jaundice and confusion. She has no known risk factors for liver disease. Physical examination shows jaundice, asterixis, and no stigmata of chronic liver disease. Which of the following would you do next?

a. Arrange laboratory work and a clinic visit the following day
b. Make arrangements for transfer to a liver transplant center
c. Arrange for immediate abdominal computed tomography
d. Administer corticosteroids intravenously
e. Start *N*-acetylcysteine therapy

47. A 45-year-old Asian man presents for evaluation of hepatitis B. He recently tried to donate blood and was found to be positive for hepatitis B core antibody. He has no knowledge of previous liver disease, although his mother died at age 50 of hepatocellular carcinoma and a younger sister has hepatitis B. He is asymptomatic. Physical examination findings are normal. Laboratory tests were normal, including a complete blood count, alanine and aspartate aminotransferase levels, bilirubin, albumin, and international normalized ratio. Hepatitis markers are as follows: positive hepatitis B surface antigen, positive IgG antibody to hepatitis B core, negative IgM antibody to hepatitis B core, negative hepatitis B e antigen, and hepatitis B virus (HBV) positive at 2,000 copies/mL. Which of the following would you recommend now?

a. Interferon
b. Adefovir
c. Lamivudine
d. Referral for liver transplantation
e. Liver ultrasonography

48. A liver transplant surgeon calls with a question about a potential liver donor. The donor is a former intravenous drug user who was involved in a motor vehicle accident and has been declared brain dead. The liver enzymes are normal

and hepatitis B surface antigen is negative, but IgG antibody to hepatitis B core and antibody to hepatitis B surface are positive. Which of the following is most correct?

a. The donor cannot transmit hepatitis B to a liver recipient
b. The donor is immune because of previous vaccination
c. The liver should not be used
d. The liver could be used for a hepatitis B-positive recipient
e. The donor likely has high levels of hepatitis B virus (HBV) DNA in the serum

49. A 53-year-old Asian man is admitted with a 1-week history of jaundice and fatigue. There is no previous history of liver disease or alcohol use. He is not aware of a family history of liver disease. He denies intravenous drug use, and he has had a long-standing monogamous relationship. His only medications are metoprolol 25 mg/d for hypertension (has been taking the medication for 2 years) and acetaminophen 1 g/d for 1 week. Laboratory studies include the following: hemoglobin 12.8 g/dL, platelets 97×10^9/L, international normalized ratio 2.4, albumin 2.8 g/dL, aspartate aminotransferase 1,048 U/L, alanine aminotransferase 948 U/L, and alkaline phosphatase 135 U/L. Hepatitis tests are as follows: positive for hepatitis B surface antigen, IgM antibody to hepatitis B core (anti-HBc), and hepatitis B e antigen; hepatitis B virus DNA 1 million copies/mL; negative for hepatitis A virus antibody and hepatitis C virus RNA. The patient's condition deteriorates, and he undergoes emergent liver transplantation. Pathology examination of the explant demonstrates cirrhosis, with a superimposed acute hepatitis and an 8-mm hepatocellular carcinoma in the peripheral right lobe. Immunostains for hepatitis B are positive. Which of the following is the most likely cause of the patient's decompensation?

a. Acute hepatitis B
b. Acute exacerbation of chronic hepatitis B
c. Hepatocellular carcinoma
d. Metoprolol-induced hepatitis
e. Acetaminophen-induced hepatitis

50. A 54-year-old man is referred because of a 6-month history of an abnormal alanine aminotransferase value. He used intravenous drugs 30 years ago. Physical examination findings are notable for splenomegaly and spider angiomas. Laboratory tests are notable for alanine aminotransferase 83 U/L, aspartate aminotransferase 62 U/L, platelets 86×10^9/L, albumin 3.6 g/dL, international normalized ratio 1.2, and positive for antibody to hepatitis C virus (HCV). Which one of the following statements is most correct?

a. Bone marrow biopsy should be performed because of the thrombocytopenia
b. Surveillance for hepatocellular carcinoma is advised
c. Splenectomy should be performed to treat thrombocytopenia
d. HCV RNA is likely to be negative
e. Hepatitis C treatment is contraindicated

51. A 38-year-old man is being treated for chronic hepatitis C, which he likely acquired 23 years ago during a brief period of intravenous drug use. His pretreatment data included the following: alanine aminotransferase (ALT) 84 U/L; normal values for bilirubin, albumin, and international normalized ratio; hepatitis C virus (HCV) genotype 1b; and HCV RNA level 857,000 U/mL. A liver biopsy specimen showed a mild lymphocytic portal infiltrate and portal (stage 1) fibrosis. After 3 months of pegylated interferon and ribavirin therapy, ALT is 75 U/L and the HCV RNA level is 700,000 IU/mL. Which of the following would you advise?

a. Continue pegylated interferon and ribavirin and check HCV RNA in 3 months
b. Stop pegylated interferon and continue ribavirin for an additional 6 months
c. Stop pegylated interferon and ribavirin, no further treatment at this time
d. Continue pegylated interferon and ribavirin, add amantadine
e. Ultrasonography and alpha fetoprotein measurement every 6 months

52. A 43-year-old man is referred for evaluation for persisting jaundice. He is a day-care employee who developed acute hepatitis A 3 months ago. At that time, his alanine aminotransferase (ALT) was 1,234 U/L, total bilirubin 4.6 mg/dL, and IgM antibody to hepatitis A virus was positive. The patient was observed and the ALT value improved, but he has continued to have hyperbilirubinemia. He is tired and has mild pruritus but otherwise feels well, with a good appetite and stable weight. He says he does not have any abdominal pain or fever. He takes no medications. Physical examination findings are notable only for jaundice. Laboratory results are as follows: ALT 236 U/L, total bilirubin 6.8 mg/dL, direct bilirubin 4.2 mg/dL, alkaline phosphatase 400 U/L, international normalized ratio 1.3, albumin 3.7 g/dL, and γ-globulin 1.3 g/dL. Ultrasonography of the liver is negative except for a small amount of sludge in the gallbladder. Which one of the following would you do next?

a. Endoscopic retrograde cholangiopancreatography
b. Magnetic resonance cholangiopancreatography

c. Endoscopic ultrasonography

d. Liver biopsy

e. Repeat laboratory tests in 1 month

53. A 53-year-old man presents with ascites. He has a history of chronic hepatitis B, and liver biopsy 10 years ago documented cirrhosis. He was given interferon therapy at that time but did not have seroconversion of hepatitis B e antigen (HBeAg). He takes no medications. Physical examination findings are notable for mild jaundice, spider angiomas, and ascites. There is no encephalopathy. Laboratory studies show the following: alanine aminotransferase 86 U/L, total bilirubin 4.3 mg/dL, direct bilirubin 2.4 mg/dL, albumin 2.9 g/dL, international normalized ratio 1.5, hemoglobin 11.8 g/dL, leukocytes 3.4×10^9/L with normal differential, and platelets 66×10^9/L. Hepatitis serologic findings are as follows: positive for hepatitis B surface antigen, IgG antibody to hepatitis B core, and HBeAg; hepatitis B virus (HBV) DNA 1.6 million copies/mL; negative for antibody to hepatitis B e and hepatitis C virus RNA. Liver ultrasonography shows a 2-cm mass worrisome for hepatocellular carcinoma. Which one of the following is most correct about this patient?

a. Liver transplantation is contraindicated

b. Interferon should be administered

c. Lamivudine or adefovir should be administered

d. Esophagogastroduodenoscopy is contraindicated

e. Use of acetaminophen is prohibited

54. A 36-year-old man with a history of intravenous drug use is found to be positive for human immunodeficiency virus (HIV) and hepatitis C virus (HCV) infection. The CD4 count is 100/µL, and he had a recent episode of *Pneumocystis carinii* pneumonia. On laboratory testing, aspartate aminotransferase is 65 U/L and alanine aminotransferase 103 U/L; liver synthetic function is normal. A liver biopsy specimen shows mild inflammation with no fibrosis. Which one of the following would you advise now?

a. Simultaneous introduction of combination antiviral therapy for HCV and highly active antiretroviral therapy (HAART)

b. Simultaneous introduction of interferon therapy for HCV and HAART

c. Combination therapy for HCV, with close follow-up of HIV RNA levels

d. HAART, with consideration for HCV therapy in 2 months

e. Interferon monotherapy for HCV, with close follow-up of HIV RNA levels

55. A 35-year-old man is referred for evaluation of hepatitis C. He is otherwise well. Hepatitis C was diagnosed 3 months ago when he attempted to donate blood. He used intravenous drugs 10 years ago. Laboratory tests are notable for the following: alanine aminotransferase 83 U/L, aspartate aminotransferase 52 U/L, and normal bilirubin, albumin, and prothrombin time. The hepatitis C viral (HCV) level is 120,000 IU/mL (600,000 copies/mL) and the HCV genotype is 3. A liver biopsy specimen demonstrates portal and periportal inflammation and incomplete septal fibrosis. Which of the following would you recommend at this point?

a. Pegylated interferon and ribavirin for 6 months

b. Pegylated interferon and ribavirin for 3 months, then check HCV level

c. Pegylated interferon and ribavirin for 12 months

d. Pegylated interferon for 1 month, then check HCV RNA by polymerase chain reaction

e. Pegylated interferon for 6 months

56. A 49-year-old woman is referred with hepatitis C, which she likely acquired 24 years earlier after receiving a blood transfusion for postpartum hemorrhage. Her complaints include fatigue, arthralgias, and mild right upper quadrant pain. Past medical history is notable for depression, which required electroconvulsive therapy. She now takes sertraline. Physical examination findings are notable only for a depressed affect. Laboratory studies show the following: hemoglobin 14 g/dL, platelets 124×10^9/L, aspartate aminotransferase (AST) 64 U/L, alanine aminotransferase (ALT) 63 U/L, total bilirubin 1.2 mg/dL, albumin 3.8 g/dL, and international normalized ratio 1.1. Other results are as follows: hepatitis C viral (HCV) level is 125,000 copies/mL, HCV genotype 2, negative for hepatitis B surface antigen and hepatitis B e antigen, positive for antibodies to hepatitis B core, undetectable hepatitis B virus DNA, negative for rheumatoid factor, and positive for antinuclear antibody at 1:40 dilution. Abdominal ultrasonography shows a coarse echotexture of liver and spleen at the limits of normal size. Which of the following would you recommend now?

a. Interferon and lamivudine combination therapy

b. Empiric course of corticosteroid therapy

c. Liver biopsy

d. Pegylated interferon and ribavirin combination therapy

e. Determination of cryoglobulins

ANSWERS

1. Answer d

She has a classic cavernous hemangioma. The abdominal pain is likely abdominal wall discomfort. Cavernous hemangiomas are seldom estrogen-sensitive, unlikely to cause symptoms, and do not pose a threat for rupture or malignant degeneration. The increased ALT level is from fatty liver. Although fine-needle aspiration can be performed without a high risk for bleeding, a histologic diagnosis is not necessary. The gallbladder mass is consistent with a benign polyp and can be observed.

2. Answer b

The lesion is classic for focal nodular hyperplasia. A central scar is present in only 20% of small lesions of this condition. The lesions are not at risk for rupture, bleeding, or malignant degeneration.

3. Answer a

The imaging characteristics and tumor marker studies demonstrated that the lesion is intrahepatic cholangiocarcinoma. No further evaluation is warranted, and resection is the best treatment option.

4. Answer d

The presence of contrast-enhancing lesions in a cirrhotic liver in conjunction with likely right portal vein tumor thrombosis is diagnostic of hepatocellular carcinoma.

5. Answer c

The patient has a liver abscess that arose from the prostatitis.

6. Answer c

The liver enzyme pattern is least consistent with alcoholic hepatitis because of the marked increase in the aminotransferase levels. With alcoholic hepatitis, the increase in aminotransferase levels is rarely more than 5 to 10 times the upper limit of normal. In alcoholics, therapeutic consumption of acetaminophen can result in acetaminophen toxicity that may be demonstrated by the laboratory test abnormalities observed in this patient. Acute hepatitis A occasionally may have a severe course, particularly in patients with underlying chronic liver disease, as suggested in this patient by the presence of spider angiomas and palmar erythema. This is the rationale for immunization against viral hepatitis in patients with chronic liver disease. However, risk factors are more supportive of acetaminophen toxicity. Alcoholics are predisposed to cardiomyopathy with low cardiac output. This suggests the possibility of a "shock liver" with markedly increased aminotransferase levels, as observed in this patient. The aminotransferase levels often improve rapidly and dramatically after correction of the hemodynamic insult in ischemic hepatitis, in contradistinction to viral hepatitis and toxic hepatitis, in which aminotransferases remain at high levels. However, hypotension is not described in this patient. Pancreatic cancer may be present with biliary obstruction and back pain, but the high aminotransferase levels do not support this diagnosis.

7. Answer c

This patient most likely has mild alcoholic hepatitis. The case reflects the difficulty often encountered in obtaining an accurate history of alcohol use. The CAGE questionnaire can be useful in such situations. Despite the absence of histologic confirmation in this case, the physical examination laboratory findings are most consistent with alcoholic hepatitis. Positivity for antibodies to hepatitis C virus is prevalent among patients with alcohol abuse. However, in this case, the aminotransferase ratio is more suggestive of alcoholic hepatitis than viral hepatitis, although further serologic testing for metabolic and viral disease should be performed. However, without an increase in prothrombin time and only a mild increase in the bilirubin level, corticosteroid therapy is not indicated. Although alcohol abuse reduces the threshold for acetaminophen toxicity, the aminotransferase pattern in this case is not very high or consistent with the diagnosis of acetaminophen toxicity. The most important treatment options for this patient focus on achieving and maintaining abstinence, nutritional assessment and support, and observation for deterioration in clinical status.

8. Answer e

Valproic acid can cause fatty liver, and the pattern is distinctly microvesicular and not macrovesicular. Wilson's disease occurs because of excess copper accumulation in hepatocytes and may produce various histologic patterns, including macrovesicular steatosis. Fatty liver from an alcohol binge also produces a macrovesicular pattern. Both obesity and diabetes are associated with nonalcoholic fatty liver, a condition with macrovesicular steatosis.

9. Answer a

The serum level of creatinine is highly predictive of survival for patients with liver disease, particularly alcoholic hepatitis. Other predictive blood tests include the international normalized ratio and bilirubin, although these choices are not provided. Other liver enzymes, such as AST, ALT, alkaline phosphatase, and GGT, have no prognostic usefulness in alcoholic hepatitis.

10. Answer d

Computed tomography demonstrates three classic features of focal nodular hyperplasia: 1) hyperintense on arterial phase (focal nodular hyperplasia is hypointense without contrast and isointense on the portal venous phase), 2) central scar, and 3) a lead vessel. As many as 98% of cases are asymptomatic. Complications such as rupture, bleeding, and malignancy probably never occur. Surgery is indicated if the diagnosis is uncertain or if patient has abdominal pain due to the mass. Patients may continue to take oral contraceptives, and pregnancy is not contraindicated if the diagnosis of focal nodular hyperplasia is certain.

11. Answer b

Surgical portosystemic shunts are contraindicated in the presence of a low pressure gradient (< 10 mm Hg) between the portal vein and infrahepatic inferior vena cava (because the shunt is not likely to function). Shunt surgery is also contraindicated in patients with acute Budd-Chiari syndrome, pronounced ascites, or Child-Pugh Class C liver disease because of the increased mortality risk. Surgical shunts are best placed in patients in whom the underlying thrombophilia has an excellent long-term prognosis.

12. Answer b

There are only two clear indications for antibiotic prophylaxis for spontaneous bacterial peritonitis in patients with cirrhosis: 1) for patients with gastrointestinal tract bleeding with or without ascites (norfloxacin 400 mg twice daily for 7 days) and 2) for patients who have previously had spontaneous bacterial peritonitis (norfloxacin 400 mg once daily indefinitely or until liver transplantation). In up to 50% of patients with bleeding, gram-negative infections occur at 1 week and are associated with increased rebleeding risk and mortality. Ascitic fluid albumin concentration < 1 g/dL is not a definite indication for antibiotic prophylaxis.

13. Answer d

The patient is excreting 120 mEq of sodium daily in urine. Therefore, the diuretic dose is adequate (target sodium excretion should be about 120 mEq/d on a 90-mEq sodium-restricted diet to ensure weight loss of about 250 g/d). The patient is gaining weight because of noncompliance with sodium restriction, the most common cause of increasing ascites.

14. Answer b

Before the availability of the *HFE* gene test, liver biopsy was important to confirm the diagnosis of hereditary hemochromatosis. However, with the availability of the *HFE* gene test, liver biopsy is not necessary to confirm the diagnosis of hereditary hemochromatosis in patients who are homozygous for the C282Y mutation and have increased values for serum iron studies and no risk factors for secondary iron overload. The other reason to perform liver biopsy is to exclude cirrhosis. This is important because patients with hereditary hemochromatosis and cirrhosis have a 200-fold increased risk of developing hepatocellular carcinoma. Although liver biopsy is the gold standard for determining the presence or absence of cirrhosis, several clinical and laboratory measures are fairly good at excluding cirrhosis. Cirrhosis is not usually present in C282Y homozygotes with a ferritin level < 1,000 µg/L, especially if they have normal liver tests, no hepatomegaly, and are younger than 40 years. Of all these variables, the serum ferritin level is best at predicting the absence of cirrhosis. Although the negative predictive value of these variables is good, the positive predictive value is not. That is, patients who do not meet these criteria still need liver biopsy to determine whether they have cirrhosis. Because our patient meets all the criteria to suggest a low risk of cirrhosis, liver biopsy could reasonably be avoided. Therapeutic phlebotomy is the treatment of choice for patients with hereditary hemochromatosis. It is simple, inexpensive, and effective. It is recommended in patients with hereditary hemochromatosis after their serum ferritin level increases. For this reason, our patient should begin therapeutic phlebotomy. Treatment with the iron chelator deferoxamine is more expensive, less effective, and requires subcutaneous administration. Unlike secondary iron overload due to anemias with ineffective erythropoiesis, iron chelators are rarely used to treat iron overload due to hereditary hemochromatosis.

15. Answer c

The patient has a markedly increased serum level of ferritin in the absence of a C282Y or H63D hemochromatosis gene mutation. On average, approximately 85% of patients with the clinical diagnosis of hereditary hemochromatosis are homozygous for the C282Y gene mutation. There is marked geographic variability, however, with the prevalence of homozygosity for C282Y ranging from 60% to 100%. Nearly all studies have demonstrated that clinically important iron overload can occur in the absence of *HFE* gene mutations. This could be due to undiscovered genetic mutations, environmental factors, or both. Several additional *HFE* and non-*HFE*–related genetic mutations have been discovered recently. These generally are uncommon and rarely of clinical importance. Although the results of abdominal ultrasonography and liver tests are normal, the patient still could have markedly increased total body iron stores or even cirrhosis. Although there are a few reports that MRI can detect increased hepatic iron stores, the results are sufficiently variable that currently MRI cannot be used to reliably predict hepatic iron overload. Also, MRI cannot definitely exclude cirrhosis. Therefore, liver biopsy with quantification of hepatic iron is the best answer. This will allow definitive exclusion or diagnosis of cirrhosis and also will allow hepatic iron stores to be determined. If the hepatic iron stores are markedly elevated, phlebotomy should be initiated regardless of the results of the *HFE* gene test.

16. Answer c

Hereditary hemochromatosis is diagnosed on the basis of the combination of clinical, laboratory, and pathologic criteria, including increased serum transferrin saturation. A transferrin saturation >45% is the earliest phenotypic abnormality in hereditary hemochromatosis. This occurs before an increase in the serum level of ferritin or in hepatic iron stores or other disease manifestations. The patient in this question could have hereditary hemochromatosis, with the only phenotypic abnormality being increased serum transferrin saturation. It is not uncommon for young patients with hereditary hemochromatosis (especially females, because of menstrual blood loss and pregnancies) to fit into this diagnostic category. The most appropriate next step in the evaluation would be *HFE* gene testing. Liver biopsy or abdominal ultrasonography is not necessary when the serum level of ferritin and liver tests are normal. Screening for iron overload in blood relatives may be necessary, but first the diagnosis of hemochromatosis should be confirmed with the *HFE* gene test. Therapeutic phlebotomy is reserved for hemochromatosis patients with iron overload as indicated by an increased serum level of ferritin. Even if this patient is homozygous for C282Y, therapeutic phlebotomy would not be initiated because the ferritin level is normal.

17. Answer b

The patient most likely has Wilson's disease presenting as an acute fulminant hepatitis. Wilson's disease should always be considered in children and young adults who have acute or chronic liver disease. In support of the diagnosis of Wilson's disease is the anemia, indirect hyperbilirubinemia, and low levels of uric acid and alkaline phosphatase. Patients with fulminant Wilson's disease may have a normal serum level of ceruloplasmin because ceruloplasmin is an acute phase reactant and may be increased in various inflammatory conditions. However, it is rare in this setting for ceruloplasmin levels to exceed 30 mg/dL. Kayser-Fleischer rings are not specific for Wilson's disease and can occur in conditions associated with cholestasis, such as primary biliary cirrhosis and primary sclerosing cholangitis. However, the presence of Kayser-Fleischer rings in a young patient with fulminant liver failure would make Wilson's disease likely. If Kayser-Fleischer rings are not seen on a slit-lamp examination, liver biopsy would be reasonable to consider if the patient's coagulopathy could be corrected. Because of his coagulopathy, a transjugular liver biopsy may be necessary. Liver biopsy would allow the copper level to be quantified, and this is the gold standard for confirming the diagnosis of Wilson's disease. Most patients with Wilson's disease have liver copper concentrations >250 µg/g dry weight. Normal concentration of copper in the liver would exclude the diagnosis, and values <250 µg/g dry weight would make the diagnosis of Wilson's disease less likely.

18. Answer c

The patient has alpha₁-antitrypsin deficiency. This is suggested by a history of jaundice as an infant and a family history of cirrhosis. The alpha₁-antitrypsin ZZ phenotype confirms the diagnosis. Alpha₁-antitrypsin phenotype is the appropriate test to diagnose alpha₁-antitrypsin deficiency. The alpha₁-antitrypsin level should not be used because it can be falsely increased in patients with an inflammatory disorder or malignancy or in those who are pregnant or receiving estrogen supplementation. Patients with alpha₁-antitrypsin deficiency are at risk for developing cirrhosis. The deficiency causes neonatal hepatitis in 15% to 30% of children with the ZZ phenotype. Although neonatal hepatitis tends to improve over time, it can lead to progressive liver disease and cirrhosis in approximately 10% of patients. Patients with cirrhosis due to alpha₁-antitrypsin deficiency are at greatly increased risk for the development of hepatocellular carcinoma. That this patient has mild liver test abnormalities and nearly normal ultrasonographic findings does not exclude the presence of cirrhosis. The low platelet count is a clue that he might, in fact, have cirrhosis. For this reason, liver biopsy should be performed. If cirrhosis is present, the patient should periodically have screening tests for hepatocellular carcinoma and varices. Although hemochromatosis should be considered in anyone with a family history of cirrhosis, determining serum transferrin saturation and ferritin level and not the *HFE* gene test would be the most appropriate initial test. Occasionally, infusions of alpha₁-antitrypsin are used to treat emphysema but not liver disease due to alpha₁-antitrypsin deficiency.

19. Answer d

The laboratory and histologic findings support the diagnosis of autoimmune hepatitis. Alternative diagnoses for conditions that might resemble autoimmune hepatitis have been excluded. The acute onset is compatible with the diagnosis, and the presence of ascites does not preclude responsiveness to corticosteroid therapy. Low-titer antinuclear antibodies cannot be ignored as a diagnostic clue. The decision for liver transplantation is best made after evaluating the response to treatment and can be made within 2 weeks.

20. Answer c

Autoantibodies occur in 30% of patients with chronic hepatitis C, typically in low titer (<1:320). The histologic findings of portal lymphoid aggregates, macrovesicular fat, and cholestasis suggest a viral rather than autoimmune basis for the disease despite the presence of plasma cells. The long interval between the first disease and the second make relapse of the original condition unlikely, even if it was autoimmune hepatitis. The recalcitrance to corticosteroid therapy suggests another disease process. The patient has advanced fibrosis, and immunosuppressive therapy should be withdrawn and antiviral treatment started.

21. Answer e

Male sex and lack of improvement with corticosteroid therapy diminish the likelihood of autoimmune hepatitis. Concurrent autoimmune disease (past history of Graves' disease) indicates a host predisposition for immune reactivity, but it does not compel a specific liver diagnosis. The more than threefold increase in the serum level of alkaline phosphatase is atypical of classic autoimmune hepatitis and suggests a cholestatic syndrome. Similarly, the liver biopsy findings suggest a biliary process. Classic primary biliary cirrhosis and primary sclerosing cholangitis are discounted by serologic and radiographic studies. The inability to confidently classify the disease in conventional diagnostic categories indicates a variant syndrome. The autoantibodies, history of Graves' disease, and features of cholestasis justify the diagnosis of autoimmune cholangitis. "Autoimmune cholangitis" is a generic term that encompasses antimitochondrial antibody-negative primary biliary cirrhosis, small-duct primary sclerosing cholangitis, and autoimmune hepatitis with coincidental bile duct injury, and it is destined to disappear as its components are defined.

22. Answer a

The deterioration of laboratory values despite compliance with corticosteroid treatment suggests treatment failure. The biochemical change, however, has occurred after 4 years of continuous therapy, in the absence of clinical decompensation (ascites) and in conjunction with obesity and diabetes. Another basis for the laboratory change must be considered, and liver biopsy is necessary to establish the diagnosis. The presence of nonalcoholic steatohepatitis would justify withdrawal of prednisone therapy, use of azathioprine as a corticosteroid-sparing agent, and greater effort controlling weight and diabetes.

23. Answer b

The asymptomatic state, lean body weight, and mild serum aminotransferase abnormalities do not exclude nonalcoholic steatohepatitis or autoimmune hepatitis as diagnostic possibilities. The ulcerative colitis suggests the possibility of primary sclerosing cholangitis, and the young age raises the possibility of Wilson's disease. Normal findings on ultrasonography of the liver do not exclude steatosis because 30% of hepatocytes must be involved to generate a bright image. There are no factors, such as immune deficiency or immunosuppressive therapy, that might result in a falsely negative test for hepatitis C virus antibodies. Therefore, chronic hepatitis C infection is the least likely diagnosis.

24. Answer d

Patients with amoxicillin-clavulanate hepatotoxicity have a cholestatic biochemical profile for up to 8 months before

resolution. This is nearly always a benign condition, and biliary cirrhosis has not been described as a complication of amoxicillin-clavulanate hepatotoxicity.

25. Answer e

Of patients with primary biliary cirrhosis, 7% to 9% have CREST syndrome and more than 90% have antimitochondrial antibody. CREST syndrome is characterized by the presence of the anticentromere antibody, although this is not diagnostic of the liver disease.

26. Answer a

Cystic fibrosis involves a secretion defect in the biliary epithelium, which causes small ducts to fill and become obstructed with a mucinlike material. This often forms what is called "focal biliary cirrhosis," which is characteristic of cystic fibrosis, particularly in an older child.

27. Answer c

Currently, no data show that ursodiol retards or prevents the progression of disease, nor does it have any effect on symptoms related to chronic ulcerative colitis. Several reports suggest that it may reduce the risk of both colonic and bile duct neoplasia.

28. Answer d

Test for endomysial antibody because up to 7% of patients with primary biliary cirrhosis have associated celiac disease. Celiac disease is also more common in patients with an Irish or Scottish background, and although pancreatic insufficiency is a possibility, the rash is consistent with dermatitis herpetiformis, which is commonly associated with celiac disease. The symptoms, including malabsorption and dermatitis herpetiformis, respond to a gluten-free diet, which has no effect on primary biliary cirrhosis.

29. Answer b

Acute viral hepatitis is the commonest cause of jaundice in a pregnant patient; the high aminotransferase levels are consistent with this diagnosis. Hyperemesis gravidarum is excluded by the lack of intractable vomiting that requires intravenous hydration. The liver tests and clinical picture are not typical of acute cholecystitis or urinary infection.

30. Answer c

This patient has gallstones and has had several episodes of pain consistent with biliary colic. She now has acute pancreatitis and abnormal liver tests suggestive of gallstone pancreatitis. She is in the second trimester of pregnancy, with 22 weeks to term. Biliary colic tends to continue once it starts in pregnancy (30% recurrence), and now that pancreatitis is present, it would be considered an indication to proceed to cholecystectomy. Pancreatitis has high maternal (10%) and fetal (13%) mortality in pregnancy. Cholecystectomy is best performed in the second trimester, and doing it now would avoid the high risk of recurrence of symptoms before the pregnancy is over. The procedure can be done safely either laparoscopically or by open method if needed.

31. Answer e

The criteria for HELLP are the presence of all three of the following: 1) hemolysis, with an abnormal blood smear, increased lactate dehydrogenase level, and an increase in indirect bilirubin (but rarely >5 mg/dL); 2) aspartate aminotransferase >70 U/L; and 3) platelet count <100 × 10^9/L. Only the abnormal blood smear is essential from the above list, although preeclampsia is common (80%), as are computed tomographic abnormalities.

32. Answer d

The clinical picture of postpartum occurrence of hepatomegaly and ascites with high aminotransferase levels of sudden onset is typical of Budd-Chiari syndrome. The other diagnoses do not fit the entire picture described here.

33. Answer d

Ursodiol has been shown in small, randomized trials to improve both pruritus and liver tests. ICP recurs in only 45% to 70% of pregnancies. Its main danger is to the fetus, and it can cause acute fetal death. The alkaline phosphatase level is generally unhelpful; the most specific biochemical marker is increased bile acid levels. LCHAD deficiency occurs in babies of mothers with acute fatty liver of pregnancy.

34. Answer d

In a patient with newly diagnosed HIV and HCV coinfection, the priority is to treat the HIV infection, especially because in this patient the hepatitis C is mild-moderate with little fibrosis here. Because HAART is often associated with liver abnormalities, it is less confusing clinically to initiate therapy sequentially, obtain a response in terms of HIV viral load, and follow this as anti-HCV therapy is introduced.

35. Answer d

In a patient with established AIDS, as here (CD4 count 36/μL), the chronic course and liver tests with normal bilirubin level but increased alkaline phosphatase level are typical of AIDS cholangiopathy; jaundice is rare; computed tomographic findings are abnormal in only about 70% of cases; and ERCP is essential. Bacterial cholangitis is unusual unless the biliary tree has been instrumented.

36. Answer a

The risk of acquisition of HCV and HIV are independent of each other. Vaccination against hepatitis B virus is successful in at least 50% of patients and, thus, should be done; there is no substantial contraindication. HIV does not worsen hepatitis C, but there is no substantial evidence that HCV worsens the progression of HIV infection. At most, 20% of HCV patients will have worsening test results because of antiretroviral medications, although hepatitis C may temporarily worsen, with increased alanine aminotransferase level and increased HCV viral loads. Drug combinations should be limited to agents least likely to produce liver abnormalities.

37. Answer b

Patients with cirrhosis must have at least 7 Child-Pugh-Turcotte points to be listed for liver transplantation (minimal listing criteria) unless they have hepatocellular carcinoma. Fatigue is not an indication for liver transplantation, particularly in patients with hepatitis C who will experience recurrence of infection after transplantation.

38. Answer b

Liver biopsy is required to confirm or exclude the diagnosis of rejection in this patient. These symptoms, signs, and timing are suggestive of acute cellular rejection. In this setting, other tests may be performed in addition to, but not in lieu of, biopsy.

39. Answer d

Both of these calcineurin inhibitors are nephrotoxic, but nephrotoxicity is more prevalent with tacrolimus.

40. Answer d

The patient has the clinical, biochemical, and radiologic features typical of nonalcoholic fatty liver disease (NAFL). NAFL is a common cause of abnormal liver tests, especially in obese patients or in those with diabetes mellitus. Although prevalence figures vary, probably 20% of obese patients and 2% of lean patients have clinically important fatty liver. Nonalcoholic steatohepatitis (NASH), a subset of NAFL, is characterized by the histologic finding of macrovesicular fatty degeneration with inflammation in a patient with negligible ethanol intake. Most patients will have a moderate increase in aminotransferase levels and, occasionally, in alkaline phosphatase. Bilirubin, albumin, and prothrombin time are usually normal unless decompensated cirrhosis is present. In contrast, alcoholic steatohepatitis is often accompanied by hyperbilirubinemia and synthetic dysfunction of the liver. Histologically, NASH can mimic alcoholic hepatitis, even exhibiting Mallory bodies. An AST:ALT ratio >2 may also favor alcoholic hepatitis, but there is enough overlap for this to be of little use in an individual patient. Good natural history data about NASH are not available, but it has been estimated that 10% to 20% of patients will develop cirrhosis. A recent randomized clinical trial failed to show any beneficial effect of ursodiol. An increase in γ-globulin would be characteristic of autoimmune hepatitis. Celiac sprue can be associated with diabetes and steatosis but would not be likely in an obese patient.

41. Answer a

Abnormal liver enzymes occur during INH treatment in up to 30% of patients. The abnormalities are usually mild and improve despite continuation of therapy. More severe acute liver injury occurs in a small fraction of patients and can mimic acute viral hepatitis. Patients at high risk for severe liver injury due to INH include those of older age or those with excessive alcohol use. INH treatment should be discontinued for patients with symptoms of acute hepatitis or progressive increase of liver enzymes. In this patient, therapy can be continued, with follow-up observation of liver enzymes and symptoms. There is no need to perform blood tests or ultrasonography in this patient who previously had normal liver enzyme levels and has a potential cause for the mild increase. Liver biopsy is not indicated.

42. Answer d

The patient's symptoms, transient increase in liver enzyme and amylase levels, and presence of gallbladder stones are consistent with passage of a common bile duct stone. Preoperative imaging of the bile duct with magnetic resonance cholangiopancreatography, endoscopic retrograde cholangiopancreatography, or endoscopic ultrasonography may be considered but most authorities would suggest cholecystectomy with intraoperative cholangiography. Steatosis is probably an incidental finding, and liver biopsy is not necessary because the liver tests are now normal. Atorvastatin may cause abnormal liver tests but is not likely to cause this pattern this late after introduction of the drug. The patient feels well now and has no symptoms that would warrant esophagogastroduodenoscopy. Observation would put the patient at risk for further complications of gallstone disease.

43. Answer e

This patient presents with clinical evidence of advanced liver disease that could be related to alcohol or hepatitis C or both. The pattern of increased aminotransferase levels may favor alcoholic hepatitis. There is nothing to suggest acetaminophen hepatotoxicity, and the low doses used are unlikely to cause problems, even in an alcoholic patient. A liver biopsy specimen almost certainly will show cirrhosis, but biopsy would carry some risk because of the low platelet count and the results are not likely to change management. The marked thrombocytopenia would be a contraindication to hepatitis C treatment.

The presence of cirrhosis due to hepatitis C and alcohol would mandate surveillance for hepatocellular carcinoma.

44. Answer b

The clinical picture is most consistent with infectious mononucleosis, and a mononucleosis screen should be the next test. Liver test abnormalities occur in 90% of cases of infectious mononucleosis, although jaundice is unusual. The other diagnoses are all possible but would not account for the other clinical findings and history.

45. Answer a

The histologic features are those of vitamin A toxicity, which can be seen in persons who ingest more than 25,000 U/d over a prolonged period. The clinical findings are relatively nonspecific, although the liver biopsy findings are characteristic.

46. Answer b

The patient has the characteristic clinical features of fulminant liver failure and should be transferred to a center with expertise in liver transplantation. The other options are not appropriate given the urgency of the clinical presentation.

47. Answer e

The patient has a low level of HBV DNA and normal aminotransferase levels; thus, he has inactive chronic hepatitis B (so-called "healthy" carrier). HBV DNA is found in nearly all patients with hepatitis B and is found more frequently because of increased test sensitivity. Generally, patients with an HBV DNA level $< 10^5$ copies/mL are considered to have low levels and are not treated. The patient's age, likely neonatal acquisition, and family history of hepatocellular carcinoma would make surveillance advisable for hepatocellular carcinoma. Ultrasonography would be advised.

48. Answer d

The donor is considered immune to hepatitis B, and the serologic profile is that of someone with natural immunity from previous infection. Nevertheless, donors with this profile may have low levels of HBV DNA in serum or liver tissue and transmit hepatitis B to the recipient and generally are used only for recipients with hepatitis B.

49. Answer b

The presence of cirrhosis and acute hepatitis suggest an acute exacerbation of chronic hepatitis B. Acute "flares" of disease may be associated with seroconversion or mutations in the hepatitis B virus. Patients with acute flares of disease may have reappearance of IgM anti-HBc. The same serologic picture could be seen with a recently acquired acute hepatitis B, but such a patient would not have cirrhosis. The small peripheral hepatocellular carcinoma would not cause acute deterioration and is likely an incidental finding. Acetaminophen toxicity should not occur with such low doses, especially in the absence of alcohol excess. Metoprolol is a rare cause of acute hepatitis.

50. Answer b

The patient presents with a hepatitis C antibody and clinical findings of cirrhosis with portal hypertension (spider angiomas and splenomegaly). Patients with hepatitis C and cirrhosis are at substantial risk for hepatocellular carcinoma, and screening is advised for patients who are candidates for treatment such as liver transplantation. The patient has a risk factor for hepatitis C; therefore, it is extremely unlikely HCV RNA will be negative. Splenomegaly with mild pancytopenia is common in patients with portal hypertension, and bone marrow biopsy is not necessary. Splenectomy should be avoided in patients with cirrhosis and portal hypertension. Patients with HCV and compensated cirrhosis may be considered for therapy against HCV, although it would have to be administered carefully because of the thrombocytopenia.

51. Answer c

The combination of pegylated interferon and ribavirin is standard treatment for hepatitis C. Nearly all patients who achieve a sustained response to treatment will have a 2-log decrease in HCV RNA level after 3 months of treatment. Therefore, in this patient, treatment should be discontinued. Treatment with ribavirin alone has not shown long-term benefit and is generally not advised. In some studies, amantadine has shown added benefit to interferon and ribavirin but is not generally advised outside of a clinical trial. Screening for hepatocellular carcinoma with ultrasonography and alpha fetoprotein is advised only for patients with hepatitis C who have cirrhosis (stage 4 fibrosis).

52. Answer e

This patient has prolonged cholestasis associated with hepatitis A. Occasionally, patients will have a recurrence of hepatitis with increasing aminotransferase levels during the cholestatic period. These flares are associated with detection of hepatitis A virus in stool. Cholestatic hepatitis A has a good prognosis, and complete recovery is the rule. Observation is recommended. There is no need for other tests given the history of hepatitis A, prolonged period of the patient's symptoms, and the lack of important findings such as hypergammaglobulinemia or ductal dilatation on liver ultrasonography.

53. Answer c

The patient has chronic hepatitis B with cirrhosis. He has

evidence of decompensation, both clinically and biochemically, and imaging studies consistent with hepatocellular carcinoma. In addition, he has serologic evidence of active viral replication, with positivity for both HBeAg and HBV DNA. Patients with decompensated hepatitis B should be referred for liver transplantation. In addition, treatment with lamivudine or adefovir is advised because it can result in clinical improvement. Patients with hepatitis B and cirrhosis should have screening tests for hepatocellular carcinoma, usually incorporating both alpha fetoprotein and liver ultrasonography. Interferon may induce a flare of acute hepatitis when administered to patients with chronic hepatitis B and should not be given to patients with decompensation. Patients with cirrhosis should have endoscopy to search for esophageal varices. Low doses of acetaminophen are acceptable for patients with cirrhosis.

54. Answer d

HCV and HIV coinfection is common, especially in intravenous drug users. Patients with HIV infection have an increased risk for vertical and sexual transmission of HCV compared with non-HIV–infected patients. HIV may accelerate progression of HCV-associated liver disease. Generally, it is reasonable to consider treatment against HCV for patients whose HIV infection is well controlled, with CD4 counts >200/μL. In this patient with a recent infection and a low CD4 count, it would be best to treat the HIV first, especially with the mild histologic changes of HCV infection.

55. Answer a

Patients with hepatitis C genotypes 2 and 3 only need treatment for 6 months, and response rates are high enough that determining HCV RNA levels during therapy are not routinely recommended. Combination therapy results in higher treatment responses than pegylated interferon monotherapy and is advised unless ribavirin is contraindicated.

56. Answer c

The patient presents with hepatitis C. She has severe depression, which is a strong relative contraindication to therapy. There are hints of advanced liver disease, including a borderline albumin value, AST higher than ALT, and spleen at upper limit of normal size. Empiric therapy can be considered for patients without contraindications to therapy who are genotype 2. In this patient with marked depression, liver biopsy should be the next step. Cryoglobulinemia is extremely unlikely in the absence of rheumatoid factor and a characteristic rash. Because there is no indication that this is hepatitis B or autoimmune hepatitis, lamivudine or corticosteroid therapy would not be advised.

SECTION VIII

Pancreas and Biliary Tree

CHAPTER 41

Acute Pancreatitis

Todd H. Baron, Sr., M.D.
Santhi S. Vege, M.D.

Approximately 210,000 new cases of acute pancreatitis occur annually in the United States and the incidence is increasing in and outside the United States. Of the new cases, about 80% are the interstitial (edematous) variety and the rest are the necrotizing variety. Necrotizing pancreatitis accounts for most of the morbidity and nearly all the mortality associated with acute pancreatitis.

ETIOLOGY

Gallstones and alcohol are the most common causes of acute pancreatitis in the United States (Table 1). Gallstones are the most common cause in affluent populations, and alcohol, in lower socioeconomic populations. Other causes include hyperlipidemia, hypercalcemia, drugs (Table 2), trauma, postoperative states, infections by various agents, and endoscopic retrograde cholangiopancreatography (ERCP). About 20% of the cases of acute pancreatitis are classified as idiopathic because no cause is found even after extensive testing. Debated causes of acute pancreatitis are sphincter of Oddi dysfunction and pancreas divisum.

Gallstones are thought to produce acute pancreatitis because they pass into the common bile duct and obstruct the channel shared by the bile duct and pancreatic duct. Patients with gallstone pancreatitis frequently have abnormal liver enzyme levels.

PATHOLOGY

The two forms of acute pancreatitis defined by inflammatory changes in the pancreatic parenchyma are "interstitial" and "necrotizing." In interstitial pancreatitis, edema and inflammation of the pancreatic parenchyma occur without death of pancreatic acini. In necrotizing pancreatitis, there is extensive parenchymal destruction, frequently with peripancreatic fat necrosis.

CLINICAL PRESENTATION

The clinical presentation of acute pancreatitis ranges from mild, nonspecific epigastric pain to a catastrophic acute medical illness. Pain occasionally is absent (especially in acute pancreatitis that occurs after renal transplantation and cardiac surgery), and sometimes acute pancreatitis is diagnosed only at autopsy. Patients with interstitial acute pancreatitis have a clinically mild presentation.

Patients usually present with epigastric or left upper quadrant pain that may radiate to the back. Nausea and vomiting are nearly always present. In the severe form, the patient is systemically ill with fever, tachycardia, tachypnea, and hypotension. Although the findings of ecchymoses in the periumbilical area (Cullen's sign) or on the flanks (Grey Turner's sign) have received much attention, they are uncommon.

The differential diagnosis of acute pancreatitis is broad and includes atypical presentation of myocardial infarction, peptic ulcer disease, symptomatic cholelithiasis, small-bowel obstruction, and small-bowel ischemia.

SEVERITY STRATIFICATION

Several severity-of-illness classifications for acute pancreatitis are used to identify patients at risk for the development of complications. The Ranson score consists of 11 clinical signs with prognostic significance: 5 criteria are measured at the

Table 1. Causes of Acute Pancreatitis

Most common
>   Choledocholithiasis
>   Ethanol
>   Idiopathic

Less common
>   Endoscopic retrograde cholangiopancreatography
>   (especially for suspected sphincter of Oddi
>   dysfunction)
>   Pancreatic ductal obstruction (pancreatic carcinoma,
>   intraductal mucinous papillary tumor)
>   Hyperlipidemia (types I, IV, and V)
>   Hypercalcemia
>   Drugs (see Table 2)
>   Pancreas divisum (?)
>   Abdominal trauma

Least common
>   Viral infection
>   Parasitic infestation of pancreatic duct
>   Hereditary (familial)

Modified from Baron TH, Morgan DE: Acute necrotizing pancreatitis. N Engl J Med. 1999;340:1412-7. Used with permission.

Table 2. Drugs Associated With Acute Pancreatitis

Likely association	Possible association
α-Methyldopa	Amiodarone
Asparaginase	Ampicillin
Azathioprine	Anticholinesterases
Cimetidine	Carbamazepine
2',3'-Dideoxycytidine	Cisplatin
2',3'-Dideoxyinosine	Colchicine
Estrogens	Corticosteroids
Furosemide	Cyclosporine
6-Mercaptopurine	Cytarabine
Metronidazole	Delavirdine
Pentamidine	Diazoxide
Salicylates	Diphenoxylate
Sulfasalazine	Enalapril
Sulfonamides	Ergotamine
Sulindac	Erythromycin
Tetracyclines	Ethacrynic acid
Valproic acid	Ganciclovir
	Gold compounds
	Indinavir
	Interleukin-2
	Isotretinoin
	Ketoprofen
	Lisinopril
	Mefenamic acid
	Metolazone
	Nelfinavir
	Nevirapine
	Nitrofurantoin
	Octreotide
	Oxyphenbutazone
	Paracetamol
	(acetaminophen USP)
	Phenformin
	Phenolphthalein
	Piroxicam
	Procainamide
	Ranitidine
	Ritonavir
	Roxithromycin
	Stavudine
	Tretinoin
	Tryptophan

time of admission, and 6 criteria are measured between admission and 48 hours later (Table 3). The number of Ranson signs and the incidence of systemic complications and presence of pancreatic necrosis are correlated. The Acute Physiology and Chronic Health Evaluation (APACHE) II score is a grading system based on 12 physiologic variables, patient age, and previous history of severe organ system insufficiency or immunocompromised state (Table 4). It allows stratification of illness severity on admission and may be recalculated daily. The main problem with the Ranson score is that it may not be completed until 48 hours. The APACHE II scoring system has the advantage of being completed at the initial presentation and being repeated daily, but it is cumbersome to use.

The Atlanta classification is the most widely used clinical system for acute pancreatitis and recognizes mild and severe types. It classifies an attack of acute pancreatitis as severe if any of the following criteria are met: 1) organ failure with one or more of the following—shock (systolic blood pressure <90 mm Hg), pulmonary insufficiency (PaO_2 ≤–60 mm Hg), renal failure (serum creatinine level >2 mg/dL after rehydration), and gastrointestinal bleeding (>500 mL in 24 hours); 2) local complications such as pseudocyst, abscess, or pancreatic necrosis; 3) three or more Ranson criteria; or 4) eight or more APACHE II criteria. Terms such as phlegmon, hemorrhagic pancreatitis, infected pseudocyst, and persistent pancreatitis were omitted because of the confusion they caused.

Various biochemical markers have been evaluated to predict the severity of acute pancreatitis. C-reactive protein is the standard for predicting the severity of acute pancreatitis; a value of more than 150 mg/L is considered diagnostic of severe acute pancreatitis when determined 48 hours after onset of symptoms. Hemoconcentration with an admission hematocrit value of 44%

or more, serum trypsinogen activation peptide, polymor-phonuclear elastase, carboxypeptidase activation peptide, interleukin-6, interleukin-8, and procalcitonin are the other potential predictive markers of severity that are being evaluated.

LABORATORY FINDINGS

The diagnosis of acute pancreatitis requires one of the following criteria: a serum level of amylase or lipase 3 times or more the upper limit of normal for that particular laboratory assay, definite findings on abdominal ultrasonography or computed tomography (CT), or surgical or autopsy confirmation.

The two major pitfalls of the serum amylase assay are 1) it is a sensitive but not specific test and 2) various intra-abdominal diseases included in the differential diagnosis of acute

Table 3. Ranson Criteria of Severity

At admission	During initial 48 hours
Age > 55 years	Hematocrit decreases > 10%
Leukocytes > 16 × 10⁹/L	Blood urea nitrogen
Blood glucose > 200 mg/dL	increases > 5 mg/dL
Serum lactate dehydrogenase > 350 IU/L	Serum calcium < 8 mg/dL
	Arterial PaO₂ < 60 mm Hg
Serum aspartate aminotrans-ferase > 250 IU/L	Base deficit > 4 mEq/L
	Fluid sequestration > 6 L

Modified from Banks PA. Practice guidelines in acute pancreatitis. Am J Gastroenterol. 1997;92:377-86. Used with permission.

Table 4. APACHE II Scoring System*

Physiology points	4	3	2	1	0	1	2	3	4
Rectal temperature, °C	≥41.0	39.0-40.9		38.5-38.9	36.0-38.4	34.0-35.9	32.0-33.9	30.0-31.9	≤29.9
Mean blood pressure, mm Hg	≥160	130-159	110-129		70-109		50-69		≤49
Heart rate, beats/min	≥180	140-179	110-139		70-109		55-69	40-54	≤39
Respiratory rate, breaths/min	≥50	35-49		25-34	12-24	10-11	6-9		≤5
Oxygenation (kPa)†									
FIO₂ ≥50% A-aDO₂	66.5	46.6-66.4	26.6-46.4		<26.6				
FIO₂ <50% PaO₂					>9.3	8.1-9.3		7.3-8.0	<7.3
Arterial pH	≥7.70	7.60-7.59		7.50-7.59	7.33-7.49		7.25-7.32	7.15-7.24	<7.15
Serum sodium, mmol/L	≥180	160-179	155-159	150-154	130-149		120-129	111-119	≤110
Serum potassium, mmol/L	≥7.0	6.0-6.9		5.5-5.9	3.5-5.4	3.0-3.4	2.5-2.9		<2.5
Serum creatinine, mmol/L	≥300	171-299		121-170	50-120		<50		
Packed cell volume, %	≥60		50-59.9	46-49.9	30-45.9		20-29.9		<20
White blood cell count, × 10⁹/L	≥40		20-39.9	15-19.9	3-14.9		1-2.9		<1

*APACHE II score = acute physiology score + age points + chronic health points.
†If fraction of inspired oxygen (FIO₂) is ≥50%, the alveolar-arterial gradient (A-a) is assigned points. If fraction of inspired oxygen is <50%, partial pressure of oxygen is assigned points.
Other points
   Glasgow coma scale: score is subtracted from 15 to obtain points.
   Age < 45 years = 0 points, 45-54 = 2, 55-64 = 3, 65-75 = 5, > 75 = 6.
Chronic health points (must be present before hospital admission): chronic liver disease with hypertension or previous liver failure, encephalopathy, or coma; chronic heart failure (New York Heart Association class IV); chronic respiratory disease with severe exercise limitation, secondary polycythemia, or pulmonary hypertension; dialysis-dependent kidney disease; immunosuppression—e.g., radiation, chemotherapy, recent or long-term high-dose corticosteroid therapy, leukemia, acquired immunodeficiency syndrome. 5 points for emergency surgery or nonsurgical patient, 2 points for elective surgical patient.
Modified from Banks PA. Practice guidelines in acute pancreatitis. Am J Gastroenterol. 1997;92:377-86. Used with permission.

pancreatitis may cause an increase in the serum level of amylase. Another problem is the falsely low serum amylase level in hyperlipidemia. Although the serum lipase assay was developed in an attempt to have a more specific test, it appears to have only marginally better sensitivity and specificity.

Increase of the alanine transaminase value by threefold or more suggests biliary origin of acute pancreatitis. Fasting triglyceride value of more than 100 mg/dL or persistent increase after resolution of the attack suggests hyperlipidemia as the cause and not the effect of acute pancreatitis. It is important to measure serum calcium after resolution of the attack because the level can be spuriously low during an attack and hypercalcemia as the cause can be missed.

The serum levels of creatinine and glucose may be increased. Decreases in total serum calcium are more likely related to low serum levels of albumin than to true hypocalcemia, which is reflected in measurements of ionized calcium. Hypoxemia also may be present.

ABDOMINAL IMAGING STUDIES

In acute pancreatitis, plain abdominal radiographs are frequently normal, but they are useful for excluding free perforation of intra-abdominal lumina. A nonspecific ileus may be present as well as a focally dilated small-bowel loop, the so-called sentinel loop. The colon cutoff sign is the abrupt narrowing of the gas in the transverse colon on a plain radiograph of the abdomen in the vicinity of the body of the pancreas as a result of inflammation.

Abdominal ultrasonography is frequently nondiagnostic in acute pancreatitis because overlying bowel gas may obscure the pancreas. However, ultrasonography is sensitive for detecting gallstones and thus adds clinical information about the underlying cause of the pancreatitis.

If the diagnosis is in doubt, the best imaging study is abdominal CT. It is imperative that intravenous contrast be administered (contrast-enhanced CT [CECT]) unless there is a major contraindication. Pancreatic perfusion is disrupted in the setting of pancreatic necrosis and is detectable only if intravenous contrast is given (Fig. 1 and 2). A CT classification system for severity of acute pancreatitis, based on the degree of necrosis and number of fluid collections, has been developed. High mortality can be expected if the CT severity index of Balthazar is 7 or more. Patients with acute pancreatitis who have normal CT findings have a good prognosis. The correlation between the failure of more than 30% of the pancreas to enhance on CECT and finding pancreatic necrosis at surgery or autopsy is good. As the degree of necrosis increases, there is a corresponding increase in morbidity and mortality.

It is not absolutely necessary to obtain abdominal imaging studies at presentation of acute pancreatitis unless the diagnosis is in doubt. If the diagnosis is in doubt, CECT rather than ultrasonography should be performed. If the cause is in doubt, ultrasonography is the best test to confirm gallstones. In definite

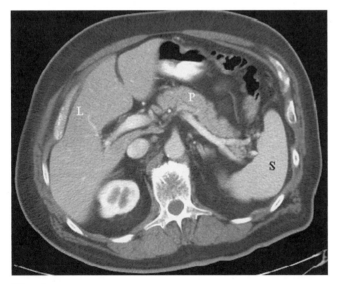

Fig. 1. Normal contrast-enhanced computed tomogram of the pancreas. Note that the pancreas (P) has a uniform enhancement intermediate between that of the liver (L) and spleen (S).

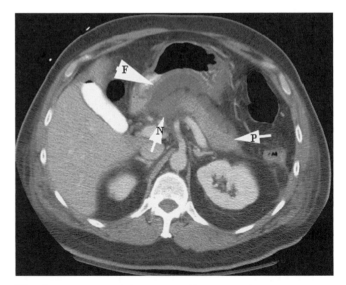

Fig. 2. Acute necrotizing pancreatitis. The patient had severe pancreatitis after endoscopic retrograde cholangiopancreatography. Note fluid collection (*arrowhead F*) near the neck of the pancreas. The density of the necrotic portion of the pancreas (*arrowhead N*) is less than that of the normal-enhancing pancreas in the tail (*arrowhead P*).

cases of acute pancreatitis, CECT can be done after 3 days if the patient is not responding, or earlier if the patient is deteriorating.

Recently, magnetic resonance imaging has been prospectively compared with CT in the setting of severe pancreatitis and found to be a reliable method for staging severity. It has predictive value for prognosis of the disease and has fewer contraindications than CT. It also can detect pancreatic duct disruption, which may occur early in the course of acute pancreatitis.

TREATMENT

Because the prognosis of interstitial pancreatitis is different from that of necrotizing pancreatitis, management of the two is discussed separately.

Treatment of Acute Interstitial Pancreatitis

Patients with interstitial pancreatitis may be managed on a general hospital ward, without need for intensive care monitoring. Often, all that is needed is to withhold oral intake and liberally administer intravenous fluids and analgesics. Nasogastric tubes should not be used routinely because they do not improve disease outcome and add to patient discomfort. However, for patients with exceptional nausea and vomiting and ileus, a nasogastric tube may improve their comfort. Empiric use of antibiotics should be avoided in interstitial pancreatitis because these agents do not alter the outcome.

If laboratory findings (increased levels of aminotransferases or bilirubin or both) and ultrasonography indicate that gallstones are the cause of the pancreatitis, cholecystectomy should be performed before hospital dismissal to prevent recurrent attacks of acute pancreatitis. If the patient is a poor surgical candidate because of severe coexisting medical illness, ERCP with biliary sphincterotomy may be a good alternative to cholecystectomy, especially if ultrasonography shows only sludge or small stones.

If the cause of pancreatitis is in doubt, the serum levels of lipids should be determined and drugs that may have caused acute pancreatitis should be reviewed thoroughly. In addition, abdominal ultrasonography should be performed. After this, if the cause is still in doubt, abdominal CT should be performed to exclude anatomical causes of pancreatic ductal obstruction, such as a pancreatic or ampullary mass lesion or suggestion of intraductal mucinous papillary tumor, especially in patients older than 50 years. For elderly patients, endoscopic ultrasonography, magnetic resonance cholangiopancreatography, or ERCP should be considered if the CT findings are negative.

Treatment of Acute Necrotizing Pancreatitis

Supportive Care

The management of patients with clinically severe pancreatitis due to pancreatic necrosis is different from that for interstitial pancreatitis. Aggressive hydration with intravenous fluids is very important. Patient-controlled analgesia for pain control requires fentanyl or morphine. There was experimental evidence that morphine caused spasm of the sphincter of Oddi, but there is no definite human evidence that morphine actually worsens the disease. Patients should be placed in the intensive care unit. In recent years, management of these patients has shifted from early surgical debridement (necrosectomy) to aggressive intensive medical care. Aggressive medical management, with an emphasis on the prevention of infection, has allowed prompt identification of complications and improvement in outcome.

Early mortality (within the first 1 or 2 weeks) is due to multisystem organ failure resulting from systemic inflammatory response syndrome. Systemic complications include adult respiratory distress syndrome, acute renal failure, shock, coagulopathy, hyperglycemia, and hypocalcemia. These complications are managed with endotracheal intubation, aggressive fluid resuscitation, fresh frozen plasma, insulin, and calcium as needed.

Antibiotics

The prevention of infection is critical because infected necrosis develops in 30% to 70% of patients with acute necrotizing pancreatitis and causes more than 80% of deaths due to acute pancreatitis. Early studies on antibiotic therapy for patients with acute pancreatitis failed to show an important benefit because of the inclusion of both patients with interstitial-edematous and those with necrotizing acute pancreatitis. In experimental acute necrotizing pancreatitis, pancreatic infection occurs primarily as a result of bacterial translocation from the colon. Human studies have shown benefits from systemic antibiotic therapy as well as "selective gut decontamination." In a prospective trial, a significant decrease in gram-negative pancreatic infection and late mortality (more than 2 weeks after onset of pancreatitis) in a group of patients with necrotizing pancreatitis was found in the selective gut decontamination group. Because selective gut decontamination antibiotics must be administered orally and rectally, this regimen may pose problems from a nursing standpoint and has not been adopted. Thus, the more commonly used approach is the systemic administration of antibiotics to prevent pancreatic infection.

Prospective and retrospective studies have shown a significant decrease in pancreatic infection in patients given imipenem-cilastatin (Primaxin) intravenously, although a reduction in mortality was not found. Fluoroquinolones should offer excellent protection against infection of necrosis; however, two randomized prospective trials using quinolone regimens in patients with severe pancreatitis suggest that these agents are not effective prophylactic agents for reducing infectious complications of acute pancreatitis.

In a recently published issue of *Cochrane Database of Systematic Reviews*, four prospective randomized trials were evaluated in which antibiotic therapy was used in patients with severe acute pancreatitis associated with pancreatic necrosis, as proved by intravenous contrast-enhanced CT. There was strong evidence that intravenous prophylactic antibiotic therapy for 10 to 14 days decreased the risk of superinfection of necrotic tissue and mortality. Currently, prophylaxis with intravenously administered antibiotics that have excellent pancreatic tissue penetration (imipenem-cilastatin) is recommended. One of the concerns with prophylactic antibiotics for severe acute pancreatitis is the development of fungal superinfection. Proposed strategies to decrease this complication include limiting the duration of the antibiotic therapy to 7 days or administering a prophylactic antifungal drug; these need to be studied in future trials. Therapy should begin as soon as severe acute pancreatitis is diagnosed. Recently, a second antibiotic (meropenem) in the same class has been shown to be equally effective for preventing septic complications of severe acute pancreatitis. Further studies are required to decide which subgroups of severe acute pancreatitis will benefit from prophylactic antibiotics.

Detection of Pancreatic Infection

Although sterile and infected acute necrotizing pancreatitis can be difficult to distinguish clinically because both may produce fever, leukocytosis, and severe abdominal pain, the distinction is important. Without intervention, the mortality for patients with infected acute necrotizing pancreatitis is nearly 100%. The bacteriologic status of the pancreas may be determined with CT-guided fine-needle aspiration of pancreatic and peripancreatic tissue or fluid. This aspiration method is safe, accurate (sensitivity of 96% and specificity of 99%), and recommended for patients with acute necrotizing pancreatitis whose condition deteriorates clinically or fails to improve despite aggressive supportive care. Ultrasonographically guided aspiration may have a lower sensitivity and specificity, but it can be performed at the bedside. Surveillance aspiration may be repeated on a weekly basis as indicated clinically.

Role of ERCP

ERCP with biliary sphincterotomy may improve the outcome of patients with severe gallstone pancreatitis. Initial studies in which urgent ERCP (within 72 hours after admission) and biliary sphincterotomy were performed in patients with acute gallstone pancreatitis and choledocholithiasis showed improved outcome for only the group of patients presenting with clinically severe acute pancreatitis. The improvement was attributed to relief from pancreatic ductal obstruction produced by an impacted gallstone in the common biliary-pancreatic channel of the ampulla of Vater. More recent studies have suggested that improved outcome after ERCP and sphincterotomy in gallstone pancreatitis may be the result of reduced biliary sepsis rather than a true improvement in pancreatitis. Therefore, for patients with severe gallstone acute pancreatitis, ERCP should be reserved for those with biliary obstruction suspected on the basis of hyperbilirubinemia and clinical cholangitis.

Nutritional Support for Acute Necrotizing Pancreatitis

To meet increased metabolic demands and to "rest" the pancreas, total parenteral nutrition has been used frequently for nutritional support of patients with acute necrotizing pancreatitis, but it does not hasten the resolution of acute pancreatitis. In randomized prospective studies of severe acute pancreatitis, comparing total parenteral nutrition with enteral feeding (through a nasoenteric feeding tube placed under radiographic guidance beyond the ligament of Treitz), patients receiving enteral feeding had significantly fewer total and infectious complications with a threefold reduction in the cost of nutritional support and improvement in acute-phase response and disease severity scores. A recent meta-analysis of enteral and parenteral nutrition in patients with acute pancreatitis found that enteral nutrition was associated with a significantly lower incidence of infections, reduced surgical interventions to control pancreatitis, and a reduced duration of hospital stay. There were no significant differences in mortality or noninfectious complications between the two groups of patients. It appears that this form of enteral feeding is preferable in patients with acute necrotizing pancreatitis and without severe ileus. Possibly, nasogastric feeding may be as safe, too, according to a small randomized study comparing nasogastric feeding with nasojejunal feeding.

Surgical Therapy for Pancreatic Necrosis

The timing and type of pancreatic intervention for acute necrotizing pancreatitis are debated, although guidelines from the International Association of Pancreatology for the surgical management of acute pancreatitis have been published. Because the mortality rate of sterile acute necrotizing pancreatitis is approximately 10% and surgical intervention has not been shown to decrease this rate, nonsurgical therapy is recommended. Conversely, infected acute necrotizing pancreatitis is considered uniformly fatal without intervention. Aggressive surgical pancreatic debridement (necrosectomy) is the standard of care and may require multiple abdominal reexplorations. Necrosectomy should be undertaken soon after infected necrosis has been confirmed. Multisystem organ failure unresponsive to maximal treatment in the intensive care unit is considered an indication for surgery. However, delaying surgical intervention beyond 14 days after the onset of acute necrotizing pancreatitis, when possible, is the present recommendation based on the recent evidence. This is related to improved demarcation between viable and necrotic tissue at the time of operation. The role of delayed necrosectomy (after multisystem organ failure has resolved) in sterile acute necrotizing pancreatitis is also debated. Some investigators advocate debridement in patients who are still systemically ill with fever, weight loss, intractable abdominal pain, inability to eat, and "failure to thrive" 4 to 6 weeks after the onset of acute pancreatitis. Others, however, argue that delayed necrosectomy is unnecessary as long as the process remains sterile. Frequently, multiple operations are required to remove the necrotic pancreatic and peripancreatic material. Abdominal zipper or open packing of the wound permits repeated explorations. If the necrosis is well contained and organized or if the patient is a poor surgical risk, minimal-access necrosectomy, either percutaneously with nephroscopes or endoscopically through the stomach, duodenum, or papilla, is the new approach. Pancreatic or gastrointestinal tract fistulas (or both) occur in up to 40% of patients after surgical necrosectomy and often require an additional procedure for closure. The mortality rate after necrosectomy for acute necrotizing pancreatitis is approximately 20%.

Prognosis

The overall mortality rate for severe acute pancreatitis has decreased as a result of improved therapies in the intensive care unit, antibiotics, and delay of surgery and is now approximately 15%. Mortality occurs in two phases: 1) early deaths (1-2 weeks after onset of pancreatitis, approximately 50% of all deaths) are due to multisystem organ failure from release of inflammatory mediators and cytokines and 2) late deaths result from local or systemic infections. As long as acute necrotizing pancreatitis remains sterile, the overall mortality rate is approximately 10%. The mortality rate at least triples if infected necrosis occurs. Patients with sterile necrosis and high severity-of-illness scores (Ranson score, APACHE II score) accompanied by multisystem organ failure, shock, or renal insufficiency have a significantly higher mortality.

Long-term Sequelae of Acute Necrotizing Pancreatitis

Despite the enormous cost of caring for patients with acute necrotizing pancreatitis, the mean quality of life outcomes up to 2 years after treatment of pancreatic necrosis are similar to those for coronary artery bypass grafting. The long-term clinical endocrine and exocrine consequences of acute necrotizing pancreatitis appear to depend on several factors: the severity of necrosis, cause (alcoholic vs. nonalcoholic), continued use of alcohol, and the degree of surgical pancreatic debridement. Sophisticated exocrine function studies have shown persistent functional insufficiency in the majority of patients up to 2 years after severe acute pancreatitis. Treatment with pancreatic enzymes should be restricted to patients with symptoms of steatorrhea and weight loss due to fat malabsorption. Although subtle glucose intolerance is frequent, overt diabetes mellitus is uncommon. Follow-up pancreatography frequently shows obstruction, disruption, or disconnection of the pancreatic duct, which may result in persistence or recurrence of fluid collections. This may require endoscopic treatment or distal pancreatic resection.

RECOMMENDED READING

Arvanitakis M, Delhaye M, De Maertelaere V, Bali M, Winant C, Coppens E, et al. Computed tomography and magnetic resonance imaging in the assessment of acute pancreatitis. Gastroenterology. 2004;126:715-23.

Baillie J. Treatment of acute biliary pancreatitis. N Engl J Med. 1997;336:286-7.

Balthazar EJ, Freeny PC, vanSonnenberg E. Imaging and intervention in acute pancreatitis. Radiology. 1994;193:297-306.

Balthazar EJ, Robinson DL, Megibow AJ, Ranson JH. Acute pancreatitis: value of CT in establishing prognosis. Radiology. 1990;174:331-6.

Banks PA. Practice guidelines in acute pancreatitis. Am J Gastroenterol. 1997;92:377-86.

Baron TH, Morgan DE. Acute necrotizing pancreatitis. N Engl J Med. 1999;340:1412-7.

Bradley EL III. A clinically based classification system for acute pancreatitis: summary of the International Symposium on Acute Pancreatitis, Atlanta, Ga, September 11 through 13, 1992. Arch Surg. 1993;128:586-90.

Buchler MW, Gloor B, Muller CA, Friess H, Seiler CA, Uhl W. Acute necrotizing pancreatitis: treatment strategy according to the status of infection. Ann Surg. 2000;232:619-26.

Dervenis C, Johnson CD, Bassi C, Bradley E, Imrie CW, McMahon MJ, et al. Diagnosis, objective assessment of severity, and management of acute pancreatitis: Santorini consensus conference. Int J Pancreatol. 1999;25:195-210.

Eatock FC, Brombacher GD, Steven A, Imrie CW, McKay CJ, Carter R. Nasogastric feeding in severe acute pancreatitis may be practical and safe. Int J Pancreatol. 2000;28:23-9.

Fan ST, Lai EC, Mok FP, Lo CM, Zheng SS, Wong J. Early treatment of acute biliary pancreatitis by endoscopic papillotomy. N Engl J Med. 1993;328:228-32.

Foitzik T, Klar E, Buhr HJ, Herfarth C. Improved survival in acute necrotizing pancreatitis despite limiting the indications for surgical debridement. Eur J Surg. 1995;161:187-192.

Folsch UR, Nitsche R, Ludtke R, Hilgers RA, Creutzfeldt W, the German Study Group on Acute Biliary Pancreatitis.

Early ERCP and papillotomy compared with conservative treatment for acute biliary pancreatitis. N Engl J Med. 1997;336:237-42.

Gerzof SG, Banks PA, Robbins AH, Johnson WC, Spechler SJ, Wetzner SM, et al. Early diagnosis of pancreatic infection by computed tomography-guided aspiration. Gastroenterology. 1987;93:1315-20.

He YM, Lv XS, Ai ZL, Liu ZS, Qian Q, Sun Q, et al. Prevention and therapy of fungal infection in severe acute pancreatitis: a prospective clinical study. World J Gastroenterol. 2003;9:2619-21.

Isenmann R, Runzi M, Kron M, Kahl S, Kraus D, Jung N, et al, German Antibiotics in Severe Acute Pancreatitis Study Group. Prophylactic antibiotic treatment in patients with predicted severe acute pancreatitis: a placebo-controlled, double-blind trial. Gastroenterology. 2004;126:997-1004.

Lobo DN, Memon MA, Allison SP, Rowlands BJ. Evolution of nutritional support in acute pancreatitis. Br J Surg. 2000;87:695-707.

Manes G, Rabitti PG, Menchise A, Riccio E, Balzano A, Uomo G. Prophylaxis with meropenem of septic complications in acute pancreatitis: a randomized, controlled trial versus imipenem. Pancreas. 2003;27:e79-83.

Marik PE, Zaloga GP. Meta-analysis of parenteral nutrition versus enteral nutrition in patients with acute pancreatitis. BMJ. 2004 Jun 12;328:1407. Epub 2004 Jun 2.

Mier J, Leon EL, Castillo A, Robledo F, Blanco R. Early versus late necrosectomy in severe necrotizing pancreatitis. Am J Surg. 1997;173:71-5.

Neoptolemos JP, Carr-Locke DL, London NJ, Bailey IA, James D, Fossard DP. Controlled trial of urgent endoscopic retrograde cholangiopancreatography and endoscopic sphincterotomy versus conservative treatment for acute pancreatitis due to gallstones. Lancet. 1988;2:979-83.

Nuutinen P, Kivisaari L, Schroder T. Contrast-enhanced computed tomography and microangiography of the pancreas in acute human hemorrhagic/necrotizing pancreatitis. Pancreas. 1988;3:53-60.

Rattner DW, Legermate DA, Lee MJ, Mueller PR, Warshaw AL. Early surgical debridement of symptomatic pancreatic necrosis is beneficial irrespective of infection. Am J Surg. 1992;163:105-9.

Rau B, Pralle U, Mayer JM, Beger HG. Role of ultrasonographically guided fine-needle aspiration cytology in the diagnosis of infected pancreatic necrosis. Br J Surg. 1998;85:179-84.

Schmid SW, Uhl W, Friess H, Malfertheiner P, Buchler MW. The role of infection in acute pancreatitis. Gut. 1999;45:311-6.

Tsiotos GG, Smith CD, Sarr MG. Incidence and management of pancreatic and enteric fistulas after surgical management of severe necrotizing pancreatitis. Arch Surg. 1995;130:48-52.

Uhl W, Warshaw A, Imrie C, Bassi C, McKay CJ, Lankisch PG, et al, International Association of Pancreatology. IAP guidelines for the surgical management of acute pancreatitis. Pancreatology. 2002;2:565-73.

Villatoro E, Larvin M, Bassi C. Antibiotic therapy for prophylaxis against infection of pancreatic necrosis in acute pancreatitis. Cochrane Database Syst Rev. 2003;(4):CD002941.

Werner J, Hartwig W, Uhl W, Muller C, Buchler MW. Useful markers for predicting severity and monitoring progression of acute pancreatitis. Pancreatology. 2003;3:115-27.

Windsor AC, Kanwar S, Li AG, Barnes E, Guthrie JA, Spark JI, et al. Compared with parenteral nutrition, enteral feeding attenuates the acute phase response and improves disease severity in acute pancreatitis. Gut. 1998;42:431-5.

CHAPTER 42

Chronic Pancreatitis

Suresh T. Chari, M.D.

Chronic pancreatitis is an often painful inflammatory condition of the pancreas characterized by progressive fibrosis that leads to irreversible destruction of exocrine and endocrine tissue and results eventually in exocrine and endocrine insufficiency. There is considerable heterogeneity in its presentation and natural history.

Chronic pancreatitis is divided broadly into "chronic calcifying pancreatitis" and "chronic obstructive pancreatitis." Chronic calcifying pancreatitis is characterized by the development of parenchymal and intraductal stones late in the course of the disease. Chronic obstructive pancreatitis is found distal (closer to the tail of the gland) to an obstruction of the pancreatic duct by any cause. It is not generally associated with stone formation. Chronic obstructive pancreatitis is commonly found distal to pancreatic tumors (ductal adenocarcinoma or intraductal papillary mucinous tumor) and postinflammatory strictures after acute pancreatitis. The rest of the discussion in this section is related to chronic calcifying pancreatitis.

ETIOLOGY OF CHRONIC CALCIFYING PANCREATITIS

Several conditions are associated with chronic calcifying pancreatitis (Table 1). The pathogenetic mechanisms of these presumed etiologic agents are generally unknown. In the West, the most common cause of chronic calcifying pancreatitis is chronic alcohol abuse.

GENETIC BASIS OF CHRONIC PANCREATITIS

Pancreatitis has so far been associated with mutations in three genes: cationic trypsinogen gene, also called *PRSS1*, the cystic fibrosis transmembrane conductance regulator gene (*CFTR*), and the pancreatic secretory trypsin inhibitor (*PSTI* or *SPINK1*) gene. Two of the mutations in *PRSS1* (R122H and N29I) are associated with the classic hereditary pancreatitis phenotype (i.e., autosomal dominant inheritance with 80% penetrance). Mutations in *CFTR* and *SPINK1* usually are associated with sporadic, idiopathic pancreatitis. Patients with pancreatitis who have *CFTR* mutations typically do not have other manifestations of classic cystic fibrosis. Mutations in *SPINK1* are present in 1% to 2% of the population but have 20% to 40% prevalence in idiopathic forms of pancreatitis.

Cationic trypsinogen, or PRSS1, is the predominant form of pro-trypsin in humans. It not only hydrolyzes dietary proteins but also activates all other digestive proenzymes. Premature activation of trypsinogen within the pancreas, with subsequent activation of other enzymes leading to pancreatic autodigestion, is believed to be central to the development of acute pancreatitis. The first line of defense against the normal intra-acinar autoactivation of small amounts of trypsinogen is SPINK1 (also known as pancreatic secretory trypsin inhibitor, PSTI), a protein co-secreted with trypsinogen by the acinar cell. SPINK1 can effectively inhibit up to 20% of potential trypsin (including mutant trypsin). Excessive trypsin activation or ineffective inhibition by mutant *SPINK1* can lead to pancreatitis by initiating the activation cascade. Autolysis of trypsin is the second line of defense and occurs by hydrolysis of the side chain connecting the two halves of the trypsin molecule at arginine 122 (R122). In hereditary pancreatitis, mutation at the R122 site (R122H) produces resistance to autolysis, leading to zymogen activation within the acinar cell with consequent

Table 1.   Causes of Chronic Calcifying Pancreatitis (CP)

Presumed cause	Salient features
Alcohol	Commonest cause of CP in the West
	CP develops in ~10% of alcoholics
	Usually after a long history of alcohol abuse
Hereditary	Mutations in cationic trypsinogen gene (R122H, N29I) associated with high penetrance (80%) autosomal dominant form of CP (see text)
	Presents at an early age (first and second decades)
	High risk of pancreatic cancer with time, especially in smokers
Idiopathic	Mutations noted in *CFTR* and *SPINK1* genes (see text)
	Early (juvenile) and late (senile) forms
	Pain a common feature of early onset
	Senile form may be painless in ~50% of patients
Hypercalcemia	Uncommon complication of hypercalcemia
Hypertriglyc-eridemia	Occurs in children with disorders of lipid metabolism
	Associated with types I, II, and V hyperlipidemia
	Triglyceride levels >1,000 mg/dL
Other	Tropical form, cause unknown
	Highest prevalence in south India
	Early age at onset (first and second decades)
	High prevalence (>80%) of diabetes and calcification at diagnosis

pancreatic autodigestion and pancreatitis. The molecular mechanism causing pancreatitis in subjects with N29I is not clear.

More than 1,000 CFTR mutations have been identified in *CFTR* which lead to minimal-to-complete loss of CFTR function. Although an association between CFTR mutations and chronic pancreatitis has been shown, how CFTR mutations might produce acute pancreatitis is unclear. A possible explanation is that the mutations are associated with production of a more concentrated and acidic pancreatic juice, leading to ductal obstruction or altered acinar cell function (e.g., reduced intracellular pH and abnormal intracellular membrane recycling or transport).

It is clear that pancreatitis is a multigenic, complex disorder in which environmental factors also play a significant role. An evolving concept is that all pancreatitis probably has a genetic basis, the strength of which varies depending on the type of pancreatitis. For example, pancreatitis in subjects with R122H and N29I mutations in *PRSS1* appears to be almost entirely explained by these gain-of-function mutations causing intrapancreatic activation of trypsinogen. Alternatively, mutations in *SPINK1* are present in 1% to 2% of the population and seem to be disease modifiers rather than causative agents. Although alcohol is a known predisposing factor for pancreatitis, the disease develops in only 5% to 10% of alcoholics, a suggestion that these persons might have a genetic predisposition for development of pancreatitis. The genetic background necessary for development of alcohol-induced pancreatitis remains to be elucidated.

The role of routine screening of subjects with pancreatitis for genetic mutations is unclear, and the clinical implications for unaffected family members of patients with low-penetrance mutations remain unknown. It is reasonable to screen subjects with early-onset (<35 years) pancreatitis, especially those with a family history.

DIAGNOSIS

Although histologic examination is the standard for diagnosing chronic pancreatitis, it often is not available. Thus, a combination of morphologic findings on imaging studies, functional abnormalities, and clinical findings is used to diagnose chronic pancreatitis. In the later stages of the disease when calcification and steatorrhea are present, the diagnosis is relatively straightforward. Difficulty arises if pancreatic structure and function are not unequivocally abnormal. The currently available diagnostic methods are not adequate for making a firm diagnosis of chronic pancreatitis without obvious changes in structure and function.

Structural Evaluation

Computed tomography (CT), endoscopic retrograde cholangiopancreatography (ERCP), endoscopic ultrasonography (EUS), and magnetic resonance imaging and cholangiopancreatography (MRI and MRCP) are four imaging procedures commonly used to evaluate structural changes in the pancreas. Pancreatic calcification suggestive but not diagnostic of chronic pancreatitis can be identified on abdominal radiographs. However, CT and EUS can detect small specks of calcification not visible on plain radiographs. Pancreatic calcification may not be visible on MRI.

Abdominal CT is a good first test in the evaluation of a patient with possible chronic pancreatitis because it is noninvasive, widely available, and has relatively good sensitivity for diagnosing moderate-to-severe chronic pancreatitis. However, the findings can be normal in early chronic pancreatitis. Chronic pancreatitis is diagnosed on CT by identifying pathognomonic calcifications within the pancreatic ducts or parenchyma or dilated main pancreatic ducts in combination with parenchymal atrophy (Fig. 1).

CT also is effective for the evaluation of pain in a patient with known chronic pancreatitis because it can identify most complications of chronic pancreatitis such as peripancreatic fluid collections, bile duct obstruction, and bowel obstruction, and it can reliably detect inflammatory or neoplastic masses larger than 1 cm.

If a tissue diagnosis is not available, ERCP is a sensitive and specific test to diagnose moderate-to-severe pancreatitis (Fig. 2). ERCP changes found in chronic pancreatitis are listed in Table 2. Minor changes in the ducts are hard to interpret and subject to interobserver variation. False-positive results may be obtained in older patients who may develop benign pancreatic duct changes without pancreatitis and in patients with recent acute pancreatitis who develop reversible or permanent pancreatic duct changes in the absence of chronic pancreatitis.

Diagnostic ERCP carries a small (2%-5%) risk of complications, including pancreatitis. Therapeutic maneuvers carry a higher risk of complications. ERCP is useful for evaluating patients when other methods are nondiagnostic or unavailable, when there is a clinical pattern of recurrent acute pancreatitis, or when a therapeutic intervention is being considered.

EUS provides high-resolution images of the pancreatic parenchyma and duct. Unlike ERCP, which can provide detailed images of changes in the pancreatic duct, EUS provides information about the pancreatic parenchyma as well as the duct. However, the role of EUS and the criteria for diagnosing chronic pancreatitis with EUS are being evaluated. Problems with interpretation may arise in older patients who have senile changes in the pancreas, in alcoholics who may have fibrosis without pancreatitis, and after a recent episode of acute pancreatitis. Interobserver variability in interpretation also is a problem. Currently, the diagnosis of chronic pancreatitis should not be made on the basis of EUS criteria alone.

Because MRCP is noninvasive, avoids ionizing radiation and the administration of a contrast agent, and does not routinely require sedation, it is the diagnostic procedure of choice for some groups of patients. It avoids the risks associated with ERCP. In combination with conventional abdominal MRI, MRCP can provide comprehensive information about the pancreas and peripancreatic tissues. Although major lesions such as grossly dilated ducts, communicating pseudocysts, and even pancreas divisum can be detected, small-duct changes and calcifications are not readily detected, and MRCP does not have therapeutic potential.

Functional Testing in the Evaluation of Chronic Pancreatitis

The pancreas has great functional reserve, so it must be damaged extensively before functional loss is recognized clinically. For example, 90% of the pancreas has to be destroyed before steatorrhea occurs. Abnormal results on function tests alone are not diagnostic of chronic pancreatitis, and diagnosis requires additional evidence of structural alteration (found on imaging studies) consistent with chronic pancreatitis. Imaging studies by themselves are usually diagnostic by the time steatorrhea develops. Invasive tests of pancreatic function (e.g., the "tubed"

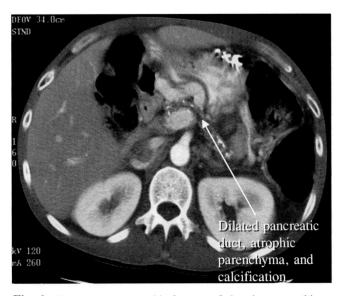

Fig. 1. Computed tomographic features of chronic pancreatitis.

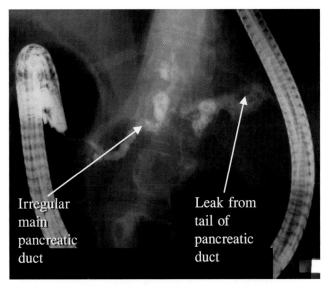

Fig. 2. Endoscopic retrograde cholangiopancreatographic findings in severe chronic pancreatitis.

Table 2.   Endoscopic Retrograde Cholangiopancreatographic Grading of Chronic Pancreatitis (Cambridge Classification)

Grade	Main duct	Side branches	Other findings
Normal	Normal	Normal	None
Mild	Normal	≥3 abnormal	None
Moderate	Abnormal—dilated, strictures	≥3 abnormal	None
Severe	Abnormal—dilated, strictures	≥3 abnormal	>1 finding—large (>10 mm) cavity, intraductal filling defects or calculi, duct obstruction, severe duct dilatation or irregularities

secretin test) show functional impairment even in the absence of steatorrhea. However, these tests are not widely available. Noninvasive pancreatic function tests have poor sensitivity for early disease.

CLINICAL FEATURES AND NATURAL HISTORY

Abdominal pain is the dominant symptom in the early part of the natural history of chronic pancreatitis, and steatorrhea and diabetes mellitus are the prominent features of late, end-stage chronic pancreatitis. Pain is often related to acute inflammatory flares. Some authors have reported a painless "burn out" of the pancreas in the late stages of the disease, but others have reported that pain continues even in late stages. Acute flares of pancreatitis or chronic fibrosis in and around the pancreas can cause complications.

The clinical features and natural history of chronic pancreatitis can differ dramatically in various forms of chronic pancreatitis. In hereditary and tropical forms of chronic pancreatitis, the onset of pain occurs at a younger age (first and second decades of life). Pain may not occur in half the patients with late-onset (senile) idiopathic chronic pancreatitis. Diabetes and calcification are uncommon at the time of diagnosis of alcoholic pancreatitis, but they are present in more than 80% of patients when tropical pancreatitis is diagnosed.

In alcoholic chronic pancreatitis, death often is related to nonpancreatic smoking- and alcohol-related complications (especially cancer). In tropical pancreatitis, the most common cause of death is diabetes-related complications, followed by pancreatic cancer. Pancreatic cancer can complicate any form of chronic pancreatitis, but it is especially common in hereditary and tropical forms, probably because of the long duration of disease.

COMPLICATIONS

Diabetes Mellitus

The progressive decrease in islet cell mass leads to diabetes in chronic pancreatitis. Although diabetes is common at

presentation in the tropical form of chronic pancreatitis, it is usually a late complication in other forms. With or without resection, diabetes eventually develops in 85% of the patients, and nonresective surgery, such as ductal drainage, does not prevent this complication.

Steatorrhea

This occurs after more than 90% of the gland has been destroyed. Treatment involves the use of oral pancreatic enzyme supplements. Patients with severe steatorrhea require 90,000 USP of lipase per meal and lesser amounts with snacks. Acid suppression may be required to prevent destruction of enzyme by gastric acid.

Pseudocyst

In early stages, pseudocysts result from a leak in the pancreatic duct after an attack of clinically acute pancreatitis (Fig. 3). In later stages, ductal dilatation can lead to leakage and the formation of pseudocysts from duct "blowout." Upstream ductal obstruction caused by a stricture often results in recurrence of pseudocyst after simple enteral drainage (e.g., endoscopic cyst drainage). This may require concomitant drainage of the main pancreatic duct (usually surgically) or resection of the diseased portion of the gland (or both).

Biliary Obstruction

This can result from edema of the head of the gland after an acute attack, compression from a pseudocyst, or bile duct entrapment in the fibrotic process involving the head of the gland. Although edema responds to conservative management and compression responds to drainage of the pseudocyst, fibrotic stricturing requires surgical biliary bypass.

Duodenal Obstruction

Potentially reversible gastric outlet obstruction can occur during an acute flare of pancreatitis as a result of peripancreatic inflammation involving the gastroduodenal region (Fig. 4). Parenteral nutrition may be required if nasojejunal feeding is not feasible to maintain nutrition during this period. Patients with

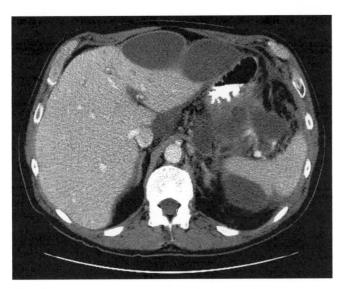

Fig. 3. Computed tomography is useful in assessing acute collections of fluid after pancreatitis.

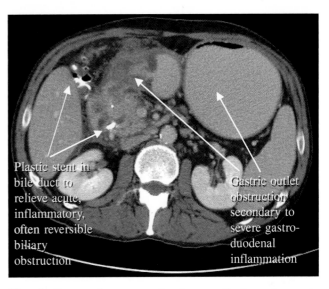

Plastic stent in bile duct to relieve acute, inflammatory, often reversible biliary obstruction

Gastric outlet obstruction secondary to severe gastro-duodenal inflammation

Fig. 4. Computed tomogram showing complications of an acute flare of pancreatitis.

a fibrotic process involving the duodenum require surgical bypass of the gastric outlet obstruction.

Splenic Vein Thrombosis

Because of the proximity of the splenic vein to the pancreas, the vein often is affected by pancreatic inflammation or fibrosis. Left-sided portal hypertension (sinistral portal hypertension) can present with gastric variceal bleeding. It is treated with splenectomy.

MANAGEMENT

Abdominal pain is the most dominant and vexing problem in the management of chronic pancreatitis. It can vary in severity from mild, intermittent pain to severe, chronic debilitating pain. Patients with alcoholic pancreatitis often are addicted to alcohol and tobacco; in addition, those with severe pain have considerable potential for narcotic addiction. It is extremely difficult to assess the true severity of the pain in patients addicted to narcotics, and often therapeutic interventions are seemingly unsuccessful because of continued dependence on narcotics. Apart from these issues, poor understanding of the pathogenesis of pain has made rational management of abdominal pain in chronic pancreatitis difficult. Despite some optimism that pancreatic pain eventually "burns out," most clinicians agree that it may be diminished but rarely disappears with time.

A stepwise approach to the management of pain in chronic pancreatitis is recommended. However, the scientific evidence to support any of the measures taken (medical, endoscopic, or surgical) is scanty, and there are few well-defined prospective trials of therapy, either in comparison with no therapy or with competing therapy.

An important first step is the assessment of pain and its nature, frequency, severity, and effect on quality of life and other activities. Patients with intermittent (once a year or less), uncomplicated episodes and full function between episodes probably are better off without a potentially injurious intervention. Regardless of the severity of pain, all patients with chronic pancreatitis should be counseled during each visit to abstain not only from alcohol but also tobacco.

Patients who have more frequent or severe pain and a tendency to take narcotics for pain control need further evaluation. An initial evaluation with imaging studies (CT) should be performed to rule out complications such as persistent acute inflammation (inflammatory mass) in the pancreas, pancreatic and peripancreatic fluid collections, biliary obstruction, or duodenal stenosis. Other diagnoses that should be considered in the appropriate clinical setting are peptic ulcer disease, gallbladder disease, and pancreatic cancer. The diagnosis of any of these should lead to appropriate intervention.

In patients without the above conditions, medical, endoscopic, and surgical options have been tried. Medical therapy includes a low-fat diet with abstinence from alcohol and a high dose of pancreatic enzymes in association with acid suppression. Endoscopic therapy includes sphincterotomy, lithotripsy, and pancreatic duct stenting. Currently, the evidence supporting the use of endoscopic therapy for pain in chronic pancreatitis is preliminary and confined largely to short-term focused observations. Although these procedures may hold promise, they need to be evaluated further in clinical trials. Celiac plexus block appears to have limited benefit in chronic pancreatitis.

Surgical therapy is an option for patients who clearly appear to have pancreas-related pain. Although no controlled trials have compared surgical treatment with medical treatment, endoscopic treatment, or no treatment, substantial experience indicates that at least some patients have lasting benefit. However, the failure rate of 20% to 40% in even the most enthusiastic reports and the potential for surgical morbidity and mortality warrant reserving surgical treatment for patients with severe pain not responsive to less invasive therapy. The choice of operation, if elected, should be predicated on the morphology of the pancreatic ducts; patients with small-duct disease undergo resection of the portion of pancreas most affected and those with large (≥7 mm) ducts are treated with drainage procedures (e.g., lateral pancreaticojejunostomy).

RECOMMENDED READING

American Gastroenterological Association Medical Position Statement. Treatment of pain in chronic pancreatitis. Gastroenterology. 1998;115:763-4.

Etemad B, Whitcomb DC. Chronic pancreatitis: diagnosis, classification, and new genetic developments. Gastroenterology. 2001;120:682-707.

Layer P, Yamamoto H, Kalthoff L, Clain JE, Bakken LJ, DiMagno EP. The different courses of early- and late-onset idiopathic and alcoholic chronic pancreatitis. Gastroenterology. 1994;107:1481-7.

Warshaw AL, Banks PA, Fernandez-Del Castillo C. AGA technical review: treatment of pain in chronic pancreatitis. Gastroenterology. 1998;115:765-76.

Witt H, Becker M. Genetics of chronic pancreatitis. J Pediatr Gastroenterol Nutr. 2002;34:125-36.

CHAPTER 43

Pancreatic Neoplasms

Randall K. Pearson, M.D.

Pancreatic neoplasms are of epithelial or nonepithelial origin (Table 1). Of all pancreatic tumors, ductal adenocarcinoma is the most important.

PANCREATIC DUCTAL ADENOCARCINOMA

Cancer of the pancreas is a fatal disease and an increasing health problem. In the United States, more than 28,000 persons die of pancreatic cancer annually. The overall survival rate with pancreatic cancer is less than 5%, the lowest 5-year survival rate of any cancer. This is due partly to the low resectability rate.

Table 1. Exocrine Pancreatic Tumors

Epithelial
  Cystic
    Microcystic (serous) cystadenoma
    Macrocystic (mucinous) cystadenoma
    Intraductal papillary mucinous tumor
    Solid-cystic (solid and papillary) tumor
  Solid
    Variants of ductal adenocarcinoma
    Adenosquamous, anaplastic, acinar cell
Nonepithelial
  Connective tissue origin
    Leiomyosarcoma
    Liposarcoma
    Rhabdomyosarcoma
    Malignant neurolemmoma
  Malignant lymphomas

Only 14% of patients are candidates for curative resection (stage I and stage II disease), and more than 50% have unresectable stage IV disease (Table 2).

Risk Factors for Development of Pancreatic Cancer

Early diagnosis of pancreatic cancer is difficult because the tumor frequently presents at a late stage, and until recent years, risk factors for development of pancreatic cancer were undefined. However, several risk factors have now been described.

Environmental Factors

Aromatic amines appear to be responsible for the increased risk of pancreatic cancer associated with environmental factors. Thus, cigarette smoking is the most important risk factor and increases the relative risk. Persons working in the chemical, petrochemical, or rubber industries and hairdressers have a greater risk of pancreatic cancer, which may be related to exposure to aromatic amines. Furthermore, animal studies indicate that aromatic amines may be a cause of pancreatic cancer.

Hereditary Pancreatitis

Two mutations of the trypsinogen gene have been described in hereditary pancreatitis. There is a high incidence of pancreatic cancer among patients with hereditary pancreatitis, but this is likely due to the duration of chronic pancreatitis rather than being related specifically to the gene mutation. The estimated cumulative risk of pancreatic cancer at age 70 is 40%. Possibly in the future, methods will be available for identifying patients at risk for pancreatic cancer, but currently no established screening techniques have proven value.

Table 2. Staging of Pancreatic Ductal Adenocarcinoma

Definition of TNM

Primary tumor (T)

TX Primary tumor cannot be assessed

T0 No evidence of primary tumor

Tis In situ carcinoma

T1 Tumor limited to pancreas, ≤2 cm in greatest dimension

T2 Tumor limited to pancreas, >2 cm in greatest dimension

T3 Tumor extends directly into any of the following: duodenum, bile duct, peripancreatic tissues, portal or superior mesenteric vessels

T4 Tumor extends directly into any of the following: stomach, spleen, colon, adjacent large arterial vessels

Regional lymph nodes (N)

NX Regional lymph nodes cannot be assessed

N0 No regional lymph node metastasis

N1 Regional lymph node metastasis

Distant metastasis (M)

MX Distant metastasis cannot be assessed

M0 No distant metastasis

M1 Distant metastasis

Stage grouping

Stage 0	Tis	N0	M0
Stage I	T1	N0	M0
	T2	N0	M0
Stage II	T3	N0	M0
Stage III	T1	N1	M0
	T2	N1	M0
	T3	N1	M0
Stage IVA	T4	Any N	M0
Stage IVB	Any T	Any N	M1

Chronic Pancreatitis

According to a multinational study, patients with chronic pancreatitis have a cumulative risk of 2% per decade and a relative risk (the ratio of observed-to-expected cases) of 16. However, chronic pancreatitis is relatively uncommon and does not contribute significantly to the population of patients with pancreatic cancer.

Intraductal Papillary Mucinous Tumors (see "Cystic Pancreatic Tumors")

This disease was first recognized in Japan in 1982 and increasingly is recognized in the United States. At Mayo Clinic, this condition has been identified in more than 100 patients. In about 25% to 50% of patients, invasive cancer is found at surgery (in some patients, it is not suspected preoperatively). Therefore, intraductal papillary mucinous tumor is a premalignant lesion, and surgical excision at presentation is the treatment of choice.

Diabetes Mellitus

More than 50% of patients who present with pancreatic cancer have diabetes mellitus, and in most patients, diabetes is diagnosed within 2 years after the diagnosis of cancer. Some but not all of the patients are insulin-dependent, and in some, diabetes is diagnosed at the same time as pancreatic cancer. The precise risk of pancreatic cancer in patients with new-onset diabetes is not well defined, but according to a meta-analysis, the risk of pancreatic cancer developing in patients who have had diabetes for more than 1 year is doubled.

Inheritance

The evidence is consistent that 6% to 8% of patients who present with pancreatic cancer have a family history of pancreatic cancer in a first-degree relative, which represents a 13-fold increase over controls. Also, well-defined syndromes are associated with an increased incidence of pancreatic cancer, including Peutz-Jeghers syndrome and familial atypical multiple mole melanoma syndrome. Germline *BRCA2* mutations contribute to 5% to 10% of pancreatic adenocarcinomas and currently are the most common known inherited predisposition to pancreatic cancer.

It is not known at what age screening should begin or indeed whether any screening technique can detect early pancreatic cancer or improve prognosis. General guidelines include performing spiral computed tomography (CT) or endoscopic ultrasonography (EUS) at regular intervals, but there are no data to support this recommendation. Tumor markers, including K-*ras* and CA 19-9, are too insensitive and nonspecific.

Pathology

About 70% of pancreatic ductal adenocarcinomas occur in the head of the pancreas. Histologically, the tumors may vary from well-differentiated tumors that exhibit glandular structures in a dense stroma to poorly differentiated tumors that exhibit little or no glandular structure or stroma. Lymphatic spread appears to occur earlier than vascular invasion, which is present in more advanced lesions. Metastatic disease occurs mainly to the liver and lungs but also to the adrenals, kidneys, bone, brain, and skin.

Diagnosis

Patients with pancreatic cancer usually present with symptoms of pain, jaundice, weight loss (with or without anorexia), and early satiety. The most common symptom is abdominal pain, which occurs in up to 80% of patients. The presence of pain, particularly pain radiating through to the back, is associated with advanced lesions with a poor prognosis, the implication being that the tumor has spread beyond the pancreas.

Jaundice is the second most common presentation and occurs in about 50% of patients. For patients with cancer of the head of the pancreas, painless jaundice is the symptom most frequently predictive of resectability.

Overt steatorrhea is a far less common presenting symptom, even in patients with overt weight loss, and when present alone, it has been associated with longer survival.

Tumor Markers for Diagnosis

Various tumor markers are increased in pancreatic cancer, but all lack sufficient sensitivity and specificity to be used as either diagnostic or screening tests. CA 19-9 has the greatest sensitivity, of about 70%, and specificity, of about 87%, when the cutoff value is 70 U/mL. If a lower cutoff value is used, sensitivity is higher, without much effect on specificity. However, the test is not useful if the biliary tract is obstructed, because even benign biliary tract obstruction can cause a marked increase in CA 19-9.

Genetic markers are present in patients with pancreatic cancer, and the most common of these are the K-*ras* mutation in 90% of patients, *p53* tumor cell suppressor gene in 50% to 70%, and reduced expression of the *DCC* gene in about 50%. Other gene deletions are less common.

Although the K-*ras* mutation can be detected in pancreatic or duodenal juice or stool from patients with pancreatic cancer, it is present less frequently than in the tumor itself and thus is not a useful test because of low sensitivity. Furthermore, lack of specificity is an important issue because K-*ras* can be detected in chronic pancreatitis.

Islet amyloid polypeptide, a hormonal factor secreted from pancreatic beta cells, is increased in patients with pancreatic cancer who have glucose intolerance. Currently, it has no proven clinical application.

Imaging Testing for Diagnosis

Spiral CT should be the primary imaging study for evaluation of patients with symptoms suggestive of pancreatic cancer. It is the appropriate study because it is not only diagnostic but also can be used to stage the tumor. The increase in sensitivity (about 85%) of dual-phase spiral CT is an important improvement over the ability of conventional CT (about 50% to 60%) to diagnose pancreatic tumors. This sometimes leads to misconceptions about the role of dual-phase CT when researching the older literature about the importance of CT in diagnosis. For tumors smaller than 15 mm in diameter, however, the sensitivity of spiral CT is 67%.

EUS has been described as the most accurate imaging test for diagnosing pancreatic cancer, being more accurate than transabdominal ultrasonography or CT. However, triple-phase

CT has "altered the equation," and currently the role of EUS is in identifying small tumors and in performing fine-needle aspiration (FNA) of the primary tumor or lymph nodes. Although EUS-guided FNA is a safe and effective method to diagnose pancreatic cancer, we rarely perform FNA in patients with evidence of resectable pancreatic cancer because the results do not affect our clinical decision to proceed with surgery. Thus, the role for EUS FNA is limited mainly to patients with unresectable lesions, and whether it should be performed needs to be balanced against obtaining histologic material by percutaneous biopsy assisted by either ultrasonography or CT.

Staging Pancreatic Tumors

CT should be the initial test not only for diagnosis but also for staging of pancreatic cancer because it may provide evidence of distant metastases or clear vascular involvement, making further staging unnecessary (Fig. 1 and 2). Magnetic resonance imaging (MRI) may be as accurate as spiral CT, but generally it is not as readily available and there is not the same expertise in interpreting the findings. EUS may be the most accurate method for staging the local extent (T staging) (Fig. 3) and nodal status (N staging). Correct interpretation of resectability by both CT and EUS varies depending on the study. For EUS, operator experience and the size of the tumor are important variables. Specifically, the area of interest relative to vascular invasion

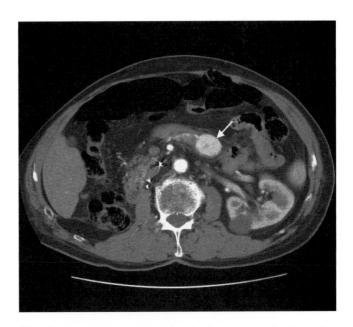

Fig. 1. Computed tomogram showing hyperattenuating lesion in the body of the pancreas (*arrow*). Primary pancreatic adenocarcinoma is usually hypoattenuating. This lesion would also be consistent with an islet cell tumor. The right kidney is absent. This lesion is a metastatic renal cell carcinoma.

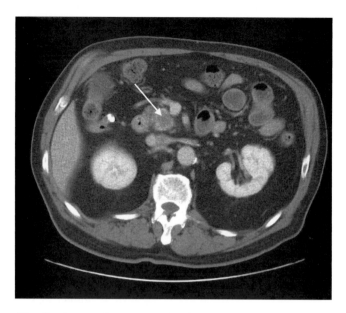

Fig. 2. Computed tomogram showing pancreatic cancer. Small hypoattenuating lesion is in the head of the pancreas (*arrow*). The superior mesenteric vessels are not involved by the tumor, which is resectable.

requires imaging through the entire extent of the tumor, and with current equipment (either radial or curved linear scanning transducers), resolution progressively deteriorates with increasing depth of imaging. Whether advances in EUS technology will improve its ability to determine resectability when CT (or MRI) findings are equivocal is unclear.

Small liver or peritoneal metastases usually are not seen on preoperative imaging studies. Laparoscopy has been recommended by some authors for viewing the liver and peritoneal surfaces preoperatively. About 10% to 15% of patients have these small metastases. Most centers do not routinely perform laparoscopy during preoperative assessment, but it can be argued that laparoscopy is indicated when the likelihood of unresectability is high. This would include all patients with cancer of the pancreatic body or tail, which has a very low chance of being resected and virtually no chance of cure, or patients with ascites, which is usually related to peritoneal metastases.

Treatment

Surgery

Most patients who undergo operative resection for pancreatic cancer ultimately die of the disease, but the only chance of cure, albeit slim, is resection. For this reason, most major centers continue to endorse the surgical approach.

Preoperative biopsy or FNA of a pancreatic mass is not required in most instances because the findings do not alter the decision to resect. Of the patients who have the typical clinical presentation and preoperative imaging results, about 90% have pancreatic cancer at surgery. The other 10% usually have chronic pancreatitis, but it is not possible to confidently exclude tumor preoperatively, and therefore it is appropriate to perform a Whipple procedure. In 10% to 15% of patients, pancreatic cancer may produce a desmoplastic response and tumor tissue may be difficult to procure with needle biopsy or FNA.

If surgical resection is not preceded by laparoscopy, the surgeon usually examines the peritoneal cavity and its contents carefully for obvious small metastases and then assesses vascular involvement, which requires mobilization of the tumor by dissection. The standard operation for pancreatic cancer is

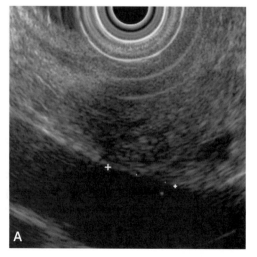

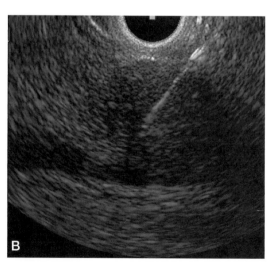

Fig. 3. *A*, Endoscopic ultrasonogram of the pancreatic head shows a poorly defined hypoechoic mass that impinges on the portal vein for a distance of 11 mm (see markers). Surgical resection confirmed portal vein invasion. *B*, Fine-needle aspirate of mass shown in *A*.

pancreaticoduodenectomy (Whipple procedure), which involves cholecystectomy and removing a portion of the stomach (at least antrectomy), the distal bile duct, head of the pancreas, the duodenum, proximal jejunum, and regional lymph nodes. Reconstruction with gastrojejunostomy, hepaticojejunostomy, and pancreaticojejunostomy is required. Results are good and mortality is low when the operation is performed by an experienced surgeon.

Alternative operations include a pylorus-preserving Whipple resection. This preserves the stomach and is a less extensive operation. It has been assumed that this operation, compared with the Whipple procedure, would improve outcome. However, the results that have been reported are not clear, so many surgeons perform either procedure depending on the situation, including the size and extent of the tumor. An extended or radical Whipple resection has been reported in the Japanese literature to provide better results, but these results have not been confirmed by studies in the United States or Europe; indeed, four prospective, randomized trials have been performed and failed to find an advantage for the more extensive procedure.

Surgery is the only chance for cure, but median survival is only about 18 months and the 5-year survival rate is about 10%. Higher survival rates have been reported, and it appears that the different rates depend on the tumor size, nodal status, and completeness of resection. For example, patients with tumors smaller than 2 cm have a reported survival rate of 20%, compared with only 1% for patients with tumors larger than 3 cm. The hypothesis that surgical treatment of early pancreatic cancer improves prognosis is based on these data.

At presentation, most patients have pancreatic cancer that is unresectable because of distant metastases or local extension. Because biliary obstruction can be relieved by endoscopic stenting, surgical management of biliary obstruction usually is limited to patients with a concomitant gastric outlet obstruction. Biliary diversion is achieved by cholecystenterostomy (but only when the cystic duct enters the common bile duct at a distance from the tumor) or by choledochoenterostomy. Because duodenal obstruction develops in less than 20% of patients before they die, it is our policy—and that of nearly all centers—not to perform prophylactic gastrojejunostomy. In some patients, neuropathy due to infiltration of the plexus by tumor, and not obstruction, may cause vomiting and slow gastric emptying; thus, a drainage procedure will not be helpful in these patients.

Most patients who have jaundice and unresectable pancreatic cancer should have endoscopic stent placement. The preferred endoscopic prosthesis for palliation is an expandable metal stent, which is less likely to become occluded than plastic stents. Percutaneous transhepatic stenting has a lower success rate and a higher 30-day mortality rate and is not the procedure of choice. According to recent reports and our experience, endoscopically placed expandable metal prostheses can successfully alleviate gastric outlet or duodenal malignant obstruction, but these new procedures require further evaluation before they can be recommended for routine use.

Palliation of pain is a major problem in pancreatic cancer. Chemical intraoperative splanchnicectomy or celiac plexus block performed percutaneously or with EUS reportedly has reduced pain markedly and, according to one report, has prolonged survival. The advantage of plexus block is that it produces fewer complications related to narcotic use, namely, constipation, nausea, and vomiting. Although no controlled trial has tested the efficacy of celiac plexus block against oral pharmacologic therapy, the current bias is that celiac block provides better pain control.

If oral analgesia is used to control pancreatic cancer pain, the type and dose of medication should depend on the severity of pain. For example, mild pain may be controlled with an acetaminophen (325 mg)-oxycodone (5 mg) combination, one or two tablets every 4 to 6 hours, whereas more severe pain may require a slow-release morphine compound, usually starting at a dose of 30 mg twice daily and increasing to a dose as high as 600 mg twice daily to achieve pain control. A short-acting liquid morphine compound may be useful to control breakthrough pain. Alternatively, a fentanyl (Duragesic) patch, 25 to 100 µg per hour, is effective in some patients.

Exocrine Pancreatic Insufficiency

Patients with cancer of the pancreatic head who have weight loss and stools suggestive of malabsorption should receive treatment with pancreatic enzymes. Available data suggest that pancreatic steatorrhea can be corrected with pancreatic replacement therapy. Our practice has been to prescribe pancreatin (Viokase), eight tablets with meals (two after a few bites, four during a meal, and two at the end of the meal), to correct steatorrhea.

Chemotherapy and Radiotherapy

Chemotherapy

No single or combination chemotherapy is highly effective for pancreatic cancer. Only 5-fluorouracil (5-FU) and gemcitabine have been associated with survival longer than 5 months. 5-FU has been administered as a bolus or short-term continuous infusion or protracted infusion to treat many tumors. However, protracted infusion of 5-FU in combination with other chemotherapeutic agents does not appear to be advantageous. Gemcitabine has a low objective response rate and, compared with 5-FU, a small statistically significant improvement in overall survival (5.7 vs. 4.4 months). One-year survival with gemcitabine treatment was 18%, compared with 2% for 5-FU.

Radiotherapy

Radiation is used in two situations. 1. It is used as adjuvant therapy after resection for cure. Until recently, the only randomized trial showed that radiotherapy in combination with 5-FU had a 2-year actuarial survival rate of 43% compared with an 18% rate for the control group (resection only). However, a recently published European study found no significant advantage. 2. In unresectable locoregional pancreatic cancer, combined chemoradiation therapy, with 5-FU and radiation, was superior to radiation alone, with a median survival of 42 versus 23 weeks.

CYSTIC PANCREATIC TUMORS

Serous Cystadenoma

Classically, these tumors are described to present as large, sometimes palpable, asymptomatic upper abdominal masses, but in our experience, they more frequently are small lesions in the head, body, or tail of the pancreas that are discovered incidentally on imaging studies (Fig. 4). They occur equally in males and females and constitute up to 10% of all cystic lesions of the pancreas. Histologically, the tumors consist of multiple tiny cysts containing watery fluid. Their cut surface shows a typical stellate scar (which is also evident on imaging). The malignant potential is almost zero (only a few case reports of malignancy have been published), and in elderly asymptomatic patients, these tumors frequently are simply observed.

Mucinous Cystadenoma and Cystadenocarcinoma

These tumors occur predominantly in persons 40 to 60 years old, and the female:male ratio is 6:1. They account for 1% to 2% of all pancreatic exocrine tumors. Foci of malignancy in many

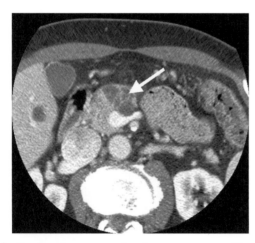

Fig. 4. Computed tomogram showing a serous cyst. The mass lesion in the head of the pancreas consists of multiple small cystic lesions (*arrow*). The findings are typical of serous cystadenoma.

of the cysts and reports of ostensibly benign resected cystadenomas later presenting with metastatic disease have led to the concept that these lesions have a high malignant potential.

The tumors consist of multiple cysts (larger than those in serous cystadenomas) containing sticky mucus. As with serous cystadenomas, these lesions are often identified as a small cystic lesion in patients having CT for another reason.

Intraductal Papillary Mucinous Tumor

This group of tumors, originally described in Japan, consists of intraductal papillary growth of mucin-producing columnar epithelium. These changes can occur in the main pancreatic duct or in side ducts and may involve a small portion of the pancreas or the entire gland. As a consequence of these changes, obstructive pancreatitis frequently occurs, with atrophy of the gland. Malignant transformation of the papillary growth occurs in up to 30% to 50% of patients at the time of diagnosis, about one-half of whom have evidence of metastatic disease.

Frequent clinical presentations include recurrent episodes of pancreatitis, abdominal pain, or steatorrhea. Jaundice and diabetes are less common. The diagnosis is suspected when a dilated pancreatic duct or side ducts are seen on CT. The chief differential diagnosis is chronic pancreatitis. At endoscopic retrograde cholangiopancreatography, about one-half of patients have the diagnostic finding of a patulous papilla extruding mucus. EUS may be helpful in making the diagnosis.

Solid-Cystic (Papillary-Cystic) Tumor

This tumor, which has various names, has a striking female predominance and usually occurs in adolescence. The histogenesis is unclear, but histologically, pseudopapillary and microcystic changes are present. Most patients present with abdominal pain. The treatment for these often large tumors is excision. The prognosis is good, and most of the tumors can be considered benign, but occasionally metastatic disease occurs.

Approach to Small, Incidentally Observed Cystic Tumors of the Pancreas

When cystic tumors of the pancreas are small, CT and ultrasonography may not be able to resolve the nature of the cyst, and EUS has an important role in defining its structure. For example, what may appear to be a unilocular simple cyst on CT may be seen on EUS to be a complex cyst with septations. Although aspiration of the cyst is a simple procedure, it is not clear whether analysis of the cystic fluid for carcinoembryonic antigen or mucin and cytologic examination for malignancy alter the decisions about management for most patients.

Generally, if the nature of a cyst cannot be determined precisely and the patient is elderly, the practice is to observe the cyst and to perform imaging studies at regular intervals to ensure that it is not rapidly increasing in size.

ACKNOWLEDGMENT

Jonathan E. Clain, M.D. is gratefully acknowledged as author of this chapter in the previous edition of the book (parts of which appear in this edition).

RECOMMENDED READING

Brugge WR, Lauwers GY, Sahani D, Fernandez-del Castillo C, Warshaw AL. Cystic neoplasms of the pancreas. N Engl J Med. 2004;351:1218-26.

DiMagno EP, Reber HA, Tempero MA, American Gastroenterological Association. AGA technical review on the epidemiology, diagnosis, and treatment of pancreatic ductal adenocarcinoma. Gastroenterology. 1999;117:1464-84.

Pearson RK, Clain JE, Longnecker DS, Reber HA, Steinberg WM, Barkin JS, et al. Controversies in clinical pancreatology: intraductal papillary-mucinous tumor (IPMT): American Pancreatic Association Clinical Symposium. Pancreas. 2002;25:217-21.

CHAPTER 44

Gallstones

Bret T. Petersen, M.D.

Gallstones are extremely common, occurring in 10% to 20% of women and 5% to 10% of men in Western cultures. They generate an enormous medical and financial burden. More than 500,000 cholecystectomies are performed each year in the United States. An understanding of the physiology, presentation, and efficient approaches to management is therefore important. Optimal clinical approaches vary considerably depending on the presentation.

BILE PHYSIOLOGY

The major components of bile are water, inorganic solutes, and organic solutes. The organic solutes include miscellaneous proteins, bilirubin, bile acids, and the biliary lipids. Bilirubin is a degradation product of heme and usually is present as conjugated water-soluble diglucuronide. The unconjugated form of bilirubin precipitates, contributing to pigment or mixed cholesterol stones. Bile acids are bipolar water-soluble molecules synthesized from cholesterol. When present above the *critical micellar concentration*, they self-associate to form micelles capable of solubilizing hydrophobic lipid molecules in bile or intestinal chyme. Their primary function is to facilitate fat digestion and absorption. The *primary* bile acids (cholic and chenodeoxycholic acid) are made in the liver. They are converted to *secondary* bile acids (deoxycholic and lithocholic acid) by bacteria in the gut. The major biliary lipids, cholesterol and lecithin (phospholipid), are insoluble in water. They are secreted into bile as lipid vesicles and are carried both in vesicles and in mixed micelles.

In health, the gallbladder concentrates bile 10-fold for efficient storage during fasting. Intraduodenal protein and fat release cholecystokinin (CCK), which stimulates gallbladder contraction, sphincter-of-Oddi relaxation, and bile flow to the intestine. More than 90% of bile acids are actively absorbed in the terminal ileum. This enterohepatic circulation cycles 4 to 12 times per day, slowing during fasting and accelerating greatly after meals (Fig. 1).

GALLSTONE PATHOGENESIS AND EPIDEMIOLOGY

Gallbladder stones are predominantly made of cholesterol in 80% of patients and of bilirubin pigment in 20% (Fig. 2). Cholesterol stones contain a mixture of 50% to 99% cholesterol by weight, a glycoprotein matrix, and small amounts of calcium and bilirubin. Development of overt stones requires three critical defects related to bile saturation, crystal nucleation, and gallbladder motility.

Cholesterol supersaturation can occur as a result of deficient bile acid secretion or hypersecretion of cholesterol. Bile acid secretion may be diminished because of reduced synthesis, as occurs with age or liver disease, or because of reduced enterohepatic circulation, as occurs with motor disorders, hormonal defects, and increased gastrointestinal losses from bile acid sequestrant therapy or terminal ileal disease, resection, or bypass. Cholesterol secretion is increased with hormonal stimuli (female sex, pregnancy, exogenous estrogens, and progestins), obesity, hyperlipidemia, age, chronic liver disease, and sometimes with excessive dietary polyunsaturated fats or calorie intake.

In a supersaturated environment, initial gallstone crystal formation occurs as a result of an excess of nucleating versus antinucleating effects of the various proteins in bile.

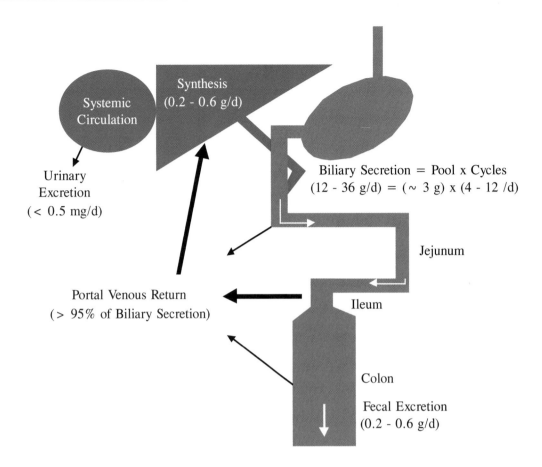

Fig. 1. Enterohepatic circulation. A pool of 3 g of bile acids cycles 4 to 12 times per day. Ileal absorption returns 97% of intraluminal bile acids back to the circulation. Ninety percent of bile acids are extracted from the portal system on their first pass through the liver. In health, hepatic synthesis of bile acids is equivalent to enteric losses. (Modified from Zucker SD, Gollan JL. Physiology of the liver. In: Haubrich WS, Schaffner F, Berk JE, editors. Bockus gastroenterology. Vol 3. 5th ed. Philadelphia: WB Saunders Company; 1995. p. 1858-1904. Used with permission.)

Gallbladder dysmotility results in inadequate clearance of crystals and nascent stones. Motility is reduced in the presence of supersaturated bile even before stone formation. Reduced motility is a dominant contributing factor to stone development during pregnancy, prolonged total parenteral nutrition, somato-statin therapy, or somatostatinoma.

The prevalence of cholesterol gallstones varies with geography and ethnicity. They are rare in populations of Africa and most of Asia, are common in most Western populations (15%-20% in women, 5%-10% in men), and almost uniformly occur in North and South American Indians (70%-90% in women). For all populations, the prevalence increases with age and is approximately twice as high in women as in men.

Black and brown pigment stones occur as a result of increased amounts of unconjugated insoluble bilirubin present in bile, often due to infection or hepatic secretion. Black stones originate in the gallbladder. They are small, irregular, dense, and insoluble aggregates or polymers of calcium bilirubinate. They may occur with cirrhosis or chronic hemolysis but usually

have no identifiable cause (Fig. 3). Brown pigment stones primarily occur in the bile ducts, where they are related to stasis and chronic bacterial colonization—as may occur above strictures or duodenal diverticuli, after sphincterotomy, or in association with biliary parasites. Brown stones are 10% to 30% cholesterol. They are softer than black pigment stones and may soften or disaggregate with cholesterol solvents (Fig. 4).

BILIARY IMAGING

Numerous methods are available for imaging the biliary tree. Some are used primarily to assess the gallbladder or the bile ducts, and others provide more general assessment of the abdomen, as in patients with undefined pain.

Abdominal plain radiography detects only 10% to 15% of gallstones, which are calcified sufficiently to appear radiopaque (Fig. 5). Abdominal radiography also detects aerobilia and porcelain gallbladder. Air within the biliary tree implies the presence of a biliary-enteric anastomosis or fistula or an

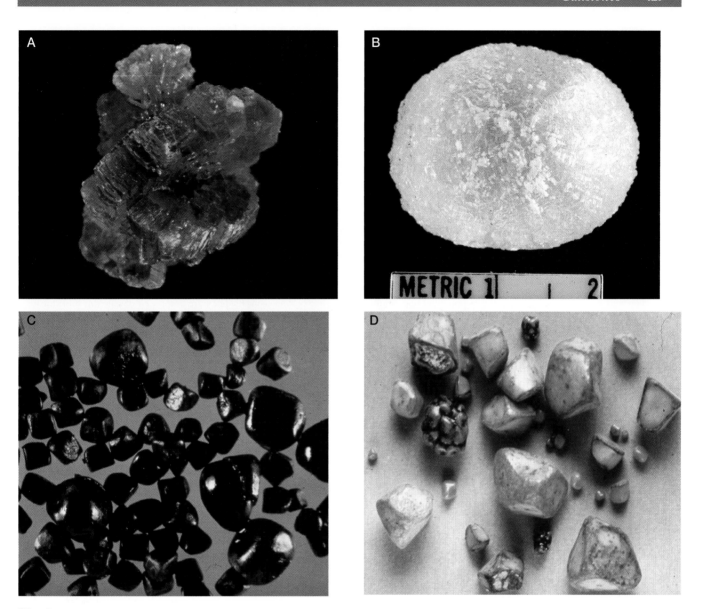

Fig. 2. Variations in morphologic findings of cholesterol gallstones. *A*, Nearly pure 97% cholesterol crystalline stone on a pigmented central nidus. *B*, Pure 99+% cholesterol stone in conformation of mothball. *C*, Faceted cholesterol stones with external shell of black pigment and calcification. *D*, Several morphologic features of mixed, predominantly cholesterol stones from one patient.

incompetent sphincter, as may occur with duodenal Crohn's disease, duodenal diverticuli, or other periampullary disease. Porcelain gallbladder refers to radiographically detectable deposition of calcium within the gallbladder wall. It has a considerable association with progression to gallbladder cancer and is therefore an indication for elective prophylactic cholecystectomy.

Oral cholecystography involves standard x-ray filming of the right upper quadrant after oral administration of a contrast agent (Fig. 6). Normal imaging during oral cholecystography necessitates ingestion, intestinal absorption, hepatic uptake, biliary excretion, and gallbladder concentration of an iodinated radiodense contrast agent. Sixty to eighty percent of gallbladders opacify after a single oral dose and 85% to 90% opacify after a second or double dose. Nonvisualization of the gallbladder after a reinforced 1- or 2-day study is 95% predictive of gallbladder disease. The use of oral cholecystography in clinical practice has diminished because it is less sensitive (65%-90%) than ultrasonography for gallbladder stones and it is not indicated when acute cholecystitis is suspected. It may be useful when ultrasonography fails to image the gallbladder or fails to demonstrate stones despite a strong clinical suspicion and for demonstration of cystic duct patency in potential candidates for nonsurgical therapies.

Transabdominal ultrasonography is the first choice for evaluation of jaundice and right upper quadrant pain and when cholangitis or cholecystitis is suspected because it is portable,

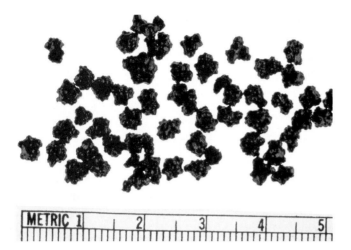

Fig. 3. Black pigment gallstones, formed primarily in the gallbladder and made of dense and insoluble polymers of calcium bilirubinate. They constitute 20% of gallbladder stones. They are associated with increasing age, cirrhosis, and hemolysis but usually are idiopathic.

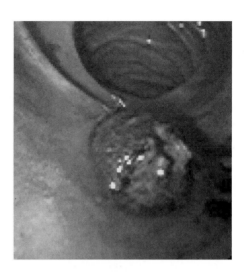

Fig. 4. Brown pigment gallstones are formed in the ducts as primary duct stones. They are composed of calcium bilirubinate and about 30% cholesterol. They are softer and more amorphous than cholesterol or black pigment stones. They are associated with strictures, stasis, duodenal diverticuli, and infection. Here, a brown stone is seen in the lumen of the duodenum after extraction from the bile duct at endoscopic retrograde cholangiopancreatography.

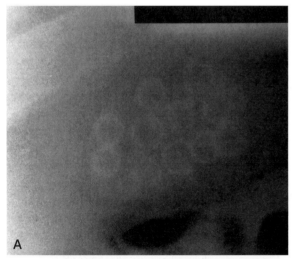

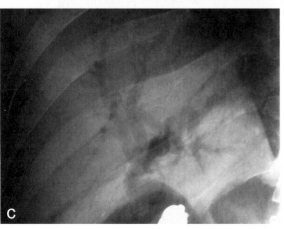

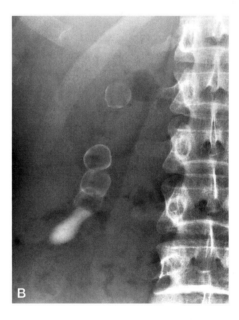

Fig. 5. Abdominal plain radiography. *A*, Radiopaque gallstones; 15% are detected on plain radiography and 50% on computed tomography. No relationship to symptoms. *B*, Radiopaque bile. So-called milk-of-calcium bile is attributed to chronic gallbladder obstruction and is likely related to symptoms when seen. Here, it is seen below four radiopaque obstructing stones. *C*, Aerobilia, indicative of past sphincterotomy or biliary-enteric anastomosis or fistula. It is sometimes seen with Crohn's disease, diverticula, or other periampullary disease.

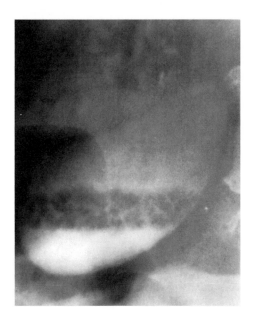

Fig. 6. Oral cholecystography. Floating cholesterol gallstones layering at interface of contrast and bile.

requires no specific preparation, and uses no radiation (Fig. 7). The examinations are analogous to a physical examination and hence are somewhat subjective and operator-dependent. They are compromised by obesity and interfering shadows caused by, for example, ribs, scars, and bowel gas. Ultrasonography is highly sensitive for dilated ducts; however, ducts may be normal in 25% to 35% of patients with choledocholithiasis, particularly when the presentation is acute or associated with biliary fibrosis. The sensitivity of ultrasonography for identification of common duct stones is widely variable (20%-80%). It is most sensitive (90%-98%) for detection of gallbladder stones that are identified as mobile, intraluminal, echogenic, shadowing particles. Cholecystitis is identified by gallbladder contraction or marked distention with surrounding fluid or wall thickening. Gallbladder thickening also may be due to portal hypertension, ascites, and hypoalbuminemia.

Endoscopic ultrasonography (EUS) is highly sensitive for intraductal stones and slightly less so for gallbladder stones, depending on anatomy. It is an optimal screening tool when the

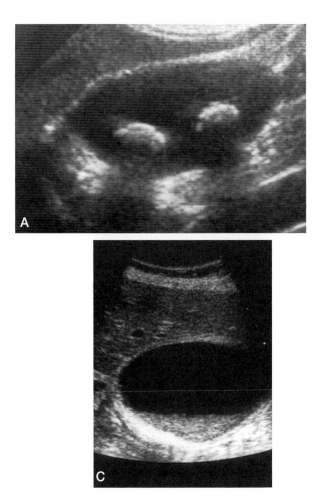

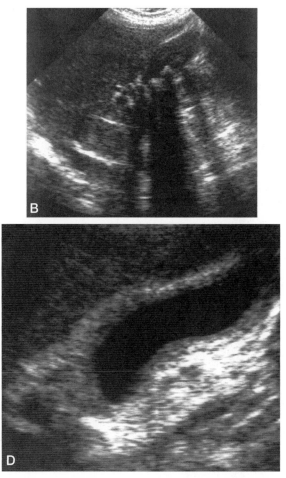

Fig. 7. Gallbladder ultrasonography. *A*, Shadowing, mobile, echodense gallstones in a normal lumen. *B*, Tightly packed and less discrete stones in a contracted gallbladder. *C*, Gallbladder sludge composed of cholesterol crystals and mucus and seen during prolonged gallbladder stasis, as with total parenteral nutrition or during pregnancy. *D*, Thick, edematous gallbladder mucosa sometimes seen with acute cholecystitis, portal hypertension, ascites, or hypoalbuminemia.

suspicion for bile duct stones is low to moderate, endoscopic examination of the upper gut is also needed, other extraluminal questions exist, or the expense and risk of endoscopic retrograde cholangiopancreatography (ERCP) are unacceptable. Compared with magnetic resonance cholangiopancreatography (MRCP) and ERCP, EUS is the most cost-effective first study for suspected stones when the pre-test probability is less than 55% to 60%. ERCP becomes cost-effective above this level, which largely includes only patients with distinctly abnormal liver enzyme values. EUS also can identify gallbladder sludge and microlithiasis in symptomatic patients with negative transabdominal ultrasonography. Patients must be safe candidates for both endoscopy and sedation.

Radionuclide biliary scanning, or hepatobiliary iminodiacetic acid scanning, involves noninvasive scanning of gamma emissions after intravenous administration, hepatic uptake, and biliary excretion of technetium iminodiacetic acid derivatives. Failure to visualize the gallbladder by 4 hours after injection is indicative of cystic duct obstruction. The primary clinical indication is for the diagnosis of acute cholecystitis. Nonvisualization of the gallbladder is 97% sensitive and 96% specific for acute calculous cholecystitis. False-negative results occur in acalculous cholecystitis, whereas false-positive results occur in chronic cholecystitis, in chronic liver disease, and during total parenteral nutrition or fasting states. The test is also useful for noninvasive confirmation of intra-abdominal bile leakage.

Abdominal computed tomography (CT) is the best imaging method for evaluation of possible complications of biliary stone disease if ultrasonography is compromised or suboptimal, as in patients with fever, right upper quadrant pain, and associated jaundice (Fig. 8). Bowel gas and ribs do not interfere, and CT is better than ultrasonography for obese patients, in whom imaging is improved by discrete fat planes. The test is not appropriate for the diagnosis of uncomplicated stone disease or evaluation of biliary colic, because half of all gallstones are radiolucent on CT.

Cholangiography can be accomplished either invasively or noninvasively. Selection of percutaneous transhepatic cholangiography, ERCP, or MRCP is largely based on institutional expertise, therapeutic goals, and the clinical setting.

ERCP is favored in patients with ascites or coagulation defects, suspected periampullary or pancreatic neoplasia, nondilated ducts, anticipated need for therapeutic maneuvers (stone removal, stenting), hypersensitivity to contrast agents, or failure of percutaneous routes (Fig. 9). Purely diagnostic use is rapidly diminishing because EUS and MRCP serve this purpose more safely in most patients. Endoscopic retrograde cholangiography is successful in more than 95% of diagnostic applications, 90% to 95% of sphincterotomies and overall stone extraction, and 90% of procedures for stenting of malignant obstruction. The overall risk of the test is 2% to 7% for diagnostic procedures and 7% to 10% for therapy. Risks include death, pancreatitis, infection, sedation or cardiovascular events, hemorrhage, and perforation.

Percutaneous transhepatic cholangiography may be favored in patients with more proximal obstruction (hilar or above), surgically distorted gastroduodenal anatomy (especially Roux limbs, but also Whipple or Billroth II anatomy), and after failure of prior ERCP. It is almost uniformly successful in patients with dilated ducts and in 75% to 95% of those with nondilated ducts. Overall risk is 3% to 8% and includes death, sepsis, bile leaks, and intraperitoneal bleeding.

MRCP is favored in frail patients who are not candidates for conscious sedation and in those with coagulopathy or a need for concurrent staging or evaluation of the hepatic parenchyma

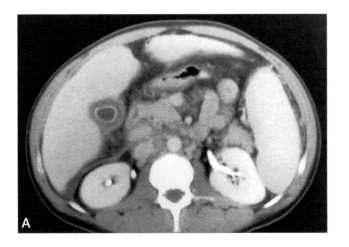
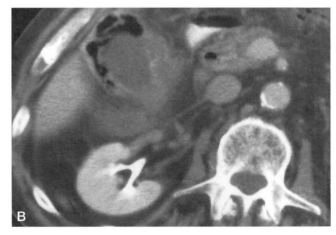

Fig. 8. Computed tomography of complicated biliary stone disease. *A*, Thickened gallbladder wall, as seen on ultrasonogram in Figure 7 *D*. *B*, Emphysematous cholecystitis due to *Clostridium* species and others presents in toxicity as a medical and surgical emergency.

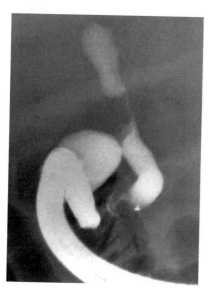

Fig. 9. Endoscopic retrograde cholangiography. Contrast-filled bile duct demonstrates Mirizzi's syndrome, recognized by the unusual eccentric stricture in the mid duct with nonvisualization of the cystic duct and gallbladder.

or other organs, especially when there is little likelihood for therapeutic intervention.

GALLSTONE CLINICAL PRESENTATIONS AND MANAGEMENT

Asymptomatic gallstones are a common incidental discovery in the course of varied abdominal imaging procedures. Gallstones remain asymptomatic long-term in 70% to 80% of patients. When gallstones eventually become symptomatic, only 2% to 3% of patients present initially with acute cholecystitis or other complications. Asymptomatic stones generally do not require therapy. However, prophylactic cholecystectomy should be considered in patients before extended travel to remote areas (e.g., Antarctica) and in American Indian populations, in whom the relative risk for stone-associated gallbladder carcinoma is 20-fold higher than in those without stones. Cholecystectomy also should be considered during weight loss operations, even without existing stones, because their subsequent development can be anticipated. Cholecystectomy is not recommended for patients with asymptomatic stones who have diabetes or sickle cell disease if they have usual access to medical care.

Biliary colic is a relatively specific form of pain that usually develops rapidly in the epigastrium or right upper quadrant and lasts more than 15 minutes but not more than 4 to 6 hours. A careful history is required to differentiate alternative causes of pain. After the development of symptoms, a similar pattern is likely to continue. The likelihood of experiencing a severe event or complication is approximately 1% per year, prompting recommendation for surgical therapy of symptomatic stones. Most patients with recurrent biliary colic have chronic cholecystitis histologically. Patients with uncomplicated colic require episodic pain management and dietary moderation emphasizing self-selection rather than strict exclusion of fat or other food types. Laparoscopic cholecystectomy is now the standard and most widely used therapy. There is a learning curve of at least 10 to 25 procedures, during which time the duration of the procedure and complications are considerably greater. The major risk is for serious duct injuries, which occur in less than 1 in 400 cases. Open cholecystectomy is necessary in less than 5% of initial laparoscopic procedures. Conversion itself is usually not considered a complication but an appropriate change in technique based on intraoperative findings. The risk for conversion is higher with acute cholecystitis.

Nonoperative therapy of gallbladder stones is largely of historical interest. A general requirement for all nonsurgical therapies is patency of the cystic duct, as determined with oral cholecystography or radionuclide biliary scanning. Stones that are seen to float above a contrast layer during oral cholecystography are high in cholesterol and very amenable to dissolution (Fig. 6). The major shortcoming of all nonsurgical therapies is the potential for gallstone recurrence, which occurs in 10% to 20% of patients per year and up to 40% to 60% overall for patients with multiple stones. Oral bile acid therapy with ursodeoxycholic acid (7-8 mg/kg per day) dissolves 30% to 80% of radiolucent stones less than 15 mm in diameter over 6 to 24 months. Repeat cholecystography is performed after 6 to 12 months, and therapy is discontinued if no dissolution is evident or if overt rim calcification has developed. Side effects of therapy are infrequent and include diarrhea in 3% to 5% of patients. Extracorporeal shock wave lithotripsy is more commonly performed in Europe than in the United States. A single machine has been approved for duct stone applications only, and no machine is approved for gallbladder stones in the United States. Extracorporeal shock wave lithotripsy is generally safe and well tolerated. Success depends on fragmentation plus either passage or dissolution of resulting debris. Optimal results are achieved with single radiolucent stones less than 20 mm in diameter, for which clearance is achieved in 70% to 95% after 12 to 24 months of full-dose bile acid therapy. Rapid dissolution of gallstones over 6 to 12 hours can be accomplished by delivery of a cholesterol solvent such as methyl-*tert*-butyl ether into the gallbladder through a transhepatic catheter. Cholesterol stones that are radiolucent by CT are predictably soluble, independent of their size or number.

Complications of gallstone disease include acute cholecystitis, Mirizzi's syndrome, gallbladder perforation, cholecystoenteric fistulas, "gallstone ileus," and gallstone or biliary pancreatitis.

Acute cholecystitis presents with biliary colic that usually lasts more than 4 to 6 hours and spreads to involve the parietal surfaces, with evolution from a nonspecific visceral character to a more localized right upper quadrant pain. There may be associated nausea, vomiting, jaundice, fever, and tenderness. The laboratory results are nonspecific and may include a leukocytosis and modest increases of aminotransferases, alkaline phosphatase, and amylase. Management of acute cholecystitis includes administration of antibiotics, hydration, analgesia, nasogastric suction as needed for comfort, and removal or drainage of the obstructed gallbladder. Gallbladder decompression with percutaneous cholecystostomy tube placement is efficacious in patients with substantial operative risk. After days to weeks of antibiotic therapy and passive drainage, subsequent operative or nonoperative management can be pursued electively. Endoscopic drainage also has been described.

Mirizzi's syndrome involves gallbladder obstruction plus obstructive jaundice from stone impaction in the distal cystic duct with inflammatory compression of the common hepatic duct. The clinical and cholangiographic findings must be differentiated from those of other benign and malignant duct strictures. Treatment is generally surgical, although endoscopic palliation with stenting and stone removal has been described.

Gallbladder perforation from stone-induced inflammation generally is contained locally and rarely is free within the abdomen. Perforation with abscess formation occurs especially with minimally symptomatic smoldering disease in elderly patients.

Cholecystoenteric fistulas can develop as a result of gallbladder perforation and decompression into any neighboring viscus. They usually involve the duodenum or the hepatic flexure of the colon. When fistulas develop to the colon, patients may present with new onset of watery bile acid diarrhea or cholangitis from colonic contamination of a diseased gallbladder.

"Gallstone ileus" results after stone passage through a fistula with subsequent obstruction in a narrow downstream section of gut. This is most common in the terminal ileum. Gallstone ileus occurs especially in elderly women. The clinical presentation is that of intestinal obstruction with aerobilia on plain radiography or CT. Management is surgical.

Gallstone or biliary pancreatitis presents acutely as a result of temporary stone impaction or traversal through the sphincter of Oddi. The best indicator of a biliary cause is acute increases in aminotransferase values (more than threefold) at initial presentation. Corroborating findings include a dilated bile duct and stones within the gallbladder.

CHOLEDOCHOLITHIASIS

Most bile duct stones originate in the gallbladder, and 5% to 15% of patients undergoing cholecystectomy have concurrent duct stones. Coexistent duct and gallbladder stones generally have the same composition: 70% are cholesterol stones, 30% pigment stones. Primary duct stones are brown pigment stones, which differ from the smaller, harder, black pigment stones found in the gallbladder.

Duct stones present in various ways, ranging from few or no symptoms to overt cholangitis or pancreatitis. The development of secondary biliary cirrhosis related to ductal pressure rarely occurs in the absence of clinical symptoms or laboratory abnormalities. Stone-related obstruction is classically recurrent and incomplete. Increases in bilirubin and alkaline phosphatase levels are less marked than those for fixed malignant obstruction; the bilirubin level usually peaks at 12 to 14 mg/dL. Ninety percent of obstructing duct stones are located distally near the ampulla, where visualization with ultrasonography and CT is difficult. Their definitive identification necessitates cholangiography. Once identified, duct stones should be removed, usually through ERCP with sphincterotomy. Extracorporeal shock wave lithotripsy of duct stones is clinically approved and feasible. It is usually coupled with ERCP removal of stone debris. Stones identified at operation can be removed through percutaneous T-tube tracts 4 to 6 weeks postoperatively. This is successful in 96% of patients, and the morbidity rate is 4%. There is no primary dissolution therapy for common duct stones, although reports of softening or disaggregation of brown pigment stones occasionally prompts use of ursodeoxycholic acid before repeat ERCP.

Optimal management for healthy patients with concurrent gallbladder and bile duct stones is incompletely defined. Current usual practice combines therapeutic ERCP with laparoscopic cholecystectomy. Laparoscopic duct exploration is still not widespread, although data suggest it is associated with lower morbidity and incurs lower costs than postoperative ERCP.

Elective management of *gallbladder* stones after resolution of cholangitis and endoscopic clearance of duct stones is somewhat controversial. For the high-risk patient, clearance of duct stones alone often is adequate. Experience suggests relative safety for observation alone. In 15% to 20% of patients, biliary colic or cholecystitis necessitating therapy subsequently develops. This risk justifies prophylactic elective cholecystectomy in average-risk patients.

CHOLANGITIS

Acute bacterial cholangitis is due to infection in obstructed bile ducts. It is most commonly caused by obstructing stones and occurs only infrequently with benign or malignant strictures. Charcot's triad (fever and chills, jaundice, and abdominal pain) is present in perhaps 60% of cases. Diagnosis may be difficult in elderly patients, in whom jaundice or pain may be absent. Acute cholangitis is a medical emergency when fever exceeds 40°C or is associated with sepsis, hypotension, peritoneal signs, or a bilirubin value more than 10 mg/dL. CT or ultrasonography is supportive for diagnosis. Most episodes are due to coliforms such as *Escherichia coli*, *Klebsiella* (70%), *Enterococcus*, and anaerobes (10%-15%). Initial therapy includes empiric use of antibiotics, including broad-spectrum agents such as ampicillin plus an aminoglycoside, extended-spectrum penicillins, or third-generation cephalosporins, with or without the addition of specific anaerobic coverage. In 85% to 90% of patients, there is a response to initial antibiotics and supportive therapy before biliary intervention. Biliary drainage is mandatory, however. Its urgency depends on the initial response to antibiotics and supportive care. ERCP with nasobiliary drain placement, stent, or sphincterotomy and duct clearance is associated with considerably lower morbidity and mortality than traditional surgical management. If endoscopy fails to achieve access, subsequent percutaneous or surgical decompression should be pursued, depending on the clinical urgency.

Recurrent pyogenic cholangitis, or oriental cholangiohepatitis, presents with recurrent progressively severe and frequent attacks of cholangitis with associated extensive stone disease, especially of the intrahepatic ducts. Secondary duct dilation, stricture formation, and further stone formation become self-perpetuating. This form of cholangitis occurs especially in the Asian-Pacific basin. It has an uncertain pathogenesis; however, postulated causes include primary congenital biliary strictures and cysts, biliary parasitic infection (*Ascaris* or *Clonorchis*), and chronic intrahepatic bacterial colonization from unclear sources. Therapy is directed toward duct decompression, drainage, stone clearance, and occasionally lobar or segmental resection for isolated intrahepatic disease. This is most common in the left hepatic ductal system.

BILIARY STRICTURES

Iatrogenic bile duct strictures develop after 1 in 200 to 1 in 1,000 cholecystectomies. Presentation may be months to years after the injury. When duct injury is recognized intraoperatively, the ideal management is primary surgical repair with choledochojejunostomy. When treated at first presentation with a surgical Roux-en-Y hepaticojejunostomy, 85% to 90% of patients have good long-term results. Endoscopic therapy is now common, however, and 75% to 85% of patients have good results 5 to 10 years later. Recent series report better results with maximal caliber dilation and stenting for 6 to 12 months. Anastomotic bile duct strictures are treated much like other iatrogenic lesions, with endoscopic dilation and stenting when accessible.

Inflammatory bile duct strictures occur with primary sclerosing cholangitis and acute or chronic pancreatitis. Those related to chronic fibrotic pancreatitis are best treated surgically with a biliary enteric anastomosis. Strictures from acute pancreatitis usually can be palliated with endoscopic stenting until the acute inflammatory phase resolves. The optimal management of primary sclerosing cholangitis-related dominant strictures is controversial, but it generally involves endoscopic balloon dilation with or without stent placement rather than operation. Intervention is used only for stricture or stone-related clinical decline such as cholangitis, pain, or jaundice.

Relative indications for endoscopic or percutaneous treatment of biliary strictures include recurrence after operative repair, poor operative risk, portal hypertension, high stricture with little or no proximal extrahepatic duct (type 3 or 4), absence of proximal dilation, dominant stricture of primary sclerosing cholangitis (potential liver transplantation), and short-term palliation of acute or chronic pancreatitis-induced stricture.

ELUSIVE BILIARY-TYPE PAIN SYNDROMES

When patients present with recurrent right upper quadrant pain, often subsequent to cholecystectomy, several potential causes must be considered.

Nonbiliary sources of pain, such as functional or irritable bowel syndrome, non-ulcer dyspepsia, gastroesophageal reflux, pancreatic disease, or even cardiac disease, may present with features suggesting a biliary source. When treated with cholecystectomy, they typically recur. Diagnosis is largely through careful history and selective use of diagnostic testing.

Gallbladder dyskinesia, sometimes termed "cystic duct syndrome" in the surgical literature, refers to a poorly contractile gallbladder as demonstrated by CCK-stimulated radionuclide biliary scanning or ultrasonographic volumetric studies. The pathogenesis of pain is uncertain, but it may be related to a diseased gallbladder wall or a small duct relative to gallbladder size. Data suggest that cholecystectomy affords pain relief to patients with markedly diminished stimulated ejection fractions. Reproducibility of testing has been demonstrated only for gallbladder contractions with use of weight-based CCK infusions rather than bolus injections or alternative means of stimulation.

Microlithiasis refers to the presence and symptomatic passage of small crystalline aggregates or stones that go undetected on ultrasonography. A patient's stone-forming disposition can be inferred from identification of cholesterol crystals or calcium bilirubinate aggregates during polarized microscopy of a centrifuged bile pellet (Fig. 10). Positive microscopy is considered an indication for cholecystectomy, or for sphincterotomy if the gallbladder has already been removed. Sludge or microlithiasis also may be demonstrable by EUS when transabdominal imaging is normal.

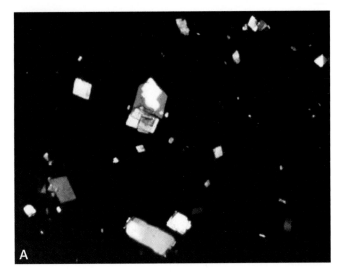
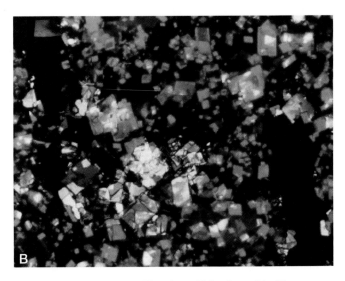

Fig. 10. Polarized microscopy of bile. *A* and *B*, Microscopic examination of sediment after centrifugation of bile shows birefringent rectangular notched crystals. Their identification confirms stone-forming physiology and the potential for an association between gallstones and the patient's symptoms. In *B*, the amorphous golden material is aggregated bilirubinate salts, which may occur with cholesterol crystals or alone. They also indicate a stone-forming propensity.

Sphincter-of-Oddi dysfunction refers to a continuum of stenosing or hypertonic abnormalities of the biliary or pancreatic sphincter. It is presumptively diagnosed on the basis of specific symptoms and laboratory criteria. *Type I* is sometimes referred to as papillary stenosis. Features include pain, dilated ducts, pain-associated aminotransferase abnormalities, and delayed drainage during cholangiography. It can be treated with sphincterotomy without prior confirmatory tests. *Type II* features pain and one or two of the associated features of type I. Type II is commonly confirmed manometrically before therapy by demonstration of intercontractile resting sphincter pressures more than 40 mm Hg. Semi-empiric sphincterotomy probably can be justified for patients with classic recurrent short-lasting increases in aminotransferase levels during pain. Presumptive *type III* is associated with pain alone and none of the more objective supporting features. Type III should not be investigated with manometry before a thorough search for alternative causes of pain and trials of medical therapies directed toward functional syndromes. ERCP should not be performed to exclude stones or other abnormalities without the availability of manometry. Hence, EUS or MRCP may be preferable early investigations in most patients. It should not be treated with

sphincterotomy in the absence of abnormal manometry results. Manometry results are abnormal in 15% to 60% of patients, depending on selectivity of testing, and response to sphincterotomy is about 70% in patients with abnormal pressures.

BILIARY LOOK-ALIKES

Intravenous ceftriaxone may lead to formation of crystalline biliary precipitates of drug. Ceftriaxone crystals can induce all potential complications of small bile duct stones, including biliary colic and pancreatitis.

Erythromycin hepatotoxicity presents with a syndrome of pain, fever, and cholestatic hepatitis which mimics acute cholecystitis. It is important to elicit an antibiotic history during evaluation of symptoms. A consistent history and associated eosinophilia may assist in identifying the syndrome.

Leptospirosis can present in a severe form termed Weil's syndrome, which is characterized by fever, jaundice, azotemia, and right upper quadrant pain. The presentation may mimic that of acute bacterial cholangitis. Clues to the diagnosis include a history of exposure risk, myalgias, ocular pain, photophobia, azotemia, and an abnormal urinalysis.

Pancreas and Biliary Tree

Questions and Answers

QUESTIONS

Multiple Choice (choose the one best answer)

1. A 25-year-old obese woman presents with a 24-hour history of nausea, vomiting, escalating epigastric pain radiating to the back, and fever to 101.3°F. Examination findings include a tender epigastrium and right upper quadrant tenderness. Laboratory study findings are as follows: amylase 14,500 U/L, lipase 9,300 U/L, aspartate amino-transferase 500 U/L, alanine aminotransferase 449 U/L, alkaline phosphatase 420 U/L, bilirubin 2.5 mg/dL, leukocytes 16×10^9/L, serum calcium 9.7 mg/dL, and triglycerides 430 mg/dL. The patient is not taking any medications. Abdominal ultrasonography shows a solitary gallbladder polyp but without evidence of cholelithiasis. What is the most likely cause of the patient's pancreatitis?
   a. Hypertriglyceridemia
   b. Alcohol abuse
   c. Choledocholithiasis
   d. Hypercalcemia
   e. Idiopathic acute pancreatitis

2. For the patient described in question 1, all of the following are viable management options in the evaluation or treatment of the suspected underlying cause of pancreatitis *except*:
   a. Contrast-enhanced abdominal computed tomography (CT)
   b. Empiric cholecystectomy
   c. Repeat transabdominal ultrasonography
   d. Endoscopic ultrasonography (EUS)

   e. Endoscopic retrograde cholangiopancreatography (ERCP) with biliary sphincterotomy

3. An 80-year-old man is admitted to the hospital for his second bout of acute pancreatitis. Admission laboratory values include amylase 3,200 U/L, lipase 2,700 U/L, aspartate aminotransferase 21 U/L, alanine aminotransferase 19 U/L, alkaline phosphatase 80 U/L, bilirubin 0.7 mg/dL, and normal serum calcium, phosphorus, and triglyceride values. The serum albumin value is low at 3.0 g/dL. Transabdominal ultrasonography of the right upper quadrant and chest and abdominal radiography are all unremarkable. The patient denies a history of abdominal trauma or alcohol use. He takes no medications. What is the next best investigation for the cause of this patient's pancreatitis?
   a. Magnetic resonance cholangiopancreatography (MRCP)
   b. Endoscopic retrograde cholangiopancreatography (ERCP)
   c. Abdominal computed tomography (CT) with thin cuts through the pancreas
   d. Determination of the serum macroamylase level
   e. Endoscopic ultrasonography (EUS)

4. A 65-year-old man is admitted to the intensive care unit for management of severe acute pancreatitis due to hyper-lipidemia with a Ranson score of 6. During the first 2 weeks of hospitalization, he continues to spike high fevers and maintain a marked leukocytosis. Blood cultures are negative. He has been receiving total parenteral nutrition and imipenem since admission. Urine cultures are growing

fungus. Computed tomography shows acute pancreatic necrosis estimated at 50%. What is the next most appropriate step in management?

a. Continued observation
b. Institution of antifungal agents
c. Surgical debridement
d. Computed tomography-guided fine-needle aspiration of the pancreatic bed
e. Endoscopic retrograde cholangiopancreatography

5. Which of the following is most likely to have the greatest positive impact in the early management of patients with severe acute necrotizing pancreatitis?

a. Total parenteral nutrition
b. Somatostatin
c. Endoscopic retrograde cholangiopancreatography (ERCP)
d. Surgical debridement
e. Enteral feeding by nasojejunal tube placed beyond the ligament of Treitz

6. A 35-year-old woman has a 5-year history of bouts of pancreatitis. Recent computed tomography has shown calcification in the head and body of the gland. From a search on the Internet, she learns that pancreatic cancer is a deadly complication of chronic pancreatitis. She is now very concerned and seeks your opinion regarding her risk for development of pancreatic cancer. She has a history of alcohol abuse for the past 15 years. She smokes 2 packs of cigarettes a day and has done so since high school. She has no family history of pancreatic disease or cancer. Which of the following statements is true?

a. Alcohol is a known pancreatic carcinogen, and alcoholics with pancreatitis have the highest risk of pancreatic cancer
b. The presence of calcification is a risk factor for development of pancreatic cancer in chronic pancreatitis
c. Smoking significantly increases the risk of pancreatic cancer in chronic pancreatitis
d. The patient should undergo yearly endoscopic ultrasonography and CA 19-9 measurements for surveillance
e. Persons with hereditary chronic pancreatitis have a low lifetime risk for development of pancreatic cancer

7. A 55-year-old woman with long-standing idiopathic chronic calcific pancreatitis seeks your opinion regarding management of diarrhea. She has 6 to 8 bowel movements a day which are loose, foul-smelling, and hard to flush. She often sees oil droplets in the stool, especially when she consumes a high-fat diet. She has a voracious appetite but is not gaining weight. A 72-hour fecal fat study done while the patient consumes 100 g of fat a day had 43 g of fat a day. An upper gastrointestinal series and small-bowel biopsy are unremarkable. The computed tomography scan is shown below. Which of the following is the most appropriate intervention?

a. Restrict fat intake to 10 g/day
b. Start a course of metronidazole for bacterial overgrowth
c. Perform endoscopic sphincterotomy and stone removal to relieve pancreatic duct obstruction
d. Start pancreatic enzyme supplements at 40,000 to 60,000 units of lipase/meal and less with snacks
e. Begin insulin therapy

8. A 45-year-old man with alcoholism seeks your help to manage abdominal pain associated with chronic calcific pancreatitis. He has had bouts of pancreatitis for the past 2 years. In the past 6 months, he has had three episodes of pancreatitis requiring hospitalization. He now has abdominal pain every day with worsening after meals. He uses 5 mg of oxycodone three times daily for partial relief of pain. He has a good appetite but has lost 10 lb during the past 6 months. His computed tomogram is shown on the next page. What is the most appropriate intervention?

a. Lateral pancreaticojejunostomy
b. Endoscopic sphincterotomy
c. Celiac plexus block
d. Pancreatic enzyme supplementation
e. Increase in the dose of narcotics

9. A 29-year-old man with chronic calcific pancreatitis is referred for evaluation. He has a history of attacks of pancreatitis since 16 years of age. His mother, maternal aunt, and maternal grandfather also had pancreatitis, and

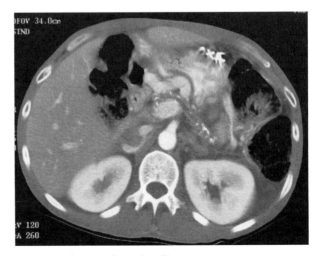

Question 7

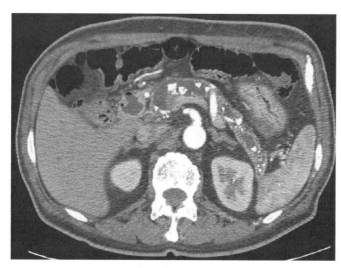

Question 8

his grandfather died of pancreatic cancer at age 50 years. He smokes 1 pack of cigarettes a day and has been drinking a case of beer every week for the past year. The physical examination of the patient is unremarkable. Serum triglyceride and calcium values are normal. Computed tomography of the abdomen shows extensive pancreatic calcification. What is the most likely cause for the pancreatitis?

a. Mutation in the *CFTR* gene
b. Chronic alcohol abuse
c. Mutation in the cationic trypsinogen gene
d. Mutation in the *SPINK1* gene
e. Mutation in the mesotrypsinogen gene

10. A 45-year-old man with alcoholism complains of abdominal pain present for the past 3 months. At the onset of his illness, he had a bout of pancreatitis requiring a 5-day admission to the hospital. Since then he has daily abdominal pain requiring narcotics at least twice a week. He has foul-smelling oily stools. He has lost 20 lb in weight since the onset of his illness. His past history includes laryngectomy for squamous cell carcinoma of the larynx 10 years ago. He smokes 2 packs of cigarettes a day and has done so for 25 years. On examination he is thin. His vital signs are stable. Abdominal examination reveals a scaphoid abdomen without organomegaly or ascites. His computed tomography (CT) scan is shown on this page. Which of the following is true?

a. The patient needs drainage of the pseudocysts complicating the chronic pancreatitis
b. The CT findings are consistent with an intraductal papillary mucinous neoplasm (IPMN)
c. The differential diagnosis includes mucinous cystic neoplasm

d. The patient needs total parenteral nutrition and bowel rest and imaging should be done again in 4 weeks
e. The differential diagnosis includes serous cystadenoma

11. A 68-year-old man has a 3-month history of dyspeptic symptoms and a 15-lb weight loss. He had normal results of upper endoscopy and has had no improvement after taking a proton pump inhibitor for 6 weeks. For 3 days he has had dark urine and pale stools and is brought to the emergency department by his family when they note scleral icterus. On examination he is comfortable and afebrile with normal vital signs. He is visibly jaundiced but his examination is otherwise normal. On biochemical studies, the bilirubin value is 10 mg/dL (direct, 6 mg/dL) and aminotransferases and alkaline phosphatase are increased threefold. What should you recommend?

a. Immediate admission to the hospital for observation and intravenous antibiotics if blood cultures are positive
b. Urgent endoscopic retrograde cholangiopancreatography (ERCP) and bile duct decompression
c. Viral serologic tests, discontinue use of the proton pump inhibitor, and referral of the patient to a hepatologist
d. Contrast-enhanced computed tomography (CT) of the abdomen
e. Referral to a surgeon for a cholecystectomy

12. A 40-year-old woman has crampy abdominal pain on a daily basis, a 25-lb weight gain, and alternating constipation and diarrhea, all since age 30 years. Abdominal computed tomography with contrast shows a 3-cm cyst in the pancreatic neck. The cyst is well circumscribed and is composed of innumerable smaller cysts no bigger than 3 to 4 mm. There is a central calcification, but the pancreas is otherwise normal, including the main pancreatic duct where seen. What do you advise?

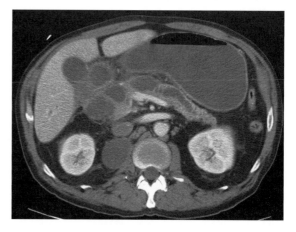

Question 10

a. This is at least a premalignant process and a Whipple resection is advised

b. This process is benign and will never change in size or ever cause problems

c. This is an incidental finding and can be managed conservatively

d. The calcium deposit indicates chronic pancreatitis and you admonish the patient to absolutely abstain from alcohol

e. Endoscopic retrograde cholangiopancreatography (ERCP) is indicated for further evaluation

13. A 45-year-old woman has had three discrete episodes of acute pancreatitis in 12 months that are well-characterized biochemically, self-limited, and uncomplicated. Her gallbladder was removed at age 40 years and an intraoperative cholangiogram was normal. She drinks alcohol three times a year. Blood test results, including triglycerides, serum calcium, and liver biochemistry values, are normal during these episodes. She takes estrogen replacement therapy and an angiotensin-converting enzyme (ACE) inhibitor. Abdominal computed tomography (CT) performed during the first episode of acute pancreatitis shows mild peripancreatic inflammation and a 2-cm cyst in the uncinate process. Subsequent CT imaging shows no change in the cyst and resolution of the inflammatory process. Endoscopic retrograde cholangiopancreatography (ERCP) done elsewhere shows a normal cholangiogram; the cyst fills off a branch of the uncinate process with a filling defect in the main pancreatic duct on the pancreatogram. Increased pressure at manometry is followed by an uneventful biliary sphincterotomy 1 month before her last attack of acute pancreatitis. What is the next *best* diagnostic test?

a. Follow-up CT imaging in 6 months

b. Magnetic resonance cholangiopancreatography

c. Endoscopic ultrasonography with cyst puncture

d. Determination of CA 19-9 level; if normal, follow-up CT in 6 months

e. Repeat ERCP and pancreatic sphincter manometry

14. For the patient described in question 13, what are the most likely diagnosis and management?

a. Idiopathic recurrent pancreatitis; she should be referred for a pancreatic sphincterotomy

b. Drug-induced pancreatitis with a pseudocyst; use of estrogen and the ACE inhibitor should be stopped

c. Recurrent biliary pancreatitis; repeat ERCP

d. Intraductal papillary mucinous neoplasm (IPMN); pancreatic resection

e. Chronic pancreatitis with a pseudocyst; cystic fibrosis gene testing and alcohol abstinence

15. A 65-year-old man has biopsy-proven adenocarcinoma of the pancreatic head. On contrast-enhanced computed tomography the lesion is locally unresectable because of encasement of the superior mesenteric vein; no liver metastases are seen. His performance status is good and he has obstructive jaundice. Which of the following is true?

a. He should be referred to a surgeon for palliative surgery of the biliary tree and gastrojejunostomy to prevent gastric outlet obstruction

b. He should be referred for endoscopic retrograde cholangiopancreatography (ERCP) and placement of a plastic biliary stent because the mean survival is less than 3 months

c. He should be referred for ERCP and placement of a self-expanding metal stent (SEMS)

d. Therapy with a combination of 5-fluorouracil and external beam radiation is associated with 10% long-term survival

e. A normal CA 19-9 level predicts a better prognosis

16. A 35-year-old woman with Crohn's disease of the terminal ileum and intermittent episodes of partial bowel obstruction presents with episodic right upper quadrant pain. Ultrasonography shows gallbladder stones. Which of the following statements best describes the likely nature of her gallstones?

They are likely to be:

a. Pigment stones due to her systemic chronic inflammatory disease

b. Cholesterol stones related to ileal disease and diminished bile acid absorption, enterohepatic circulation, and biliary secretion

c. Cholesterol stones related to hypercholesterolemia due to Crohn's disease

d. Pigment stones related to an imbalance of biliary nucleating and antinucleating factors

e. Mixed-character stones related to gallbladder dysmotility

17. Which of the following statements regarding pigment gallstones is true?

a. Brown pigment stones form primarily in the gallbladder and tend to be soft and partially soluble in cholesterol solvents

b. Black pigment stones form primarily in the bile duct and tend to be small, hard, and insoluble

c. Ninety percent of stones found in the bile duct are pigment stones

d. Duodenal diverticula predispose to pigmented bile duct stones by causing relative incompetence of the biliary sphincter

e. Ten percent of stones found in the bile duct are pigment stones

18. A 52-year-old man undergoes a cholecystectomy for symptomatic gallstones. Several months later he presents with several similar but milder episodes of pain. His laboratory test results are virtually normal, and right upper quadrant ultrasonography shows mild dilatation of his extrahepatic duct alone. What is the most cost-effective approach to excluding a common duct stone?
    a. Prompt endoscopic retrograde cholangiopancreatography (ERCP)
    b. Magnetic resonance cholangiopancreatography (MRCP)
    c. Endoscopic ultrasonography
    d. Observation alone
    e. Serial laboratory testing and abdominal computed tomography (CT) or repeat ultrasonography

19. Which of the following statements regarding treatment of gallbladder stones is correct?
    a. After the occurrence of biliary colic, approximately 50% of patients with gallbladder stones have subsequent acute complications such as pancreatitis, acute cholecystitis, or cholangitis in a year, and for this reason cholecystectomy should be performed prophylactically
    b. Calcified gallbladder stones should be removed independent of symptoms, because they are associated with a greater risk of both gallbladder cancer and biliary colic
    c. Asymptomatic stones can be observed, because their likelihood of eventually inducing symptoms is only about 20%
    d. When gallbladder stones are identified in patients with dyspepsia, fatty food intolerance, or gastroesophageal reflux disease, cholecystectomy is the second-line therapy, after a trial of proton pump inhibitors
    e. Large gallbladder stones are more likely to cause pancreatitis than small ones

20. Elective cholecystectomy should be entertained in which of the following patients with asymptomatic gallbladder stones?
    a. Adults with brittle diabetes
    b. Any patient with large stones more than 8 mm in diameter
    c. Any patient with small stones less than 5 mm in diameter
    d. American Indians with numerous stones of any size
    e. African-Americans with sickle cell disease

ANSWERS

1. Answer c

Gallstones remain the most common cause of acute pancreatitis (45% of all cases). Increased bilirubin, alkaline phosphatase, and aminotransferase values in the setting of markedly increased amylase and lipase values are strongly suggestive of biliary and pancreatic duct obstruction due to common bile duct stones. Despite improvements in sonographic technology, detection of small gallstones remains difficult in some cases. Adherent gallstones can mimic gallbladder polyps. The false-negative rate for detection of gallstones is 1% to 2%. Alcohol abuse, although a very common cause of acute pancreatitis, is unlikely to cause such a severe increase in the aminotransferase levels. Hypercalcemia is a cause of acute pancreatitis, but this patient has a normal calcium level. Hypertriglyceridemia is also a cause of acute pancreatitis, but a level of 430 mg/dL is insufficiently increased to cause this patient's pancreatitis, and the triglyceride level can be increased in the setting of acute pancreatitis from other causes.

2. Answer a

In this case, the clinical suspicion of cholelithiasis as a cause of pancreatitis is so high that an empiric cholecystectomy could be justified. Alternatively, repeat transabdominal ultrasonography, EUS, or biliary crystal analysis could be performed to diagnose cholelithiasis definitively. When the diagnosis of pancreatitis is in doubt or the suspicion for gallstone-induced pancreatitis is low, contrast-enhanced CT is the single-best study to evaluate the abdomen and pancreas. However, the sensitivity of CT for diagnosing cholelithiasis or choledocholithiasis is not as good as that of ultrasonography. Given the patient's classic presentation of acute pancreatitis, there is no need to perform contrast-enhanced abdominal CT. EUS is not only more sensitive than transabdominal ultrasonography for diagnosing cholelithiasis but also significantly more sensitive than transabdominal ultrasonography and CT for detecting choledocholithiasis, which may be present in this case. ERCP with sphincterotomy is an option in this patient, although in a young operative candidate it is not recommended as an alternative to cholecystectomy.

3. Answer c

In an elderly patient with first onset of pancreatitis, absence of risk factors for pancreatitis, and no evidence of gallstones on ultrasonography, the suspicion for a pancreatic ductal obstruction due to pancreatic carcinoma, ampullary carcinoma, or intraductal papillary mucinous neoplasm is high. Repeat transabdominal ultrasonography would be indicated if the clinical suspicion for gallstones were high, because a second ultrasonography may show small stones that were not initially seen. CT will give the best information of the pancreatic anatomy and will show either a mass or pancreatic ductal dilatation or both if pancreatic carcinoma is responsible for his pancreatitis. ERCP and MRCP are not indicated until after high-quality CT has been performed. Although EUS is very sensitive for evaluating the pancreas, it cannot be recommended before obtaining a good-quality CT scan of the abdomen.

4. Answer d

Continued systemic illness suggests possible infected pancreatic necrosis. In a recent study of patients with documented pancreatic fungal infection, positive urine cultures were frequent. The use of total parenteral nutrition and broad-spectrum antibiotics may also play a role in the development of pancreatic fungal infections. Because infected necrosis cannot be diagnosed on clinical grounds, fine-needle aspiration is indicated.

5. Answer e

The management of patients with severe acute necrotizing pancreatitis has shifted from early surgical debridement to intensive supportive care. Prevention of pancreatic infection has become paramount, because patients with sterile necrosis may be managed without operation. Of the choices given, enteral feeding is the most likely to have an impact, because it helps maintain gut integrity, improves severity scores, and decreases infection compared with total parenteral nutrition. Somatostatin has not been proved beneficial for the treatment of acute pancreatitis. Although total parenteral nutrition is widely used for support of patients with severe necrotizing pancreatitis, it also has never been shown to improve the outcome of acute pancreatitis. ERCP is helpful in only a subset of patients whose pancreatitis is caused by gallstones.

6. Answer c

Pancreatic cancer is a fatal complication of chronic pancreatitis. The forms of pancreatitis at highest lifetime risk for development of pancreatic cancer are the hereditary and tropical forms, which often manifest in childhood. Alcohol is not a proven pancreatic carcinogen. Although pancreatic calcification often is present in chronic pancreatitis complicated by pancreatic cancer, this is not an independent risk factor. Smoking is a well-known risk factor for ductal adenocarcinoma of the pancreas, and it significantly increases the risk of pancreatic cancer in chronic pancreatitis. There is no good surveillance regimen for detecting pancreatic cancer in chronic pancreatitis. Endoscopic ultrasonography is not helpful in the presence of extensive pancreatic calcification, and CA 19-9 measurement is not sensitive for detection of early pancreatic cancer.

7. Answer d

The patient clearly has pancreatic steatorrhea due to advanced chronic pancreatitis and consequent loss of pancreatic parenchyma. This condition will not respond to relief of ductal obstruction by removal of pancreatic duct stones. The first step in management is to initiate pancreatic enzyme therapy at the appropriate dose and to be taken with meals and snacks. Drastic restriction of fat is not necessary and may hamper weight gain. Although bacterial overgrowth can complicate pancreatic steatorrhea, therapy for this is appropriate only in patients not responding to enzyme supplements. There is no indication of diabetes mellitus requiring insulin therapy.

8. Answer a

This patient has disabling chronic calcific pancreatitis complicated by frequent acute flares of pancreatitis and chronic narcotic-requiring pain. Celiac plexus block and pancreatic enzyme supplements have been tried in the setting of chronic pain and do not prevent acute flares of pancreatitis. Endoscopic sphincterotomy is unlikely to be helpful in the setting of multiple stones throughout a dilated pancreatic duct. Lateral pancreaticojejunostomy can help the chronic pain and acute flares that the patient is experiencing. Increasing the dose of narcotics is a poor long-term choice.

9. Answer c

The patient's family history and early onset of chronic pancreatitis strongly suggest a hereditary cause for chronic pancreatitis. To date, mutations in three genes have been associated with chronic pancreatitis. Mutations in the cationic trypsinogen gene cause an autosomal dominant form of chronic pancreatitis. Mutations in *CFTR* and *SPINK1* genes are mostly found in apparently sporadic forms of pancreatitis because they have a low penetrance. The *mesotrypsinogen* gene is not implicated in pancreatitis. Alcohol is unlikely to be the cause of the pancreatitis because the alcohol history is short and the pancreatitis pre-dates the alcohol use.

10. Answer b

The CT scan shows a markedly dilated pancreatic duct throughout the gland with cystic lesions in the head of the pancreas. This could be pseudocysts complicating the chronic pancreatitis, but the possibility of IPMN needs to be excluded because it would significantly alter the management. Mucinous cystic neoplasm occurs in middle-aged women in the body and tail of the pancreas and does not cause marked dilatation of the pancreatic duct. This is not the radiologic picture of a serous cystadenoma. The patient needs diagnostic testing to exclude IPMN, including endoscopic retrograde cholangiopancreatography and cyst aspiration to look for mucin. If IPMN is excluded, drainage of pseudocysts may be considered.

Pseudocysts associated with chronic pancreatitis are unlikely to resolve with bowel rest and total parenteral nutrition.

11. Answer d

This is a classic presentation of painless obstructive jaundice due to pancreatic carcinoma of the head. Affected patients rarely have cholangitis despite an obstructed biliary tree and generally can be evaluated on an outpatient basis. ERCP is rarely needed as a diagnostic test and should be reserved for palliation of biliary obstruction in patients who cannot have surgical resection because of comorbid health conditions or locally advanced or metastatic cancer. CT of the abdomen is a highly sensitive test for establishing a dilated biliary tree, identifying the primary mass (likely pancreatic), and accurately staging the cancer.

12. Answer c

The patient's symptoms likely reflect a functional disorder, possibly irritable bowel syndrome, and have none of the features suggestive of a pancreatic disease. Incidentally noted pancreatic cysts are becoming increasingly common as transaxial abdominal imaging becomes more frequent and precise. The lesion described is a classic description of a serous cystadenoma or microcystic adenoma. This includes the central calcification and cluster of small cysts, clinically and morphologically distinct from the calcifications and pseudocyst formation common in chronic pancreatitis. Microcystic adenomas are entirely benign and unrelated to alcohol or other risk factors for pancreatitis. Found in both men and women, they are neoplastic and can grow, uncommonly causing symptoms from a mass effect. The approach to an indeterminate pancreatic cyst would generally place endoscopic ultrasonography ahead of ERCP in the diagnostic algorithm.

13. Answer c

See discussion in the answer to question 14.

14. Answer d

Discussion for Questions 13 and 14:

This patient likely has IPMN. IPMNs are ductal epithelial tumors arising in the main pancreatic duct or its major branches. The clinical presentation ranges from an incidental cyst to chronic pancreatitis with gland failure. An important clinical presentation is recurrent idiopathic acute pancreatitis, accounting for about one-third of patients. This patient's cyst likely involves the uncinate branch (branch duct IPMN), and the recurrent pancreatitis is due to obstruction from secreted mucin (also likely responsible for the filling defect seen on the pancreatogram). Mild acute pancreatitis would be unlikely to lead to an inflammatory pseudocyst, and the cyst was observed on the initial imaging study, suggesting the possibility of causality. Although estrogens are linked to pancreatitis, the cases involve induction of hyperlipidemia. ACE inhibitors also are linked to pancreatitis, but it is an extremely rare association and the astute clinician would be considering the cystic neoplasm as a far more likely mechanism than either drugs or sphincter of Oddi dysfunction. Endoscopic ultrasonography with cyst puncture can aid in the diagnosis by showing mural nodules (papillary projections) within the cyst and by biochemically characterizing the cyst fluid (mucinous with a high carcinoembryonic antigen level). IPMN is frankly malignant in about a third of patients at presentation. The prognosis of noninvasive intraductal papillary neoplasms is favorable when they are completely excised, including adenomas, neoplasms with moderate dysplasia, and noninvasive carcinomas. Resection of the tumor can be expected to relieve or eliminate the pancreatitis and prevent invasive cancer from developing.

15. Answer c

Endoscopic palliation for obstructive jaundice complicating inoperable pancreatic cancer is superior to surgical palliation from morbidity and cost perspectives. Furthermore, gastric outlet obstruction is an uncommon complication (5% of patients or less) and endoscopic therapies with SEMS are becoming available. Choosing between a plastic stent and a SEMS from a cost perspective is based on expected survival; locally unresectable pancreatic cancer with a good performance status would be expected to be associated with a survival longer than 6 months; the SEMS is associated with a much less likely need for repeat ERCP and thus is cost-effective. Although chemoradiation for locally advanced cancer is the standard of care in the United States, it is associated with a modest increase in survival (mean duration of survival, about 1 year) with no realistic chance of cure. Finally, about 5% of the population do not express the CA 19-9 antigen, and testing for it has limited use in the diagnosis and management of pancreatic cancer.

16. Answer b

Ileal resection or chronic disease reduces the efficiency of bile acid absorption. If absorption is significantly diminished, losses exceed the liver's capacity to synthesize more bile acids. In this setting, cholesterol supersaturation may occur. Diminished bile acid secretion is not necessary for cholesterol stone formation. Cholesterol supersaturation often occurs in the setting of cholesterol hypersecretion with *normal* bile acid secretion. Nucleating and antinucleating factors contribute to a more rapid "nucleation time" in gallstone formers, and gallbladder dysmotility precludes daily clearance of crystals and nascent stones.

17. Answer d

Brown pigment stones are primary duct stones, which indeed are more soft and partially soluble than black stones.

They form as a result of bacterial contamination, stasis, and bilirubin deconjugation. Black pigment stones are found in the bile ducts as "secondary duct stones," following formation in the gallbladder and migration through the cystic duct. They are small, hard, and insoluble. About half of stones in the duct are primary and pigment in nature. The other half reflect the nature of gallbladder stones, which are 70% cholesterol. Therefore, overall, 60% to 70% of duct stones are pigment stones. Duodenal diverticula predispose to primary duct stone formation by causing incompetence of the sphincter, resulting in reflux of duodenal contents, bacterial colonization of the duct, and subsequent bilirubin deconjugation.

18. Answer c

Endoscopic ultrasonography is highly sensitive for common duct stones and either equal to or better than ERCP in most published studies. For diagnostic purposes it is more cost-effective when the likelihood of stones varies between 13% and 55% to 60%. Observation is most cost-effective when the likelihood is very low. The sensitivity of MRCP is approximately equivalent to that of ERCP in many studies, but perhaps not uniformly across the United States. ERCP is most cost-effective when the likelihood of stones exceeds 55% to 60%, because it includes the therapeutic ability for their removal, whereas identification of stones in all other scenarios leads to a subsequent ERCP. CT and abdominal ultrasonography are not highly sensitive for common duct stones.

19. Answer c

Approximately 20% of patients with asymptomatic stones eventually go on to have symptoms of uncomplicated biliary colic. After presentation of colic, patients with stones continue with a similar frequency of colic, progressing to acute complications in only a small minority. Development of cancer is not related to stone calcification but does correlate with stone size; the risk is much greater in patients with stones more than 2 cm in diameter. The only symptom that is reliably relieved with cholecystectomy is of classic biliary colic, identified as episodic abrupt and significant epigastric or right upper quadrant pain lasting 15 minutes to several hours. Nausea and dyspeptic symptoms occasionally occur with stones, but the association is hard to make and symptom relief cannot be anticipated with surgery.

20. Answer d

The risk of gallbladder cancer is significantly increased in American Indians with gallstones, and prophylactic cholecystectomy should be entertained in this group. Brittle diabetes is not a risk factor for progression to symptomatic stone disease. Current-day medical care can deal with symptoms when they occur, and the presence of diabetes or sickle cell disease alone should not prompt performance of prophylactic cholecystectomy. Stones more than 2 to 3 cm in diameter are associated with a higher incidence of cancer and should be considered for cholecystectomy, but not all those more than 8 mm. Small stones are at greater risk of migration to the duct, with subsequent occurrence of cholangitis or pancreatitis, but there are no data to suggest small stones should be removed prophylactically.

INDEX